Trauma Computed Tomography

Friedrich Knollmann
Editor

Trauma Computed Tomography

Springer

Editor
Friedrich Knollmann
Department of Medical Imaging
Penn Presbyterian Medical Center
Philadelphia, PA, USA

ISBN 978-3-031-45745-6 ISBN 978-3-031-45746-3 (eBook)
https://doi.org/10.1007/978-3-031-45746-3

This Springer imprint is published by the registered company Springer Nature Switzerland AG
The registered company address is: Gewerbestrasse 11, 6330 Cham, Switzerland

Paper in this product is recyclable

Contents

Contributors

Suehyb Alkhatib Department of Radiology, Perelman School of Medicine at the University of Pennsylvania, Philadelphia, PA, USA

Raisa Amiruddin Department of Radiology, Children's Hospital of Philadelphia, Philadelphia, PA, USA

Linda J. Bagley Division of Neuroradiology, Department of Radiology, Perelman School of Medicine at the University of Pennsylvania, Philadelphia, PA, USA

Laura De León Benedetti Department of Radiology, Children's Hospital of Philadelphia, Philadelphia, PA, USA

Jeremy W. Cannon Division of Traumatology, Surgical Critical Care and Emergency Surgery, Surgery at the Hospital of the University of Pennsylvania and the Presbyterian Medical Center of Philadelphia, Philadelphia, PA, USA

Kyle Costenbader Department of Diagnostic Radiology and Nuclear Medicine, University of Maryland School of Medicine, Baltimore, MD, USA

Francis Deng Department of Radiology, Johns Hopkins University, Baltimore, MD, USA

Achala Donuru Department of Radiology, Hospital of the University of Pennsylvania, Philadelphia, PA, USA

David Dreizin Trauma and Emergency Radiology, Department of Diagnostic Radiology and Nuclear Medicine, R Adams Cowley Shock Trauma Center, University of Maryland School of Medicine, Baltimore, MD, USA

Mohamed Elbanan Division of Abdominal Imaging, Department of Radiology, Hospital of the University of Pennsylvania, Philadelphia, PA, USA

Division of Abdominal Imaging, Department of Radiology, University of Missouri, Columbia, MO, USA

Joanie Garratt Department of Radiology, University of Pennsylvania, Philadelphia, PA, USA

Antje Greenfield Department of Radiology, University of Pennsylvania, Philadelphia, PA, USA

Akshya Gupta Department of Radiology, University of Rochester, Rochester, NY, USA

Mauro Hanaoka Department of Radiology, Perelman School of Medicine at the University of Pennsylvania, Philadelphia, PA, USA

Mathew Hensley Department of Radiology, University of Pennsylvania, Philadelphia, PA, USA

Paul Hill Department of Radiology, Winchester Radiologists, Winchester, VA, USA

Jay Im Department of Radiology, University of Rochester, Rochester, NY, USA

Christina L. Jacovides Division of Trauma, Acute Care Surgery, Surgical Critical Care, and Burn Surgery, Philadelphia, PA, USA

Neal Joshi Department of Radiology, Thomas Jefferson University Hospital, Philadelphia, PA, USA

Vinay Kandula Department of Medical Imaging, Nemours Children's Hospital, Wilmington, DE, USA

Riti Kanesa-thasan Department of Radiology, University of Pennsylvania, Philadelphia, PA, USA

Friedrich Knollmann Department of Medical Imaging, Penn Presbyterian Medical Center, Philadelphia, PA, USA

Maruti Kumaran Department of Radiology, Temple University Hospital, Philadelphia, PA, USA

Robert Kurtz Department of Radiology, Perelman School of Medicine at the University of Pennsylvania, Philadelphia, PA, USA

Suyash Mohan Department of Radiology, Perelman School of Medicine at the University of Pennsylvania, Philadelphia, PA, USA

Rahul Nikam Department of Medical Imaging, Nemours Children's Hospital, Wilmington, DE, USA

Abass M. Noor Department of Radiology, Hospital of the University of Pennsylvania, Philadelphia, PA, USA

Michael R. Rudnick Renal-Electrolyte and Hypertension Division, Perelman School of Medicine, University of Pennsylvania, Philadelphia, PA, USA

Hersh Sagreiya Division of Abdominal Imaging, Department of Radiology, Hospital of the University of Pennsylvania, Philadelphia, PA, USA

Kathleen E. Schenker Department of Medical Imaging, Nemours Children's Hospital, Wilmington, DE, USA

J. Eric Schmitt Departments of Radiology and Psychiatry, University of Pennsylvania, Philadelphia, PA, USA

Elana B. Smith Trauma and Emergency Radiology, Department of Diagnostic Radiology and Nuclear Medicine, R Adams Cowley Shock Trauma Center, University of Maryland School of Medicine, Baltimore, MD, USA

Ryan Spiardi Renal-Electrolyte and Hypertension Division, Perelman School of Medicine, University of Pennsylvania, Philadelphia, PA, USA

Taylor Standiford Department of Radiology, Temple University Hospital, Philadelphia, PA, USA

Joel M. Stein Division of Neuroradiology, Department of Radiology, Perelman School of Medicine at the University of Pennsylvania, Philadelphia, PA, USA

Kalpana Suresh Department of Radiology, University of Pennsylvania, Philadelphia, PA, USA

Nnamdi D. Udeh Department of Radiology, Hospital of the University of Pennsylvania, Philadelphia, PA, USA

The Evolving Role of Computed Tomography (CT) in Trauma Care

1

Christina L. Jacovides, Nnamdi D. Udeh, Jeremy W. Cannon, and Friedrich Knollmann

Introduction

Since its invention, computed tomography (CT) has played a critical and increasingly important role in the workup and management of acutely injured patients. As an adjunct to trauma protocols and algorithms, in hemodynamically stable patients, CT provides rapid assessment and diagnosis of injuries in multiple body cavities, guiding additional triage of injuries and therapeutic interventions. The following chapters will focus on the specific roles for CT within individual body regions, discuss the role for CT in specific patient populations (e.g., children, patients with renal failure), and discuss new developments on the horizon as CT technology and image interpretation continue to evolve. The goal of this chapter is to introduce the role of CT within the larger trauma system and to establish the historical context in which modern CT finds itself. Understanding how CT fits into overall trauma algorithms and how its role has changed over time sets the stage for its continued evolution.

C. L. Jacovides (✉)
Division of Trauma, Acute Care Surgery, Surgical Critical Care, and Burn Surgery, Temple University Hospital, Philadelphia, PA, USA
e-mail: Christina.Jacovides@tuhs.temple.edu

N. D. Udeh
Department of Radiology, Hospital of the University of Pennsylvania, Philadelphia, PA, USA
e-mail: Nnamdi.Udeh@Pennmedicine.upenn.edu

J. W. Cannon
Division of Traumatology, Surgical Critical Care and Emergency Surgery, Surgery at the Hospital of the University of Pennsylvania and the Presbyterian Medical Center of Philadelphia, Philadelphia, PA, USA
e-mail: Jeremy.Cannon@pennmedicine.upenn.edu

F. Knollmann
Department of Medical Imaging, Penn Presbyterian Medical Center, Philadelphia, PA, USA
e-mail: Friedrich.Knollmann@pennmedicine.upenn.edu

History of ATLS

Understanding how CT fits into the overall workup of injured patients requires an understanding of trauma algorithms and systems. Trauma is not a new pathology—patients have presented for medical care for injury for thousands of years. However, the last 50 years have witnessed the growing development of and protocolization of trauma care, starting with the establishment of trauma algorithms and the development of trauma systems.

In 1976, a tragic plane crash resulted in serious injuries to orthopedic surgeon Dr. Jim Styner and his family. He felt that the trauma care they received was inadequate based on the standards of the day, and he originated the first Advanced Trauma Life Support (ATLS) course in 1978 to standardize the practice of trauma resuscitations [1]. In the years since the establishment of the ATLS course and protocols, trauma care in the

F. Knollmann (ed.), *Trauma Computed Tomography*, https://doi.org/10.1007/978-3-031-45746-3_1

first hour after trauma has changed significantly worldwide. Since the development of ATLS, there has been increasing focus on and interest in the development of trauma centers and trauma systems to optimize the immediate stabilization and long-term complex care of injured patients.

The major tenet of ATLS is that patients who present to a trauma center with traumatic injuries should be rapidly evaluated and resuscitated by a trauma team. This resuscitation is algorithmic, focusing first on the most life-threatening injuries (e.g., establishing an airway, confirming that the patient has bilateral breath sounds, and evaluating the extremities for pulses and the presence of exsanguinating hemorrhage). In the process of this evaluation, trauma surgeons and emergency personnel use adjunctive imaging modalities for rapid assessment of the patient's condition. These include focused abdominal ultrasound in trauma (FAST) exams as well as plain films of the chest, abdomen, pelvis, head/neck, and extremities, as indicated. Once physical exam and initial adjuncts are completed, the trauma team determines the next best location for the patient, depending on the injury complex identified at initial presentation [2].

Following the initial resuscitation, patients either undergo treatment for their injuries or additional diagnostic studies to better define those injuries. Patients who are too unstable for additional imaging may be taken directly to the operating room for operative exploration to better define and address their injuries. Patients who are stable and have clearly defined injuries based on plain films and physical exam may be treated for their injuries. The many patients in the middle ground who are clinically stable and for whom additional diagnostic modalities may better clarify their injury patterns undergo additional imaging. In many cases, this additional imaging involves CT [2].

The Development of Trauma Systems

ATLS defines the actions of individual providers to stabilize injured patients within the first hour after injury, but trauma care cannot exist in a vacuum. Successful stabilization of injured patients requires not only immediate provider input, but a robust trauma system to support the ongoing care of injured patients. As ATLS has been disseminated worldwide, there has been a concurrent expansion and formalization of trauma systems to mobilize the resources required to care for injured patients.

In the USA, trauma centers are designated at five levels. These range from Level 1 trauma centers, which are comprehensive tertiary referral centers that serve as regional resources in the overall trauma system and can provide total trauma care to the injured patient, to Level 5 trauma centers, which can provide basic initial evaluation and stabilization of injured patients prior to transfer for definitive care. These five levels are designated by state and local entities and the specific details of these designations vary from state to state. Nationally, however, the American College of Surgeons (ACS) has the role of verifying that designated trauma centers at each level have the appropriate resources required for their level [3]. It is through a combination of excellent ATLS care delivered within this network of trauma centers that injured patients may be acutely stabilized and provided with the long-term specialty care that their injuries require for management.

While patients with more trivial traumatic injuries may not necessarily benefit from referral to higher level trauma centers, survival and outcomes tend to be better for patients with major trauma who are treated in an advanced level trauma center [4–6].

History of CT and Its Role in Trauma Systems

The role of CT has evolved greatly since it was first introduced in the setting of trauma. CT was first invented in 1967 by Sir Godfrey Hounsfield, with the first patient CT scan (a brain CT) performed in 1971. CT scanners became much more prevalent during the 1980s and 1990s, and as technology has developed, new techniques have improved CT image quality, reduced time to image acquisition, and reduced radiation doses [7]. These developments have resulted in an evolution in the use of CT in trauma. Early use of CT was limited in trauma to only those patients who were truly stable enough for imaging and who also would have non-subtle findings on thick-slice CT. With modern CT scanners, the decreased time to image acquisition and the significant improvement in resolution of images means that more trauma patients are candidates for imaging prior to definitive intervention. As a result, there have been significant shifts in the use of CT in trauma as well as in patterns of interventions in trauma patients.

As CT technology improves, moreover, the indications for appropriateness of CT imaging in trauma patients continue to expand. The tenets of good trauma care remain in place—e.g., only patients who are stable enough to be in a CT scanner should undergo imaging—but because CTs may be obtained much more rapidly with newer scanners, more patients are stable enough for CT now than there were in the early years of CT. Moreover, with newer scanners has come finer resolution on CT imaging and nuanced protocols that allow for the visualization of injury patterns which previously not routinely imaged. As a result, there has been a growing use of CT in the evaluation of injured patients.

By definition, level 1 trauma centers must also have 24-h availability of CT imaging [3, 8]. While CT is now widely available across most developed countries, the degree of specialization of the radiologist providing the interpretation of imaging results in increased rates of identification of both diagnoses that alter patient care and those that do not (e.g., incidental findings) [9]. As many centers move toward specialization and subspecialization of imaging interpretation, the interaction between different specialists contributes to the ongoing education of the next generation of radiologists.

Following the same principle, the practice of diagnostic radiology has also steered toward higher degrees of specialization, with the expectation that a sufficient clinical practice base and subspecialization allow for higher quality of patient care. Accordingly, subspecialization in radiology has progressed especially in large academic medical centers, which also share the academic mission that is bestowed upon the level 1 trauma center.

In an ideal world, the most advanced imaging services would be immediately available at all times and could be immediately correctly interpreted to the benefit of the patient. The current concept of a level 1 trauma center with 24-h availability of CT comes closest to this ideal situation. Sharing the diagnostic experience from subspecialities aids in disseminating the resultant insights.

However, there is always the risk of over-utilization of advanced imaging services and the identification of incidental findings that may have no bearing on a patient's clinical state or may prompt additional invasive procedures to the patient's detriment.

Appropriateness Criteria in a Trauma Setting

The problem of potential over-utilization has been addressed by the American College of Radiology (ACR) through development of appropriateness criteria [10]. These criteria are established using available literature and categorize available imaging in multiple modalities as either "Usually appropriate," "May be appropriate," or "Usually not appropriate" in a variety of clinical settings. For major blunt trauma in hemodynamically unstable patients, they note that plain films and ultrasound are usually appropriate, and that CT whole body with or without IV contrast may be appropriate. In hemodynamically stable patients with major blunt trauma, CT whole body with IV contrast is extended to be considered "usually appropriate." The ACR also provides guidance on imaging for patients with major blunt polytrauma in situations in which specifically facial, extremity, bowel, and genitourinary injury is suspected, as well as guidance for the imaging of pregnant patients. Separate guidance is given for patients with penetrating trauma to the lower abdomen and pelvis [11], although this is the only guidance given for patients with penetrating injury. The ACR also provides guidance on the appropriateness of imaging studies used in a variety of other suspected trauma pathologies, including blunt chest trauma with suspected cardiac injury [12], extremity/joint trauma [13–17], spine trauma [18], head trauma [19, 20], facial trauma [21], as well as trauma in children (head and spine) [22, 23].

Recommendations about the appropriateness of imaging options in traumatically injured patients come from these summary documents from the ACR but also from a variety of surgical and trauma perspectives from various entities. The American College of Surgeons (ACS)'s Trauma Quality Improvement Program (TQIP) has put forth guidelines for best practices guidelines in imaging [8]. The Eastern Association for the Surgery of Trauma (EAST) trauma practice management guidelines include commentary on overall evaluation and treatment of a variety of trauma pathologies, including guidance on appropriateness of various diagnostic and therapeutic imaging modalities [24]. The Western Trauma Association (WTA) has established algorithms for defining appropriateness in workup and management of traumatic injuries [25].

The ACS TQIP imaging guidelines state that trauma centers should all have multidetector computed tomographic (MDCT) trauma protocols established for each body region. CT imaging must be readily available in trauma centers. Additionally, they recommend that the CT scanner be as close to the trauma bay as possible, that trauma patients receive priority imaging ahead of patients with conditions that are not life-threatening, and that trauma imaging be interpreted promptly with information relayed back to the trauma team expeditiously to allow for rapid decision-making. In order to obtain high-quality vascular imaging with CTA and reconstruction for definitive care of patients with vascular injuries (e.g., at level 1 and 2 trauma centers), they recommend a 64-channel scanner. For more routine imaging or in trauma centers that typically transfer more critically injured patients, 16-channel scanners may be adequate.

The ACS TQIP guidelines make additional commentary on the need to consider radiation exposure risk (particularly in children and pregnant patients) in determining the appropriate CT studies ordered. It is important to note that one of the basic tenets of care of the pregnant trauma patient is that the pregnant patient should receive the same treatment as the non-pregnant patient since excellent trauma care for the pregnant patient optimizes outcomes for the fetus. Moreover, most diagnostic imaging modalities used in trauma provide radiation doses far below the level that has been associated with increased rate of development of fetal anomalies or of fetal death [26]. The guidelines also comment on contrast considerations including the need for intravenous contrast for the purposes of assessing for contrast blush and solid organ injury, as well as the potential but low risk for contrast nephropathy, which is typically discounted given the significant increase in diagnostic yield of contrast-enhanced imaging. Finally, they discuss the importance of adequate sedation in the agitated or pediatric patient for various imaging modalities and make the important point that trauma resuscitation should be continued during imaging acquisition, if necessary [8].

Controversies in Trauma CT

As with any evolving technology in an evolving field, there remain numerous points of ongoing research and investigation regarding best practices in the utilization of CT imaging in trauma patients. We highlight here some of the more notable ongoing controversies in CT imaging in trauma patients.

Whole-Body CT Scan Versus Selective CT Scan

The introduction of multidetector CT technology has greatly accelerated the ease with which whole-body CT images may be obtained. Early studies suggested that whole-body CT, obtained using a streamlined image acquisition protocol to depict the head, neck and torso, may improve patient survival in severely injured patients [27].

The subsequently performed REACT-2 study randomized severely injured patients to either "conventional" organ-focused CT vs. whole-body CT did not demonstrate this survival benefit—even after post hoc analysis of patients with polytrauma presentation and traumatic brain injury [28]. Nevertheless, the widespread availability of accelerated techniques for whole-body imaging has contributed to a dramatic increase in the usage of CT in trauma patients in recent years [29].

The potential harms associated with whole-body CT include the increased radiation exposure inherent in whole-body scanning as opposed to selective scanning, and the fact that whole-body imaging results in the identification of incidental findings which may be clinically insignificant, but which may result in invasive and risky diagnostic procedures to determine their implications. While there is some concern that whole-body CT might also be associated with increased cost, the REACT-2 study did not find that whole-body CT increased costs [28].

The presumptive benefit of whole-body CT is that standardized rapid imaging can result in earlier identification of injuries and fewer missed injuries. However, care must be taken in assessing the value of whole-body CT in comparison to selective CT. For example, while several observational studies report a mortality benefit with whole-body CT, Gupta et al. noted that patients who undergo whole-body CT have injury severity scores (ISS, a trauma scoring system typically used to determine the extent and clinical significance of a patient's injuries) that are twice that of those who undergo selective CT only, but that if "unnecessary" CT scans are excluded, the two groups have similar ISS scores [30]. Moreover, in one recent investigation, about 75% of trauma CT studies did not result in any injury diagnosis [31]. Efforts to identify clinical criteria that qualify a patient for whole-body CT will increase diagnostic yield and prevent over-utilization.

In addition to optimizing patient selection, there is nuance in the whole-body versus selective CT scan options in terms of the specific techniques used to obtain each set of images. Guidelines specify many details of the imaging technique [32] and ongoing technological developments such as spectral imaging continue to expand the usage of CT in trauma care while decreasing total radiation dose and improving overall image quality [33]. With every new technology comes the need for balance—modern CT scanners have incredible capabilities, but we must still employ this technology cautiously, always keeping in mind the risk/benefit ratio for use in each individual patient.

An example of a whole-body CT protocol is reproduced in Table 1.1.

Table 1.1 Whole-body CT protocol

Protocol name	Trauma one run
Indication	Polytrauma
Protocol designed for (scanner model)	GE revolution apex
Patient preparation	Arms to be elevated after second series
First series	Head non contrast
Oral contrast	NA
IV contrast	NA
Tube settings	
kV	120
mA	550
Dose modulation	Off
Scan type	Axial
Tube rotation time (s)	0.6 s
Table speed (mm/s)	
Slice collimation	
Reconstructed slice thickness	5 mm
Anatomical coverage	Vertex to C1
Reconstruction kernel	STND, ASIR 50%
Breath hold	NA
Window settings	100/30
Post processing	0.625 ax, 3 cor, 2 mm ax
Other	
Typical dose	
CTDIvol	
DLP	
Eff. Dose	
Second series	C-spine
Oral contrast	NA
IV contrast	NA
Tube settings	
kV	120
mA	SmartmA, 220–400 mA

(continued)

Table 1.1 (continued)

Protocol name	Trauma one run
Dose modulation	SmartmA, noise index 12
Tube rotation time (s)	0.7 s
Table speed (mm/s)	56.25 mm/s
Slice collimation	
Reconstructed slice thickness	2.5 mm
Anatomical coverage	Above odontoid to T1
Reconstruction kernel	STND, ASIR 50
Breath hold	NA
Window settings	350/50
Post processing	2.5 bone, 2 mm sag
Other	
Typical dose	
CTDIvol	
DLP	
Eff. Dose	
Third series	Chest-abdomen-pelvis
Oral contrast	NA
IV contrast (mL, mL/s)	70/3, 55/2, 20 NaCl 2 cc/s
	Delay: 65 s
Tube settings	
kV	120
mA	SmartmA 120–550
Dose modulation	SmartmA, noise index 12
Tube rotation time (s)	0.5 s
Table speed (mm/s)	158.75 mm/s
Pitch	0.992
Slice collimation	0.625 mm
Reconstructed slice thickness	5 mm
	0.625 TrueFidelity
Anatomical coverage	C-A-P
Reconstruction kernel	STND, ASIR 50
Breath hold	Inspiration
Window settings	400/40
Post processing	1 mm STND, lung, 3 mm STND, lung, 2 mm sag and Cor
Other	
Typical dose	
CTDIvol	
DLP	
Eff. Dose	

Optimizing Imaging Protocols for Injured Patients

Given the risks of increased contrast load and radiation exposure as well as the goal of reducing the time required to obtain appropriate diagnostic imaging in acutely injured patients, there are continued debates about the optimal protocols for CT imaging. Numerous authors have proposed a variety of different protocols for CT by varying patient positioning [34], timing of contrast bolus, use of enteric (e.g., oral and/or rectal contrast) [35, 36], and various maneuvers/protocols for evaluation of specific injuries (e.g., CT cystogram for evaluation of bladder injuries) [37]. The overall goal is to obtain imaging that has the best possible diagnostic yield in the shortest amount of time while exposing the patient to the least risk from contrast, radiation, or overdiagnosis. By combining the expertise of trauma surgeons and radiologists, we can hope to optimize the most important factors for critically injured patients for whom accurate, timely diagnosis is crucial for appropriate treatment.

In trauma, patient positioning and cooperation may add time to the acquisition of imaging data. Although placing both arms above the head during whole-body CT has been shown to reduce overall patient dose and increase image quality rating compared to one or two arms in the gantry [38], there are often factors that may limit a patient's ability to be appropriately positioned. Depending on the mechanism of injury, a patient may only be able to have one arm or neither arm outside of the gantry. Though not ideal, this compromise has still been shown to be effective in detecting life-threatening injuries [39]. As an alternative to having both arms up, Studer et al. propose a protocol in which the patient's arms are placed on a ventral pillow rather than above their heads and note that this adjustment reduces the overall time required for scan [34], with subsequent studies showing that image quality is also improved with this technique [40]. In critically ill patients for whom CT has been deemed appropriate but who may be clinically tenuous, reducing the time required to obtain accurate imaging by even a few minutes may have a significant clinical impact.

In addition to varying patient positioning, CT protocols may vary the timing and amount of contrast dye injection as well as the timing and number of images obtained after injection. This allows for multi-phase imaging that makes diagnosis of arterial, venous, solid organ, liver/portal vein, genitourinary injury, etc. possible. Numerous authors have proposed a variety of protocols for optimizing these imaging techniques [41–43].

System-Based Staffing Considerations

All trauma centers must find a way to balance their available resources to provide the best possible care for patients at all times. Finding ways to creatively deploy available resources while still ensuring excellent care regardless of time of day or day of week is a crucial part of the development of a trauma center. Any trauma centers that leverage trainee assistance in interpretation of images must have an established protocol for rapid and accurate interpretation of imaging to provide timely and appropriate care to all trauma patients. This is particularly true for and important at level 1 trauma centers, since education and research are at the forefront of their mission [3]. Several authors have investigated the degree of discrepancy between resident reads of trauma scans and attending radiologists' reads, with overall findings of low discrepancy rates. Moreover, they note that some of these discrepancies are related to perceived complexity of a case and that even attending radiologists disagree about final findings in many of these cases. They note, moreover, low rates of additional intervention as a result of these discrepancies [44, 45].

Some trauma centers, to cover staffing needs, have turned to teleradiologist support instead of or in addition to in-house resident or attending interpretation of images. The potential benefit of teleradiologists is that they are attending radiologist with more experience than trainee radiologists; the downside is that they are remote, they have less interaction with the trauma patient and trauma team caring for the patient, and they may have slower turnaround times for imaging reads since they are not in-house. Yeates et al. found that residents tend to have more overcalls and shorter turnaround time for image interpretation, while teleradiologists had more discrepancies (as compared to a final attending radiologist's interpretation) and more missed injuries but fewer overcalls. They concluded that the combination of resident and teleradiologists interpretations together reduced the overall chance of missed injuries and reduced discrepancies [46].

Conclusion

As CT technology continues to improve, the role for CT in the immediate and ongoing evaluation of the injured patient continues to evolve. With faster acquisition and higher resolution of imaging has come increased utilization of CT. There remains a need to balance the basic tenets of trauma care (e.g., that unstable patients require immediate intervention rather than ongoing non-therapeutic diagnostic workup) with the potential benefits of imaging to guide targeted interventions. The remaining chapters will elaborate further on specific controversies and important questions for consideration in the imaging of various organ systems and structures and will delve further into some of the current controversies in each of these areas. CT remains a powerful tool in the armamentarium of the modern trauma surgeon and system. Understanding the nuances in image acquisition and interpretation as well as the strengths and weaknesses of different imaging protocols gives the trauma surgeon the clearest understanding of potential injuries and the best guidance for necessary interventions in the critically injured patient.

References

1. About advanced trauma life support. ACS [cited 2023 Jan 26]. https://www.facs.org/quality-programs/trauma/education/advanced-trauma-life-support/about/.
2. American College of Surgeons. Atls course administration and faculty guide. 10th ed. Chicago, IL: American College of Surgeons; 2017.
3. Trauma Center Levels Explained-American Trauma Society. [cited 2023 Jan 26]. https://www.amtrauma.org/page/traumalevels.
4. Dakessian A, Bachir R, El Sayed MJ. Association between trauma center designation levels and survival of patients with motor vehicular transport injuries in the United States. J Emerg Med. 2020;58(3):398–406.
5. Mehta VV, Grigorian A, Nahmias JT, Dolich M, Barrios C, Chin TL, et al. Blunt trauma mortal-

ity: does trauma center level matter? J Surg Res. 2022;276:76–82.
6. Bukur M, Felder SI, Singer MB, Ley EJ, Malinoski DJ, Margulies DR, et al. Trauma center level impacts survival for cirrhotic trauma patients. J Trauma Acute Care Surg. 2013;74(4):1133–7.
7. Half a century in CT: how computed tomography has evolved. ISCT 2016 [cited 2023 Jan 26]. https://www.isct.org/computed-tomography-blog/2017/2/10/half-a-century-in-ct-how-computed-tomography-has-evolved.
8. Ball JW. Best practices guidelines in imaging. American College of Surgeons, trauma quality improvement program; 2018 [cited 2023 Feb 2]. https://www.facs.org/media/oxdjw5zj/imaging_guidelines.pdf.
9. Bell ME, Patel MD. The degree of abdominal imaging (AI) subspecialization of the reviewing radiologist significantly impacts the number of clinically relevant and incidental discrepancies identified during peer review of emergency after-hours body CT studies. Abdom Imaging. 2014;39(5):1114–8.
10. ACR Appropriateness Criteria. American College of Radiology; [cited 2023 Jan 31]. https://acsearch.acr.org/list.
11. Expert Panel on Urological Imaging, Heller MT, Oto A, Allen BC, Akin O, Alexander LF, et al. ACR appropriateness criteria® penetrating trauma-lower abdomen and pelvis. J Am Coll Radiol. 2019;16(11S):S392–8.
12. Expert Panels on Cardiac Imaging and Thoracic Imaging, Stojanovska J, Hurwitz Koweek LM, Chung JH, Ghoshhajra BB, Walker CM, et al. ACR appropriateness criteria® blunt chest trauma-suspected cardiac injury. J Am Coll Radiol. 2020;17(11S):S380–90.
13. Bancroft LW, Kransdorf MJ, Adler R, Appel M, Beaman FD, Bernard SA, et al. ACR appropriateness criteria acute trauma to the foot. J Am Coll Radiol. 2015;12(6):575–81.
14. Expert Panel on Musculoskeletal Imaging, Smith SE, Chang EY, Ha AS, Bartolotta RJ, Bucknor M, et al. ACR appropriateness criteria® acute trauma to the ankle. J Am Coll Radiol. 2020;17(11S):S355–66.
15. Expert Panel on Musculoskeletal Imaging, Taljanovic MS, Chang EY, Ha AS, Bartolotta RJ, Bucknor M, et al. ACR appropriateness criteria® acute trauma to the knee. J Am Coll Radiol. 2020;17(5S):S12–25.
16. Expert Panel on Musculoskeletal Imaging, Torabi M, Lenchik L, Beaman FD, Wessell DE, Bussell JK, et al. ACR appropriateness criteria® acute hand and wrist trauma. J Am Coll Radiol. 2019;16(5S):S7–17.
17. Tuite MJ, Kransdorf MJ, Beaman FD, Adler RS, Amini B, Appel M, et al. ACR appropriateness criteria acute trauma to the knee. J Am Coll Radiol. 2015;12(11):1164–72.
18. Expert Panel on Neurological Imaging and Musculoskeletal Imaging, Beckmann NM, West OC, Nunez D, Kirsch CFE, Aulino JM, et al. ACR appropriateness criteria® suspected spine trauma. J Am Coll Radiol. 2019;16(5S):S264–85.
19. Expert Panel on Neurological Imaging, Shih RY, Burns J, Ajam AA, Broder JS, Chakraborty S, et al. ACR appropriateness criteria® head trauma: 2021 update. J Am Coll Radiol. 2021;18(5S):S13–36.
20. Shetty VS, Reis MN, Aulino JM, Berger KL, Broder J, Choudhri AF, et al. ACR appropriateness criteria head trauma. J Am Coll Radiol. 2016;13(6):668–79.
21. Expert Panel on Neurological Imaging, Parsons MS, Policeni B, Juliano AF, Agarwal M, Benjamin ER, et al. ACR appropriateness criteria® imaging of facial trauma following primary survey. J Am Coll Radiol. 2022;19(5S):S67–86.
22. Expert Panel on Pediatric Imaging, Ryan ME, Pruthi S, Desai NK, Falcone RA, Glenn OA, et al. ACR appropriateness criteria® head trauma-child. J Am Coll Radiol. 2020;17(5S):S125–37.
23. Expert Panel on Pediatric Imaging, Kadom N, Palasis S, Pruthi S, Biffl WL, Booth TN, et al. ACR appropriateness criteria® suspected spine trauma-child. J Am Coll Radiol. 2019;16(5S):S286–99.
24. Trauma Practice Management Guidelines. [cited 2023 Jan 31]. https://www.east.org/education-career-development/practice-management-guidelines/category/trauma.
25. Western Trauma Association Algorithms-Western Trauma Association. [cited 2023 Jan 31]. https://www.westerntrauma.org/western-trauma-association-algorithms/.
26. Raptis CA, Mellnick VM, Raptis DA, Kitchin D, Fowler KJ, Lubner M, et al. Imaging of trauma in the pregnant patient. Radiographics. 2014;34(3):748–63.
27. Huber-Wagner S, Lefering R, Qvick LM, Körner M, Kay MV, Pfeifer KJ, et al. Effect of whole-body CT during trauma resuscitation on survival: a retrospective, multicentre study. Lancet. 2009;373(9673):1455–61.
28. Sierink JC, Treskes K, Edwards MJR, Beuker BJA, den Hartog D, Hohmann J, et al. Immediate total-body CT scanning versus conventional imaging and selective CT scanning in patients with severe trauma (REACT-2): a randomised controlled trial. Lancet. 2016;388(10045):673–83.
29. Salastekar NV, Duszak R, Santavicca S, Horný M, Balthazar P, Khaja A, Hughes DR, Hanna TN. Utilization of chest and abdominopelvic CT for traumatic injury from 2011 to 2018: evaluation using a National commercial database. AJR Am J Roentgenol. 2023;220(2):265. [cited 2023 Feb 15]. https://pubmed.ncbi.nlm.nih.gov/36000666/.
30. Gupta M, Gertz M, Schriger DL. Injury severity score inflation resulting from pan–computed tomography in patients with blunt trauma. Ann Emerg Med. 2016;67(1):71–75.e3.
31. Hansen CK, Strayer RJ, Shy BD, Kessler S, Givre S, Shah KH. Prevalence of negative CT scans in a level one trauma center. Eur J Trauma Emerg Surg. 2018;44(1):29–33.
32. Wirth S, Hebebrand J, Basilico R, Berger FH, Blanco A, Calli C, et al. European Society of Emergency Radiology: guideline on radiological polytrauma

imaging and service (short version). Insights Imaging. 2020;11(1):135.
33. Kahn J, Fehrenbach U, Böning G, Feldhaus F, Maurer M, Renz D, et al. Spectral CT in patients with acute thoracoabdominal bleeding-a safe technique to improve diagnostic confidence and reduce dose? Medicine (Baltimore). 2019;98(25):e16101.
34. Studer S, van Veelen NM, van de Wall BJM, Kuner V, Schrading S, Link BC, et al. Improving the protocol for whole-body CT scans in trauma patients. Eur J Trauma Emerg Surg. 2022;48(4):3149–56.
35. Paes FM, Durso AM, Pinto DS, Covello B, Katz DS, Munera F. Diagnostic performance of triple-contrast versus single-contrast multi-detector computed tomography for the evaluation of penetrating bowel injury. Emerg Radiol. 2022;29(3):519–29.
36. Durso AM, Paes FM, Caban K, Danton G, Braga TA, Sanchez A, et al. Evaluation of penetrating abdominal and pelvic trauma. Eur J Radiol. 2020;130:109187.
37. Haroon SA, Rahimi H, Merritt A, Baghdanian A, Baghdanian A, LeBedis CA. Computed tomography (CT) in the evaluation of bladder and ureteral trauma: indications, technique, and diagnosis. Abdom Radiol (NY). 2019;44(12):3962–77.
38. Brink M, de Lange F, Oostveen LJ, Dekker HM, Kool DR, Deunk J, et al. Arm raising at exposure-controlled multidetector trauma CT of thoracoabdominal region: higher image quality, lower radiation dose. Radiology. 2008;249(2):661–70.
39. Kahn J, Grupp U, Maurer M. How does arm positioning of polytraumatized patients in the initial computed tomography (CT) affect image quality and diagnostic accuracy? Eur J Radiol. 2014;83(1):e67–71.
40. Karlo C, Gnannt R, Frauenfelder T, Leschka S, Brüesch M, Wanner GA, et al. Whole-body CT in polytrauma patients: effect of arm positioning on thoracic and abdominal image quality. Emerg Radiol. 2011;18(4):285–93.
41. Kim SJ, Ahn SJ, Choi SJ, Park DH, Kim HS, Kim JH. Optimal CT protocol for the diagnosis of active bleeding in abdominal trauma patients. Am J Emerg Med. 2019;37(7):1331–5.
42. Flammia F, Chiti G, Trinci M, Danti G, Cozzi D, Grassi R, et al. Optimization of CT protocol in polytrauma patients: an update. Eur Rev Med Pharmacol Sci. 2022;26(7):2543–55.
43. Baghdanian AH, Armetta AS, Baghdanian AA, LeBedis CA, Anderson SW, Soto JA. CT of major vascular injury in blunt abdominopelvic trauma. Radiographics. 2016;36(3):872–90.
44. Chung JH, Strigel RM, Chew AR, Albrecht E, Gunn ML. Overnight resident interpretation of torso CT at a level 1 trauma center an analysis and review of the literature. Acad Radiol. 2009;16(9):1155–60.
45. Carney E, Kempf J, DeCarvalho V, Yudd A, Nosher J. Preliminary interpretations of after-hours CT and sonography by radiology residents versus final interpretations by body imaging radiologists at a level 1 trauma center. AJR Am J Roentgenol. 2003;181(2):367–73.
46. Yeates EO, Grigorian A, Chinn J, Young H, Colin Escobar J, Glavis-Bloom J, et al. Night radiology coverage for trauma: residents, teleradiology, or both? J Am Coll Surg. 2022;235(3):500–9.

Head CT in Trauma

2

Linda J. Bagley and Joel M. Stein

Societal Impact of Traumatic Brain Injury

Traumatic brain injury is a major public health issue. In the USA, approximately 2.8 million people sustain a traumatic brain injury (TBI) each year. Of those individuals, approximately 2.5 million will be evaluated in an emergency department, more than 200,000 will be hospitalized, and likely greater than 50,000 will die (64,362 in 2020) [1]. Motor vehicle accidents are the leading cause of moderate to severe TBI in young adults with falls being the most frequent cause in the elderly and children. Additional causes include sports related injuries and penetrating trauma [2]. Risks of hospitalization and death are greatest in patients over age 75, with men more than two times more likely to be hospitalized than women and more than three times as likely to die [3]. The risks of sustaining moderate to severe head trauma have been somewhat mitigated in recent years with improvements in and increased utilization of motor vehicle safety devices, increased severity of penalties for driving while intoxicated, and development of more sophisticated helmets and other protective gear. It is estimated that 5.3 million Americans suffer with long term disabilities related to traumatic brain injury. Individual and societal costs are staggering. The CDC previously estimated the lifetime societal economic costs of TBI, including lifetime medical expenses, in and outpatient rehabilitation costs and lost wages to exceed $76 billion in 2010 dollars [4]. The unemployment rate within 2 years of a traumatic brain injury is approximately 60% [5], and more than 50% of homeless individuals have been affected by TBI [6].

Primary traumatic brain injuries may be direct (due to impact with possible resultant intracranial hemorrhage) or indirect (related to contracoup injury or to rotational or acceleration-deceleration injuries with resultant axonal disruption) [7, 8]. Secondary effects of traumatic brain injuries include increased intracranial pressure with resultant herniation syndromes, hypoxic and ischemic sequelae, and secondary infections. Long-term sequelae include focal encephalomalacia, diffuse volume loss, hydrocephalus, epilepsy, and chronic traumatic encephalopathy (CTE) as well as osseous and soft tissue deformities [9].

Multiple clinical trials including those examining the roles of hypothermia, neurostimulants, and neuroprotective agents (including cell cycle inhibitors, estrogen related agents, and erythropoietin) have yielded disappointing results for improvement of outcomes in TBI. Mortality sta-

L. J. Bagley (✉) · J. M. Stein
Division of Neuroradiology, Department of Radiology, Perelman School of Medicine at the University of Pennsylvania, Philadelphia, PA, USA
e-mail: Linda.Bagley@pennmedicine.upenn.edu; Joel.Stein@pennmedicine.upenn.edu

F. Knollmann (ed.), *Trauma Computed Tomography*, https://doi.org/10.1007/978-3-031-45746-3_2

tistics have somewhat improved, however, since the 1950s, largely related to improved monitoring and treatment of increased intracranial pressure, specifically related to the earlier detection of injuries and earlier neurosurgical intervention including hematoma evacuation and decompressive craniectomies [10].

Central Role of CT in Imaging Head Trauma

Multiple advantages of computed tomography (CT) make it the primary imaging modality for assessing head trauma. With a single scan, CT rapidly generates whole head volumetric density data that can be reconstructed in multiple planes, variable resolutions, and different kernels emphasizing osseous details or soft tissue contrasts. Modern scanners enable protocols with fast helical acquisitions and superb resolution (Table 2.1). CT exquisitely depicts bony anatomy including skull fractures. At the same time, CT provides sufficient soft tissue contrast resolution to demonstrate superficial soft tissue injuries and critical intracranial findings, including hemorrhage, brain edema, infarction, mass effect, herniation and hydrocephalus.

Intracranial assessment by CT is facilitated by the anatomy and physical properties of the brain and its supporting structures, and in particular the density differences between bone, gray matter, white matter, cerebrospinal fluid (CSF), and hematomas of different ages. Appropriate window levels (Table 2.1) should be used and adjusted to accentuate these differences visually. Critically, acute clotted blood whether in the epidural, subdural, subarachnoid, intraventricular, or intraparenchymal spaces appears hyperdense to brain tissue on CT. As hematomas soften, sediment and resorb, their density approaches that of brain tissue in the subacute phase (days to weeks) and CSF in the chronic phase (weeks to months). Furthermore, the density difference between brain and CSF in ventricles, sulci, and cisterns makes mass effect in the intracranial space readily apparent. With the use of iodinated intravenous contrast, CT also delivers excellent depiction of the intracranial arterial and venous vasculature. Three-dimensional post-processing techniques including volume rendering and maximum intensity projection facilitate visualization of vascular structures. Dual-energy CT scanners permit one to distinguish acute hematoma from iodinated contrast.

The main disadvantage of CT is its use of ionizing radiation, although head CTs impart lower effective dose than body imaging studies [11], and techniques such as dose modulation and iterative reconstruction help to decrease dose. Lower dose protocols may also be used for follow-up scans. CT provides less soft tissue contrast including lower sensitivity for ischemic stroke than MRI. CT

Table 2.1 Typical protocol for unenhanced head CT in trauma

Protocol name	Unenhanced head CT
Indication	Trauma, stroke, headache, altered mental status
Protocol designed for (scanner model)	Siemens
Patient preparation	All metal, glasses, hats, clips, jewelry taken off prior to scan
Patient positioning	Head first, chin slightly tilted towards chest, supine
Oral contrast	None
IV contrast	None
Acquisition mode	Helical
Tube settings	
kV	120
mA	400
Dose modulation	Yes
Tube rotation time (s)	1
Table speed (mm/s)	2.75
Slice collimation (mm)	5
Reconstructed slice thickness (mm)	5 (soft tissue), 2 (bone)
Anatomical coverage	Top of skull to orbital meatal line
Reconstruction kernel	Hc40 (soft tissue), Hr68 (bone)
Breath hold	No
Window level settings (HU center:Width)	40:80 (soft tissue), 444:1500 (bone), 30:30 (stroke)
Post processing	Coronal 3 mm sections (soft tissue), thin 1 mm sections as needed
Typical dose (mGy)	38.64–60.41
CTDIvol (mGy)	45.98–56.30
DLP (mGycm)	974.8
Eff. Dose (eff. mAS)	332

images can be degraded by beam hardening artifact from dense bone or streak artifact from metallic objects such as ballistic fragments, dental amalgam, aneurysm clips or coils, and support devices overlying the patient. On the other hand, there is no safety risk from ferromagnetic materials as with MRI. Due to its efficiency and general utility, CT is widely available in emergency departments and medical centers worldwide.

CT scanning has proven instrumental in the rapid detection of conditions, namely intracranial hematomas, fractures, hydrocephalus and mass effect/herniation, amenable to neurosurgical intervention. In recent years, artificial intelligence tools have been developed to allow automated detection of intracranial hemorrhage. These tools have been reported to have approximately 93% accuracy with lower rates of detection for subdural and subarachnoid hemorrhage and false positives occurring in the settings of artifacts and neoplastic lesions. Nonetheless, these tools can be used to draw the attention of the reading radiologist to "flagged" studies with hemorrhage, have been shown to reduce report turn-around times by approximately 10% [12–14], and may become a larger part of radiologic practice over time.

Additionally, utilization of portable head CT has increased the efficiency of imaging critically ill inpatients, while also improving the safety of imaging such patients. Multidetector portable CT scanners (Fig. 2.1), typically weighing

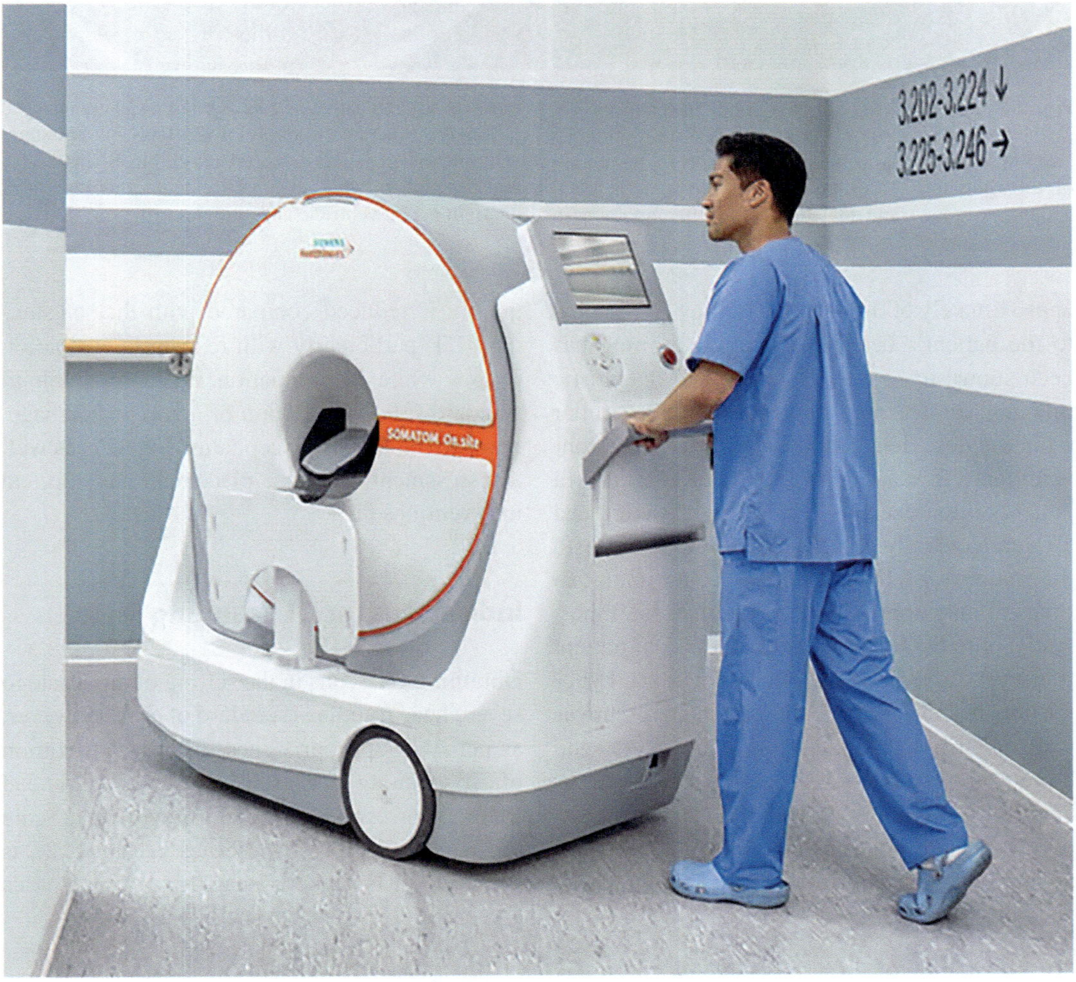

Fig. 2.1 Portable CT scanner. Portable unit is moved through hospital hallway

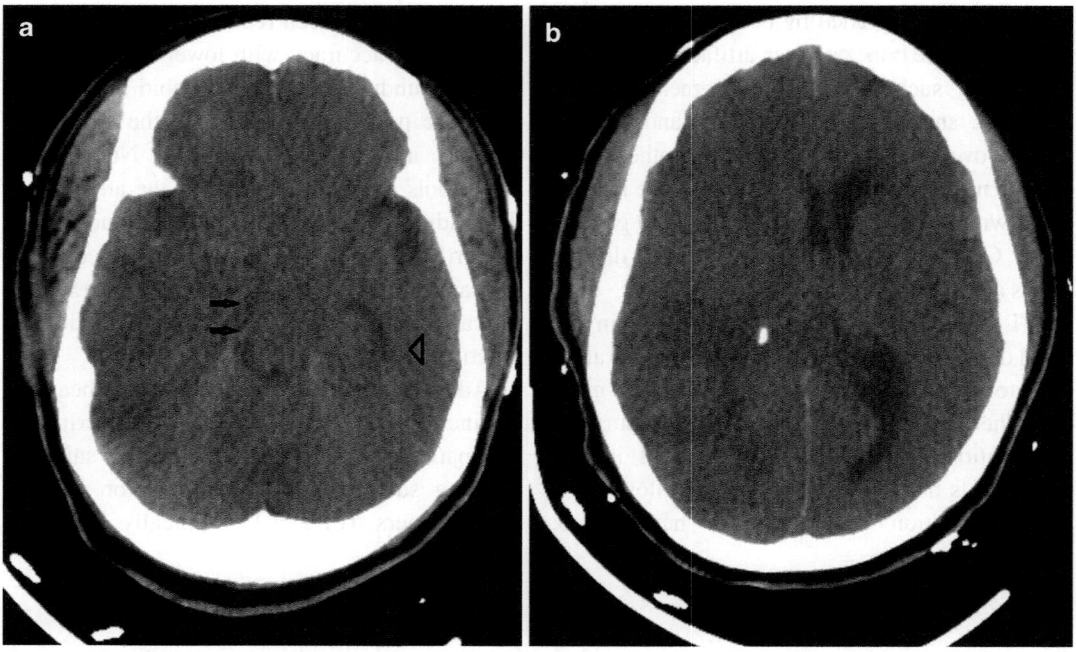

Fig. 2.2 Portable head CT. (**a**) Axial unenhanced CT image generated portably demonstrates disproportionate swelling with edema in the right hemisphere, herniation of the right uncus, compression of the right cerebral peduncle (arrows), and dilatation of the left temporal horn (arrowhead), indicative of trapping. (**b**) Axial unenhanced CT image generated portably at the level of the lateral ventricles again demonstrates edema within the right cerebral hemisphere with sulcal effacement, compression of the right lateral ventricle and midline shift

approximately 500–750 pounds, may be wheeled to the patient's bedside. Portable scanning has been shown to be cost effective, and diagnostic imaging studies may be obtained with similar radiation dose delivered as would be with a conventional CT scanner. Transport of critically ill patients often exceeds 1 h, while portable head CTs are generally completed within 20 min with the majority of time spent in set up and scan times of only approximately 3 min. Most importantly, portable CT eliminates the risks of patient transport. Adverse events such as hypoxia, hypotension, and elevations in intracranial pressure as well as dislodgement of tubes, catheters, and monitoring devices have been reported to occur between 15 and 70% of the time during transport. Despite limitations, portable CT is of diagnostic quality in >95% of cases. Though image quality is reduced compared with that of standard CT, particularly with respect to evaluation of grey white differentiation, it is comparable to standard CT for detection of acute hemorrhage, mass effect, and hydrocephalus (Fig. 2.2) as well as assessment of device placement and surgical interventions [15].

Indications for CT Scanning

Obtaining CT scans in the setting of moderate to severe head trauma is standard of care. However, as per ACR appropriateness criteria, utilization of CT scanning in the setting of acute mild head trauma, corresponding to Glasgow Coma Scale (GCS) scores of 13–15 (Tables 2.1 and 2.2), is generally of low yield with 10% or fewer cases demonstrating positive findings and 1% or less prompting surgical intervention [16–18]. Both the Canadian CT Head Rule and The New Orleans Criteria have validated clinical decision making in the setting of minor head trauma (typically manifest with no or brief loss of consciousness or other symptoms of concussion). New Orleans Criteria apply to patients who sustained blunt head trauma within 24 h of presentation, who experienced loss of consciousness, definite amnesia or witnessed disorientation (Table 2.3). These criteria state that head CT is indicated in such patients when one or more of the following criteria are met: Age over 60, headache, vomiting, intoxication, persistent anterograde amnesia, seizure, or visible trauma above the clavicle [19]. The Canadian CT Head rule excludes patients with GCS scores <13, age < 16 years, on blood thinners, or with visible open skull fractures. Otherwise, the rule indicates that head CT is only warranted for minor head injuries when one or more of the following criteria are present: GCS not returned to baseline after 2 h, age > 65, suspected open or depressed skull fractures, signs of skull base fractures (hemotympanum, CSF rhinorrhea or otorrhea, "Battle's sign" or raccoon eyes), two or more episodes of vomiting, retrograde amnesia for 30 min or more, or dangerous mechanism (pedestrian struck by motor vehicle, motor vehicle ejection, fall down five or more steps or from greater than 3 ft.) [20].

Table 2.2 Glasgow coma scale

Eye opening score	
No eye opening	1
Opens eyes to verbal stimulus	2
Opens eyes to painful stimulus	3
Opens eyes spontaneously	4
Verbal score	
No verbal response	1
Makes incomprehensible sounds	2
Says inappropriate words	3
Confused	4
Oriented to person, place, and time	5
Motor score	
Motionless	1
Abnormal extensor posturing	2
Abnormal flexion	3
Withdraws from painful stimuli	4
Localizes to painful stimuli	5
Follows commands	6

Table 2.3 Grading of TBI

Classification	GCS	Duration of loss of consciousness	Duration of post-traumatic amnesia
Mild	13–15	< 30 min	< 24 h
Moderate	9–12	30 min–24 h	1–7 days
Severe	3–8	>24 h	> 7 days

Predictors of Outcome

CT findings at presentation not only often dictate management but have been shown to contribute to prognostication of patient outcome. Clinical predictors of outcome include age, socio-economic status, race, ethnicity, Glasgow Coma Scale score, duration of post traumatic amnesia, mechanism of injury, underlying psychiatric disease, intoxication, and presence of hypotension, hypoxia, hypothermia, hyperglycemia, and thrombocytopenia [21]. Imaging characteristics most predictive of outcome include the status of the basilar cisterns (normal, compressed or absent), presence of midline shift >5 mm, presence of epidural hematoma, and presence of subarachnoid and/or intraventricular hemorrhage. A quantitative Rotterdam score can be calculated based on these characteristics, with the lowest Rotterdam score (1) associated with no mortality and highest Rotterdam score (6) associated with greater than 60% mortality [22].

Primary Injuries

Again, primary injuries refer to the direct effects of head trauma, including skull fractures and hemorrhage in different anatomic compartments. As described in detail in the following paragraphs, intracranial hemorrhage occurs in distinct locations due to different pathological mechanisms and relationships between skull, arteries, venous sinuses, meningeal layers, and brain, resulting in different imaging patterns, evolution over time, and clinical impact. Often, traumatic intracranial hemorrhage will be identified in multiple compartments and complex trauma cases present numerous important findings. Thus, it is important to develop a thorough search pattern, optimize images and approach for detecting pathology, learn to distinguish between hemorrhage in different locations, and avoid common pitfalls in trauma head CT interpretation (Table 2.4).

Epidural hematomas (Fig. 2.3) are most often seen in young patients, ages 20–30, are associ-

Table 2.4 Tips for avoiding common pitfalls in trauma head CT interpretation

Pitfalls	Tips and explanations
Missed findings in cases with multiple abnormalities (i.e., satisfaction/ exhaustion of search)	Develop a systematic search pattern or checklist
Missed fracture, hemorrhage or infarct	Use appropriate kernels and window levels
Missed fractures (especially nondisplaced or in-plane)	Use thin section reconstructions and multiplanar reformats Look near sites of scalp swelling or pneumocephalus
Missed skull base or temporal bone fractures	Clear the paranasal sinuses and temporal bone air spaces Look near sites of pneumocephalus
Normal sutures misinterpreted as fractures	Appreciate normal locations, symmetry, zigzag shape and corticated margins of calvarial sutures
Beam hardening artifact misinterpreted as blood	Use thin section reconstructions and multiplanar reformats Appreciate artifact typical locations and non-anatomic pattern Remove overlying material when possible, prior to scanning
Partial volume through bone misinterpreted as blood	Use thin section reconstructions and multiplanar reformats
Missed small intracranial hematomas	Use thin section reconstructions and multiplanar reformats Look for hemorrhage subjacent to scalp swelling and fractures
Missed subdural hematomas isodense to brain	Follow sulci out to the inner table of the calvarium
Missed subdural collection hypodense to brain	Look for displacement of cortical veins
Contusions misinterpreted as extra-axial blood	Look for hypodense edema around parenchymal hemorrhage Look for expansion of hemorrhagic contusions over 24–48 h

Table 2.4 (continued)

Pitfalls	Tips and explanations
Epidural versus subdural confusion	Subdural hematomas may appear lentiform, especially on coronal images. Vertex, occipital posterior fossa and anterior middle cranial fossa epidural hematomas are typically venous and displace adjacent dural venous sinuses Epidural collections are typical beneath craniotomy flaps
Mixed density hematomas	Mixed density hematomas often reflect acute or subacute on chronic hemorrhage but low density can reflect unclotted hyperacute hemorrhage, coagulopathy or CSF mixing
Transiently hyperattenuating subdural hygromas	Patients often receive additional contrast-enhanced trauma imaging after unenhanced head CT; previously hypodense subdural hygromas may increase attenuation transiently on follow-up scans due to contrast diffusing into these collections

ated with skull fractures in 75–90% of cases, and are classically related to injuries of the middle meningeal artery though may also be seen in the setting of injury to a dural venous sinus. They are classically lentiform in shape and typically do not cross suture lines (though this rule may be violated in the setting of fractures as well as surgically created calvarial defects). As the calvarium typically absorbs the brunt of impact, there may be little underlying brain injury, and prognosis in the setting of an isolated promptly detected epidural hematoma may be quite good. As epidural hematomas result from major vascular injury (85% associated with arterial injuries), they have the potential for rapid expansion [23]. Mixed attenuation or presence of a swirling effect within an epidural hematoma is highly suggestive of active hemorrhage [24]. Surgical intervention is warranted in these situations as well as in the setting of poor neurologic status, focal neurologic deficit, midline shift greater than 5 mm, and hematoma volume exceeding 30 mL. Hematoma volume can be calculated by the ellipsoid method, multiplying the three dimensions of the hematoma and dividing by two. Conservative manage-

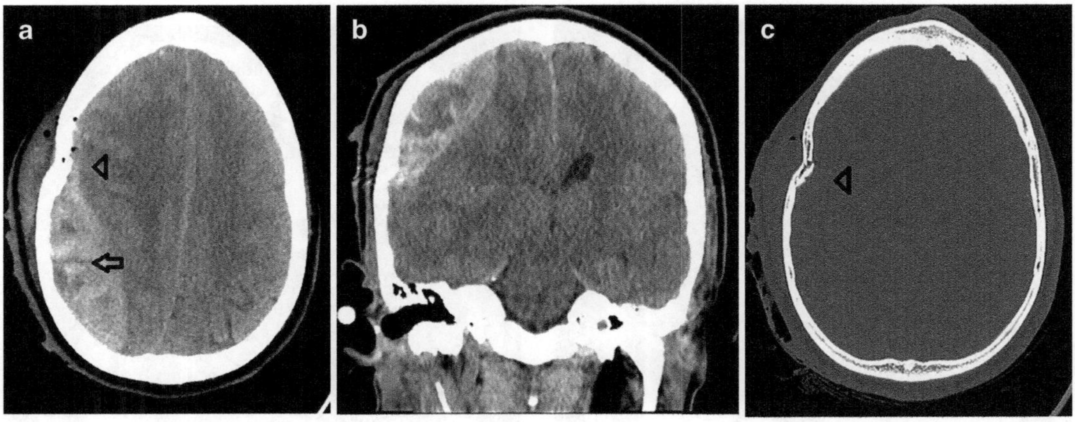

Fig. 2.3 Epidural hematoma. (**a–c**) Axial and coronal unenhanced CT scans reconstructed in soft tissue and bone algorithms (**c**) demonstrate a large, lentiform epidural hematoma. Mixed attenuation within the collection is suggestive of active hemorrhage (arrow). The collection exerts significant mass effect upon the underlying brain parenchyma with associated compression of the right lateral ventricle and minimal midline shift to the left. The collection appears to originate adjacent to a fracture extending through the squamous portion of the right temporal bone with associated probable injury to the right middle meningeal artery (arrowhead at the level of the groove within which the artery travels along the inner table of the calvarium)

ment to include frequent neurological examinations and follow-up head CTs at 6–8 h intervals is reasonable in the absence of the above-described conditions. Venous epidural hematomas are less common but occur in characteristic locations usually due to fractures traversing the major dural venous sinuses, that is at the vertex (superior sagittal sinus), occipital posterior fossa (transverse sinus), and anterior middle cranial fossa (sphenoparietal sinus). These hematomas typically displace the involved sinus from the overlying bone, crossing the midline at the vertex (Fig. 2.4) or the posterior margin of the tentorium (Fig. 2.5). In these cases, it is always imperative to search for associated venous sinus thrombosis. Anterior middle cranial fossa epidural hematomas tend not to enlarge or cause significant mass effect and often can be managed conservatively (Fig. 2.6) [25].

Subdural hematomas (Fig. 2.7) are typically venous in etiology, attributed to torn bridging veins, and often associated with brain parenchymal injury. They are associated with high morbidity and mortality, particularly in the elderly. These hematomas are typically crescentic in

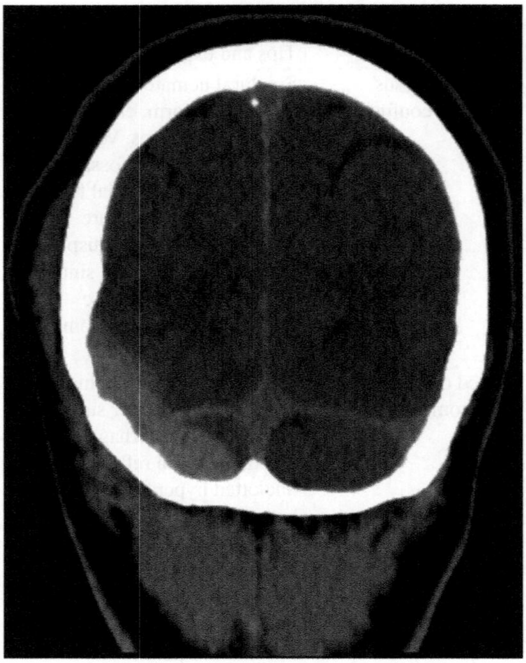

Fig. 2.5 Occipital posterior fossa epidural hematoma. Coronal unenhanced CT scan demonstrates an acute venous hematoma due to a skull fracture crossing the transverse sinus. The hematoma displaces the sinus and tentorium, extending between the occipital convexity and posterior fossa

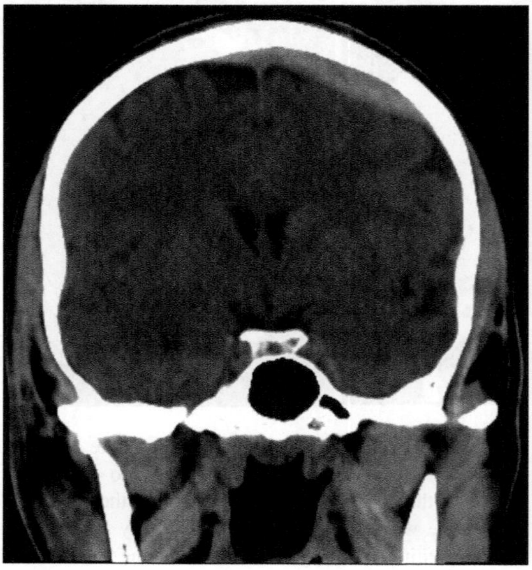

Fig. 2.4 Vertex epidural hematoma. Coronal unenhanced CT scan shows an acute venous hematoma at the left vertex due to a skull fracture traversing the superior sinus. The hematoma displaces the sinus and crosses the midline to the right

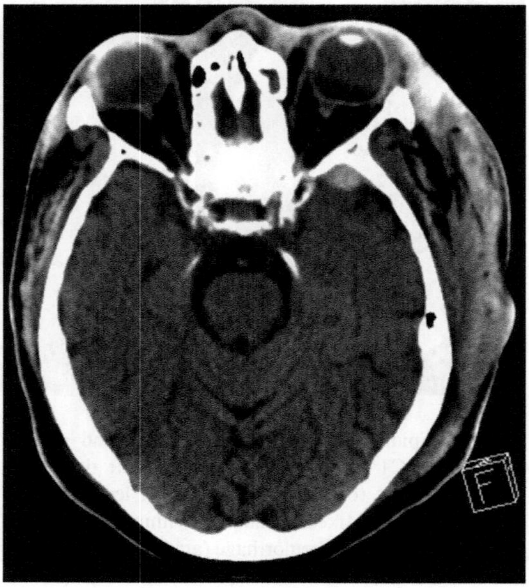

Fig. 2.6 Anterior middle cranial fossa epidural hematoma. Axial unenhanced CT scan shows a typical benign acute venous hematoma along the left greater sphenoid wing

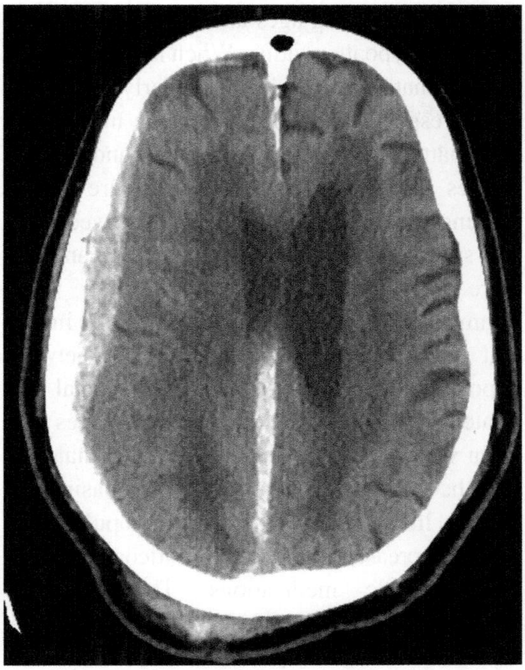

Fig. 2.7 Acute subdural hematoma. Axial unenhanced CT scan demonstrates an acute subdural hematoma along the right cerebral convexity, exerting mild mass effect upon the right cerebral hemisphere, manifest by sulcal effacement, compression of the right lateral ventricle, and minimal midline shift to the left. There is also acute subdural hemorrhage seen along the falx. There is posterior scalp soft tissue injury. Hypoattenuation in the white matter likely reflects sequela of small vessel and/or perfusional ischemic disease

shape and are not bounded by calvarial sutures lines. However, they do not cross the midline as they are bounded by the falx. They may occur or extend along the interhemispheric fissure or tentorium (Fig. 2.8) [23].

Acute subdural hematomas may not always be hyper-attenuating. They may be iso or hypo-attenuating due to decreased iron content in the setting of severe anemia (Fig. 2.9) or due to mixing with CSF when there has been disruption of the arachnoid membrane. Subdural hygromas, hypodense collections of CSF in the subdural space, may also occur in the acute setting, again typically attributed to tears in the arachnoid membrane. Trauma imaging often includes enhanced chest, abdomen and pelvis CT studies after the initial unenhanced head CT. Due to iodinated contrast diffusing into the subdural space, hygromas may show transiently increased attenuation on short-term follow-up CT scans and be confused with new acute hematomas (Fig. 2.10). In such cases, look back for a hygroma on the initial scan, stable in size but uniformly increased in attenuation on the subsequent exam, and rapidly decreasing in attenuation on further follow-up.

Subdural hematomas may also present in the subacute and chronic phases, containing blood

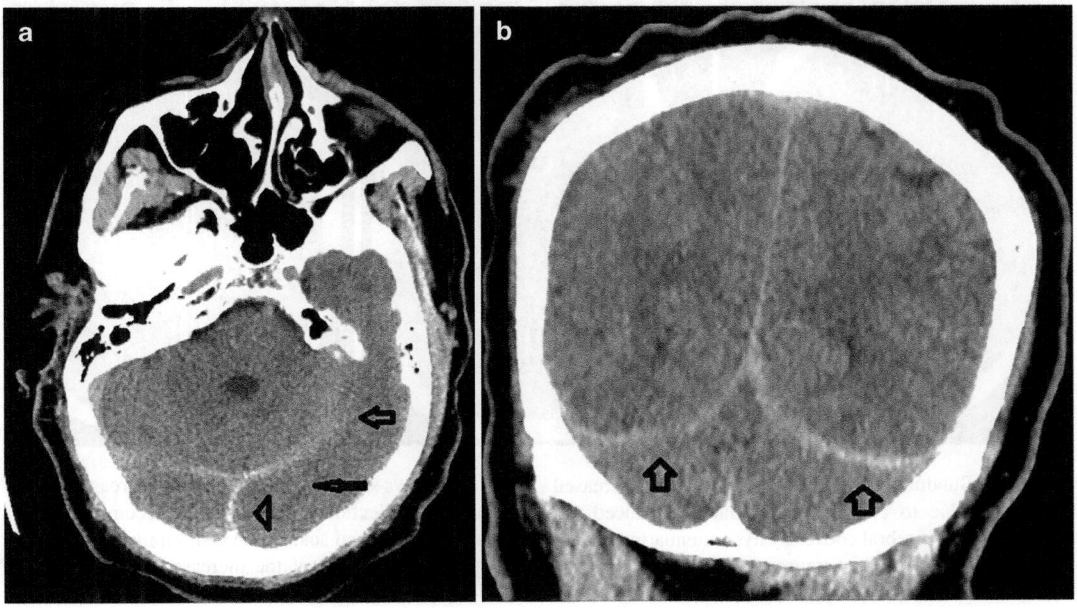

Fig. 2.8 Acute subdural hematoma (Tentorium and Falx). (**a**) Axial unenhanced CT scan is notable for ill defined, hyper-attenuating acute subdural hemorrhage, layering along the tentorial leaflets (arrows) and posterior falx (arrowhead). (**b**) Coronal image better demonstrates small left larger than right subdural hematomas (arrows)

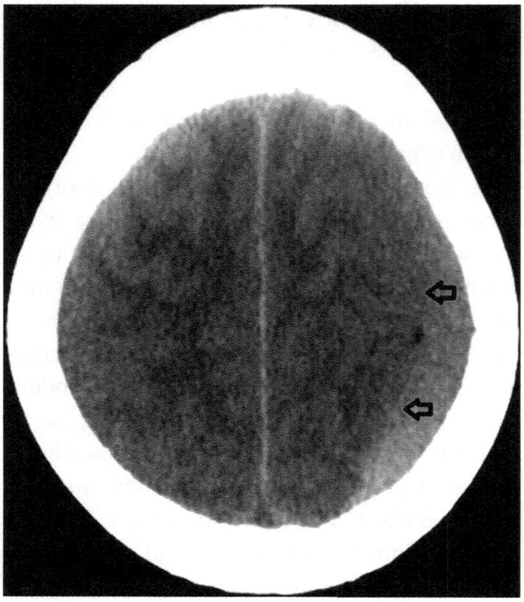

Fig. 2.9 Isodense subdural hematoma. Axial unenhanced CT scan obtained in a markedly anemic patient with leukemia reveals a large, approximately 1.4 cm in maximal width, subdural hematoma overlying the left convexity. The hematoma is of mixed density with largely isodense component. Although the collection in part has similar attenuation characteristics to normal brain, it is amorphous; note that the normal gyral pattern of the brain is displaced medially by the collection (arrows) and does not extend to the inner table of the calvarium

products of varying ages and hence also appearing iso or hypoattenuating. When iso-attenuating, these hematomas may be particularly difficult to detect, especially if bilateral. Again multiplanar reformatted images are essential, and all CT images should be scrutinized to ensure that an isodense collection is not present between gyri and sulci and the calvarial inner table, and that there is no displacement of cortical veins. Examination of cortical veins is especially important in older patients to distinguish between hypodense subdural collections and normal age-related enlargement of subarachnoid spaces with brain volume loss. Chronic subdural hematomas have been seen with significantly increasing frequency, likely related to the aging population as well as increased utilization of anticoagulant and antithrombotic medications. They typically develop over a period of weeks. Components of acute hemorrhage may be present within them, and membranes may form (Fig. 2.11). Re-accumulation of fluid and blood products within these collections is common (generally estimated at 10–30% following surgical evacuation), and often makes their management troublesome. Recently, middle meningeal artery embolization has been utilized for treatment of chronic subdural hematomas. A meta-analysis of

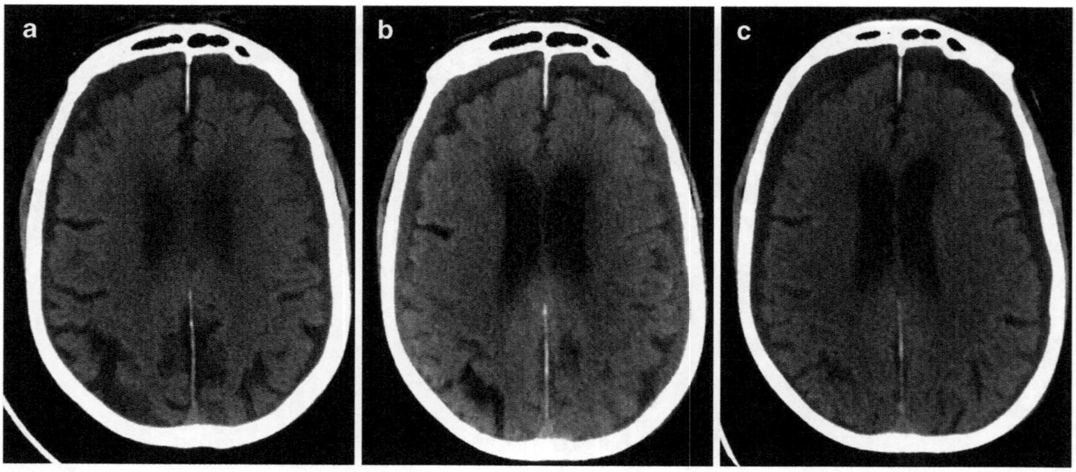

Fig. 2.10 Subdural hygromas with transiently increased attenuation due to contrast. (**a**) Axial unenhanced CT shows bilateral cerebral convexity hypoattenuating collections consistent with post-traumatic hygromas. Note the inward displacement of cortical veins. (**b**) Axial scan 1 day later shows stable size but uniformly increased attenuation of the collections due to contrast accumulated from an interval enhanced scan. (**c**) Axial scan yet another day later shows resolution of the increased attenuation seen the day before

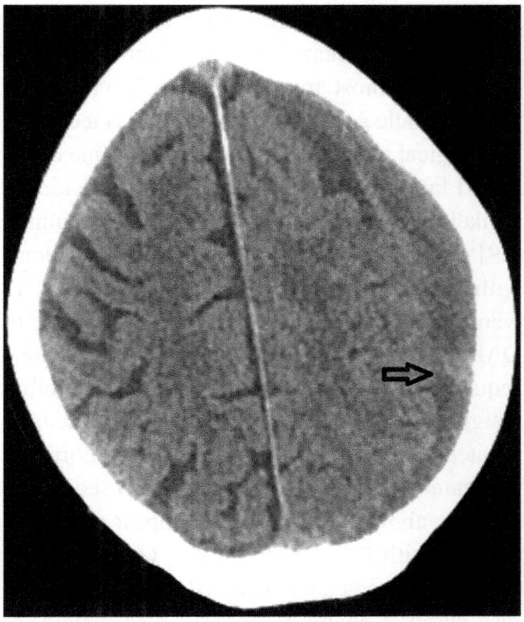

Fig. 2.11 Chronic subdural hematoma. Axial unenhanced CT scan reveals a predominantly hypo-attenuating chronic subdural hematoma along the left convexity with small components of acute hemorrhage (hyper-attenuating focus seen posteriorly) (arrow) and internal membranes. There is associated mass effect upon the left hemisphere as manifest by sulcal effacement

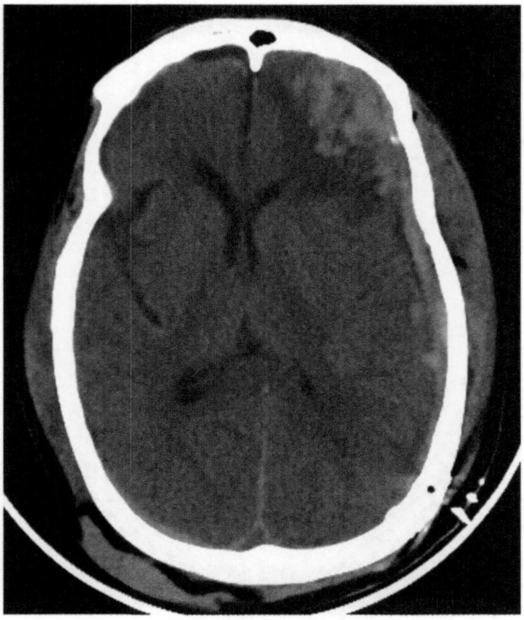

Fig. 2.12 Contusion. Axial image demonstrates parenchymal hemorrhage and surrounding edema, representing contusion in the left frontal lobe. Hemorrhage in this case is multi-compartmental, including subdural hemorrhage along the left convexity and posterior interhemispheric fissure. Note mass effect upon the left cerebral hemisphere, and prominent left scalp soft tissue swelling

several case series reported recurrence rate of only 2.1% following middle meningeal artery embolization [26].

Cortical contusions (Fig. 2.12) may be bland or hemorrhagic, with scattered petechial hemorrhage within surrounding edematous brain (in contradistinction to subarachnoid hemorrhage, not typically associated with edema) or with development of frank, space occupying hematomas. They may be coup (occurring at the site of impact) or contrecoup (occurring opposite to the site of impact). They most commonly occur at sites where brain impacts the calvarium or skull base. As such, the most frequently affected areas are the inferior frontal lobes which impact the cribriform plate and planum sphenoidale and the anterior temporal lobes which impact the sphenoid wings. Delayed hemorrhage and/or worsening edema, typically manifesting within the first 24–72 h, occurs in approximately 40–50% of cases. Male patients, elderly patients, and those with coagulopathy are at increased risk for delayed hemorrhage. Risk of death and disability are correlated with initial hematoma volume as well as hematoma growth [27].

Intraventricular and subarachnoid hemorrhage may also be present with intraventricular hemorrhage occurring in approximately up to 35% of cases of moderate to severe TBI [28]. Intraventricular hemorrhage may result from extension of an intraparenchymal hematoma or may result from rotationally induced tears of subependymal veins. It is seen in approximately 60% of cases with corpus callosal injuries. Trauma is the most common cause of subarachnoid hemorrhage. When traumatic in etiology, subarachnoid hemorrhage is typically peripherally located, scattered, and seen in association with multi-compartmental hemorrhage as well as external signs of trauma (Fig. 2.13). In some cases, particularly when the mechanism of injury is unclear, it may be difficult to distinguish traumatic from aneurysmal subarachnoid hemorrhage and angiographic imaging may be required.

Diffuse axonal injury (DAI) is typically clinically manifest by immediate and often prolonged

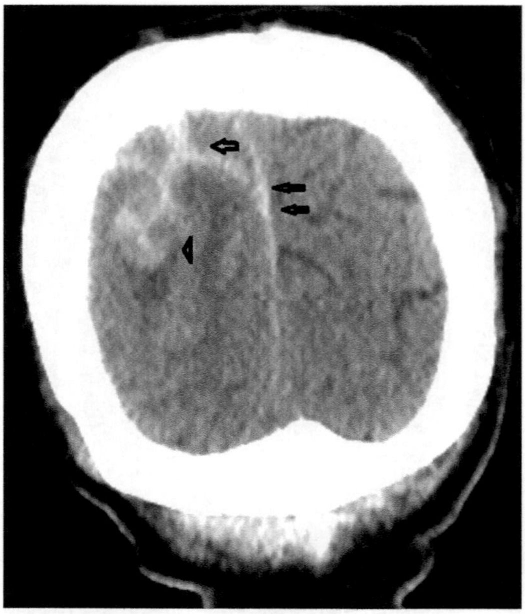

Fig. 2.13 Subarachnoid hemorrhage. Coronal CT scan reveals subarachnoid hemorrhage within right parietal sulci (arrow). Additionally, there is a small amount of parenchymal hemorrhage seen inferiorly (arrowhead), and there is subdural hemorrhage along the falx (double arrow)

loss of consciousness and is caused by rapid acceleration/deceleration and/or rotational movements. It is most frequently seen in victims of motor vehicle accidents but has been detected on histological analysis even in those who have sustained falls from a standing height. Its incidence is likely grossly underestimated by CT scanning [29]. In one study, approximately 30% of patients with mild head trauma and normal head CTs were shown to have abnormalities indicative of DAI on MRI obtained with gradient echo sequences [30]. Furthermore, susceptibility weighted sequences demonstrate significantly greater sensitivity for intracranial hemorrhage compared to traditional gradient echo sequences [31]. As above, head CTs may appear normal in patients with DAI. Alternatively, CT scans may demonstrate petechial hemorrhages and/or diffuse cerebral edema with associated paucity of sulci, ventricular, and cisternal effacement and loss of grey-white differentiation. Typically affected areas include the grey-white junctions (Grade 1), the splenium of the corpus callosum (Grade 2), and the brainstem (Grade 3)—most often the dorsal midbrain (Fig. 2.14). Neurologic

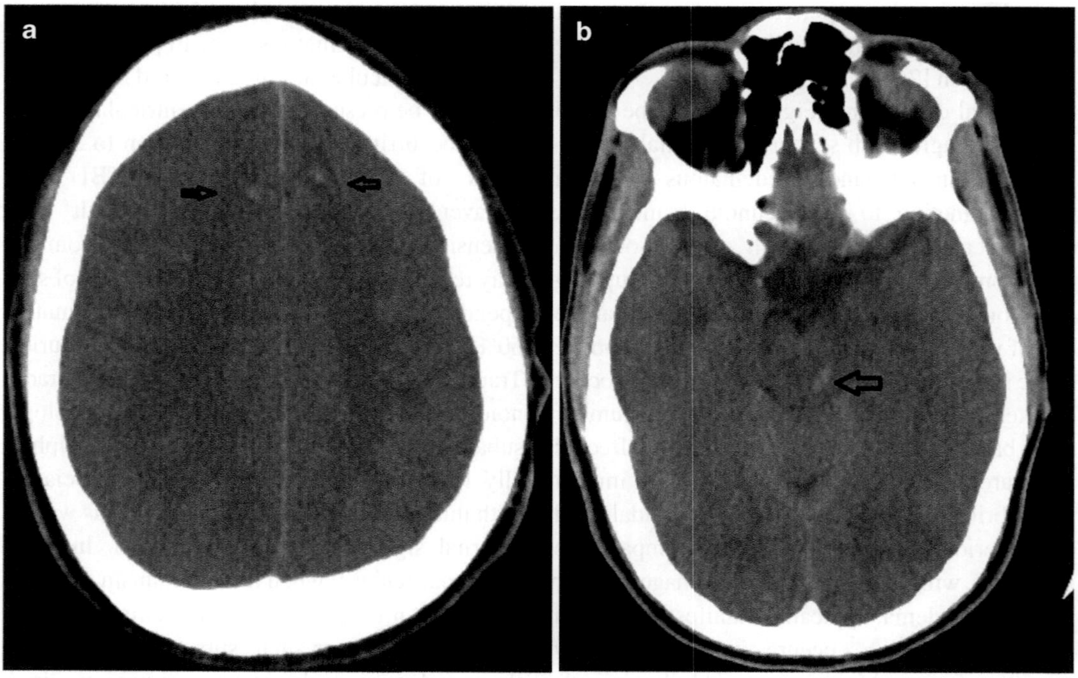

Fig. 2.14 Diffuse axonal injury. (**a**) Axial image demonstrates small regions of hemorrhagic shear injury in the bilateral frontal lobes with mild surrounding edema (arrows). (**b**) Axial unenhanced head CT demonstrates acute linear hemorrhage in the dorsal midbrain on the left (arrow)

prognosis has been correlated with both extent and location of shear injuries—with worsening prognosis associated with higher grades of injury [32].

Penetrating trauma may produce parenchymal hematomas and/or lacerations and is often associated with vascular injuries including dissections, transections, and/or arterial or venous occlusion (Fig. 2.15) and formation of aneurysms, pseudoaneurysms (Fig. 2.16), and arteriovenous fistulas. Initial screening is generally performed with CT angiography (CTA). Patients may be further studied with conventional angiography when non-invasive methods are equivocal or when there is a suspected need for endovascular intervention, such as vessel sacrifice or occlusion of a vascular abnormality [33].

Images reconstructed in bone algorithm with creation of 2D and 3D reformatted images aid in the detection of calvarial fractures

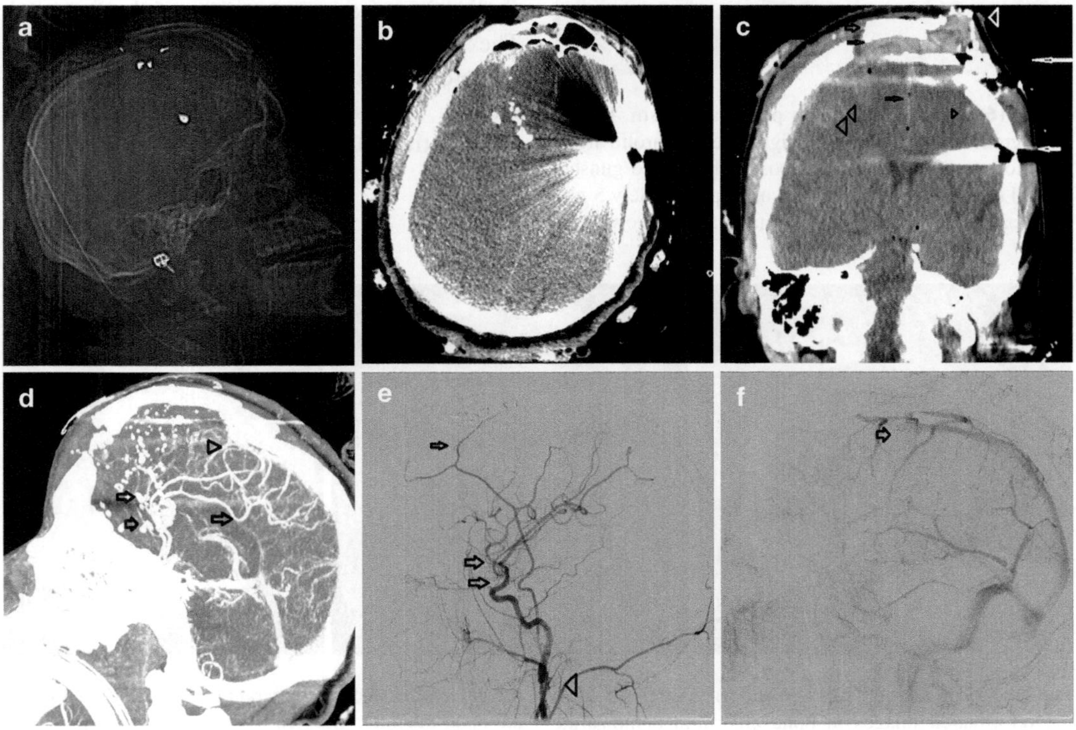

Fig. 2.15 Penetrating trauma. (**a**) Lateral scout topogram demonstrates numerous ballistic fragments projected over the skull with marked displacement and elevation of calvarial fracture fragments. (**b** and **c**) Axial and coronal CT scans redemonstrate the multiple ballistic fragments with associated streak artifact (white arrows). Images are also notable for multiple associated injuries including comminuted and displaced calvarial fractures (double black arrows), subdural hemorrhage along the falx (black arrows), scattered parenchymal (black arrowhead) and subarachnoid (black double arrowheads) hemorrhage, and external herniation of brain contents through the calvarial fractures (white arrowhead). (**d**) Sagittal maximal intensity projection (MIP) image from CT angiogram demonstrates irregularity of anterior cerebral artery branches (arrows) with paucity of vasculature in the frontal lobe. The superior sagittal sinus (arrowhead) is occluded anteriorly at the site of the fractures and reconstituted beyond the fractures. (**e**) Lateral view of cerebral angiogram obtained following left common carotid artery injection (arterial phase) is notable for relatively poor intracranial flow as manifest by earlier opacification of external carotid artery branches, e.g., the superficial temporal artery (arrow) than internal carotid artery branches (double arrow). This is likely secondary to a combination of proximal stenosis—see narrowing of left internal carotid artery secondary to dissection or vasospasm (arrowhead) and increased intracranial pressure. (**f**) Lateral view of cerebral angiogram obtained following left common carotid artery injection (venous phase) is notable for occlusion of the anterior portion of the superior sagittal sinus at the site of multiple calvarial fractures

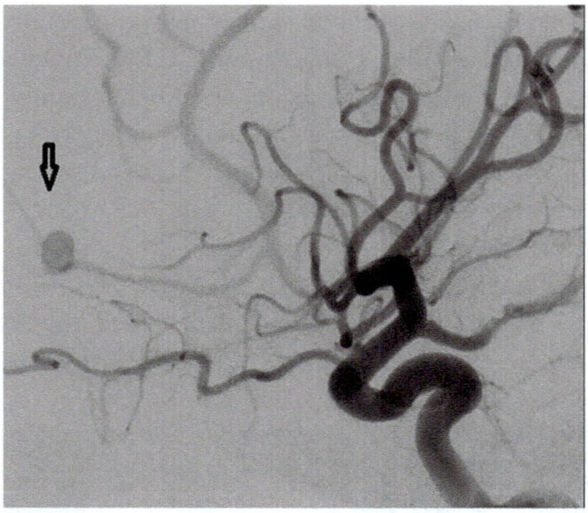

Fig. 2.16 Penetrating trauma pseudoaneurysm. Lateral angiogram obtained following right internal carotid artery injection in this patient status post self-inflicted gunshot wound to the head demonstrates an approximately 5 mm pseudoaneurysm of the orbitofrontal branch (arrow)

(Fig. 2.17) which carry associated risks of cosmetic deformity, infection (meningitis, cerebritis, brain abscess), and CSF leak with possible resultant intracranial hypotension in addition to brain injuries and intracranial hemorrhage. Repair of a depressed calvarial fracture is indicated when depression exceeds 1 cm or the width of the adjacent calvarium, when there is gross cosmetic deformity, when the fracture communicates with the paranasal sinuses, and when there is dural injury or pneumocephalus (indicative of an open nature of the fracture). The presence of a significant intracranial hematoma or the development of active intracranial infection also necessitates surgical intervention [34].

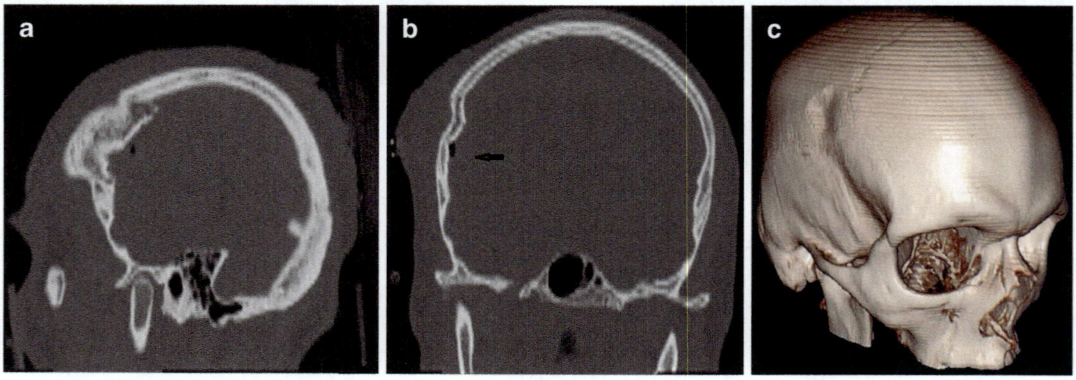

Fig. 2.17 Calvarial fractures. (**a** and **b**) Sagittal and coronal reformatted images in bone algorithm demonstrate comminuted depressed fracture of the frontal bone. Major fragments are depressed by approximately the width of the calvarium. Foci of intracranial air indicate that this is an open fracture. Surgical repair is indicated. (**c**) 3D reconstructed CT scan highlights the cosmetic deformity associated with the fracture

Secondary Injuries

Direct injuries to the brain can lead to cellular swelling (cytotoxic edema), disruption of the blood–brain barrier, and loss of autoregulation, all of which may contribute to increased intracranial pressure with subsequent potential development of herniation syndromes (Figs. 2.18, 2.19, 2.20, and 2.21), including subfalcine herniation, uncal or transtentorial herniation, central herniation, external herniation, tonsillar herniation, and upward cerebellar herniation [35]. Vascular displacement and compression may occur in association with these herniation syndromes with resultant infarction. Midline shift is always present when there is subfalcine herniation, though the converse is not necessarily true. Subfalcine herniation is defined by herniation of the cingulate gyrus beneath the falx (Fig. 2.19). Both the anterior cerebral arteries and the internal cerebral veins may be compressed in this setting, and images should be carefully examined for parasagittal and basal ganglionic infarctions as well as trapping of the contralateral lateral ventricle.

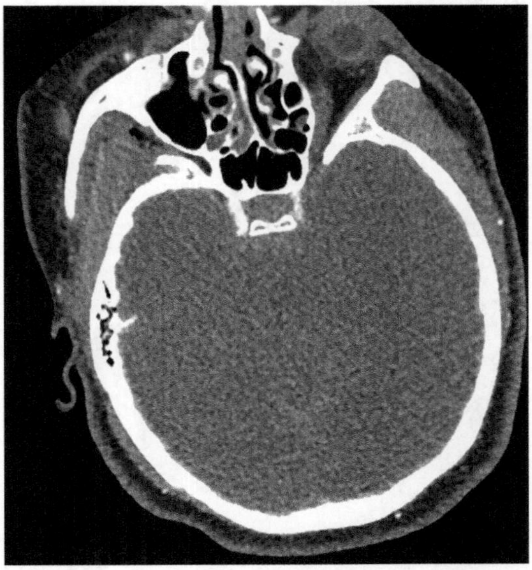

Fig. 2.18 Central herniation and diffuse cerebral edema. Axial unenhanced CT scan demonstrates diffuse loss of grey-white differentiation. No sulci are visible. Additionally, there is complete effacement of the basilar cisterns. Findings are indicative of diffuse cerebral edema with associated herniation

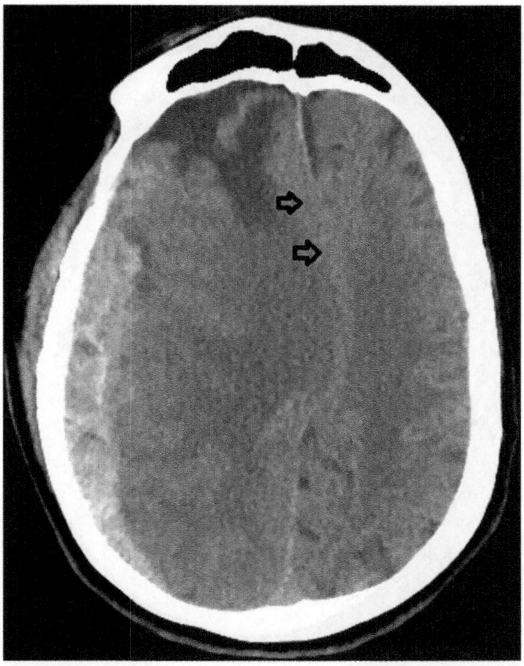

Fig. 2.19 Subfalcine herniation. Axial unenhanced CT scan in this patient with an acute right convexity subdural hematoma and evidence of prior traumatic brain injury with right frontal encephalomalacia reveals midline shift to the left with herniation of the cingulate gyrus beneath the falx (arrows)

Uncal or transtentorial and central herniation syndromes lead to compression of the brainstem, notably the cerebral peduncle(s), and the oculomotor (third cranial) nerves as well as the posterior cerebral and anterior choroidal arteries with resultant territorial infarctions involving the parietal, occipital and posterior temporal lobes and the globus pallidus, genu of the internal capsule, and mesial temporal lobe, respectively, ocular motor palsies, fixed and dilated ("blown") pupils, hydrocephalus, and abnormal "coned" configuration of the brainstem (Fig. 2.20). Ascending transtentorial (Fig. 2.21), or upward herniation of the cerebellum/vermis, is seen in the context of posterior fossa mass effect with associated compression of the fourth ventricle, basilar cisterns and aqueduct of Sylvius and resultant hydrocephalus. The foramen magnum should be carefully examined on all studies and should contain CSF. Crowding at the foramen magnum is seen with tonsillar herniation (Fig. 2.22) [35].

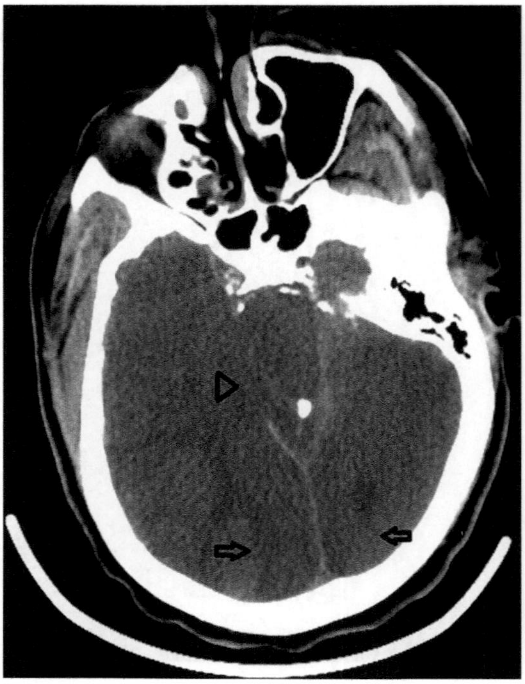

Fig. 2.20 Uncal herniation and resultant posterior cerebral artery territory infarction. Axial unenhanced CT scan reveals marked paucity of sulci. The right uncus has herniated over the tentorial incisura (arrowhead). There is complete effacement of the basilar cisterns bilaterally with abnormal configuration of the brainstem ("coned appearance"). Due to bilateral posterior cerebral artery compression, there are bilateral, right larger than left, posterior cerebral artery territory infarctions (arrows), manifest by loss of grey-white differentiation

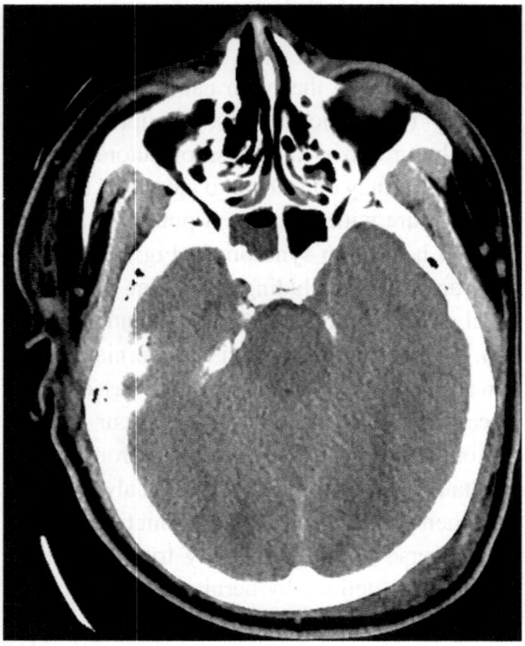

Fig. 2.21 Ascending herniation. Axial unenhanced CT scan at the level of the brainstem demonstrates ascending herniation of the cerebellar vermis with associated effacement of the basilar cisterns and deformation of the brainstem

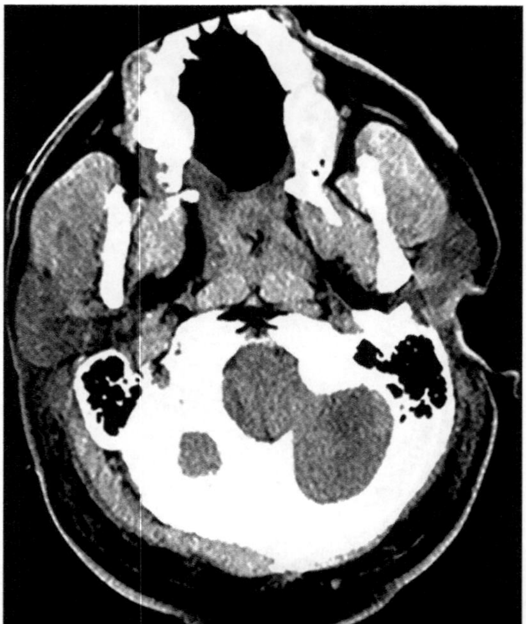

Fig. 2.22 Tonsillar herniation. Axial CT scan is notable for herniation of the cerebellar tonsils through the foramen magnum. There is near complete effacement of CSF space within the foramen magnum, and there is mild compression of the cervicomedullary junction

Victims of traumatic brain injury are at risk for development of numerous long-term sequelae. Those with subarachnoid and/or intraventricular hemorrhage may develop hydrocephalus (distinguished from central volume loss by disproportionate enlargement of the temporal horns, "ballooned" configuration of the frontal horns, and a relatively acute callosal septal angle) (Fig. 2.23) [36]. Volume loss may be diffuse, profound, and at times relatively rapid, particularly in association with diffuse axonal injury. There may be preferential neuronal loss within the limbic system with associated dramatic hippocampal atrophy. Focal encephalomalacia is most often seen at sites of prior contusional injuries; again, typically the inferior frontal lobes and the temporal lobes (Fig. 2.24). These encephalomalacic lesions may serve as seizure foci, and up to 20%

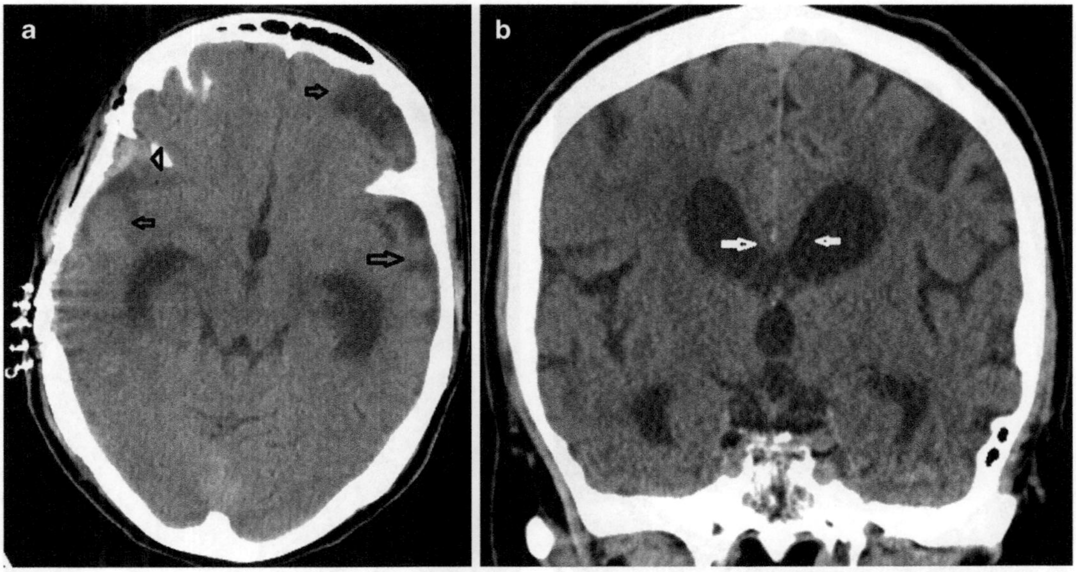

Fig. 2.23 Hydrocephalus. (**a**) Axial unenhanced CT scan demonstrated disproportionate enlargement of the temporal horns as well as mild dilatation of the third ventricle. Exam is also notable for regions of evolving encephalomalacia in the bilateral temporal lobes and the left frontal lobe (arrows). The patient is status post right craniotomy. A small amount of extra axial hemorrhage is present along the right convexity (arrowhead). (**b**) Coronal image demonstrates dilated ventricles with an acute callososeptal angle (arrows)

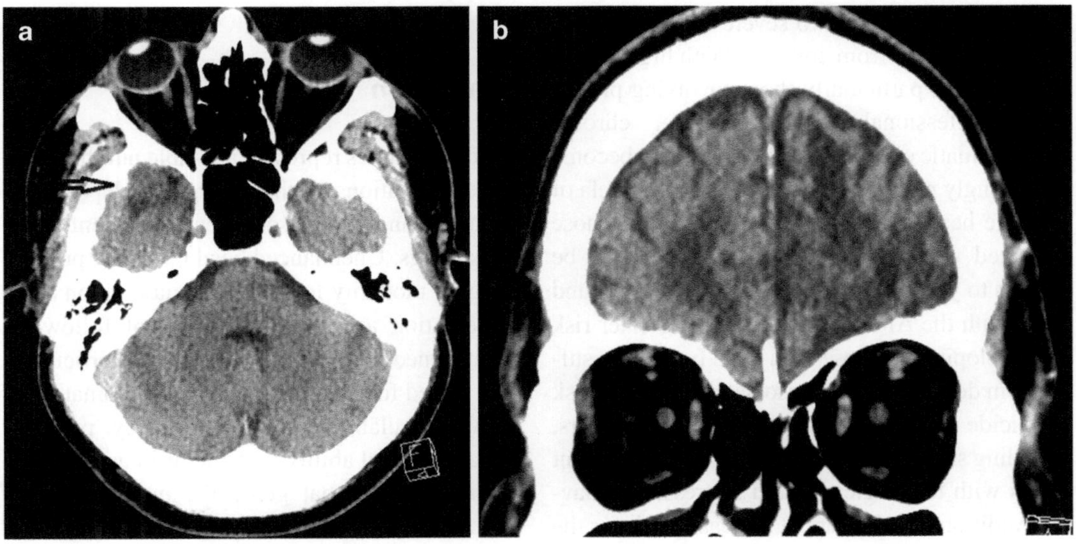

Fig. 2.24 Post traumatic encephalomalacia. (**a**) Axial unenhanced CT scan reveals post traumatic encephalomalacia at site of prior contusional injury in the right anterior temporal lobe (arrow). (**b**) Coronal unenhanced CT scan demonstrates extensive left greater than right bifrontal post-traumatic encephalomalacia

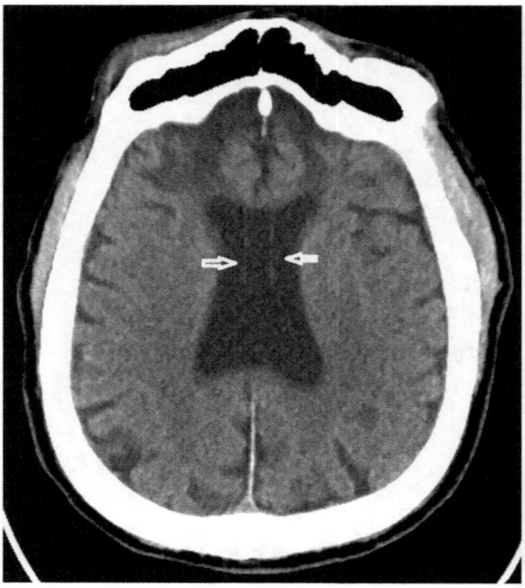

Fig. 2.25 Acquired cavum. Axial unenhanced head CT is notable for a dilated cavum septum pellucidum et vergae (arrows) in this patient with bilateral frontal post traumatic encephalomalacia

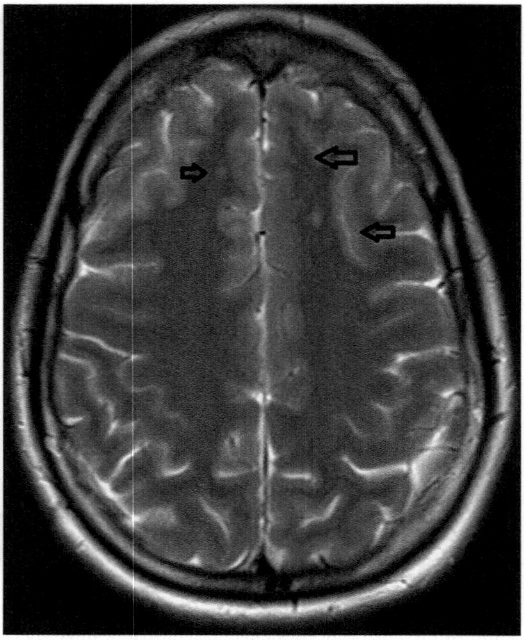

Fig. 2.26 MRI white matter abnormalities. Axial T2 weighted MR image demonstrates small foci of signal abnormality in the frontal subcortical white matter (arrows) of this young patient

of victims of moderate to severe traumatic brain injury will suffer from epilepsy. With highly publicized cases, particularly those involving prominent professional athletes [37], chronic post-traumatic encephalopathy (CTE) has become increasingly recognized as a long-term sequela of multiple head injuries/concussions such as those sustained with contact sports. Its onset may be months to years following the injury/injuries, and those with the APOE e4 allele are at greater risk for developing it. Those with CTE frequently suffer from depression with associated increased risk of suicide as well as other psychiatric disorders, including substance abuse and anger management issues with tendencies toward aggressive behavior. Additionally, they are at increased risk for the development of Parkinsonism and dementia [38–42]. Imaging findings include volume loss, acquired cava, which may be septated (Fig. 2.25), and nonspecific white matter lesions, typically frontal and subcortical in location, better demonstrated on MRI (Fig. 2.26).

Conclusion

Head CT studies represent a sizable number of all CT examinations in the emergency department, inpatient, and to a lesser extent outpatient imaging settings. Unenhanced head CT is the primary imaging modality for head trauma both on acute presentation and during subsequent follow-up. As outlined in this chapter, CT is particularly well suited for this role due to its combination of relative availability, speed, efficiency, potential portability, and ability to depict primary and secondary injuries that guide the management of patients with TBI. At the same time, CT should be used judiciously, following appropriateness criteria guidelines, and can be complemented by MRI depending on the clinical scenario and question. Radiologists and other health care providers should be well versed in trauma head CT findings and their implications for TBI, including classic imaging appearances, less common variations, and potential pitfalls for image interpretation described herein.

References

1. Centers for Disease Control and Prevention. National center for health statistics: mortality data on CDC WONDER. [cited 2023 Mar 26]. https://wonder.cdc.gov/mcd.html.
2. Kraus JF, McArthur DL. Epidemiologic aspects of brain injury. Neurol Clin. 1996;14(2):435–50.
3. Bell JM, Breiding MJ, DePadilla L. CDC's efforts to improve traumatic brain injury surveillance. J Saf Res. 2017;62:253–6.
4. Finkelstein EA, Corso PS, Miller TR. Incidence and economic burden of injuries in the United States. Oxford, NY: Oxford University Press; 2006. p. 208.
5. Cuthbert JP, Harrison-Felix C, Corrigan JD, Bell JM, Haarbauer-Krupa JK, Miller AC. Unemployment in the United States after traumatic brain injury for working-age individuals: prevalence and associated factors 2 years postinjury. J Head Trauma Rehabil. 2015;30(3):160–74.
6. Stubbs JL, Thornton AE, Sevick JM, Silverberg ND, Barr AM, Honer WG, et al. Traumatic brain injury in homeless and marginally housed individuals: a systematic review and meta-analysis. Lancet Public Health. 2020;5(1):e19–32.
7. Adams JH, Graham DI, Scott G, Parker LS, Doyle D. Brain damage in fatal non-missile head injury. J Clin Pathol. 1980;33(12):1132–45.
8. Gentry LR. Imaging of closed head injury. Radiology. 1994;191(1):1–17.
9. Centers for Disease Control and Prevention. Report to congress on traumatic brain injury in the United States: epidemiology and rehabilitation. Atlanta, GA: National Center for Injury Prevention and Control; Division of Unintentional Injury Prevention; 2015.
10. Maas AIR, Roozenbeek B, Manley GT. Clinical trials in traumatic brain injury: past experience and current developments. Neurotherapeutics. 2010;7(1):115–26.
11. Smith-Bindman R, Lipson J, Marcus R, Kim KP, Mahesh M, Gould R, et al. Radiation dose associated with common computed tomography examinations and the associated lifetime attributable risk of cancer. Arch Intern Med. 2009;169(22):2078–86.
12. Seyam M, Weikert T, Sauter A, Brehm A, Psychogios MN, Blackham KA. Utilization of artificial intelligence-based intracranial hemorrhage detection on emergent noncontrast CT images in clinical workflow. Radiol Artif Intell. 2022;4(2):e210168.
13. Arbabshirani MR, Fornwalt BK, Mongelluzzo GJ, Suever JD, Geise BD, Patel AA, et al. Advanced machine learning in action: identification of intracranial hemorrhage on computed tomography scans of the head with clinical workflow integration. NPJ Digit Med. 2018;1:9.
14. O'Neill TJ, Xi Y, Stehel E, Browning T, Ng YS, Baker C, et al. Active reprioritization of the reading worklist using artificial intelligence has a beneficial effect on the turnaround time for interpretation of head CT with intracranial hemorrhage. Radiol Artif Intell. 2021;3(2):e200024.
15. Peace K, Wilensky EM, Frangos S, MacMurtrie E, Shields E, Hujcs M, et al. The use of a portable head CT scanner in the intensive care unit. J Neurosci Nurs. 2010;42(2):109–16.
16. Cushman JG, Agarwal N, Fabian TC, Garcia V, Nagy KK, Pasquale MD, et al. Practice management guidelines for the management of mild traumatic brain injury: the EAST practice management guidelines work group. J Trauma. 2001;51(5):1016–26.
17. Servadei F, Teasdale G, Merry G, Neurotraumatology Committee of the World Federation of Neurosurgical Societies. Defining acute mild head injury in adults: a proposal based on prognostic factors, diagnosis, and management. J Neurotrauma. 2001;18(7):657–64.
18. Expert Panel on Neurological Imaging, Shih RY, Burns J, Ajam AA, Broder JS, Chakraborty S, et al. ACR appropriateness criteria® head trauma: 2021 update. J Am Coll Radiol. 2021;18(5S):S13–36.
19. Ebell MH. Computed tomography after minor head injury. Am Fam Physician. 2006;73(12):2205–7.
20. Smits M, Dippel DWJ, de Haan GG, Dekker HM, Vos PE, Kool DR, et al. External validation of the Canadian CT head rule and the New Orleans criteria for CT scanning in patients with minor head injury. JAMA. 2005;294(12):1519–25.
21. Madhok DY, Yue JK, Sun X, Suen CG, Coss NA, Jain S, et al. Clinical predictors of 3- and 6-month outcome for mild traumatic brain injury patients with a negative head CT scan in the emergency department: a TRACK-TBI pilot study. Brain Sci. 2020;10(5):269.
22. Murray GD, Butcher I, McHugh GS, Lu J, Mushkudiani NA, Maas AIR, et al. Multivariable prognostic analysis in traumatic brain injury: results from the IMPACT study. J Neurotrauma. 2007;24(2):329–37.
23. Aromatario M, Torsello A, D'Errico S, Bertozzi G, Sessa F, Cipolloni L, et al. Traumatic epidural and subdural hematoma: epidemiology, outcome, and dating. Medicina (Kaunas). 2021;57(2):125.
24. Guo C, Liu L, Wang B, Wang Z. Swirl sign in traumatic acute epidural hematoma: prognostic value and surgical management. Neurol Sci. 2017;38(12):2111–6.
25. Gean AD, Fischbein NJ, Purcell DD, Aiken AH, Manley GT, Stiver SI. Benign anterior temporal epidural hematoma: indolent lesion with a characteristic CT imaging appearance after blunt head trauma. Radiology. 2010;257(1):212–8.
26. Ironside N, Nguyen C, Do Q, Ugiliweneza B, Chen CJ, Sieg EP, et al. Middle meningeal artery embolization for chronic subdural hematoma: a systematic review and meta-analysis. J Neurointerv Surg. 2021;13(10):951–7.

27. White CL, Griffith S, Caron JL. Early progression of traumatic cerebral contusions: characterization and risk factors. J Trauma. 2009;67(3):508–14; discussion 514–515.
28. Ballabh P, de Vries LS. White matter injury in infants with intraventricular haemorrhage: mechanisms and therapies. Nat Rev Neurol. 2021;17(4):199–214.
29. Adams JH, Doyle D, Ford I, Gennarelli TA, Graham DI, McLellan DR. Diffuse axonal injury in head injury: definition, diagnosis and grading. Histopathology. 1989;15(1):49–59.
30. Mittl RL, Grossman RI, Hiehle JF, Hurst RW, Kauder DR, Gennarelli TA, et al. Prevalence of MR evidence of diffuse axonal injury in patients with mild head injury and normal head CT findings. AJNR Am J Neuroradiol. 1994;15(8):1583–9.
31. Liu G, Ghimire P, Pang H, Wu G, Shi H. Improved sensitivity of 3.0 tesla susceptibility-weighted imaging in detecting traumatic bleeds and its use in predicting outcomes in patients with mild traumatic brain injury. Acta Radiol. 2015;56(10):1256–63.
32. Mesfin FB, Gupta N, Hays Shapshak A, Taylor RS. Diffuse axonal injury. In: StatPearls. Treasure Island (FL): StatPearls Publishing; 2023. [cited 2023 Mar 26]. http://www.ncbi.nlm.nih.gov/books/NBK448102/.
33. Larsen DW. Traumatic vascular injuries and their management. Neuroimaging Clin N Am. 2002;12(2):249–69.
34. Vincent A, Sokoya M, Shokri T, Gordin E, Inman JC, Manolidis S, et al. Management of skull fractures and calvarial defects. Facial Plast Surg. 2019;35(6):651–6.
35. Riveros Gilardi B, Muñoz López JI, Hernández Villegas AC, Garay Mora JA, Rico Rodríguez OC, Chávez Appendini R, et al. Types of cerebral herniation and their imaging features. Radiographics. 2019;39(6):1598–610.
36. Miskin N, Patel H, Franceschi AM, Ades-Aron B, Le A, Damadian BE, et al. Diagnosis of normal-pressure hydrocephalus: use of traditional measures in the era of volumetric MR imaging. Radiology. 2017;285(1):197–205.
37. Bracken T. Aaron Hernandez's CTE worst seen in a young person. Boston, MA: Boston University; 2020. [cited 2023 Mar 26]. https://www.bu.edu/articles/2017/aaron-hernandez-cte-worst-seen-in-young-person/.
38. Saulle M, Greenwald BD. Chronic traumatic encephalopathy: a review. Rehabil Res Pract. 2012;2012:816069, 1.
39. Stein TD, Alvarez VE, McKee AC. Chronic traumatic encephalopathy: a spectrum of neuropathological changes following repetitive brain trauma in athletes and military personnel. Alzheimers Res Ther. 2014;6(1):4.
40. Maroon JC, Winkelman R, Bost J, Amos A, Mathyssek C, Miele V. Chronic traumatic encephalopathy in contact sports: a systematic review of all reported pathological cases. PLoS One. 2015;10(2):e0117338.
41. McKee AC, Cantu RC, Nowinski CJ, Hedley-Whyte ET, Gavett BE, Budson AE, et al. Chronic traumatic encephalopathy in athletes: progressive tauopathy after repetitive head injury. J Neuropathol Exp Neurol. 2009;68(7):709–35.
42. Fesharaki-Zadeh A. Chronic traumatic encephalopathy: a brief overview. Front Neurol. 2019;10:713.

3 Navigating Complex Facial Trauma: A Comprehensive Guide to CT-Based Fracture Detection and Analysis

Mauro Hanaoka, Suehyb Alkhatib, Francis Deng, and Suyash Mohan

Imaging Technique

The standard of care imaging modality for the evaluation of facial fractures is CT. The CT acquisition parameters should be adjusted to the thinnest collimation possible, and the images reconstructed with 1 mm or less slice thickness using bone and soft tissue algorithms. The reconstructions should have a relatively limited field of view to maximize the spatial resolution. There should be multiplanar reconstructions in the coronal and sagittal planes, as complex facial fractures can occur in different directions. Three-dimensional volume surface rendering provides a bird's eye view of the anatomy that facilitates fracture pattern recognition and reconstruction planning (Fig. 3.1) [1].

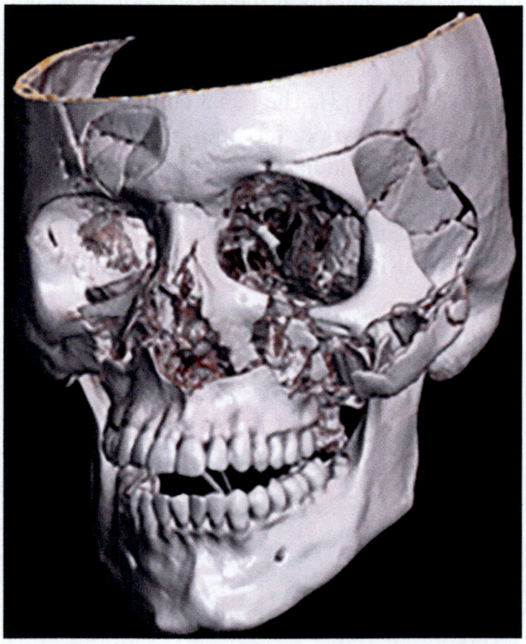

Fig. 3.1 3D reconstruction provides a bird-eye view of extensive maxillofacial fractures, including complex bilateral naso-orbital ethmoidal (NOE) fractures, and LeFort type III configuration fracture pattern of the left and LeFort type II on the right, mildly displaced fracture of the left frontal calvarium extending to the squamous temporal bone

M. Hanaoka (✉) · S. Alkhatib · S. Mohan
Department of Radiology, Perelman School of Medicine at the University of Pennsylvania, Philadelphia, PA, USA
e-mail: Hanaomauro.hanaoka@pennmedicine.upenn.edu

F. Deng
Department of Radiology, Johns Hopkins University, Baltimore, MD, USA

F. Knollmann (ed.), *Trauma Computed Tomography*, https://doi.org/10.1007/978-3-031-45746-3_3

Facial Anatomy and Clinically Directed Report Structure

The facial skeletal anatomy, also known as the viscerocranium, is composed of nine bones: five paired (zygoma, maxilla, nasal bones, inferior nasal conchae, lacrimal bones) and four unpaired bones (frontal bone, mandible, palatine bone, vomer) [2]. Due to the complexity of the facial anatomy, rather than reporting a laundry list of fractured bones, it is more helpful to the clinicians to provide a report that describes facial fractures based on their regional units. Underlying the regional anatomy is the concept of facial buttresses, which simplifies the facial skeleton into four pairs of horizontally and vertically oriented struts (Fig. 3.2) [3]. The facial buttresses provide a rigid framework for the orbital contents, sinuses, teeth, and nasal cavities. Disruption of a facial buttress can alter the face's normal function and change its dimensions, requiring surgical repair using rigid titanium plates and screws anchored in the buttress, with or without bone grafts [4].

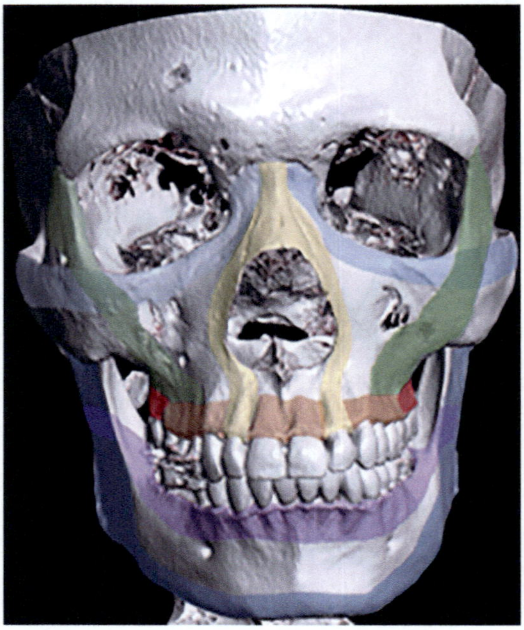

Fig. 3.2 System of facial buttresses. The horizontal buttresses are the upper transverse maxillary (light blue), lower transverse maxillary (orange), upper transverse mandibular (purple), and lower transverse mandibular (dark blue) buttresses. The vertical buttresses are the medial maxillary (yellow), lateral maxillary (green), posterior maxillary (red), and posterior vertical mandibular (dark blue) buttresses

The *"vertical buttresses"* define the height of the face and maintain normal masticatory function. The medial maxillary buttress originates from the junction of the nasofrontal suture and extends along the lateral margin of the piriform aperture and the maxillary alveolar process, projecting posteriorly to include the medial orbital wall and maxillary sinus medial wall. The lateral maxillary buttress extends across the zygomaticofrontal suture, the lateral orbital rim through the body of the zygomatic bone, the zygomaticomaxillary suture, the maxillary alveolar process close to the posterior molars, and posteriorly as the lateral orbital wall and the lateral maxillary sinus wall. The posterior maxillary buttress is comprised of the pterygoid plates of the sphenoid bone, which connect the maxilla (midface) to the skull base and are an important site of craniofacial dissociation (Le Fort) fractures. The posterior mandibular buttress courses along the posterior margin of the mandible, including portions of the angle, ramus, and condyle.

The *"horizontal buttresses"* define the width and forward projection of the face and give stability to the vertical buttresses. The upper transverse maxillary buttress extends along the nasofrontal suture, inferior orbital rim, zygomatic bone to the zygomaticotemporal suture, and posteriorly as the orbital floor. The lower transverse maxillary buttress includes the maxillary alveolar process and extends to the hard palate. The upper transverse mandibular buttress involves the mandibular alveolar process, extending along the mandibular ramus and the posterior cortical margin of the mandible. The lower transverse mandibular buttress courses along the inferior margin of the mandible.

In an alternate and still surgically useful categorization, the bony structure of the face is divided into three parts: upper, middle, and lower thirds (Fig. 3.3). The *upper third* is composed of the frontal bone and the frontal sinuses and is separated from the middle third by the superior orbital rims and orbital roofs. The *middle third* of the face, or midface, spans from the superior orbital rims downwards to the maxilla and thus incorporates the orbits, nose, and maxillary, ethmoid, and sphenoid sinuses. The middle third of the face is

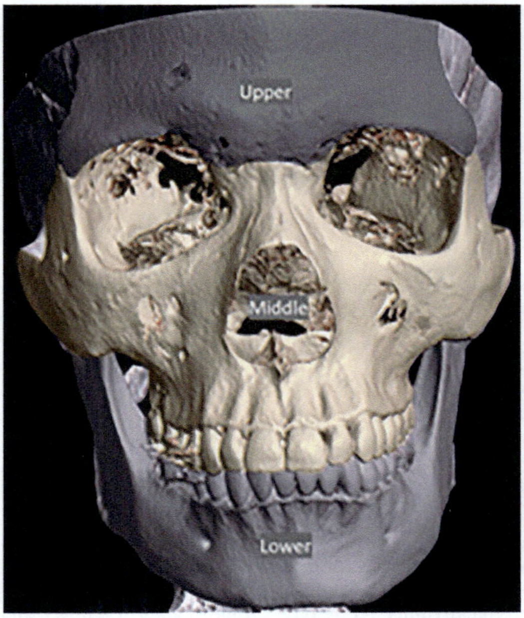

Fig. 3.3 System of facial partitions. Partition of the facial anatomy into upper (dark gray), middle (yellow), and lower thirds (light gray), which is used by ENT to describe locations of fracture in the facial anatomy

bordered posteriorly by the zygomaticotemporal sutures, which connect the midface to the calvarium, and posteromedially by the pterygoid plates, which connect it to the skull base. The midface accounts for a majority of facial fractures. The *lower third* of the face comprises the mandible.

Categorizing pan-facial fractures based on their position in the facial thirds can aid in preoperative planning because repair is often sequenced (e.g., bottom-to-top or top-to-bottom). For instance, a bottom-top approach starts with fixing the mandible, mandibulomaxillary fixation to re-establish the dental occlusion, fixation of the midface and orbital reconstruction, and then addressing frontal sinus/bone fractures.

Fracture Patterns and Expected Complications

Upper Third Facial Fractures

Frontal and Frontal Sinus Fractures

Fractures that occur in the upper third of the face usually affect the wall of the frontal bone and the frontal sinuses [5]. These fractures can involve only the anterior wall (or table) of the frontal sinus or extend into the posterior wall. When the posterior wall is involved, it creates a passage between the frontal sinus and the anterior cranial fossa, which increases the risk of complications such as intracranial hemorrhage, cerebrospinal fluid leakage, and intracranial infection. Significant posterior wall injury may require sinus obliteration or cranialization. If a fracture is displaced along the medial margin of the frontal sinus, it may obstruct the drainage of the sinus via the frontal recess (nasofrontal duct), resulting in a mucocele formation. Significant frontal recess injury may require sinusotomy or obliteration.

Middle Third Facial Fractures

Le Fort Fractures

Le Fort fractures (Fig. 3.4) are complex facial fractures that result from a forceful impact on the midface structures and are distinguished by varying degrees of craniofacial dissociation across numerous facial buttresses [6]. These fractures were initially explained by René Le Fort, a French surgeon in the early twentieth century who conducted experiments where blunt force was applied to cadavers' midfaces. Le Fort identified three common fracture patterns, each resulting from a different magnitude of force, all of which included a fracture through the pterygoid plates. Depending on the distribution of forces across the facial skeleton, various Le Fort fracture patterns may occur simultaneously, and different combinations may occur on either side of the face (for instance, type I and II fractures on the left side and type II and III fractures on the right).

A Le Fort I fracture (Fig. 3.5), also called a Guérin fracture or floating palate, occurs due to high-force impact on the midface structures and results in the separation of the hard palate (lower transverse maxillary buttress) from the remainder of the face and skull base. This fracture pattern is oriented horizontally and extends through the anterior, lateral, and medial maxillary walls, crossing the inferior margin of the piriform aperture and nasal septum and projecting posteriorly

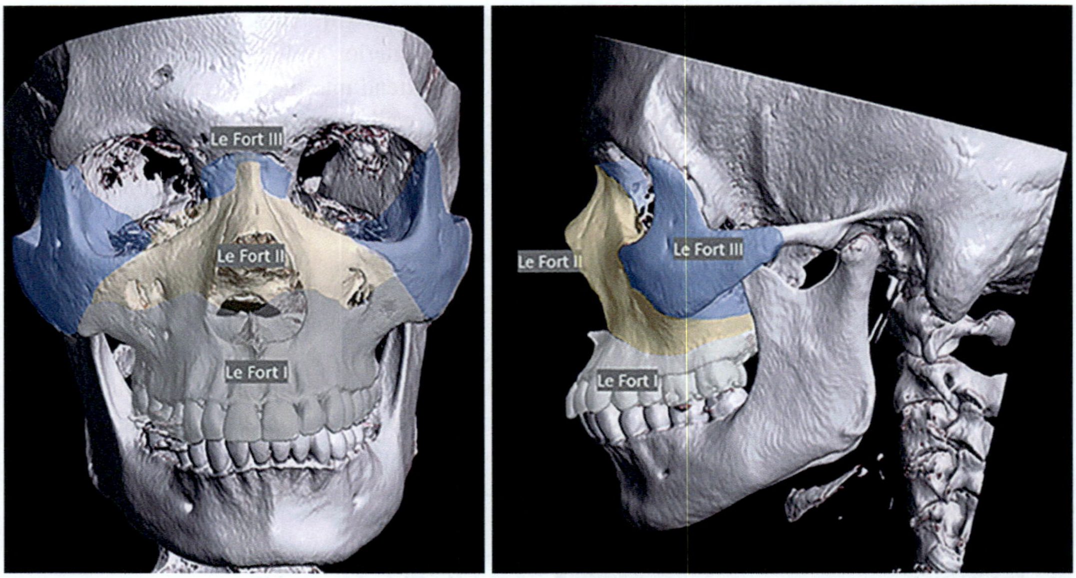

Fig. 3.4 Le Fort fractures. osseous facial structures that are typically affected by type I (blue), type II (yellow), and type III (gray) Le Fort fracture

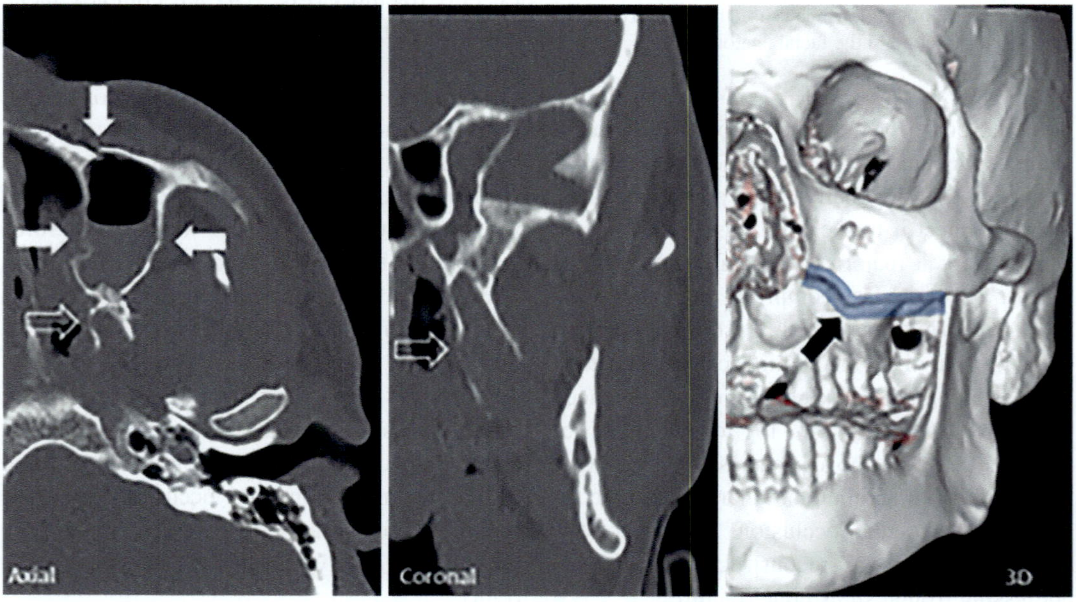

Fig. 3.5 Left LeFort type I fracture. This fracture pattern is oriented horizontally (blue line) and extends through the anterior, lateral, and medial maxillary walls (white arrows), crossing the inferior margin of the piriform aperture and nasal septum and projecting posteriorly through the pterygoid plates (hollow arrows)

through the pterygoid plates. Due to its anteroposterior extension in the axial plane, it is best visualized on coronal, sagittal, and three-dimensional surface rendered images.

A Le Fort II fractureFacial trauma: (Fig. 3.6), also called a "pyramidal" fracture, creates a pyramid-shaped maxillary bone fragment that moves separately from the rest of the midface and skull base. The top of the pyramid is located at or

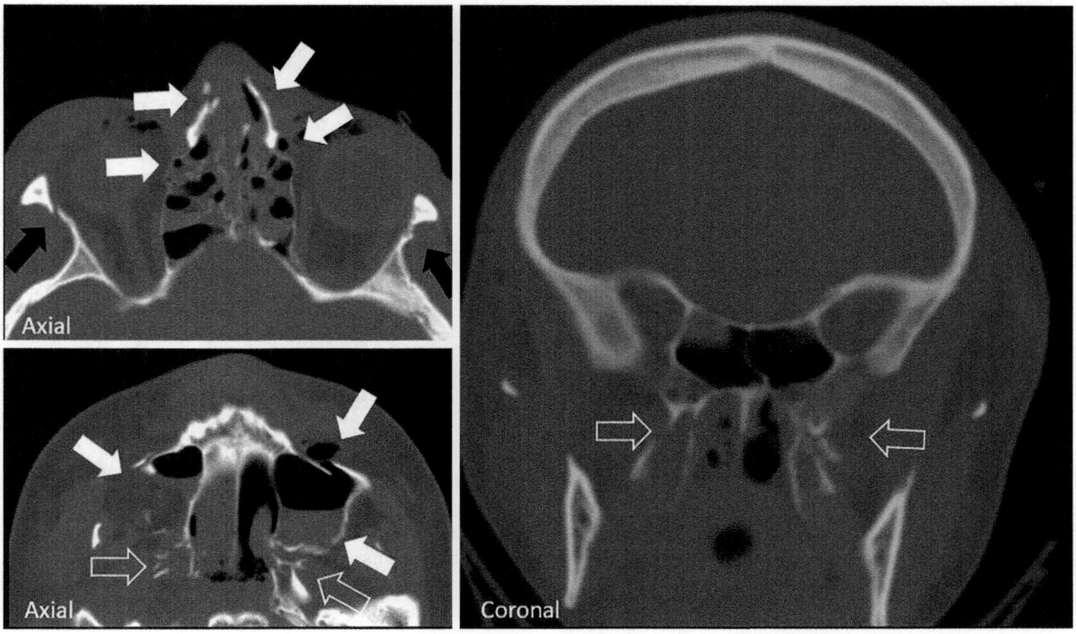

Fig. 3.6 LeFort II fractures involving the inferior, medial, and lateral orbital walls, lateral maxillary sinuses, and highly comminuted in the nasal bones

slightly below the nasofrontal suture. The oblique fracture passes through the medial orbital wall, orbital floor, and zygomaticomaxillary suture, but excludes the zygomatic bone. This fracture involves the superior medial maxillary, inferior lateral maxillary, upper transverse maxillary, and posterior maxillary buttresses. Axial and coronal reformatted images and surface renders are most useful for visualizing the extension of a Le Fort II fracture in an oblique plane through the inferior orbital rim as well as medial orbital wall and orbital floor.

A Le Fort III fracture (Fig. 3.7), also referred to as craniofacial dissociation, results in complete separation of the face from the skull base, beginning at the nasofrontal suture and extending laterally through the medial and lateral orbital walls and zygomatic arch. In contrast to types I and II, Le Fort III fractures involve the zygomatic bone, affecting the superior portions of the medial and lateral maxillary buttresses, upper transverse maxillary buttress, and posterior maxillary buttress. Accurate identification of the fracture extension to the lateral orbital wall and zygomatic arch on axial or coronal images and surface renders helps to differentiate Le Fort III from Le Fort II fracture, as both types typically involve the nasofrontal suture and medial orbital walls.

Surgical repair of Le Fort fractures involves the use of rigid plates and screws placed along the fractured facial buttresses. The surgical procedure begins with restoration of the normal configuration of the medial and lateral maxillary buttresses to permit proper alignment of the maxillary and mandibular teeth. Then, maxillomandibular fixation is done to maintain dental occlusion during the rest of the repair process. Next, the anterior parts of the facial buttresses are repaired to restore facial dimensions and provide support to the facial structure. Finally, the maxilla is reattached to the calvaria to complete the surgery.

All Le Fort fractures involve the pterygomaxillary junction located in the posterior maxillary buttress. If a fracture extends posteriorly into the sphenoid bone, it can lead to carotid artery injury or carotid-cavernous fistula. A posterior mandibular buttress fracture, especially when combined with a displaced fracture of the condylar process

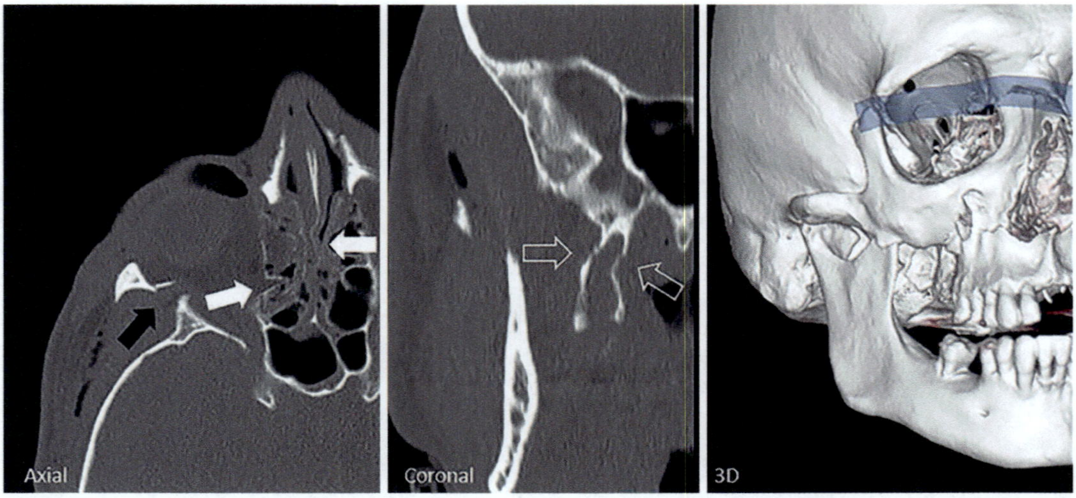

Fig. 3.7 Right LeFort type III fracture. This pattern of fracture is characterized by complete separation of the face from the skull base, beginning at the nasofrontal suture and extending laterally through the medial and lateral orbital walls (blue line) and zygomatic arch (black arrow), and extending to pterygoid plates (hollow arrows)

or temporomandibular joint dislocation, can cause malocclusion and trismus.

Nasal and Naso-Orbitoethmoid (NOE) Complex Fractures

Nasal bone fractures are a common type of injury to the facial skeleton [7]. This is due to the nose being located superficially and the bones being relatively thin. Such fractures usually result from blunt force to the front or side of the nose. The category of nasal fractures are not limited to the paired nasal bones, but also the frontal (ascending) processes of the maxillae and anterior nasal spine. A nasal fracture that extends into the nasal septum can damage the perichondrium, leading to a septal hematoma. Nasoseptal fractures can cause complications such as impaired nasal breathing, abscess formation, and necrosis, resulting in septal perforation and/or saddle nose deformity.

Naso-orbitoethmoid (NOE) complex fractures (Fig. 3.8) occur due to high-energy force applied to the nose, transmitted to the ethmoid bone. The comminution of the medial maxillary buttress results in a fracture pattern that involves the nasal bones and septum, ethmoid sinus, and medial orbital wall.

The Markowitz and Manson classification system is used to categorize fractures of the NOE complex based on the involvement of the medial canthal tendon. Type I fractures involve a single large fracture fragment with an intact medial canthal tendon. Type II fractures are comminuted, but the medial canthal tendon is still attached to a single bone fragment. Type III fractures involve comminution that extends to the insertion site of the medial canthal tendon on the lacrimal fossa of the anterior medial orbital wall, resulting in tendon avulsion. Three-dimensional volume-rendered reconstructions can be used to identify the fracture type, and the degree of comminution at the level of the lacrimal fossa can help with surgical planning for medial canthal tendon repair.

The medial maxillary buttress includes the lateral walls of the ethmoid sinuses, medial walls of the orbits, and medial walls of the maxillary sinuses, which are located close to many delicate structures such as the orbital contents, frontal recess, sphenoethmoid recess, ostiomeatal complex, lacrimal duct and sac, and medial canthal tendon. Complications such as sinus drainage blockage, medial canthal tendon damage, defects that would allow cerebrospinal fluid leakage, and lacrimal duct and sac damage should be described for appropriate management and surgical plan-

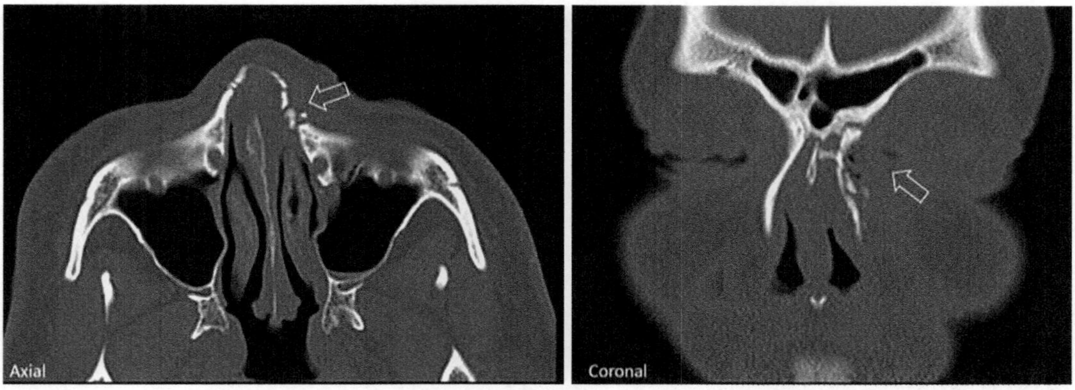

Fig. 3.8 Left-sided type II naso-orbitoethmoid complex fracture with minimal asymmetric tenting of the left medial rectus muscle but no entrapment

ning. If a medial maxillary buttress fracture extends through the cribriform plate, it can tear the underlying dura and allow cerebrospinal fluid to leak into the nasal cavity and paranasal sinuses. If the fracture extends into the paranasal sinuses, it can create a pathway for bacteria to spread into the normally sterile environment of the anterior cranial fossa, causing infections such as meningitis, epidural abscess, or cerebral abscess. If bone fragments obstruct the frontal recess, it can lead to the formation of frontal sinus mucocele, which requires surgery to open the frontal sinus. Damage to the lacrimal duct and/or sac can cause a dacryocystocele or dacryocystitis, which requires surgical correction. Medial canthal tendon injury, a common complication of NOE complex fractures, can result in telecanthus and requires surgical fixation. Changes in intraorbital volume can result in enophthalmos or exophthalmos, requiring orbital wall reconstruction.

Orbital Fractures

The orbital walls are composed of several buttresses, including the medial maxillary, lateral maxillary, and upper transverse buttresses, as well as the osseous floor of the anterior cranial fossa. Single-buttress fractures of the orbit result from direct trauma to the globe, leading to an orbital "blowout" fracture (Fig. 3.9) as the orbital wall is displaced outward away from the orbit (or more rarely, a "blow-in" fracture as the wall is displaced inward). These are known as "pure" orbital fractures, wherein the orbital rim is spared. The orbital floor is most frequently affected [8], while the medial wall is the next most commonly affected. Complications of orbital blowout fractures may include extraocular muscle herniation and entrapment, intraorbital (retrobulbar) hemorrhage, orbital emphysema, globe injury, and injury to the infraorbital nerve in the presence of an orbital floor fracture. The internal fixation of orbital blowout fractures typically involves replacement or reinforcement of the fractured part of the orbital wall with a mesh material to restore orbital volume and prevent the herniation of intraorbital contents into the paranasal sinuses.

Additionally, there are two special types of orbital fractures: the orbital rim fracture and the pediatric "trapdoor" fracture. Orbital fractures that involve an orbital rim are frequently part of other fracture patterns of the midface, such as an NOE, Le Fort, or zygomaticomaxillary complex fracture, which should be specifically sought and reported as a superceding fracture pattern. The trapdoor fracture is a type of orbital floor blowout fracture that occurs in children. In this fracture, the inferior rectus muscle or its associated fascia can herniate through the orbital floor fracture, the fracture fragment springs back into place, and the muscle becomes entrapped, resulting in ophthalmoplegia and diplopia. While clin-

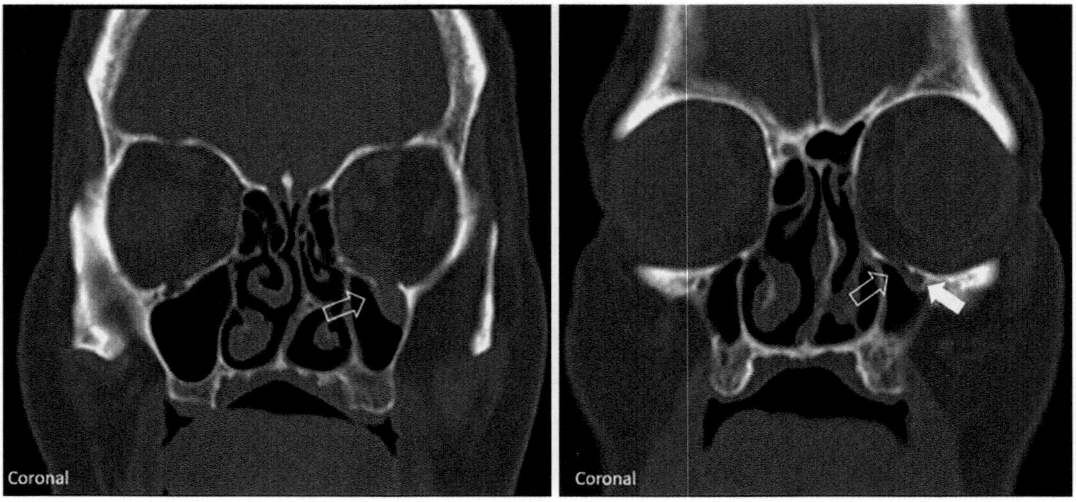

Fig. 3.9 Blowout fracture of the left orbital floor with involvement of the left infraorbital canal which may reflect injury to the left infraorbital nerve with extraconal fat herniation but no entrapment of the inferior rectus muscle

ical manifestations are primarily used to diagnose inferior rectus muscle entrapment, a rounded appearance of the muscle belly and herniation through a narrow defect can raise the suspicion for entrapment.

Injuries to the infraorbital nerve, a branch of the maxillary division of the trigeminal (cranial nerve V_2) nerve, as it passes through the infraorbital nerve canal on the orbital floor, are common complications of orbital blowout and Le Fort II fractures. Such injuries may cause temporary or permanent hypesthesia of the cheek and maxillary gingiva on the same side.

Superior orbital fissure syndrome is the result of a fracture that extends through the superior orbital fissure and leads to damage to the cranial nerves III, IV, V1 (the ophthalmic branch of the trigeminal nerve), and VI as they traverse the fissure into the orbit. This causes ophthalmoplegia or diplopia (paralysis of the extraocular muscles) and ptosis (paralysis of the levator palpebrae superioris, which is innervated by cranial nerve III). Injury to the optic nerve (cranial nerve II) at the orbital apex may result from orbital apex syndrome, which is characterized by uniocular visual loss and other signs and symptoms. Prompt surgical intervention is required for orbital apex syndrome because it is a surgical emergency that may lead to permanent blindness. Rupture of the cornea, sclera, or all layers of the globe due to trauma can lead to blindness and can be identified on a CT scan as a "flat tire" sign, intraocular gas, intraocular foreign body, or change in depth of the anterior segment of the globe, but it may require further examination by an ophthalmologist to detect more subtle disruptions.

Fractures involving the lateral aspect of upper transverse maxillary buttress may cause trismus, secondary to injury or impingement of the temporalis muscle in the infratemporal fossa.

Isolated Zygomatic Arch and Zygomaticomaxillary Complex Fracture

A zygomaticomaxillary complex fracture, which is also known as a tetrapod or quadripod fracture, happens due to direct trauma to the malar eminence. This leads to the separation of the zygomatic bone (zygoma) from its bony attachments, to the frontal, sphenoid, temporal, and maxillary bones. The zygomatic bone is part of the lateral orbital wall positioned beneath the frontal bone, roof of the maxillary sinus, and anterior to the temporal bone in the zygomatic arch. A zygomat-

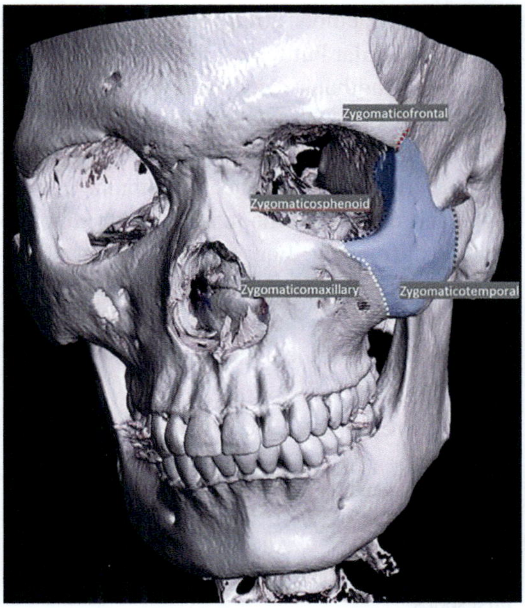

Fig. 3.10 A zygomaticomaxillary complex (ZMC) fracture, also referred to as a tetrapod or quadripod fracture, occurs as a result of direct injury to the malar prominence. This type of fracture transpires in proximity to or through the four zygomatic sutures (zygomaticofrontal, zygomaticomaxillary, zygomaticotemporal, and zygomaticosphenoid)

icomaxillary complex fracture happens through or near the four sutures of the zygoma, which was historically known as a tripod fracture in the days of radiography because only three disrupted sutures (zygomaticofrontal, zygomaticomaxillary, and zygomaticotemporal sutures) could be identified (Fig. 3.10).

An isolated zygomatic arch fracture may occur in patients with direct trauma to the posterior part of the upper transverse maxillary buttress. It is essential to distinguish this type of fracture from a zygomaticomaxillary complex fracture, which affects the lateral orbital wall and extends anteriorly. The zygomatic arch has a ring-like structure, usually resulting in a segmental fracture with mild comminution. The fracture may involve the zygomaticotemporal suture and cause depression of bone fragments into the infratemporal fossa. Displaced bone fragments may press on the temporalis muscle or adjacent mandibular coronoid process, resulting in trismus.

Alveolar Process Fracture

An alveolar process fracture is the most commonly observed fracture in the maxilla, and it primarily affects the lower transverse maxillary buttress. This fracture can occur from direct or indirect forces. Direct forces are caused by trauma to the alveolar process, while indirect forces are caused by the base of the dental crown, which acts as a fulcrum for the underlying teeth. Due to the presence of abundant bacteria in the mouth, this fracture is considered an open fracture, which requires surgical debridement and prophylactic antibiotics to prevent infection [9]. Complications may include dental root avulsion, crown or root fracture, dental intrusion or extrusion, and malocclusion.

Lower Third Facial Fractures

Mandibular Fractures

Mandibular fractures (Fig. 3.11) often, but not always, result in two discrete fractures because of

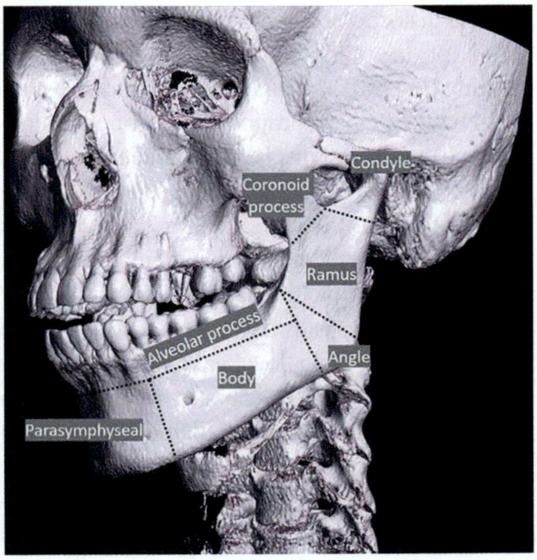

Fig. 3.11 Mandible fractures are categorized into the following regions: the alveolar process (yellow), parasymphyseal region (orange), body (red), angle (green), ramus (blue), coronoid process (purple), and condyle (bright green)

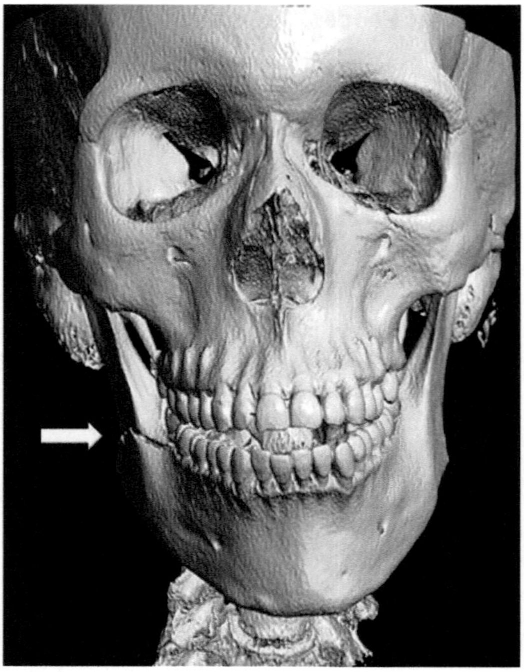

Fig. 3.12 A single fracture of the right mandible is likely due to a fracture-dislocation complex with subsequent reduction of the temporomandibular joints before imaging

its ring-like U-shaped configuration. A single fracture of the mandible on imaging is likely due to a fracture-dislocation complex with subsequent relocation of the temporomandibular joints before imaging (Fig. 3.12). Mandibular fractures are classified based on their location, degree of comminution, and presence of displaced fragments. Fractures involving the mandibular canal may result in injury to the inferior alveolar nerve. Surgical techniques for the management of mandibular fractures include external (maxillomandibular) fixation and/or open reduction with internal fixation to restore dental occlusion and allow healing of the bone by transferring the forces generated by mastication from the mandible to rigid titanium plates and screws [10–16].

Upper transverse mandibular buttress fractures and lower transverse maxillary buttress fractures have similar complications because they both involve the alveolar process. Most mandibular fractures affect both the upper and lower mandibular buttresses. Fractures that occur along the mandibular canal can injure the inferior alveolar nerve, which is a branch of the mandibular division of the trigeminal nerve (cranial nerve V_3) that runs through the mandibular ramus, angle, and body from the mandibular foramen to the mental foramen. Injury to the inferior alveolar nerve can cause numbness in the lower lip, chin, front part of the tongue, and mandibular teeth on the same side.

CT Protocol

Protocol name	CT maxillofacial
Indication	Facial trauma
Protocol designed for (scanner model)	Siemens
Patient preparation	All metal, glasses, hats, clips, jewelry taken off prior to scan
First series	
Oral contrast	None
IV contrast	None
Tube settings	
kV	120
mA	100
Dose modulation	On
Tube rotation time (s)	1.0 s
Table speed (mm/s)	5
Slice collimation	3.0 mm
Reconstructed slice thickness	3 × 3 mm, 1.0 × 0.7 mm
Anatomical coverage	Caudocranial, hard palate to top of frontal sinuses
Reconstruction kernel	Hr60, Hr38
Breath hold	None
Window settings	Bone, abdomen
Post processing	Optional
Other	3D reconstruction at radiologists or ordering provider's discretion
Typical dose	
CTDIvol	110 mGy
DLP	1600 mGy*cm
Eff. Dose	3.3 mSv

Conflict of Interest The authors have no conflict of interest.

References

1. Levy RA, Edwards WT, Meyer JR, Rosenbaum AE. Facial trauma and 3-D reconstructive imaging: insufficiencies and correctives. AJNR Am J Neuroradiol. 1992;13(3):885–92.
2. Sun JK, LeMay DR. Imaging of facial trauma. Neuroimaging Clin N Am. 2002;12(2):295–309.
3. Khan TU, Rahat S, Khan ZA, Shahid L, Banouri SS, Muhammad N. Etiology and pattern of maxillofacial trauma. PLoS One. 2022;17(9):e0275515.
4. Thoren H, Snall J, Salo J, Suominen-Taipale L, Kormi E, Lindqvist C, et al. Occurrence and types of associated injuries in patients with fractures of the facial bones. J Oral Maxillofac Surg. 2010;68(4):805–10.
5. Allareddy V, Allareddy V, Nalliah RP. Epidemiology of facial fracture injuries. J Oral Maxillofac Surg. 2011;69(10):2613–8.
6. Salentijn EG, van den Bergh B, Forouzanfar T. A ten-year analysis of midfacial fractures. J Craniomaxillofac Surg. 2013;41(7):630–6.
7. Davies R, Hammond D, Ridout F, Hutchison I, Magennis P. British Association of Oral and Maxillofacial Surgeons' National Facial Injury Surveys: hard tissue facial injuries presenting to UK emergency departments. Br J Oral Maxillofac Surg. 2020;58(2):152–7.
8. Eng JF, Younes S, Crovetti BR, Williams KJ, Haskins AD, Hernandez DJ, et al. Characteristics of orbital injuries associated with maxillofacial trauma. Laryngoscope. 2022;133:1624.
9. Luce EA. Developing concepts and treatment of complex maxillary fractures. Clin Plast Surg. 1992;19(1):125–31.
10. Alpert B, Tiwana PS, Kushner GM. Management of comminuted fractures of the mandible. Oral Maxillofac Surg Clin North Am. 2009;21(2):185–92.
11. Anderson SR, Wolsefer NS, Miremadi AR. Management of mandible angle fractures with a right angle drill: description of technique. J Craniofac Surg. 2022;33(4):e359–e60.
12. Hackenberg B, Lee C, Caterson EJ. Management of subcondylar mandible fractures in the adult patient. J Craniofac Surg. 2014;25(1):166–71.
13. Hughes D, Ng SM, Smyth D, Patel H, Kent S, Henry A, et al. Emergency versus semi-elective management of mandible fractures: a maxillofacial trainee research collaborative (MTReC) study. Ann R Coll Surg Engl. 2022;60:e98.
14. Reddy L, Lee D, Vincent A, Shokri T, Sokoya M, Ducic Y. Secondary management of mandible fractures. Facial Plast Surg. 2019;35(6):627–32.
15. Shokri T, Misch E, Ducic Y, Sokoya M. Management of complex mandible fractures. Facial Plast Surg. 2019;35(6):602–6.
16. Sudheer R, Chakravarthy BD, Vura N, Rajasekhar G. Management of angle mandible fractures by 3D rectangular grid plate: a prospective study. J Maxillofac Oral Surg. 2020;19(3):420–4.

Traumatic Injuries in the Soft Tissue Neck

4

Mauro Hanaoka and Robert Kurtz

Clinical Presentation

The signs and symptoms may vary considerably, and the severity of the clinical presentation does not always correlate with the extent of soft tissue neck injury [1, 2]. Laryngotracheal and pharyngoesophageal injuries can present with anterior neck pain, dyspnea, dysphonia, stridor, dysphagia, cough, hemoptysis, ecchymosis, hematoma, penetrating wound, tenderness to palpation, subcutaneous emphysema, mediastinal emphysema (Hamman's sign), air bubbling from a penetrating wound, or persistent pneumothorax and air leak after thoracostomy tube placement. Cervical vascular and neural injuries can present as acute stroke, cranial neuropathy, or Horner's syndrome.

Mechanisms of Injury

Traumatic injuries to the soft tissue neck can be classified as blunt or penetrating. Blunt trauma is the most common mechanism of injury [3]. Penetrating neck injuries are less common and are defined as injuries that penetrate the platysma resulting from stabbing, gunshot wound, or penetrating debris (i.e., glass or shrapnel).

The neck soft tissues are particularly vulnerable to damage in direct blows, which can occur in road traffic accidents, assaults, and sports (i.e., ice hockey, basketball, martial arts). High-energy trauma with complex mechanisms of injury can force the neck into extremes of flexion, extension, and rotation, subjecting the soft tissue structures to severe tensile and shear forces. Despite the broad spectrum of injuries, several identifiable patterns exist and correspond to specific injury mechanisms.

A direct blow to the soft tissue neck may result in fracture to the laryngeal skeleton, compromise of the laryngeal airway, laryngotracheal mucosal or ligamentous tear, pharyngoesophageal mucosal tear, and neurovascular injury, including arterial dissection or pseudoaneurysm. Aryepiglottic fold tears can also result in detachment of the epiglottis.

Hyperextension injuries result from tensile and shear forces acting on the aerodigestive tract fixed against the cervical vertebrae. Characteristic injuries include vertical laryngeal cartilage fractures and tracheal tears. In rare cases, complete laryngotracheal separation at the level of the cricoid cartilage/cricotracheal membrane can be seen, as the airway is relatively immobile at this location. The prototypical example would be a driver's hyperextended neck accelerated forward

M. Hanaoka (✉) · R. Kurtz
Department of Radiology, Perelman School of Medicine at the University of Pennsylvania, Philadelphia, PA, USA
e-mail: Hanaomauro.hanaoka@pennmedicine.upenn.edu

F. Knollmann (ed.), *Trauma Computed Tomography*, https://doi.org/10.1007/978-3-031-45746-3_4

against the steering wheel, dashboard, or windshield during a motor vehicle collision.

Increased intrathoracic or intratracheal pressure against a closed glottis during chest or lower neck blunt trauma can result in laryngotracheal rupture (barotrauma). This type of injury mechanism can occur during rapid deceleration with an inappropriately high seat belt position across the chest or lower neck.

Strangulation injuries result from compressive forces to the neck. Strangulations can be accidental, self-inflicted or related to assault or other intentional method (i.e., judicial hanging). Manual strangulation is a type of strangulation that involves the use a forced applied directly to the neck by body parts such as hands, arms, or legs. Ligature strangulation involves the use of a constricting object or a band placed around the neck that is tightened by force other than gravity. Hanging is another type of strangulation that involves the use of a constricting band placed around the neck, which constricts the due to the effect of gravity. In suicidal hangings, the forces exerted on the neck are typically lower than those seen in judicial hangings, making cervical spine injury less of a concern. However, vascular injury (i.e., carotid dissection) and fractures of the trachea, thyroid cartilage, cricoid cartilage, and hyoid bone can occur. Death from strangulation can occur from carotid sinus stimulation-induced cardiac arrest, asphyxia, vascular occlusion, and spinal cord or brainstem damage. The most common findings on clinical exam in strangulation include subcutaneous edema, lymph node or submandibular gland hemorrhage, intramuscular hematomas of the platysma and sternocleidomastoid muscles, and edema or hemorrhage of the vocal cords [4]. Horizontal fractures involving the thyroid cartilage are classically encountered. They are typically bilateral, involve the superior border of the thyroid lamina and the superior horns of the thyroid cartilage, and are often associated with hyoid bone fractures [5, 6].

Iatrogenic injuries to the soft tissues of the neck are less common. They may occur from aerodigestive tract instrumentation (endotracheal intubation, bronchoscopy, endoscopy) or intraoperatively (cricothyroidotomy, emergent tracheostomy).

Laryngotracheal Injuries

The laryngeal skeleton is comprised of six cartilages connected by membranes, ligaments, and muscles. These cartilages include the epiglottis, thyroid, cricoid, arytenoid, cuneiform, and corniculate cartilages.

Some of the cartilages in the larynx, including the epiglottis, vocal process of the arytenoids, cuneiform, and corniculate cartilages, are made of elastic fibrocartilage and do not ossify. On the other hand, the thyroid and cricoid cartilages are composed of hyaline cartilage and undergo ossification due to normal aging [7, 8] (Fig. 4.1). This process is more common in males than in females [9].

The epiglottis is a spoon shaped cartilage. It is connected to the larynx by its base, also known as the petiole, and to the hyoid bone by the hyoepiglottic ligament.

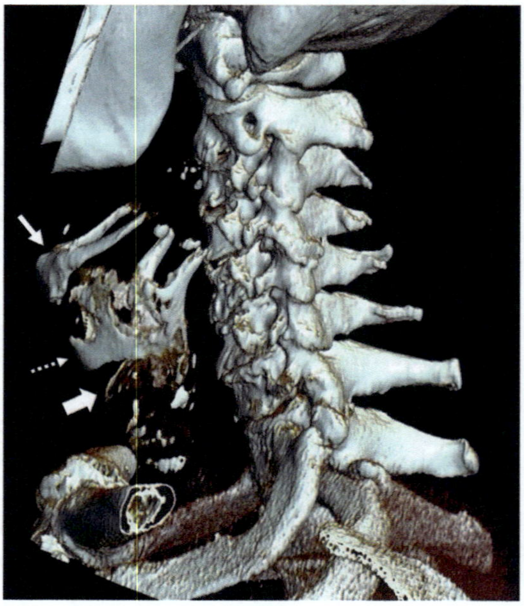

Fig. 4.1 Anatomy and anatomic relationships of the ossified structures of the larynx. 3D surface rendered images of the ossified structures of the larynx shows the hyoid bone (thin solid arrow), with a body and lesser and greater horns, the thyroid cartilage (dashed arrow) and the partially ossified cricoid cartilage (thick arrow). The arytenoid cartilages are obscured by the overlying thyroid cartilage

The thyroid cartilage has two laminae, or plates, that are fused anteriorly and has superior and inferior horns, or cornua, posteriorly. The superior horn of the thyroid cartilage is attached to the hyoid bone via the infrahyoid muscles and to the thyrohyoid membrane. The inferior horn is connected to the cricoid cartilage through the cricothyroid membrane and the sternum through the sternohyoid muscle. The thyroid cartilage often begins to ossify at the posterior inferior border and in the inferior horns in early adulthood (Fig. 4.2). The process tends to progress to the superior horns and the superior border of the thyroid laminae, although ossification is variable. By age 65, the thyroid cartilage may be fully ossified, although the median portions of the thyroid laminae may remain non-ossified. Inward bending of the superior horns is a normal anatomic variant and should not be mistaken for a fracture.

The cricoid cartilage is shaped like a signet ring with a thicker lamina posteriorly and is the only complete cartilaginous ring within the larynx. The cricothyroid membrane connects the cricoid cartilage to the thyroid cartilage superiorly, while the cricotracheal ligament anchors the cricoid cartilage to the first ring of the trachea inferiorly. Ossification begins at the cricoid cartilage's superior aspect (Fig. 4.3).

The arytenoid cartilages have a pyramidal shape, and the cartilages' base articulates with the cricoid cartilage's posterior lamina, forming the cricoarytenoid joint. The arytenoid cartilage has an anterior vocal process, which is attached to the vocal fold, and a lateral muscular process, which is the insertion of the lateral and posterior cricoarytenoid muscles. The ossification of the arytenoid cartilage may be asymmetric in 12.9% of patients [10].

The hyoid bone is comprised of a body, two greater horns, and two smaller superior/posterior projecting lesser horns. Ossification of the hyoid bone starts in the greater horns and progresses to the body and the lesser horns. Although ossification of the hyoid bone is usually completed before the second decade of life, the fibrous cartilage connecting the body and greater horn may persist and should not be mistaken as a fracture (Fig. 4.4). Injury to the suprahyoid or infrahyoid muscles may cause malpositioning of the hyoid bone, as contraction of the suprahyoid muscle results in elevation and anterior displacement of

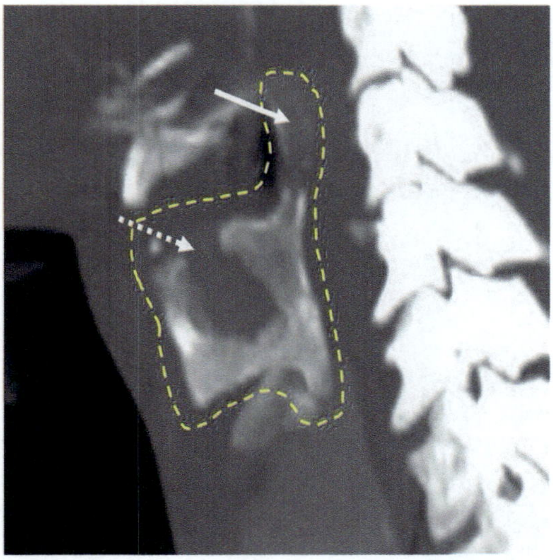

Fig. 4.2 Incomplete ossification of the thyroid cartilage in a 35-year-old male. A sagittal maximum intensity projection image of the thyroid cartilage (yellow dashed line) from a CT angiogram of the neck shows ossification of the inferior horn and inferior margin of the lamina but with lack of ossification of the superior horn (arrow) and superior border of the lamina (dashed arrow) as well as the central portion of the lamina

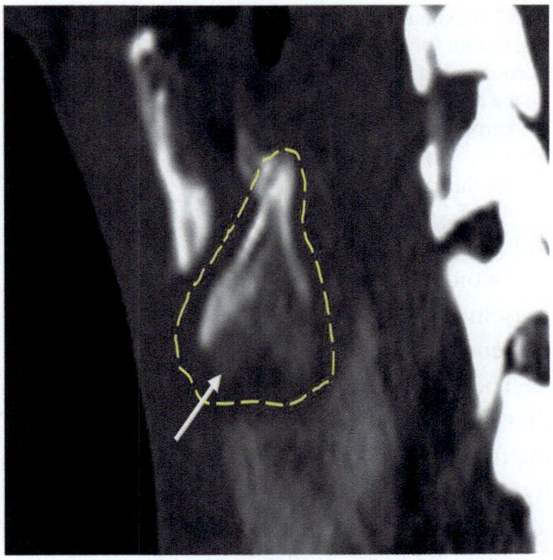

Fig. 4.3 Incomplete ossification of the cricoid cartilage in a 35-year-old male. A sagittal maximum intensity projection image of the cricoid cartilage (yellow dashed line) from a CT angiogram of the neck shows ossification of the superior margin but with lack of ossification of the more inferior aspect (arrow)

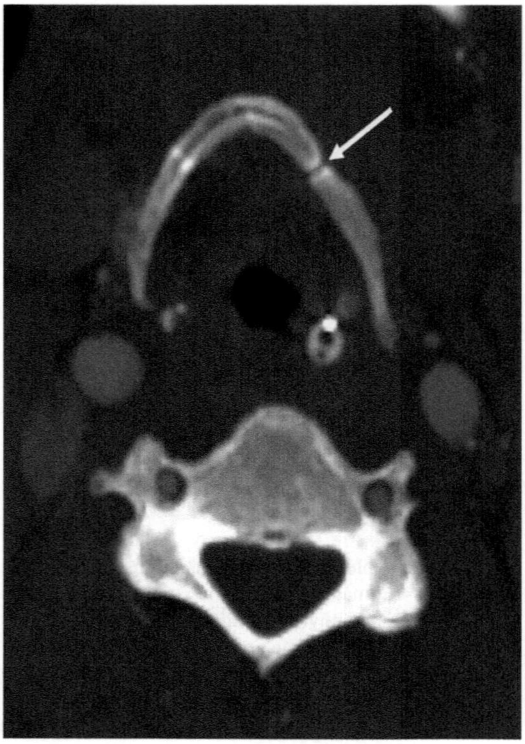

Fig. 4.4 Asymmetric ossification of the hyoid bone. Axial maximum intensity projection image from a CT angiogram of the neck shows ossification across the fibrous cartilage that connects the body to the greater horn on the right. On the left, there is lack of ossification across the cartilage (arrow). This should not be confused with a fracture, noting the well corticated margins of bone adjacent to the cartilage

the hyoid bone, and contraction of the infrahyoid muscle results in depression and posterior displacement of the hyoid bone.

The triticeal cartilages are a pair of cartilages that are located between the superior horns of the thyroid cartilage and the greater horns of the hyoid bone. The variable and asymmetric attenuation of the triticeal cartilage should not be misidentified as avulsed cartilaginous fragments, which can lead to a diagnostic pitfall (Fig. 4.5).

When a laryngeal injury is suspected or known to have occurred, the most important initial step is to assess for laryngeal patency. It may be difficult to directly visualize the larynx under laryngoscopy due to severe supraglottic edema, so CT may be the only available method for complete assessment of the airway [11]. Laryngeal compromise can be secondary to edema, intramural hematoma or extrinsic compression. If there is asymmetric thickening of the laryngeal mucosa in the absence of extrinsic compression, it is also important to carefully evaluate for the possibility of mucosal tears or lacerations.

The search pattern for laryngotracheal injuries on CT should include inspection of the neck with soft tissue and bone windows with multiplanar reconstructions. Due to wide variations in the extent of ossification of the laryngeal cartilages, it can be difficult to assess for fractures. Some useful clues to assess for that may indicate the presence of a fracture are abrupt differences in the position of ossified or non-ossified cartilage as well as flat and sharp margins between ossified portions of the cartilage. Nonfractured areas of ossification within cartilage tend to have more rounded or indistinct margins. Fractures of the thyroid cartilage are often caused by road traffic accidents and are typically vertical fractures through the lamina or midline of the cartilage (Fig. 4.6). In cases of strangulation, thyroid cartilage fractures are more likely to be horizontal, bilateral, involve the superior border of the thyroid lamina and the superior horns of the thyroid cartilage, and may be accompanied by fractures of the hyoid bone (Figs. 4.7 and 4.8). Coronal and sagittal images can be especially helpful in evaluating the extent of complex and oblique fractures (Fig. 4.9).

Injury to the cricoarytenoid joint, which is located on the superior-posterior aspect of the cricoid cartilage, can lead to subluxation or dislocation of the arytenoid cartilage. The most common type of injury to the arytenoid cartilage is anterior subluxation (Fig. 4.10). When the arytenoid cartilage is misaligned, axial images may show asymmetry of the bilateral cricoarytenoid joints and medialization of the ipsilateral true vocal folds. To accurately determine arytenoid cartilage subluxation/dislocation, it is best to view in the sagittal plane, as this type of injury may be missed on axial images. Cricoarytenoid dislocations and subluxations are treated with operative reduction, and in some cases, vocal fold injections and/or thyroplasty.

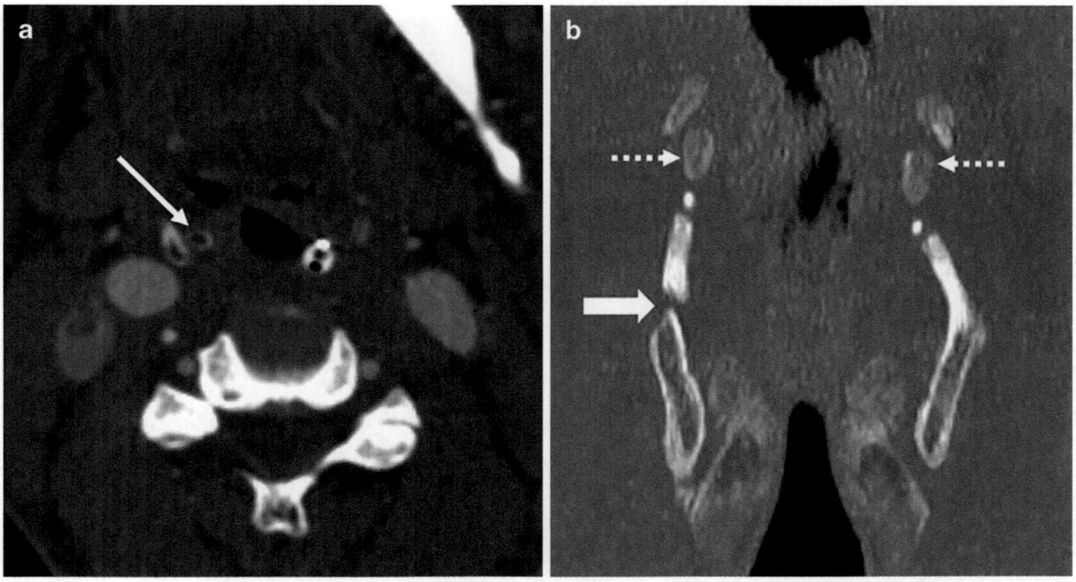

Fig. 4.5 Normal triticeal cartilages in a patient with a thyroid cartilage superior horn fracture. Axial image from a CT angiogram of the neck (**a**) shows a well corticated, oval ossified structure adjacent to the greater horn of the hyoid bone, representing a normal triticeal cartilage (thin arrow). This should not be confused with a fracture fragment from the hyoid bone or superior horn of the thyroid cartilage. Coronal maximum intensity projection CT image of the neck (**b**) shows symmetric normal triticeal cartilages (dashed arrows) located between the greater horns of the hyoid and the superior horns of the thyroid cartilage. There is a mildly displaced fracture at the base of the right superior horn of the thyroid cartilage (thick arrow). Also note the small variant ossifications at the superior margins of the thyroid cartilage superior horns

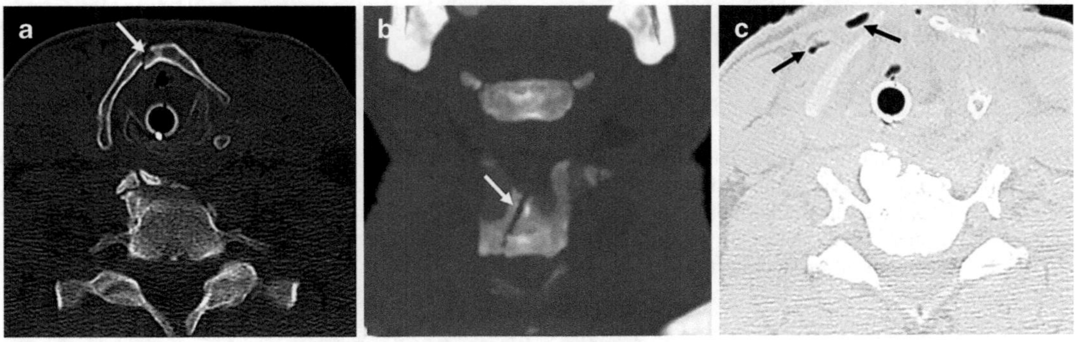

Fig. 4.6 Vertical fracture of the thyroid cartilage. (**a**) Axial CT of the neck shows a vertical fracture of the right thyroid cartilage lamina (arrow). (**b**) Coronal maximum intensity projection reformatted image shows that the fracture line extends the full height of the thyroid cartilage lamina (arrow). (**c**) Axial image in lung window shows foci of air in the soft tissues related to disruption of the laryngeal mucosa

Anterior commissure disruption results from avulsion of the vocal ligaments from the thyroid cartilage. This injury requires suturing of the anterior vocal ligament to the thyroid perichondrium to restore the normal scaphoid anatomy of the glottis.

Fractures of the cricoid cartilage often occur in more than one location and can result in collapse of the lumen of the larynx. The normal mucosal surface is thin and cannot be seen on CT or MRI. Therefore, mucosal thickening at the level of the cricoid cartilage should be considered abnormal.

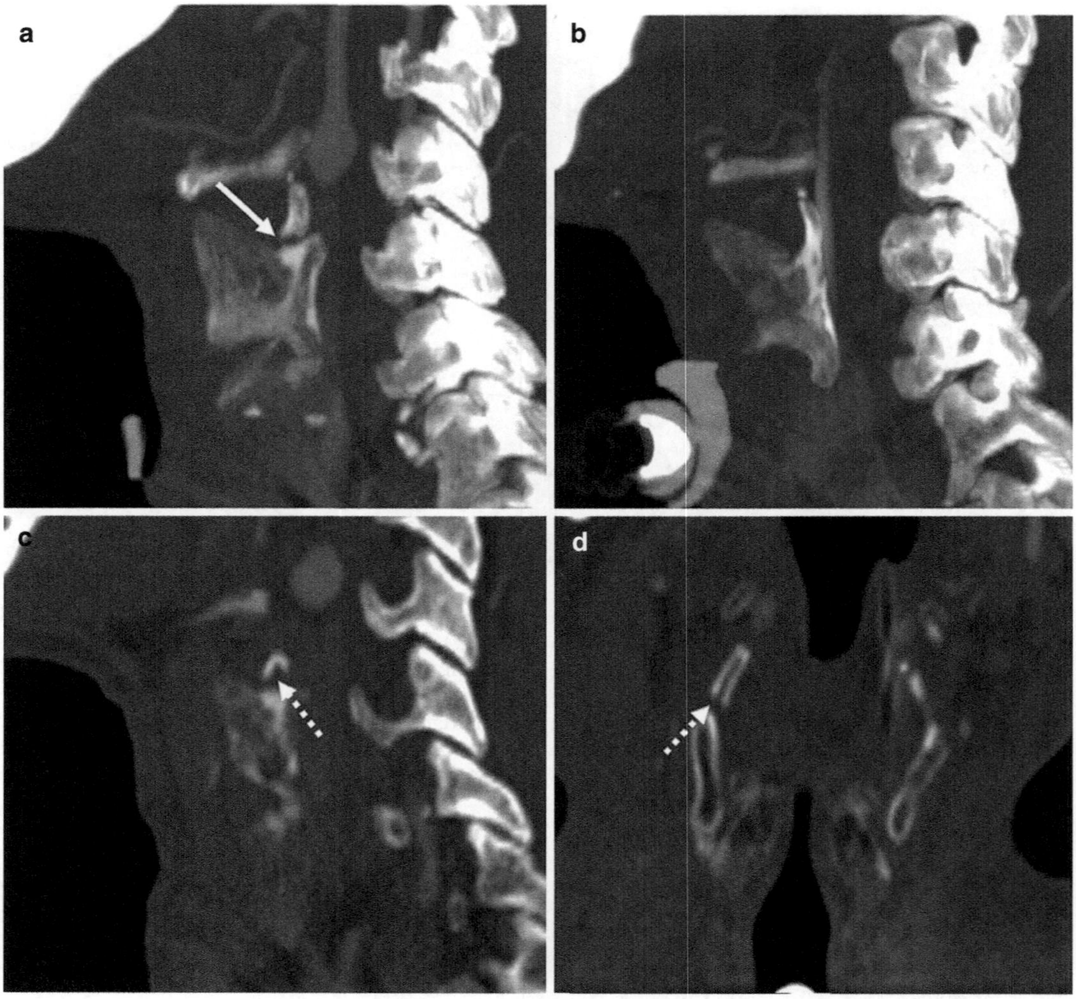

Fig. 4.7 (**a**) Sagittal maximum intensity projection image from a CT angiogram of the neck shows a fracture through the base of the superior horn of the thyroid cartilage with mild anterior displacement of the superior horn. (**b**) Sagittal maximum intensity projection image on the left shows the normal superior horn for comparison. (**c**, **d**) Sagittal (**c**) and coronal (**d**) CT images show the fracture, with lack of cortication/sclerosis along the fracture margin (dashed arrows)

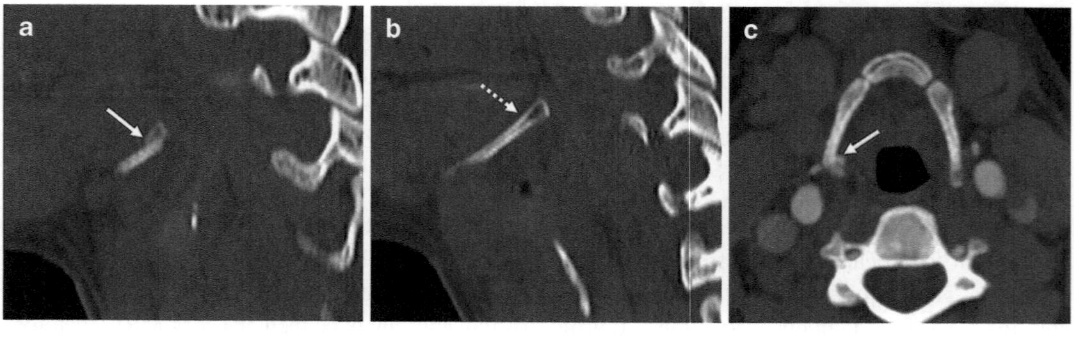

Fig. 4.8 Hyoid bone fracture in a 20 year-old-female following strangulation. (**a**) Sagittal image from a CT angiogram of the neck shows a fracture at the posterior aspect of the right greater horn of the hyoid bone, with superior displacement of the fracture fragment and mild overlapping of the fragments (arrow). (**b**) Sagittal image of the normal left hyoid bone greater horn for comparison. (**c**) Axial maximum intensity projection CT image shows the fracture fragment to also be mildly medially displaced (arrow)

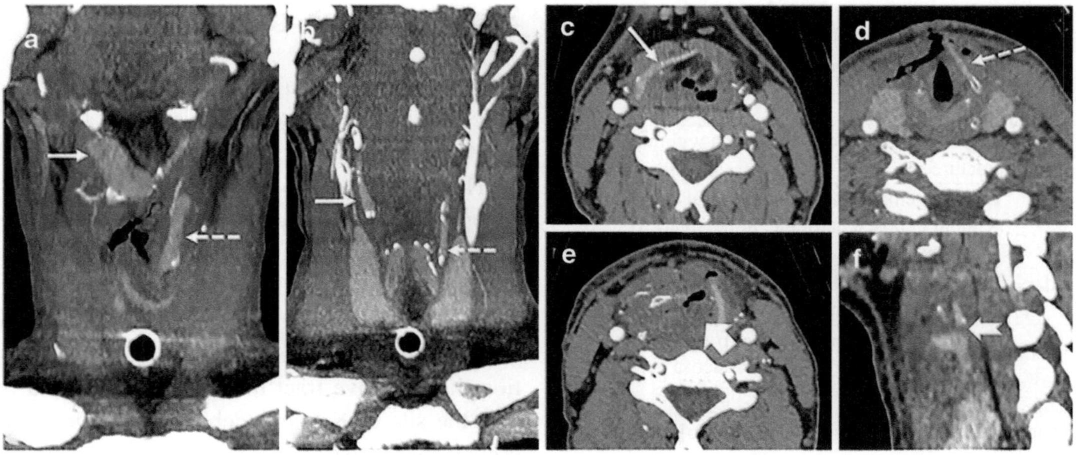

Fig. 4.9 Complex thyroid cartilage fracture/dislocation following a motorcycle accident. (**a, b**) Coronal maximum intensity projection images from a CT angiogram of the neck show a vertically oriented fracture through the left lamina of the thyroid cartilage. There is a tearing of the right thyrocricoid membrane with superior displacement of the right aspect of the thyroid cartilage (arrow) and tear of the left thyrohyoid membrane with inferior displacement of the left aspect of the thyroid cartilage (dashed arrow). (**c–e**) Axial images show medial rotation of the right thyroid cartilage lamina (arrow) and mild medial rotation of the left thyroid lamina (dashed arrow). There is edema and swelling and in the laryngeal soft tissues (thick arrow) with narrowing of the laryngeal airway. (**f**) Sagittal maximum intensity projection image shows a fracture of the non-ossified left superior horn (notched arrow)

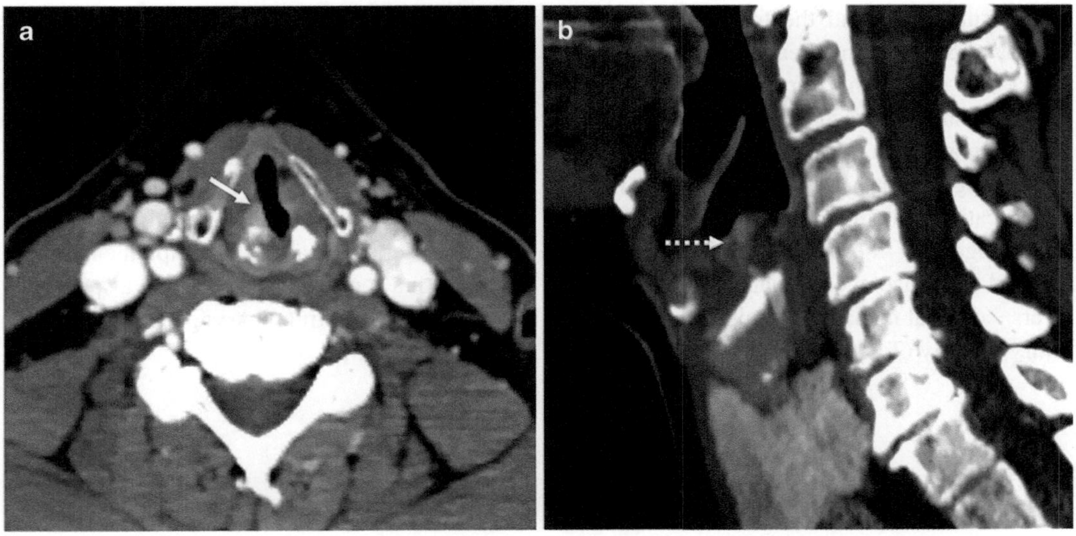

Fig. 4.10 Right arytenoid dislocation in a patient with hoarseness and dysphagia after prior intubation. (**a**) Axial contrast enhanced CT of the neck shows anterior displacement of the non-ossified right arytenoid cartilage (arrow) compared to the normally positioned, ossified left arytenoid cartilage. There is mild medialization of the right vocal fold. Note that there can be asymmetric ossification of the arytenoids. (**b**) Sagittal reformatted image shows the anterior dislocation of the arytenoid cartilage in relation to the cricoid cartilage posterior lamina

Table 4.1 Classification scheme for categorizing the severity of laryngeal injuries

Schaefer-Fuhrman classification of laryngeal injury	
Grade	Findings
I	Minor endolaryngeal hematoma without fracture
II	Edema, hematoma, minor mucosal disruption without exposed cartilage, nondisplaced fractures
III	Massive edema, mucosal tears, exposed cartilage, cord immobility
IV	Grade III with more than two fracture lines or massive trauma to laryngeal mucosa
V	Complete laryngotracheal separation

Source: Modified from Schaefer et al. [26] and Furhman et al. [27]

Laryngotracheal separation is the most severe type of laryngotracheal injury and is usually fatal unless an emergent airway is obtained immediately at the trauma scene. On imaging, there is marked soft tissue emphysema. The separation occurs at the cricotracheal ligament and can be either partial or complete. In cases of complete laryngotracheal separation, the hyoid bone is displaced superiorly, and the trachea is displaced inferiorly. Surgical intervention is typically necessary to repair the rupture and separation, although smaller tracheal lacerations (<2 cm) may be treated conservatively.

Although there are several laryngeal trauma classification systems, the American Academy of Otolaryngology—head and neck surgery has adopted the Schaefer-Fuhrman classification as it offers a clinical management algorithm based on injury severity (Table 4.1).

Pharyngoesophageal Injury

Most pharyngoesophageal injuries are caused by penetrating trauma and comprise only 1–7% of all traumatic head and neck injuries [12].

The pharynx can be divided into three parts: nasopharynx, oropharynx, and hypopharynx. The hypopharynx starts from the hyoid bone level and extends to the lower edge of the cricoid cartilage. The pharyngoesophageal junction is located in the lower hypopharynx and is the narrowest portion the digestive tract in the neck. This area is also the site of Killian's dehiscence, which is a point of weakness in the digestive tract where the pharyngeal wall consists only of mucosa and serosa without intervening muscle. As a result, this area is more prone to perforation from instrumentation and blunt trauma.

On imaging, determining the trajectory of the perforating object is important to localize the site of pharyngoesophageal injury. The region with the greatest amount of soft tissue emphysema, the presence of mural or extrinsic hematoma, or the loss of fat planes surrounding the pharynx or esophagus are also helpful to localize a perforation. Furthermore, fluoroscopic imaging with water soluble oral contrast, possibly followed by CT, can be performed to determine the site of injury (Fig. 4.11). If perforation is suspected, but unable to be localized on imaging, endoscopy is a good complement procedure, with a sensitivity of 50% and a specificity of 100% for detecting pharyngoesophageal perforation [12–15].

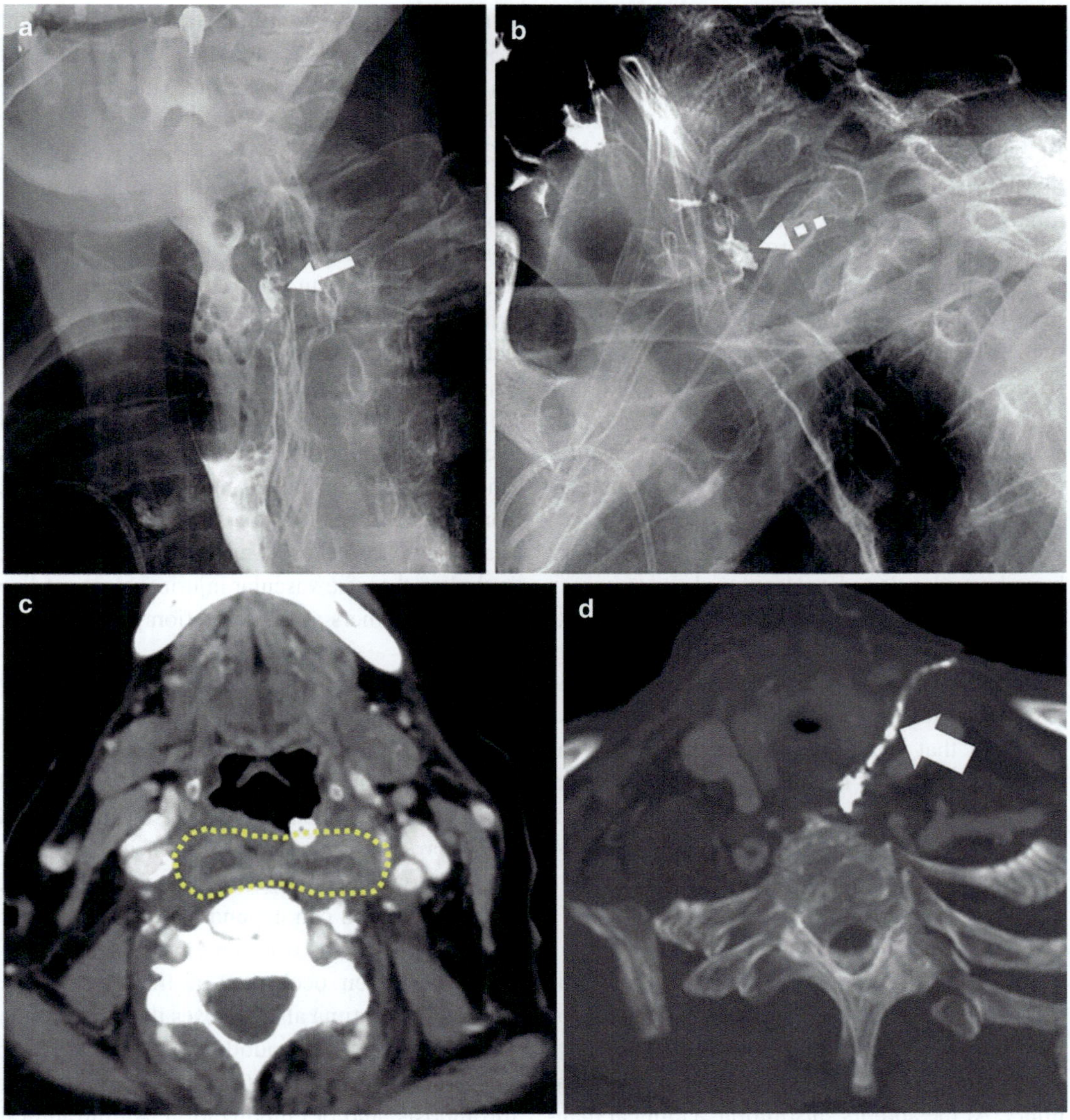

Fig. 4.11 Upper esophageal perforation following penetrating injury. (**a**) AP image from a water soluble contrast agent esophagram shows a collection of extraluminal contrast along the left side of the upper esophagus (arrow). (**b**) The extraluminal contrast is seen to persist and is located posterior to the esophagus on an oblique image (dashed arrow). (**c**) Subsequent contrast enhanced CT shows a rim enhancing retropharyngeal collection, representing an abscess (dashed circle). (**d**) Maximum intensity projection image from a later CT of the neck after drainage of the abscess and removal of the drain and immediately after a water soluble contrast agent esophagram shows persistence of leakage of contrast and extension of contrast to the skin surface along the prior drain tract (thick arrow)

Cerebrovascular Injury

Cerebrovascular injuries in the neck can occur with either blunt or penetrating trauma, with motor vehicle accidents being the most common etiology of blunt cerebrovascular injury (BCVI), causing around 50% of the injuries [16]. Traditionally, BCVIs have been underdiagnosed; however, in the past two decades, there has been substantial increase in the diagnosis of these injuries owing to increased screening of the asymptomatic trauma population, now thought to have a prevalence of approximately 1% of the screened trauma patient population [17, 18]. Untreated BCVI has high associated morbidity and mortality, with significant decrease in morbidity when rapidly diagnosed and with early institution of antithrombotic therapy [19]. There is often a short asymptomatic period from the time of injury to the development of neurologic sequelae, with most patients that develop neurologic sequelae showing symptoms within 72 h of injury [16]. This leaves a relatively narrow window from the time of injury to diagnosis and institution of therapy to decrease the risk of permanent injury and disability.

There are a number of screening protocols that have been developed to decide whom to screen for cerebrovascular injury. An appropriate screening protocol should attempt to capture a high percentage of injuries while at the same time avoid the overutilization of imaging and false positives that could lead to overtreatment, as there are mimics of BCVI on CTA, which is currently the imaging modality of choice for screening of BCVI. Common mimics of BCVI on CTA are atherosclerotic plaque and streak artifact from dental or cervical spine hardware.

One of the more commonly used screening protocols is the Denver Criteria [2, 20]. This includes a list of clinical signs and symptoms as well as radiologic findings that should trigger a request for CTA of the neck to assess for vascular injury. At the authors' institution, a clinical management guideline was developed for this purpose and is currently in use at the time of this writing. Symptomatic patients with the following signs of BCVI warrant immediate diagnosis and/or intervention: neurologic deficit that is unexplained by a diagnosed injury or incongruous with head/spine CT or MRI; arterial hemorrhage from the neck, mouth, nose, or ears; cervical hematoma; cervical bruit or thrill in a patient <50 years of age; evidence of cerebral infarction on CT or MRI. Asymptomatic patients with the following risk factors should be screened for BCVI: injury mechanism suspicious for cervical hyperextension, hyperflexion, or rotation; anterior neck "clothesline" type injury or "seat belt" abrasion with swelling, pain, or altered mental status; near-hanging with cerebral anoxia; TBI with GCS </= 6 and diffuse axonal injury; cervical spine fracture, subluxation, or ligamentous injury at any level; severe facial trauma including bilateral facial fractures, Le Fort II or Le Fort III facial fractures, or complex mandible fractures (including all subcondylar mandibular fractures); complex skull fracture, basilar skull fracture, or scalp degloving injury; major thoracic injuries, including thoracic vascular injuries, blunt cardiac rupture, or others at the discretion of the trauma surgeon.

Arterial walls are composed of three primary layers—the intima, media and adventitia. A dissection is characterized by a tear in the intima, which can result in a raised intimal flap. Blood can then dissect beneath the raised intima and cause progression of a dissection in the direction of flowing blood, creating of false lumen. The false lumen can expand and cause variable compression of the true lumen resulting in narrowing or even occlusion of the vessel. The injury to the intima also exposes the blood to the thrombogenic subendothelial extracellular matrix, which can lead to platelet aggregation, thrombosis, and/or embolization. An intramural hematoma results from injury to the vasa vasorum in the adventitial layer, with blood dissecting through the media and adventitia and can result in luminal narrowing or occlusion. A pseudoaneurysm results from injury to all three layers, with a focal vascular outpouching contained by incomplete adventitia or surrounding soft tissues [21].

Table 4.2 Classification scheme for categorizing the severity of blunt cerebrovascular injuries

Biffl scale for blunt cerebrovascular injury	
Grade	
I	Luminal irregularity or dissection with <25% luminal narrowing
II	Dissection or intramural hematoma with ≥25% luminal narrowing, intraluminal thrombus, or raised intimal flap
III	Pseudoaneurysm
IV	Occlusion
V	Transection with free extravasation

Source: Biffl et al. [22]

The Biffl (Denver) scale is a commonly used tool to evaluate the severity of cerebrovascular injury [22] (Table 4.2). Injuries are graded on a scale from I to V, with higher grades indicating a worse prognosis and a greater risk for stroke when involving the carotid arteries. Grade I injuries (Fig. 4.12) include luminal irregularity or dissection/intramural hematoma with <25% luminal narrowing (compared to the diameter of the lumen immediately proximal to the injury). These can easily be confused with atherosclerotic plaque, with the presence of calcification suggestive of atherosclerosis rather than acute injury [21]. Grade II injuries include dissection or intramural hematoma with >/= 25% luminal narrowing as well as any intraluminal thrombus or any raised intimal flap (Figs. 4.13 and 4.14). Grade III injury is a pseudoaneurysm (Fig. 4.15), grade IV injury is complete vessel occlusion (Fig. 4.16), and grade V injury is transection with free extravasation. This grading scale can be used for both carotid and vertebral artery injuries.

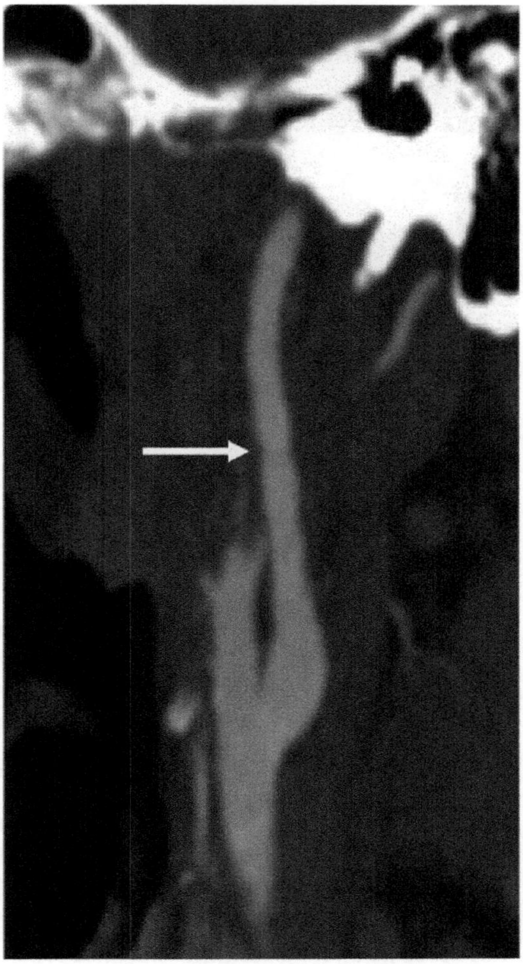

Fig. 4.12 Grade I injury of the left internal carotid artery. Sagittal image from a CT angiogram of the neck in a patient with cervical spine fractures following motor vehicle collision shows mild irregularity of the wall of the left internal carotid artery (arrow) with less than 25% narrowing of the lumen, consistent with a grade I injury

On interpretation of CTA, it is important to individually examine the aortic arch and each major vessel. The vessels should be smooth, round, and gradually taper from the main vessel moving distally. Sudden change in the vessel's caliber or shape, wall thickening, wall irregularity, intraluminal filling defect, vascular outpouching or loss of the fat plane around the vessel may indicate underlying vascular injury. In addition, close inspection should be given to vessels in the path of penetrating trauma or nearby fractures or cervical spine dislocations to assess for injury, active extravasation, transection or complete

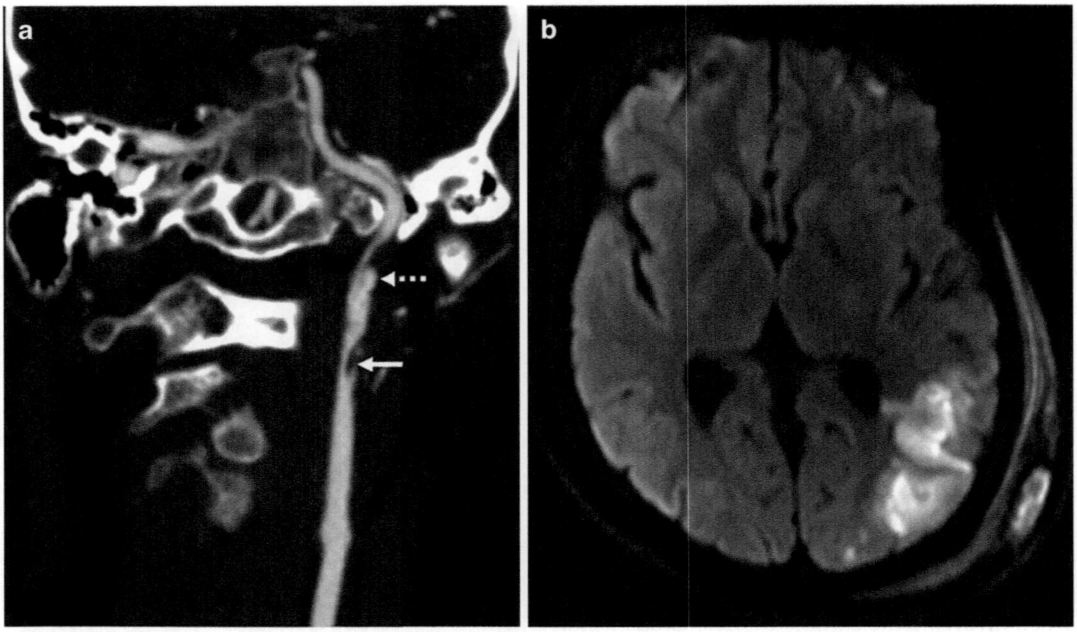

Fig. 4.13 Grade II/III injury of the left internal carotid artery. (**a**) Curved planar reformation image of a CT angiogram of the neck in a patient following motor vehicle collision with cervical spine fractures shows irregularity of walls of the mid to distal cervical left internal carotid artery. There is a curvilinear filling defect (arrow) representing a raised intimal flap, which would be consistent with a grade II injury. More superiorly in the artery is an additional raised flap, possibly with small pseudoaneurysm formation (dashed arrow), which could indicate a grade III injury. There is greater than 25% narrowing of the lumen at both sites. (**b**) Axial diffusion weighted image of the head shows an acute infarct in the posterior left MCA territory, likely the result of an embolic event from the carotid dissection, as well as a contusion/hematoma in the left posterior scalp from the preceding trauma

occlusion. In cases that are equivocal for injury or in which no injury is identified but there is persistent high clinical suspicion for injury, DSA can be performed. MRA with high resolution vessel wall imaging has also shown promise in problem cases [23], particularly for identifying intramural hematomas and distinguishing atherosclerotic plaque from dissection [21]. However, CTA remains the current standard for screening.

Antithrombotic therapy is the current standard of care for treatment of grade I through IV injuries and can consist of antiplatelet therapy or anticoagulation, most often utilizing aspirin. Use of antithrombotic therapy has been shown to significantly decrease the occurrence of secondary neurologic morbidity and mortality [19]. For grade V injuries, surgical or endovascular management should be considered depending on the clinical status of the patient [21].

Grade I through III injuries can have dynamic changes in the acute to subacute time period, therefore follow-up imaging with CTA in 7–10 days is recommended to assess for resolution or worsening of the imaging findings and is used to guide therapy [19] (Fig. 4.14). If the imaging findings resolve, then antithrombotic therapy may be discontinued, whereas if findings progress, endovascular or surgical management may be considered. Grade I injuries are more likely to heal at follow-up, whereas Grade II and III injuries have higher incidence of progression [16].

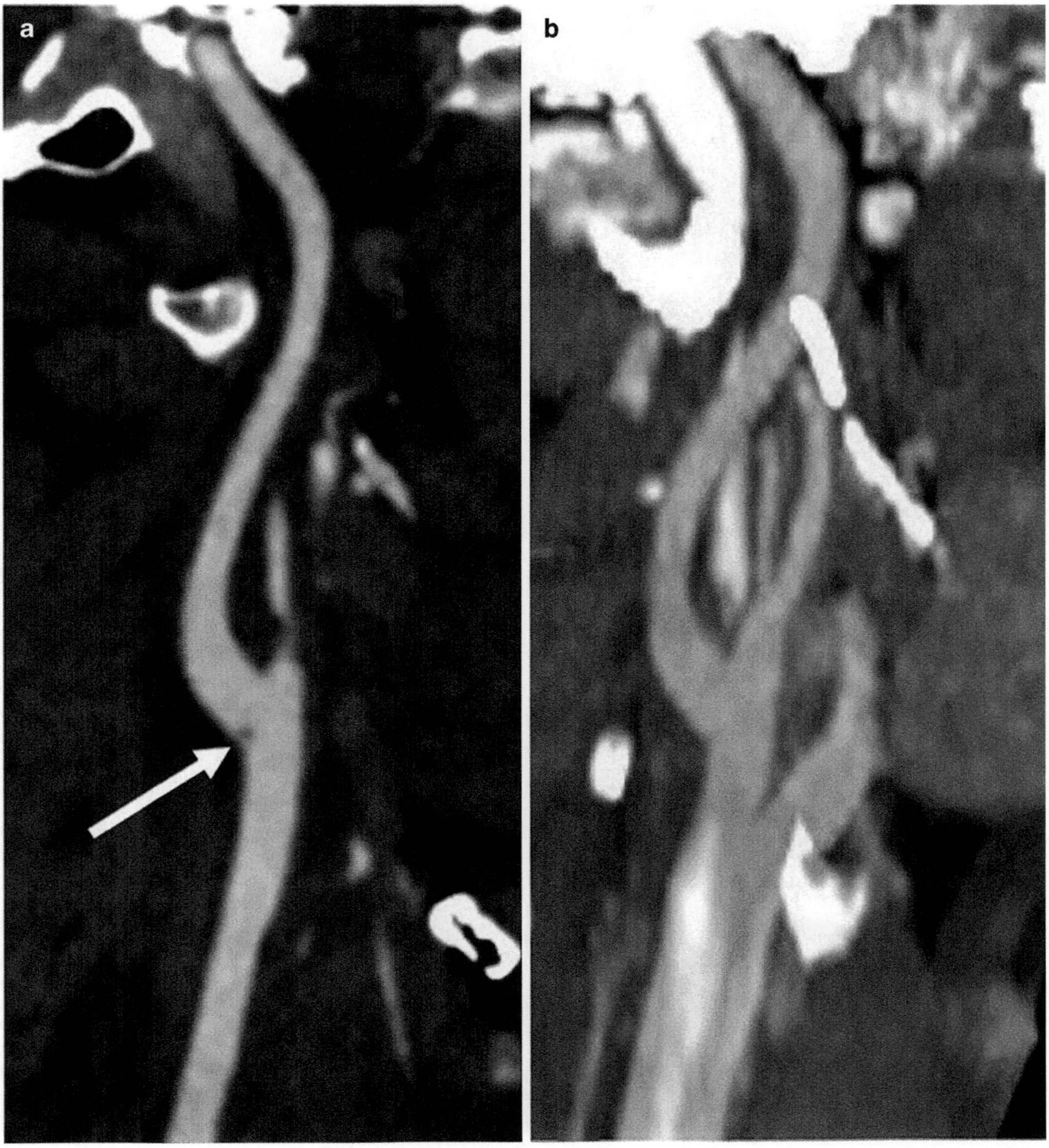

Fig. 4.14 Grade II carotid injury follow a self-inflicted stab wound. (**a**) Curved planar reformatted image from a CT angiogram of the neck shows a small filling defect along the posterior margin of the carotid bulb (arrow), which likely represented a small intraluminal thrombus. (**b**) Sagittal maximum intensity projection reformatted image from a follow-up CT angiogram of the neck 10 days later shows that the thrombus is no longer present

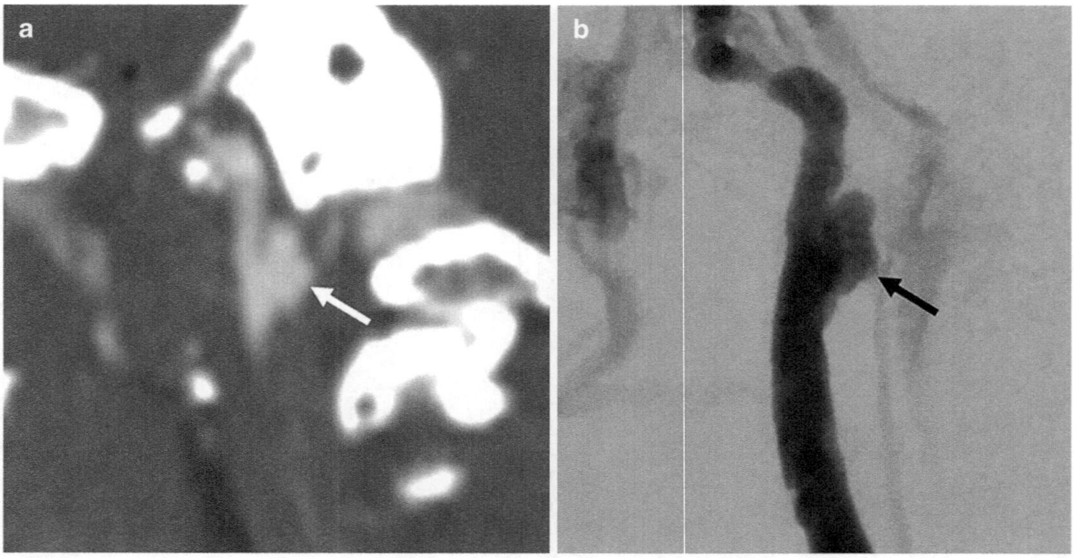

Fig. 4.15 Left carotid pseudoaneurysm/grade III injury. (**a**, **b**) Sagittal reformatted image from a CT angiogram of the neck (**a**) and DSA (**b**) show an outpouching from the left internal carotid artery just below the level of the skull base (arrows), representing a pseudoaneurysm

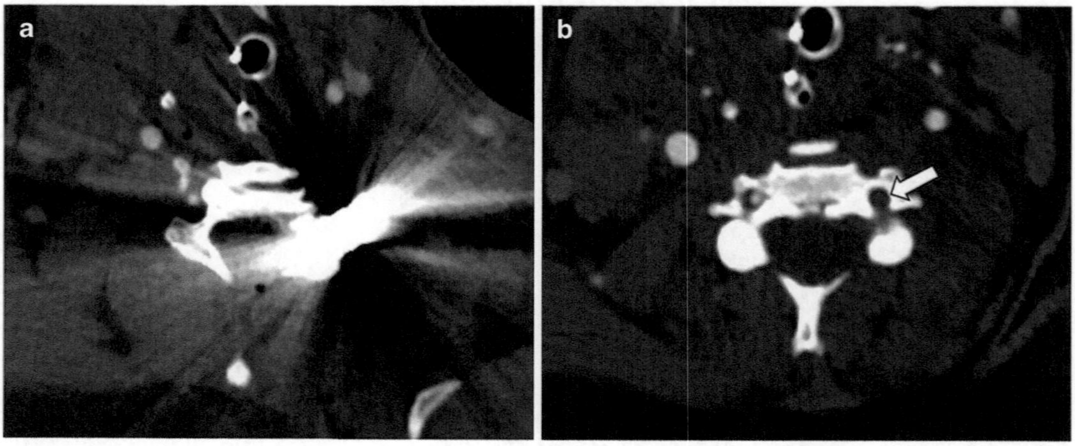

Fig. 4.16 Left vertebral artery occlusion/grade IV injury following a gunshot wound. (**a**) Axial image from a CT angiogram of the neck shows metallic artifact along the left aspect of the cervical spine from a ballistic fragment. (**b**) A more cranial image demonstrates lack of contrast filling of the left vertebral artery in the foramen transversarium (arrow), representing complete occlusion of the vessel

Salivary Gland Injury

Salivary gland traumatic injuries are rare. Parotid gland and duct injuries are more prevalent than injuries to the submandibular and sublingual glands, which are protected by the mandible [24]. Salivary gland injury can present with gland enlargement with surrounding fat stranding from edema and/or hyperattenuation from hemorrhage (Fig. 4.17). In cases of complex trauma, these injuries can be missed due to the satisfaction of search if not included into the search pattern. Salivary gland injuries can be complicated by the formation of sialoceles or fistulas, and can result in secondary infection (Fig. 4.18) [25].

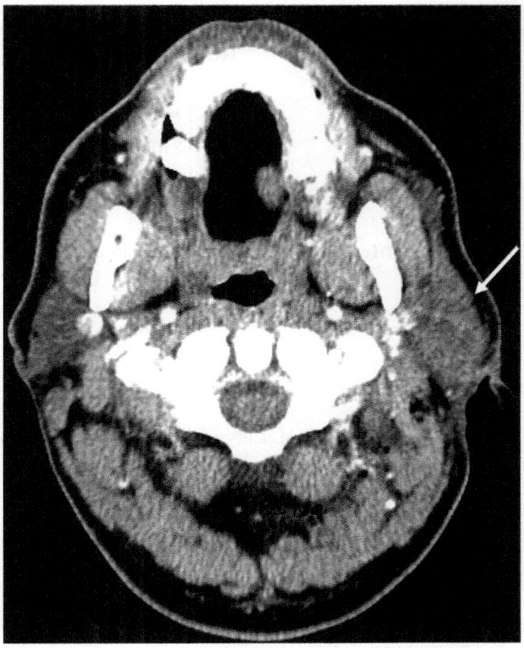

Fig. 4.17 Left parotid gland acute traumatic injury. Axial contrast enhanced CT of the neck shows asymmetric increased size and increased attenuation of the left parotid gland (arrow) compared to the right due to edema and hemorrhage in this patient who presented following penetrating trauma to the left side of the face

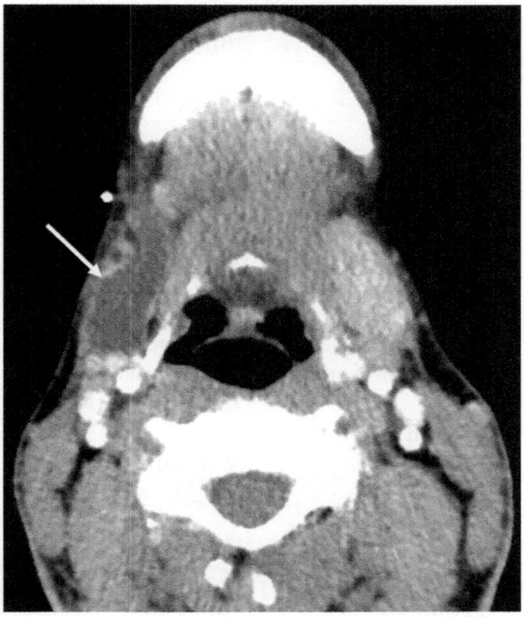

Fig. 4.18 Iatrogenic right submandibular gland sialocele. Axial contrast enhanced CT of the neck in this patient with submandibular swelling and a history of submandibular gland resection shows a somewhat tubular-shaped fluid density collection in the right submandibular space (arrow), consistent with an iatrogenic sialocele. A BB was placed on the patient's skin at the site of the palpable swelling

CT Protocols

Protocol name	CT neck with IV contrast
Indication	Trauma, mass, infection
Protocol designed for (scanner model)	GE revolution
Patient preparation	20 gauge IV catheter above wrist
First series	ST neck with
Oral contrast	N/A
IV contrast	100 mL @ 3.5 mL/s, 210 s delay
Tube settings	
kV	120 kV
mA	100–545 mA
Dose modulation	Smart mA
Tube rotation time (s)	0.5 s
Table speed (mm/s)	50 mm/s
Slice collimation	0.625 mm
Reconstructed slice thickness	2.5 mm
Anatomical coverage	Sella Turcica to carina
Reconstruction kernel	Standard fine
	Bone plus
Breath hold	None
Window settings	WW 400
	WL 40
Post processing	
Other	
Typical dose	
CTDIvol	10.23 mGy
DLP	216.1 mGy*cm
Eff. Dose	1.274 mSv

Protocol name	CTA neck
Indication	Trauma, Cspine fracture, strangulation, stroke
Protocol designed for (scanner model)	GE revolution
Patient preparation	20 gauge IV in right AC
First series	
Oral contrast	N/A
IV contrast	50 mL @ 5 mL/s
Tube settings	
kV	120 kV
mA	200–600 mA
Dose modulation	Smart mA
Tube rotation time (s)	0.5 s
Table speed (mm/s)	50 mm/s
Slice collimation	0.625 mm
Reconstructed slice thickness	1.25 mm
	5.0 mm
Anatomical coverage	Carina to Sella turcica
Reconstruction kernel	STANDARD
Breath hold	None
Window settings	WW 300, WL 30
Post processing	CPR of each vessel; sag and cor MIP
Other	Smart prep at aortic arch, with ROI in aortic arch.
	Scan when ROI reaches HU of 120
Typical dose	
CTDIvol	14.52 mGy
DLP	331.35 mGy*cm
Eff. Dose	1.95 mSv

Conflict of Interest The authors have no conflict of interest.

References

1. Mathisen DJ, Grillo H. Laryngotracheal trauma. Ann Thorac Surg. 1987;43(3):254–62.
2. Geddes AE, Burlew CC, Wagenaar AE, Biffl WL, Johnson JL, Pieracci FM, et al. Expanded screening criteria for blunt cerebrovascular injury: a bigger impact than anticipated. Am J Surg. 2016;212(6):1167–74.
3. Kiser AC, O'Brien SM, Detterbeck FC. Blunt tracheobronchial injuries: treatment and outcomes. Ann Thorac Surg. 2001;71(6):2059–65.
4. Yen K, Thali MJ, Aghayev E, Jackowski C, Schweitzer W, Boesch C, et al. Strangulation signs: initial correlation of MRI, MSCT, and forensic neck findings. J Magn Reson Imaging. 2005;22(4):501–10.
5. Kempter M, Ross S, Spendlove D, Flach PM, Preiss U, Thali MJ, et al. Post-mortem imaging of laryngohyoid fractures in strangulation incidents: first results. Leg Med (Tokyo). 2009;11(6):267–71.
6. Yen K, Vock P, Christe A, Scheurer E, Plattner T, Schön C, et al. Clinical forensic radiology in strangulation victims: forensic expertise based on magnetic resonance imaging (MRI) findings. Int J Legal Med. 2007;121(2):115–23.
7. Hatley W, Samuel E, Evison G. The pattern of ossification in the laryngeal cartilages: a radiological study. Br J Radiol. 1965;38:585–91.
8. Mupparapu M, Vuppalapati A. Ossification of laryngeal cartilages on lateral cephalometric radiographs. Angle Orthod. 2005;75(2):196–201.
9. Jurik AG. Ossification and calcification of the laryngeal skeleton. Acta Radiol Diagn (Stockh). 1984;25(1):17–22.

10. Zan E, Yousem DM, Aygun N. Asymmetric mineralization of the arytenoid cartilages in patients without laryngeal cancer. AJNR Am J Neuroradiol. 2011;32(6):1113–8.
11. Shi J, Uyeda JW, Duran-Mendicuti A, Potter CA, Nunez DB. Multidetector CT of laryngeal injuries: principles of injury recognition. Radiographics. 2019;39(3):879–92.
12. Steenburg SD, Sliker CW, Shanmuganathan K, Siegel EL. Imaging evaluation of penetrating neck injuries. Radiographics. 2010;30(4):869–86.
13. Catala J, Puig J, Munoz JM, Vivancos J, Llopart JR. Perforation of the pharynx caused by blunt external neck trauma. Eur Radiol. 1998;8(1):137–40.
14. Demetriades D, Velmahos GG, Asensio JA. Cervical pharyngoesophageal and laryngotracheal injuries. World J Surg. 2001;25(8):1044–8.
15. Soliman AM, Ahmad SM, Roy D. The role of aerodigestive tract endoscopy in penetrating neck trauma. Laryngoscope. 2014;124(Suppl 7):S1–9.
16. Biffl WL, Ray CE Jr, Moore EE, Franciose RJ, Aly S, Heyrosa MG, et al. Treatment-related outcomes from blunt cerebrovascular injuries: importance of routine follow-up arteriography. Ann Surg. 2002;235(5):699–706; discussion –7.
17. Berne JD, Reuland KS, Villarreal DH, McGovern TM, Rowe SA, Norwood SH. Sixteen-slice multi-detector computed tomographic angiography improves the accuracy of screening for blunt cerebrovascular injury. J Trauma. 2006;60(6):1204–9; discussion 9–10.
18. Schneidereit NP, Simons R, Nicolaou S, Graeb D, Brown DR, Kirkpatrick A, et al. Utility of screening for blunt vascular neck injuries with computed tomographic angiography. J Trauma. 2006;60(1):209–15; discussion 15–6.
19. Cothren CC, Biffl WL, Moore EE, Kashuk JL, Johnson JL. Treatment for blunt cerebrovascular injuries: equivalence of anticoagulation and antiplatelet agents. Arch Surg. 2009;144(7):685–90.
20. Biffl WL, Moore EE, Offner PJ, Brega KE, Franciose RJ, Elliott JP, et al. Optimizing screening for blunt cerebrovascular injuries. Am J Surg. 1999;178(6):517–22.
21. Rutman AM, Vranic JE, Mossa-Basha M. Imaging and management of blunt cerebrovascular injury. Radiographics. 2018;38(2):542–63.
22. Biffl WL, Moore EE, Offner PJ, Brega KE, Franciose RJ, Burch JM. Blunt carotid arterial injuries: implications of a new grading scale. J Trauma. 1999;47(5):845–53.
23. Hunter MA, Santosh C, Teasdale E, Forbes KP. High-resolution double inversion recovery black-blood imaging of cervical artery dissection using 3T MR imaging. AJNR Am J Neuroradiol. 2012;33(11):E133–7.
24. Lewis G, Knottenbelt JD. Parotid duct injury: is immediate surgical repair necessary? Injury. 1991;22(5):407–9.
25. Van Sickels JE. Management of parotid gland and duct injuries. Oral Maxillofac Surg Clin North Am. 2009;21(2):243–6.
26. Schaefer SD. The acute management of external laryngeal trauma: a 27-year experience. Arch Otolaryngol Head Neck Surg. 1992;118(6):598–604.
27. Fuhrman GM, Stieg FH 3rd, Buerk CA. Blunt laryngeal trauma: classification and management protocol. J Trauma. 1990;30(1):87–92.

Thoracic Trauma

5

Taylor Standiford, Maruti Kumaran,
Friedrich Knollmann, and Achala Donuru

CT Protocols

A collimation of 1.25 mm or 0.6 mm is recommended. Use of 120 Kv and 300 mA is acceptable [1]. Automatic exposure control (AEC) can be applied wherever available [2]. Ideally scans should be obtained before and after the administration of intravenous contrast, however, this is not always possible due to time constraints in a trauma situation. Majority of times, the scans are performed after intravenous contrast Table 5.1. Every attempt should be made to raise the arms above the head. Optimal opacification may be obtained with injection of 100–140 mL of iodinated contrast medium at a flow rate of 3–4 mL/s and a delay of 25–40 s. The axial thin slices can be used to create axial, coronal and sagittal reformations at 2–2.5 mm. All reformatted images should be routinely viewed at soft tissue and lung windows.

Table 5.1 Chest CT Protocol

Protocol name	Trauma one run
Indication	Polytrauma
Protocol designed for (scanner model)	GE revolution apex
Patient preparation	Arms to be elevated after CT head and CT C spine
Oral contrast	N/A
IV contrast (mL, mL/s)	70/3, 55/2, 20 NaCl 2 cc/s
Delay	If CT of the chest is part of a whole-body trauma CT, then use a 75-s delay
Tube settings	
kV	120
mA	SmartmA 120–550
Dose modulation	SmartmA, noise index 12
Tube rotation time (s)	0.5 s
Table speed (mm/s)	158.75 mm/s
Pitch	0.992
Slice collimation	0.625 mm
Reconstructed slice thickness	5 mm
	0.625 TrueFidelity
Anatomical coverage	Chest
Reconstruction kernel	STND, ASIR 50
Breath hold	Inspiration
Window settings	400/40
Post-processing	1 mm STND, lung, 3 mm STND, lung, 2 mm sag and Cor

T. Standiford · M. Kumaran
Department of Radiology, Temple University Hospital, Philadelphia, PA, USA
e-mail: Taylor.Standiford@tuhs.temple.edu; maruti.kumaran@tuhs.temple.edu

F. Knollmann
Department of Medical Imaging, Penn Presbyterian Medical Center, Philadelphia, PA, USA
e-mail: friedrich.knollmann@pennmedicine.upenn.edu

A. Donuru (✉)
Department of Radiology, Hospital of the University of Pennsylvania, Philadelphia, PA, USA
e-mail: achala.donuru@pennmedicine.upenn.edu

F. Knollmann (ed.), *Trauma Computed Tomography*, https://doi.org/10.1007/978-3-031-45746-3_5

Chest Wall Injuries

Soft Tissue Injuries

Chest wall injuries are common, seen in 36.1% of patients presenting with thoracic trauma [3] and up to 50% of patients with blunt thoracic trauma [4]. As the most external structures of the chest, the soft tissues are almost invariably injured to some degree in thoracic trauma. The thoracic soft tissues can be evaluated using a variety of modalities, but radiographs and CT are most often encountered in the setting of trauma. On plain radiographs, abnormalities of the thoracic soft tissues will be seen as areas of increased or decreased density [5]. CT is better able to characterize the nature of the chest wall injury due to high soft tissue contrast and multiplanar imaging. Ultrasound may occasionally be used in the setting of trauma to identify important injuries such as pneumothorax and hemothorax as discussed later in the chapter, but more superficial injuries such as hematomas can quickly be identified and characterized by ultrasound [6]. MRI provides the greatest soft tissue contrast and can be used to characterize chest wall lesions [5], yet it is rarely used in the setting of acute trauma because of longer exam times and decreased availability as compared to CT.

Air in the extra-thoracic soft tissues (soft tissue emphysema) is a common finding in thoracic trauma [5, 7] and can be secondary to skin or pleural disruption. In the setting of blunt trauma, pleural disruption can result from sudden increases in alveolar pressure [8] in a similar mechanism to pneumomediastinum. Subcutaneous emphysema can also be secondary to surgical pleural drain placement in the setting of hemothorax or pneumothorax [5]. Subcutaneous emphysema is readily identified on chest radiographs, classically presenting as radiolucent striations in the upper chest outlining the pectoralis musculature. Notably, extensive subcutaneous emphysema can limit evaluation of underlying structures on plain radiographs. In addition to gas within the soft tissues, apparent subcutaneous gas may also be secondary to venous gas introduced during venous cannulation and medication or contrast injection. Venous gas is a common finding, seen in up to 23% of CT's and should not be misinterpreted as being related to injury [9].

Hematomas can be seen in the subcutaneous tissues or chest wall muscles and may become life threatening in anticoagulated patients [4]. Soft tissue hematomas are encountered in both blunt and penetrating thoracic trauma and may be arterial or venous in origin. Multiphasic CT acquisitions are useful in evaluating for active bleeding, which may require endovascular or surgical intervention (Fig. 5.1). The intercostal arteries and internal mammary arteries are the most frequently injured arteries in the chest wall [10] and can lead to chest wall hematomas, extrapleural hematomas, hemothorax, or even hemoperitoneum (Figs. 5.2 and 5.3). Injury to these vessels may also present as delayed bleeding in some cases. Catheter angiography and embolization is often the procedure of choice for precise diagnosis and treatment of chest wall arterial injury. Breast hematomas are a special consideration in female patients (Fig. 5.4).

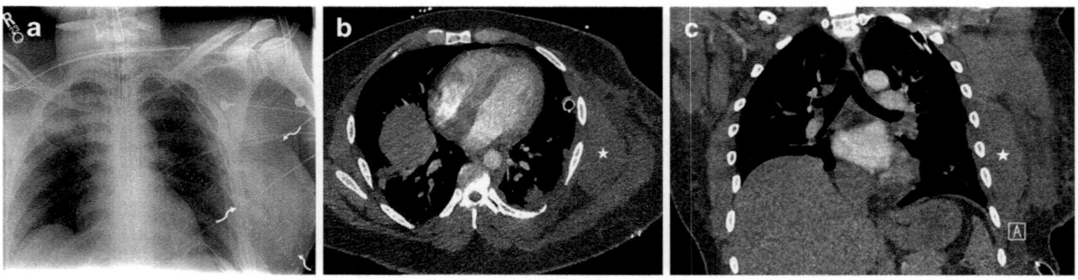

Fig. 5.1 Chest X-ray (**a**), axial (**b**), and coronal (**c**) contrast enhanced CT scan: 33-year-old male patient presented with a left chest wall stab wound. CXR demonstrates soft tissue swelling involving the left lateral chest wall (white curved arrows). Chest CT with IV contrast demonstrates a 13 cm collection in the left posterolateral chest wall representing a hematoma (white asterix)

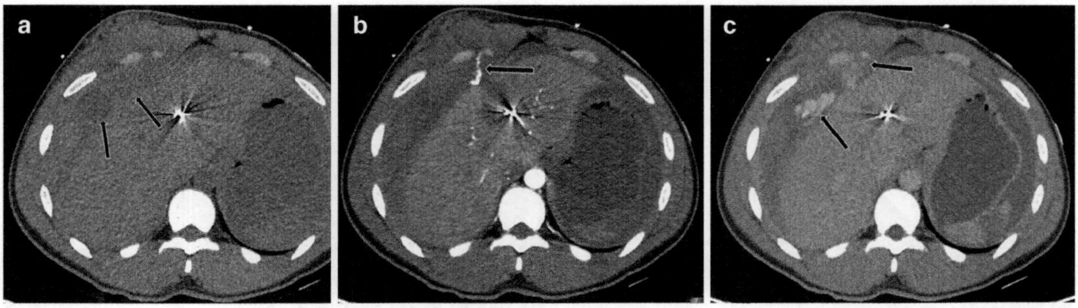

Fig. 5.2 Non-contrast (**a**), arterial phase (**b**), and delayed (**c**) axial CT scan of the chest: 28-year-old female patient presenting with a stab wound to the right upper quadrant. Patient complained of severe abdominal pain. Focus of active bleeding from the fifth intercostal artery and within the soft tissues of the right anterior chest wall noted on non-contrast, arterial phase and delayed phase CT (arrows). The patient was taken to the interventional radiology suite for angiography. The bleeding vessel was embolized

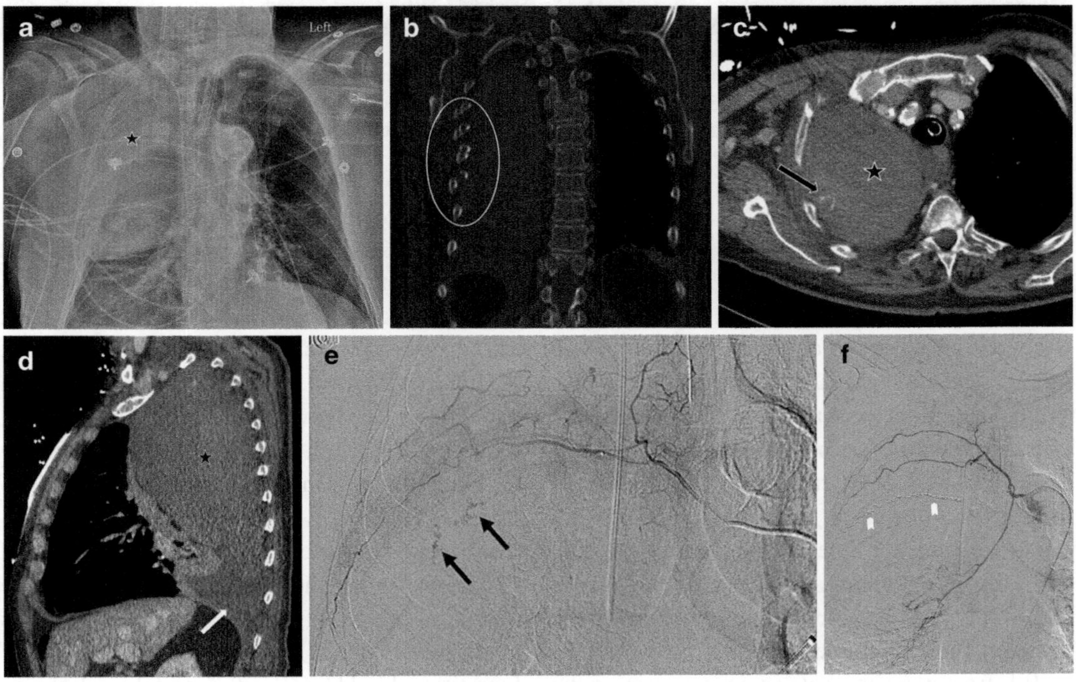

Fig. 5.3 Chest X-ray (**a**), coronal (**b**), axial (**c**), sagittal (**d**), and arteriogram (**e** and **f**): 84-year-old male presented to an outside hospital s/p fall while transferring to a chair. CXR and CT demonstrate multiple right rib fractures (white circle). Large opacity was note within the right hemithorax (black star) corresponding to an extrapleural hematoma. Linear focus of hyperattenuation (black arrows) was noted on arterial phase CT. Sagittal CT demonstrates dependent pleural effusion (white arrow) separate from the extrapleural hematoma by fat plane. Diagnostic right third intercostal arteriogram demonstrates extravasation of contrast (black arrows) into the extrapleural hematoma within the right chest. Coils were deployed into the distal portions of the right third intercostal artery (white chevron heads)

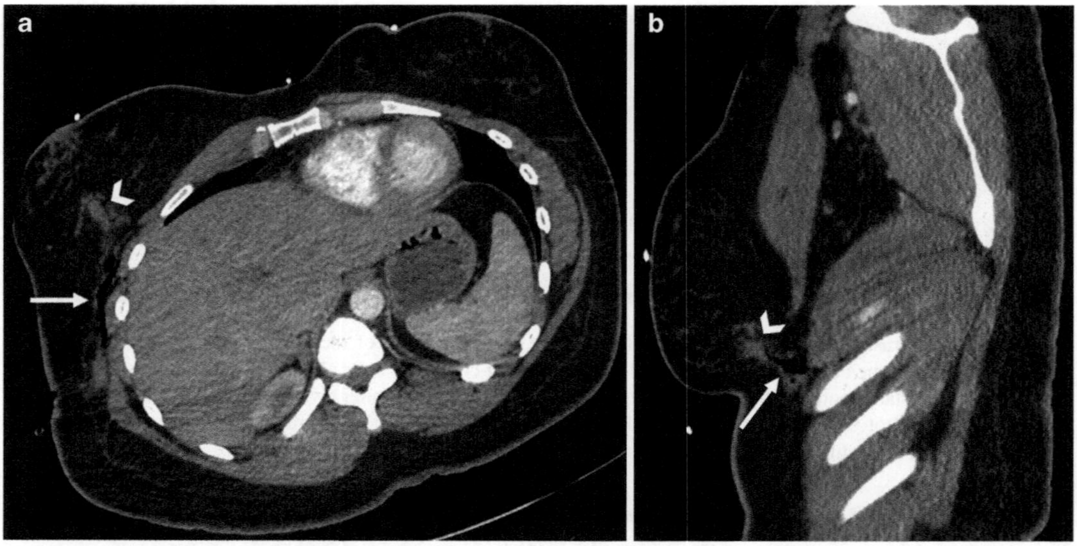

Fig. 5.4 Axial (**a**) and sagittal (**b**) contrast enhanced CT scan: 26-year-old female presented after a stab wound to her right chest. CT chest with IV contrast on soft tissue window demonstrates a small hematoma (chevron arrow) and subcutaneous emphysema (white arrow) within the soft tissues of the right breast

Fractures

Plain film radiography is often the first study obtained in the evaluation of fractures, with radiographs often obtained in the trauma bay. While plain films are sensitive for long bone fractures, rib fractures are notoriously challenging to identify on AP chest radiographs, especially if they are non-displaced. In one series, 50% of rib fractures were not detected on radiographs [3]. Therefore, CT remains a more useful modality in identifying and characterizing rib fractures in the acute post-traumatic setting.

Rib fractures can serve as an indicator of the severity of thoracic trauma. While trauma patients presenting with rib fractures have an overall mortality of approximately 4%, patients with fractures of the first or second ribs had a mortality of 36%. This reflects the significantly increased force required to fracture the relatively more protected and sturdier first and second ribs [3]. Additionally, fractures of the first ribs have the potential to injure the subclavian vessels and brachial plexus nerves. Careful attention needs to be paid to the vessels in any patient presenting with high rib injuries. Fractures of the middle ribs are more likely to be associated with pulmonary findings such as lung contusions, lacerations, and pneumothoraces. Fractures of the lowest two ribs may be associated with abdominal injuries, such as hepatic, splenic, or renal lacerations [3]. Notably, while rib fractures are common in patients presenting with thoracic trauma, almost a quarter (24.7% in one series) of patients may have intrathoracic injuries without associated rib fractures [3].

Lung herniation can occur through a congenital defect in the chest wall, but post-traumatic defects in the chest wall created by rib fractures or dislocations can also allow for herniation of lung tissue [4, 11]. CT is the modality of choice for identifying and characterizing lung herniations (Fig. 5.5).

Flail chest is a segmental disruption of the chest wall caused by the fracturing of at least three contiguous ribs in at least two places [3]. Separation of the rib at the costochondral junction can cause the same effect and is more challenging to diagnose, especially on plain radiographs (Fig. 5.6). Flail chest is more common in blunt trauma than in penetrating trauma and is often associated with pulmonary contusions, pneumothorax, and hemothorax.

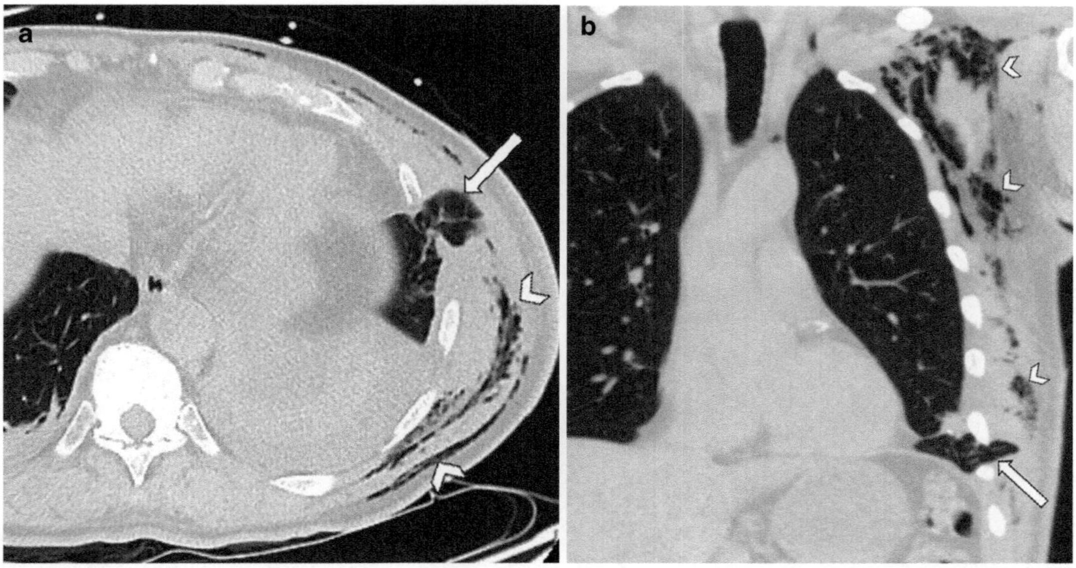

Fig. 5.5 Axial and coronal CT (**a**, **b**): 78-year-old male presented s/p mechanical fall from two flights of stairs. Axial and coronal images in lung windows from a chest CT demonstrate herniation of the lingula (arrows) and extensive subcutaneous emphysema in the left lateral chest wall (chevron arrows)

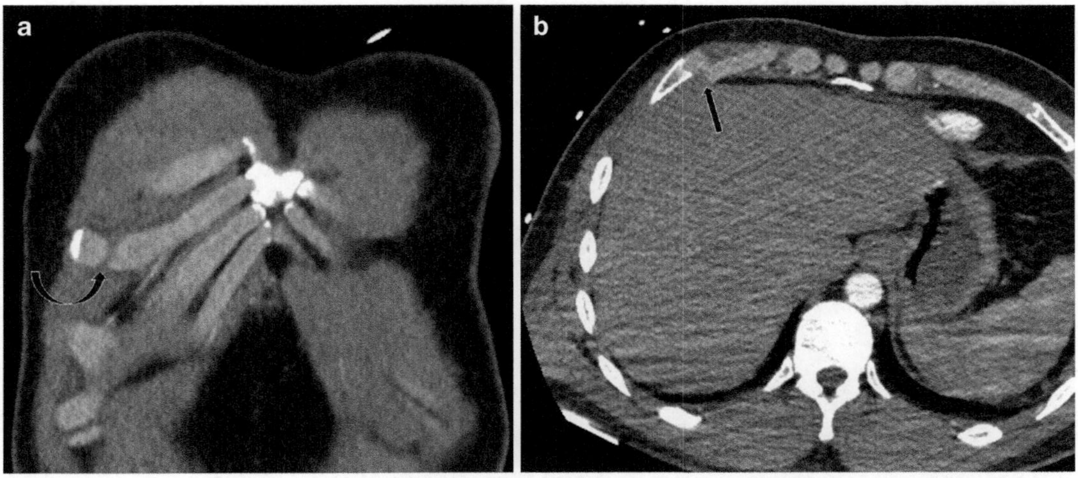

Fig. 5.6 Coronal (**a**) and axial (**b**) contrast enhanced CT scan: 31-year-old male presenting as a transfer from an outside hospital after a bull riding accident. CT chest with IV contrast in soft tissue window demonstrates right anterior fifth rib costal cartilage fracture in axial plane (straight arrow) and coronal plane (curved arrow) with overlapping fracture fragments

Sternal fractures are typically caused by anterior blunt trauma [3] and are seen in 3–8% of all chest trauma cases. Sternal fractures generally require considerable force and may be associated with or contribute to vascular, pulmonary, aortic, and cardiac injuries. Sternal fractures are almost always accompanied by anterior mediastinal hemorrhage (Fig. 5.7). It is important to distinguish between anterior mediastinal hemorrhage secondary to sternal fractures from anterior mediastinal hemorrhage caused by aortic injury. In cases of hemorrhage secondary to sternal fractures, the fat plane between the blood products and the aorta will be preserved.

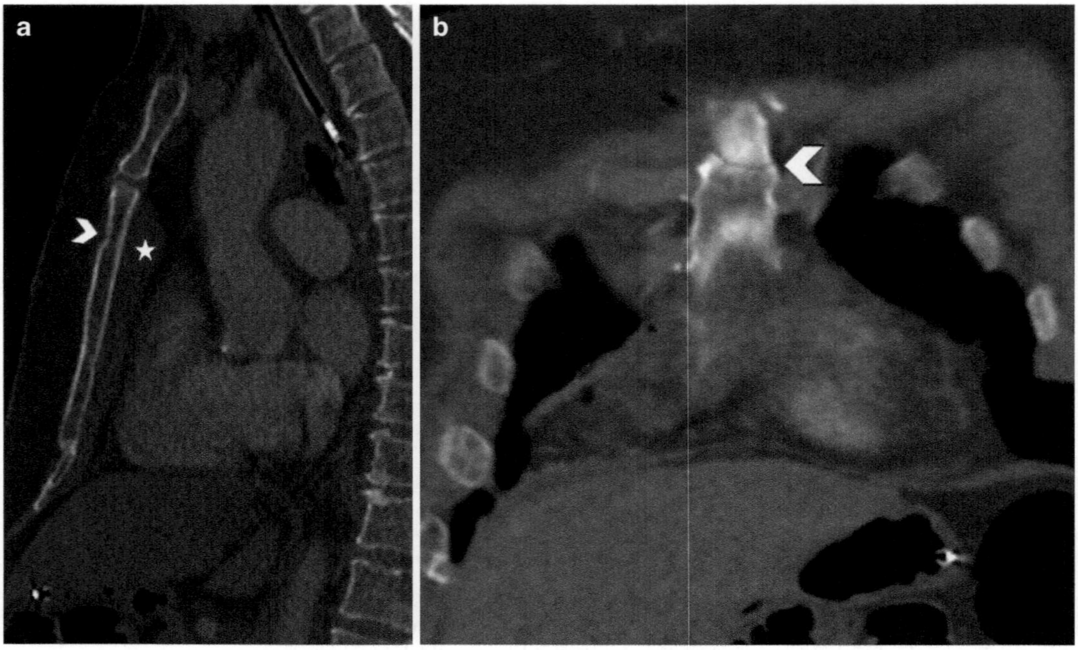

Fig. 5.7 Sagittal (**a**) and coronal (**b**) CT scans bone windows: 68-year-old female status post-trauma. Type of trauma is unknown. Patient received CPR. Coronal and sagittal images from CT chest demonstrate a sternal fracture (chevron arrow) with adjacent hematoma in the anterior mediastinum (star)

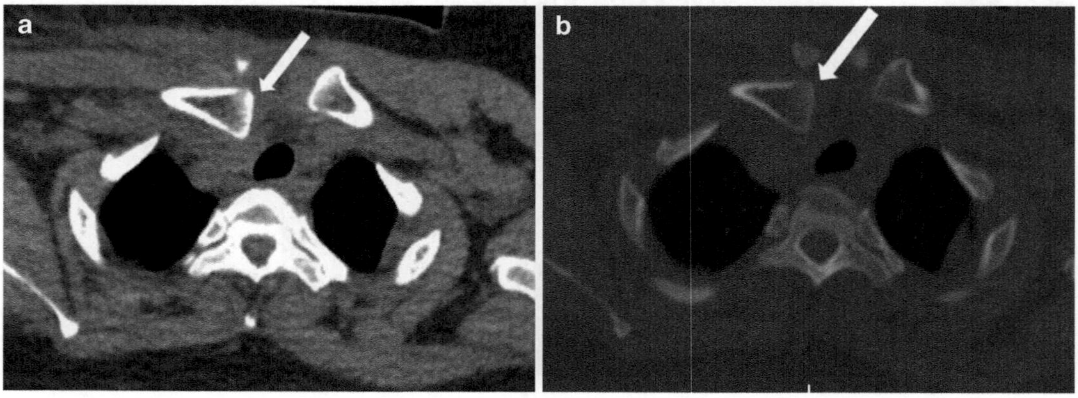

Fig. 5.8 Axial CT (**a**, **b**): A 50-year-old female presents to the emergency department status post fall. Axial images from a CT chest demonstrate posterior dislocation of the right clavicle at the sternoclavicular joint (arrows) on soft tissue and bone windows

Sternoclavicular dislocation is another uncommon yet significant thoracic injury. Anterior dislocation is more common and typically benign but suggests a high energy mechanism. Posterior dislocations are more important clinically due to the potential for injury to the mediastinal structures, including the major branches of the aorta [1, 4]. CT is the most useful modality for diagnosing sternoclavicular dislocations as these injuries are often very difficult to detect on AP radiographs of the chest (Fig. 5.8).

Thoracic spine injuries will be discussed in a separate chapter (Fig. 5.9).

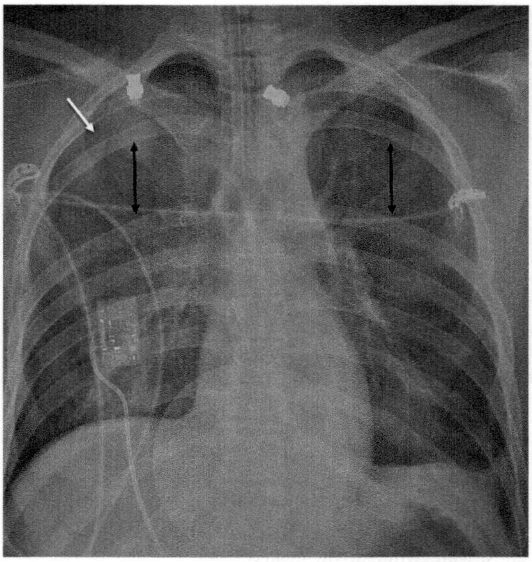

Fig. 5.9 Chest x-ray (**a**): Male patient in his mid-30s presented after falling from a bridge and secondarily being struck by an automobile. He was pulseless on the scene. Spinal distraction seen at the level of T4-T5 (double headed black arrows). Small right pneumothorax (white arrow)

Diaphragmatic Injuries

Diaphragmatic injuries can be associated with both thoracic and abdominal trauma and are often difficult to detect both clinically and radiographically, especially in patients who do not meet criteria for surgical intervention [5]. On plain radiographs, overt signs of diaphragmatic injury include herniation of abdominal structures into the chest. More subtle signs of diaphragmatic injury include basal atelectasis or consolidation, especially if new when compared to prior radiographs, as well as alterations in the diaphragmatic contour. However, the chest radiograph is normal in approximately one quarter of patients with acute diaphragmatic injury. CT is more sensitive in diagnosing diaphragmatic injuries in the acute setting. Herniation of abdominal contents into the thorax is readily identified on multiplanar CT, and the diaphragmatic defect may be directly visualized. These herniated viscera may lie dependently against the posterior thoracic wall, generating what is known as the "dependent viscera sign." Other CT findings of diaphragmatic injury include inward curling of the diaphragmatic edges, thickening of the crus, and constriction of the bowel or dome of the liver as they transit through the diaphragmatic defect [11]. Ultrasound can occasionally be used to identify diaphragmatic injuries, either by identifying abdominal structures in the thorax or directly visualizing the diaphragmatic injury; however, this is often limited by poor visualization of the diaphragm. In the setting of penetrating trauma, a wound tract that traverses the diaphragm is virtually diagnostic of diaphragmatic injury (Fig. 5.10). Bochdalek hernia the most common congenital diaphragmatic hernia demonstrates discontinuity of the posterior posteromedial diaphragm with protrusion of peritoneal or retroperitoneal fat through the defect. Herniation of colon, small bowel, liver, spleen, or kidney into the thoracic cavity is less common.

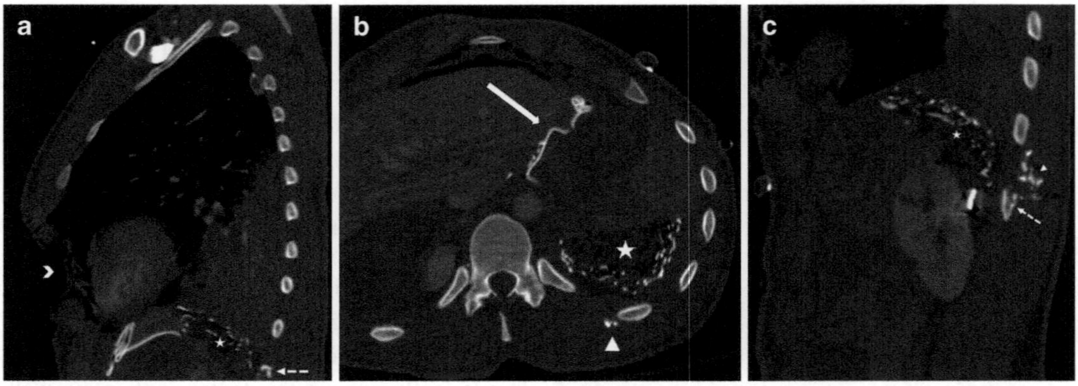

Fig. 5.10 Sagittal (**a**), axial (**b**) and oblique sagittal (**c**) Contrast enhanced CT scan: 23-year-old male was brought to the trauma bay unresponsive, apneic, and pulseless after GSW to the right chest parasternal region below the nipple line, and left chest at the posterior axillary line. The patient was unstable and therefore taken to the OR. He underwent thoracotomy (chevron white arrow) and repair of right ventricular injury (white arrow). CT chest demonstrates packing material in the left upper quadrant (white star) for left diaphragmatic tear, left rib fractures (dashed arrows) with ballistic material in the left lateral chest wall (white arrow heads)

Pneumothorax and Hemothorax

Pneumothorax is defined as air within the pleural space (between the visceral and parietal pleura) [12] and is a common complication of thoracic trauma, seen in 40–50% of thoracic traumas [13] and in approximately 5% of all trauma patients [14]. Pneumothoraces can be broken down into small (0–10%), medium (10–40%), and large (>40%) [15]. Large pneumothoraces are more likely to be immediately life threatening; however, small and medium pneumothoraces can expand, especially in patients on mechanical ventilation [15]. Therefore, it is important to detect all post-traumatic pneumothoraces.

Pneumothoraces occur by three main mechanisms in the setting of trauma. In penetrating and ballistic trauma, the projectile can disrupt the chest wall and parietal pleura, allowing outside air to enter the pleural space. Depending on the trajectory of the projectile, the visceral pleura and underlying lung may also be injured, allowing inspired air to reach the pleural space [11]. A second mechanism, occurring more often in blunt trauma, is the laceration of the pleura and underlying lung by a piece of fractured bone, typically a rib, which then allows inspired air to enter the pleural space. Finally, increased intrathoracic pressure can lead to alveolar rupture and interstitial emphysema with gas tracking to the periphery of the lung and rupturing into the pleural space [16].

A chest radiograph is the first-line imaging modality for detecting pneumothorax in a trauma patient and can be obtained in the trauma bay. If the clinical situation allows, an erect chest radiograph is preferred for the detection of pneumothoraces. The most specific sign of pneumothorax on an erect radiograph is direct visualization of the visceral pleura separating the partially collapsed lung medially from the pleural air laterally (Fig. 5.11). If there is uncertainty, the radiograph can be repeated in the expiratory phase to accentuate contrast between the lung and the pneumothorax and increase the conspicuity of small pneumothoraces [16]. The erect radiograph is sensitive for the detection of pneumothoraces (92% sensitivity) [14], but sensitivity can be degraded by skin folds, pulmonary blebs, and overlying devices/wires [17].

Due to the need for strict cervical spine immobilization as well as additional patient and technical factors, erect radiographs are not often possible to obtain in the acute trauma setting. Therefore, supine radiographs are more commonly performed. Diagnosing pneumothoraces on supine radiographs is often challenging. In one series, 55% of post-traumatic pneumothoraces were occult on initial supine radiographs

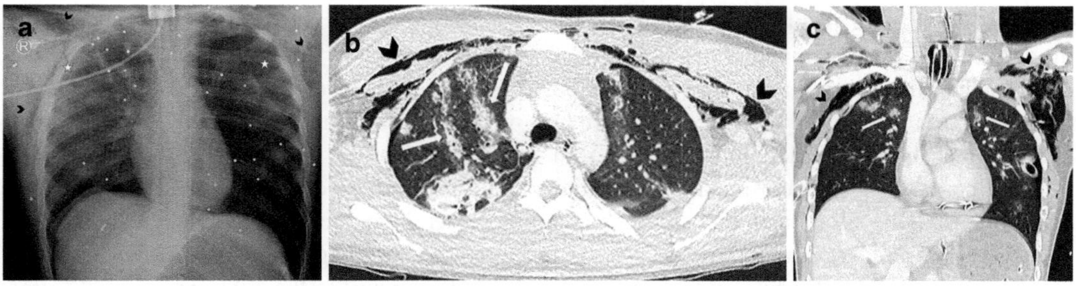

Fig. 5.11 Chest x-ray (**a**), axial and coronal CT (**b**, **c**): A 33 year old male with gun shot wound with multiple shrapnel fragments in the chest. CXR demonstrates bilateral pneumothoraces (white star). CT chest with IV contrast demonstrates patchy airspace opacities in both lungs correspond to pulmonary hemorrhage along the trajectory of bullet fragments (white arrows) in axial and coronal planes. There is extensive subcutaneous emphysema (chevron)

[18]. Supine radiographs are especially limited for the detection of small and medium pneumothoraces [19]. However, there are multiple signs on a supine radiograph that can clue the radiologist into the presence of a pneumothorax. In the supine patient, the anteromedial portion of the lung is the most nondependent. Therefore, air in a pneumothorax will collect here first. If the pneumothorax is large enough, the affected hemithorax will appear more lucent than the contralateral side [16]. Additional signs of pneumothorax on the supine radiograph include sharpening of the mediastinal borders, visualization of the dome and the anterior portion of the diaphragm on the affected side, known as the "double diaphragm" sign, and deepening and increased lucency of the lateral costophrenic sulcus, known as the "deep sulcus" sign [16].

Ultrasound is an alternative to radiographs for the diagnosis of pneumothorax in the acute setting. The advantage of ultrasound in the trauma bay is that it can be performed at the bedside with the patient in a supine position and provides better sensitivity for detecting pneumothoraces than supine radiographs (78.6% vs. 39.8% in one met-analysis) [20]. Disadvantages of ultrasound include the need for a skilled operator and longer exam times as compared to radiographs. As opposed to radiographs, imaging the patient in the supine position improves the sensitivity of ultrasound for pneumothorax. Air will rise to the least dependent portion of the chest, so in a supine patient, the anterior chest should be imaged at the second to fourth intercostal spaces in the mid-clavicular line. In a normal lung ultrasound (without pneumothorax) the lung is seen sliding against the chest wall. This pleural sliding is the most important finding in confirming the absence of a pneumothorax. A secondary sign of the normal lung is B-lines, also referred to as comet-tail artifacts. They appear as hyperechoic vertical lines extending from the pleura. These lines are created in the normal aerated lung and move with the pleura. Notably, excessive B-lines suggest pulmonary interstitial edema [15]. Pneumothorax prevents visualization of the visceral pleura, leading to a loss of the sliding pleura sign and B-lines. If lung sliding is present, pneumothorax is effectively ruled out (negative predictive value 99.2–100%), but lung sliding can be absent in a variety of other conditions, such as ARDS, pulmonary parenchymal diseases, and phrenic nerve paralysis. Therefore, correlation with additional imaging findings may be needed to confirm a pneumothorax. The specificity of lung sliding for the detection of pneumothorax is 60–99%.

Computed tomography (CT) is the gold standard for detecting pneumothoraces. CT is especially useful for identifying "occult pneumothoraces," which are pneumothoraces which were not identified on initial imaging (typical chest radiograph). Occult pneumothoraces can be seen in up to 20% of blunt trauma patients and 17% of patients with penetrating trauma [21]. CT can also be used to more accurately quantify the size of pneumothoraces and help direct clinical management. Pneumothoraces do not generally pose a diagnostic challenge on CT as long as thin slices are provided in lung kernel, but beam hardening artifact from injected contrast or adjacent metal, air in adjacent veins, and pulmonary blebs/bullae can occasionally mimic a pneumothorax.

The most important acute complication of pneumothorax in the trauma setting is tension pneumothorax. Tension pneumothorax occurs when air can enter the pleural space but cannot escape, leading to progressively increasing intrathoracic pressure. If this pressure becomes high enough, venous return to the heart becomes impaired and the patient can experience obstructive shock [21]. Tension pneumothorax is ultimately a clinical diagnosis, but it can be suggested when a pneumothorax is identified with contralateral mediastinal shift, flattening, or inversion of the ipsilateral hemidiaphragm or hyperexpansion of the ipsilateral hemithorax [22].

Hemothorax

Hemothorax is defined as blood collecting within the pleural space. Many of the same mechanisms that can cause pneumothoraces can result in hemothoraces, but abdominal visceral injuries such as liver and spleen injuries, combined with diaphragmatic injuries, may cause hemothorax without associated pneumothorax. Hemothorax is most commonly caused by rib fractures, which generally result in small to moderate hemothoraces. Moy et al. develop a classification system for pleural effusions and chose <20%, 20% to 40%, and > 40% of the hemithorax for small, moderate, and large effusions, respectively [23]. However, hemothorax can occasionally result in massive hemorrhage, which are more likely to be caused by injury to the pulmonary vessels, great vessels, or heart [21]. Massive hemothorax is hemorrhage in excess of 1 L of blood with clinical signs of shock and hypoperfusion [22]. In addition to the potential cardiovascular complications of blood loss into the pleural space, hemothoraces can lead to additional medium-to long-term complications and, therefore, are important for the radiologist to identify and relay to the treating team. Complications include empyema and fibrothorax, which can develop in 27–33% of cases where hemothorax is not adequately evacuated. Results of an Eastern Association for the Surgery of Trauma multi-institutional trial showed questionable benefit of drainage in small hemothorax <300 cc. Hemothorax is indistinguishable from other pleural fluid collections on radiographs but can be easily characterized by CT [22, 24]. Pleural fluid with attenuation between 35 and 70 HU is characteristic of blood in the pleural space. If hemothorax and pneumothorax are identified in the same hemithorax, this is termed hemopneumothorax and is subject to the complications of both conditions (Fig. 5.12).

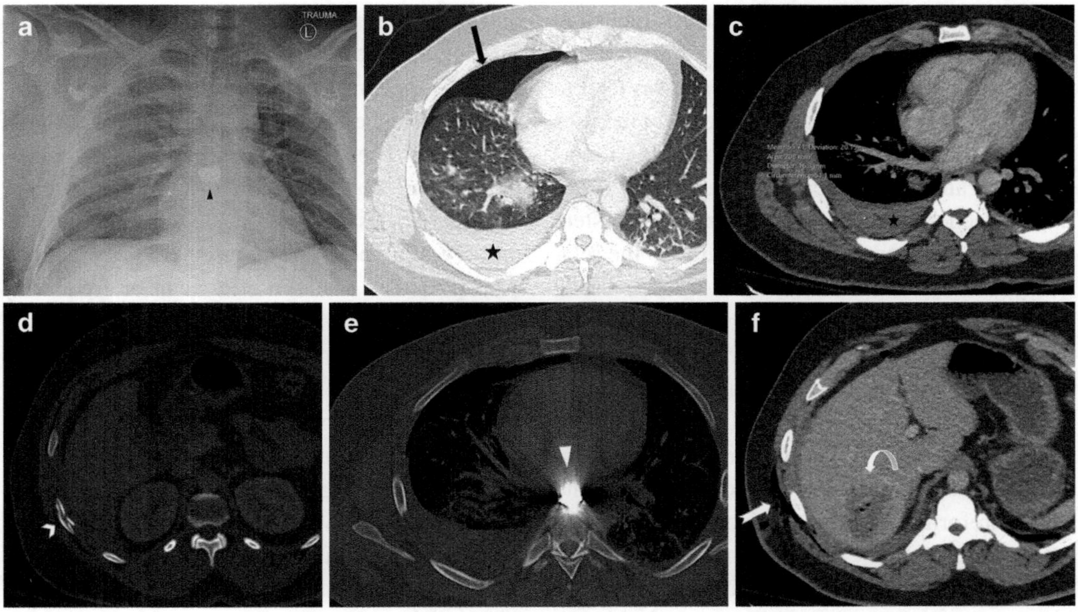

Fig. 5.12 Chest X-ray (**a**), axial CT scans (**b–f**): 35 year old male, status post gunshot wound to the right chest. Moderate right-sided hemopneumothorax noted with a high density layering fluid compatible with a hemothorax (black star) and air in the nondependent portion compatible with pneumothorax (black arrow). There is a comminuted fracture of lateral aspect of the right tenth rib (chevron white arrow). Metallic foreign body (shrapnel) is located immediately anterior to the T6-T7 disc space, to the right of the descending thoracic aorta and posterior to the left atrium (white arrowhead). Subcutaneous emphysema noted along the right side of the chest wall (notched white arrow). Heterogeneous low attenuation area containing multiple gas foci in the right hepatic lobe is consistent with liver laceration (curved white arrow)

Airway and Parenchymal Injuries

Tracheobronchial Injuries

Tracheal injuries in trauma are rare, but are serious and often fatal injuries. Approximately 30–80% of patients with tracheobronchial injuries die before reaching the hospital, often due to other significant injuries that are often associated with tracheobronchial injuries [25]. Overall, tracheobronchial injuries are suspected to occur in 0.5–2% of patients who sustain trauma to the neck or chest [26]. These injuries are important to detect early in the patient's clinical course as the knowledge of these injuries often shapes clinical management. Early treatment is often essential in avoiding complications.

Understanding the imaging findings of tracheobronchial injuries is aided by knowledge of tracheal anatomy. Tracheal support and protection are provided by D-shaped cartilaginous "rings" that span the anterior and lateral aspects of the trachea. As the posterior portion of the trachea lacks cartilaginous support, it is more susceptible to injury, especially in cases of penetrating trauma. Right-sided tracheal injuries are more common than left-sided injuries. This is hypothesized to be due to protective effects from the aorta and the proximity of the right mainstem bronchus to the vertebral bodies [25]. As the aortic arch shifts the trachea to the right, the left mainstem bronchus travels a longer distance within the mediastinum than the right mainstem bronchus. Consequently, injuries to the right mainstem bronchus tend to result in pneumothorax as well as pneumomediastinum while injuries to the left mainstem bronchus are more likely to produce pure pneumomediastinum.

Injuries to the cervical trachea are more likely to be secondary to penetrating trauma due to the anterior and superficial location of the trachea in this location, making it particularly vulnerable to stab type injuries. Blunt trauma can also lead to injury of the cervical trachea, especially in cases of cervical hyperextension, which leads to tearing of the anterior trachea. However, injury to the distal trachea, carina, and proximal mainstem bronchi is more common. This is due to the relatively fixed position of the distal trachea in the mediastinum [25]. It is important to differentiate a tracheal diverticulum and a Zenker's diverticulum from airway injuries. The relationship between the tracheal diverticulum with tracheal lumen and Zenker's diverticulum with the esophagus can be demonstrated by axial, coronal, and sagittal reformat multiplanar images [27]. A third mechanism of injury to the tracheobronchial tree is barotrauma, which occurs most commonly in blunt trauma, where thoracic compression in the setting of a closed glottis increases pressure within the tracheobronchial tree, leading to rupture. Iatrogenic airway injury occurs after tracheotomy, endotracheal intubation, and rigid bronchoscopy.

As discussed previously, chest radiographs are typically the first-line imaging for patient presenting with thoracic trauma. The most common findings of tracheobronchial injury on chest radiographs are subcutaneous emphysema, pneumothorax, and pneumomediastinum. Pneumothorax is seen in 17–70% of patients with tracheobronchial injury. An abnormal tracheal contour or positioning of the endotracheal tube outside of the expected course of the trachea are suggestive of tracheal injury or rupture, but these findings are rare. Even though tracheobronchial injuries are serious injuries with profound consequences, 10–20% of these injuries may be occult on initial chest radiographs [26].

CT is more sensitive for detecting tracheobronchial injuries; however, the primary injury may still be occult, necessitating the use of secondary signs to suggest underlying injury. Findings suggestive of tracheobronchial injury include pneumomediastinum, pneumothorax, and subfascial emphysema in the upper chest and neck [22]. The Macklin effect is linear collections of air contiguous to the bronchovascular sheaths on chest CT. The air dissects into the pulmonary hila and from there enters the mediastinum [28]. The Macklin effect can be frequently observed on the MDCT images of patients with spontaneous pneumomediastinum not associated with trauma (Fig. 5.13). In cases of bronchial transection at the pulmonary hilum, the lung will often collapse inferiorly and posteriorly toward the pulmonary ligaments instead of collapsing more centrally toward the pulmonary hilum as is seen in cases of bronchial obstruction [26]. This is known as the "fallen lung" sign [29] (Fig. 5.14). In the setting of penetrating trauma, the trajectory of the missile must be scrutinized, and the possibility of tracheobronchial injury may be suggested even if an injury is not directly visualized. In these cases, bronchoscopy may be pursued for further evaluation. While bronchoscopy remains the gold standard for diagnosing injuries to the tracheobronchial tree, advanced CT techniques such as virtual bronchoscopy may improve noninvasive detection of these injuries.

Timely diagnosis of tracheobronchial injuries is important due to the potential immediate and more distant complications. Complications arising early in patient care can include persistent air leaks and tension pneumomediastinum, which can lead to respiratory and cardiovascular compromise [25]. If a defect in the trachea or mainstem bronchi allow secretions to enter the mediastinum, mediastinitis and sepsis can result [30]. Long-term complications of these injuries include airway stenosis or obstruction, and patients may represent with respiratory complications including recurrent infections.

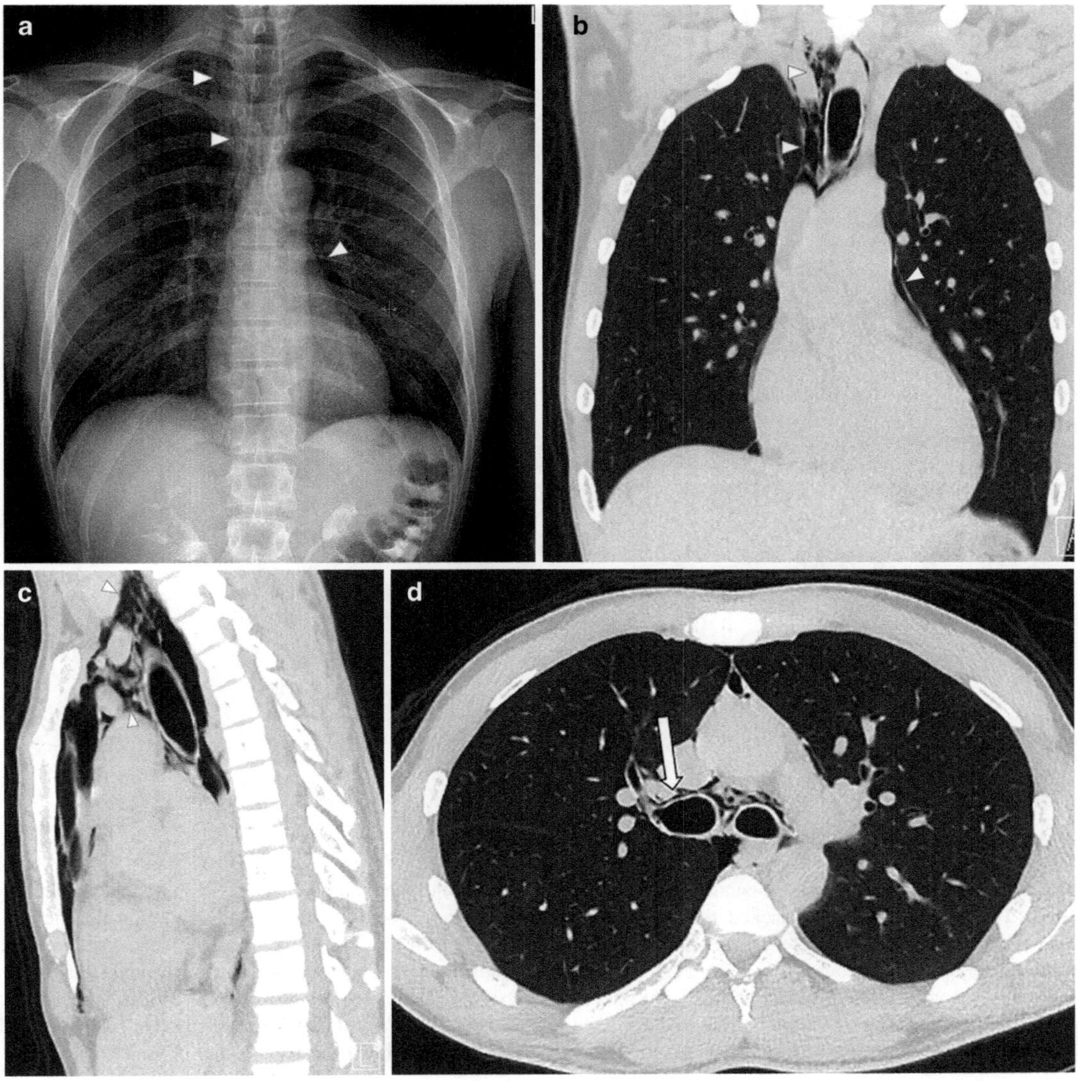

Fig. 5.13 Frontal x-ray (**a**), coronal (**b**), sagittal (**c**) and axial (**d**): 40-year-old male presented to ED with chief complaint of back pain and abdominal pain for 2 days. There was no history of trauma. CXR and Chest CT demonstrate moderate pneumomediastinum (white arrowheads). Air noted dissecting along the bronchovascular sheath (white arrow), known as the Macklin effect

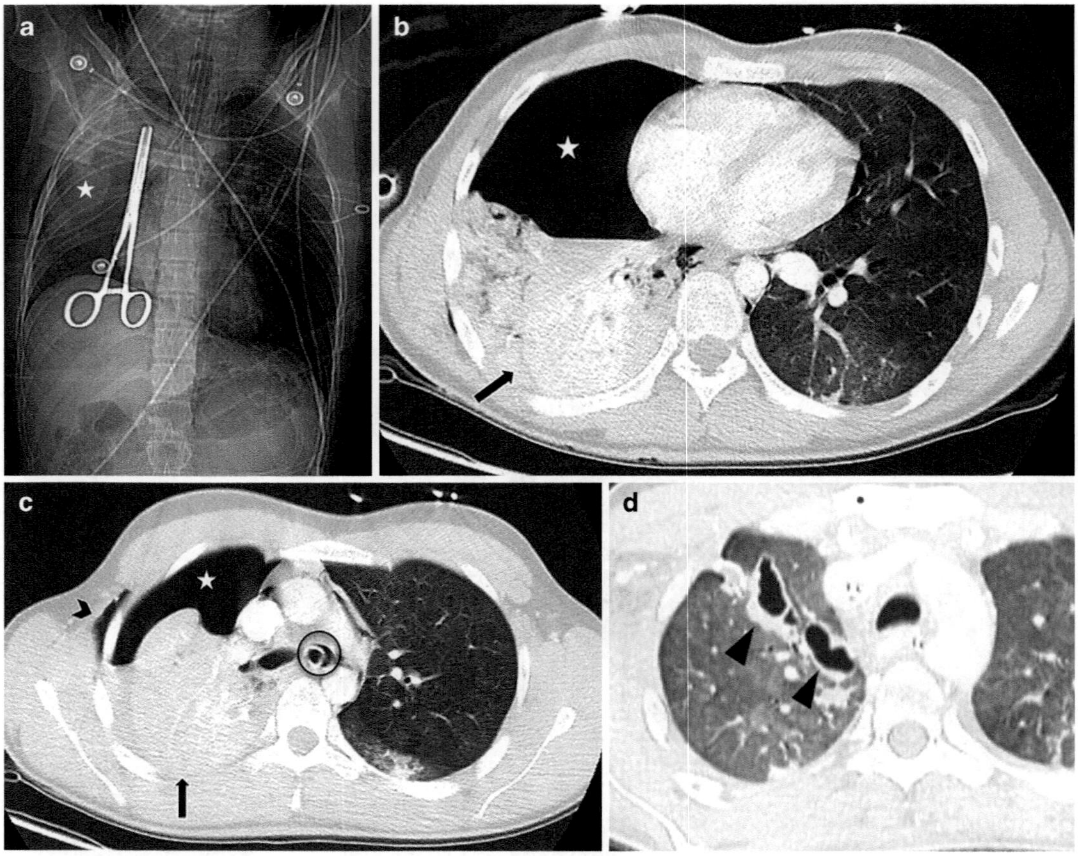

Fig. 5.14 Chest X-ray (**a**), axial contrast enhanced CT (**b–d**): 18-year-old male was carjacked, then run over with his car, suffered from bronchial injury, pneumothorax and multiple rib fractures. Scout image from a CT and Chest CT with IV contrast demonstrates a large right pneumothorax (white star). The right lung is collapsed in a dependent position, hanging on the hilum only by its vascular attachments compatible with fallen lung. Subcutaneous emphysema noted in the right lateral chest wall (chevron black arrow). 11 days status post bronchus intermedius repair, there is improved aeration of the right lung with residual pneumatoceles in the right upper lobe (black arrowheads). Patient had a left main stem intubation on the Chest CT (black circle)

Pulmonary Parenchymal Injuries

Pulmonary contusions are the most common pulmonary parenchymal injury in blunt chest trauma, occurring in up to 75% of cases [12]. Pulmonary contusions are typically seen within the first 12 h after trauma [16] as blood and edema fill the alveoli. Chest radiographs will demonstrate focal or diffuse, nonsegmental airspace opacities [12]. These opacities become more consolidative over time, typically stabilizing by 24 h [16] and gradually resolving over a period of 1 to 2 weeks. Pulmonary contusions that fail to resolve are suspicious for superimposed ARDS or infection. CT is more sensitive for the diagnosis of pulmonary contusion than chest radiographs, but contusions seen on CT that are not demonstrated on radiographs may not be clinically important [12]. On CT, pulmonary contusions are typically seen as ground glass opacities with subpleural sparing. Pulmonary contusions are most frequently seen at the site of injury, but contra-coup contusions can also occur in the lung as it decelerates against the chest wall. Pulmonary contusions are more common at the lung bases, where the lung is more mobile [12] (Fig. 5.15).

In the initial trauma setting, aspiration pneumonia/pneumonitis can often mimic pulmonary contusions, but a clinical history of hemoptysis

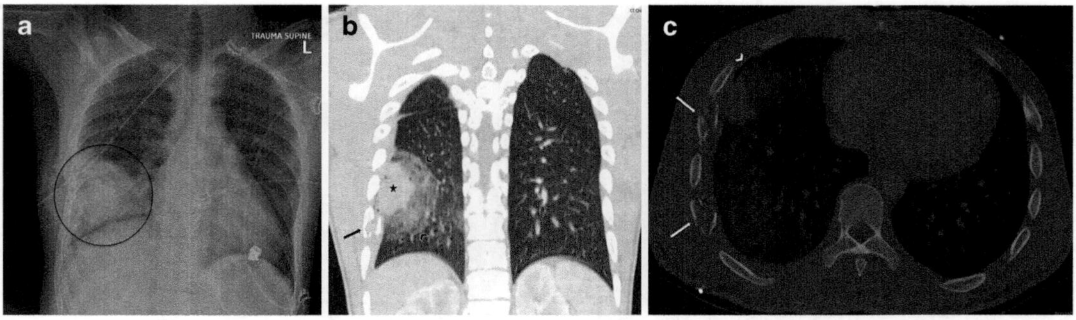

Fig. 5.15 Chest X-ray (**a**), coronal and axial CT (**b**, **c**): 19-year-old male presented after GSW to the right chest. Chest radiograph demonstrates an airspace opacity with surrounding ground glass opacity in the right lower zone (black circle). CT chest demonstrates localized displaced fracture deformities involving the lateral right seventh, eighth, and ninth ribs (arrows). Large air space opacity noted in the right lung consistent with pulmonary contusion (star). Extensive surrounding parenchymal ground glass opacities in keeping with intrapulmonary hemorrhage (chevron black arrows). Small right pneumothorax noted (chevron white arrow)

or blood suctioned from the endotracheal tube favor a diagnosis of pulmonary contusion [16]. Additionally, ground glass opacities developing more than 48 h after patient presentation are suspicious for ARDS over pulmonary contusion [16].

Pulmonary lacerations occur frequently in penetrating thoracic trauma but can also occur in blunt trauma and are often associated with pulmonary contusions [22]. In penetrating trauma, pulmonary lacerations are directly caused by the penetrating object traveling through the lung parenchyma. In blunt trauma, lacerations occur secondary to shearing forces in the lung. The elastic recoil of the lung parenchyma leads to separation of the lung along the laceration and a typical elliptical appearance of pulmonary lacerations (Fig. 5.16). The cavity formed when the two edges of the lung pull away from one another can fill with air (pneumatocele) due to disruption of small airways, blood (hematocele/pulmonary hematoma) due to disruption of pulmonary capillaries, or both. Pulmonary lacerations are slower to heal than pulmonary contusion, often taking weeks to months to resolve. Complications of pulmonary lacerations can include abscess formation and bronchopleural fistula, resulting in persistent pneumothorax [12].

Pulmonary lacerations in the setting of nonpenetrating thoracic trauma can be grouped into four categories based on mechanism and radiologic findings according to the findings of Wagner et al. [31]. Type 1 lacerations are the most common. They occur when thoracic compression generates enough pressure within the lungs to rupture the pulmonary parenchyma. These lacerations generally occur centrally in the lung, but can occasionally extend into the periphery and even into the pleural space, leading to pneumothorax. A type 2 laceration occurs when the lung parenchyma compresses and shears across the vertebral column. Therefore, these injuries are seen in the paraspinal regions of the lungs. Type 3 lacerations occur secondary to penetration from a fractured rib and are frequently associated with pneumothorax. Type 4 lacerations occur secondary to pleural disease which fixes the lung in position and prevents motion of the lung in the thoracic cavity, leading to increased shearing forces.

Traumatic pneumatocele is a rare complication of blunt chest trauma. It represents air trapped within a pulmonary laceration. Chest X-ray has a low sensitivity of 24% in diagnosing traumatic pneumatoceles. CT is much more accurate, with a reported sensitivity of 96%. The typical appearance of traumatic pneumatocele on CT is a round or oval thin-walled cavitary lesion with air-fluid levels (Fig. 5.17) [32]. Post-traumatic pulmonary pneumatoceles usually resolve spontaneously but can be complicated and can require surgery.

The American Association for the Surgery of Trauma (AAST) has published a scoring scale for

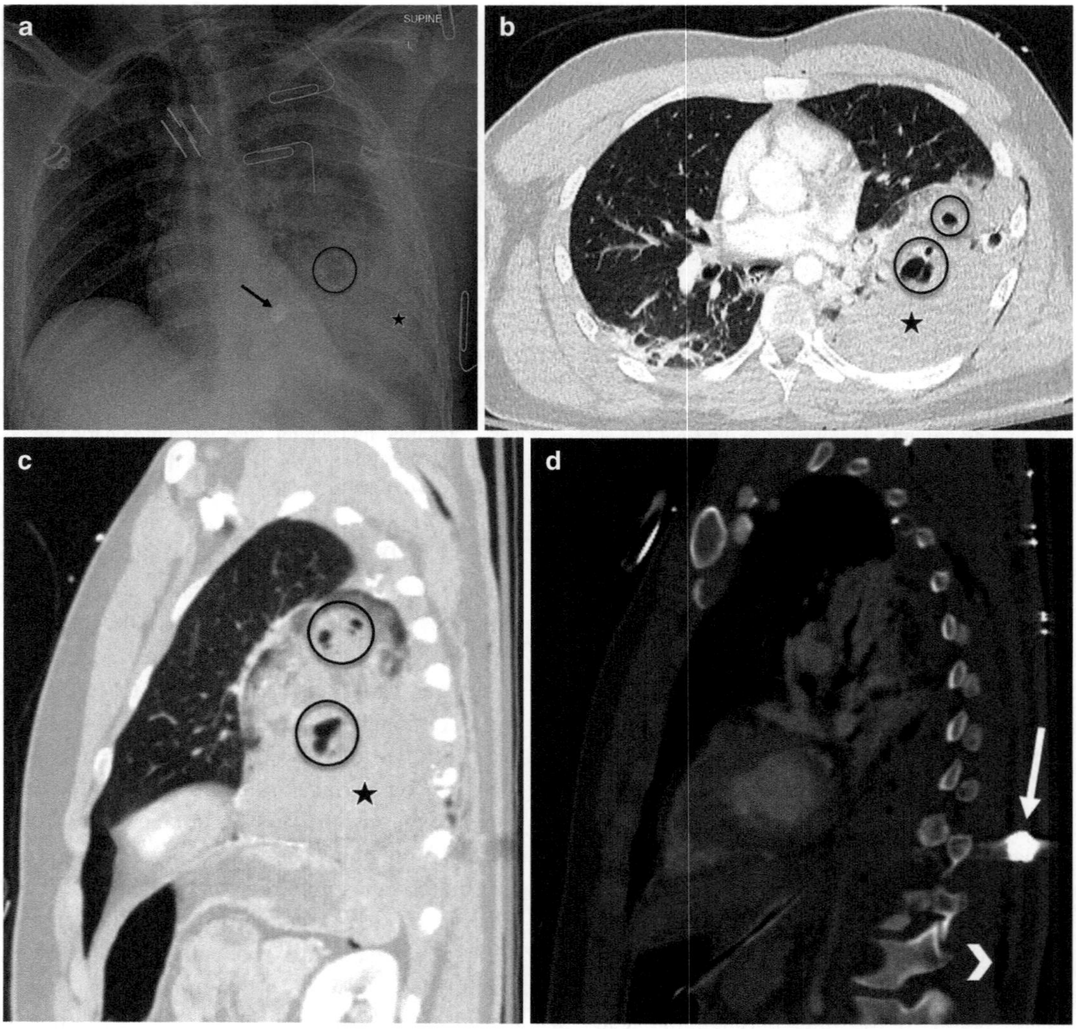

Fig. 5.16 Chest X-ray (**a**), axial and sagittal CT (**b**, **c**, **d**): 18-year-old male presented with a gun shot injury to the left chest. CXR demonstrates the ballistic fragment over lying the mediastinum (black arrow), with extensive opacification of the left lung compatible with pulmonary contusion (black star). Lucencies noted within the consolidation corresponds to pulmonary lacerations (black circles). Chest CT confirms the findings noted on CXR. Subcutaneous emphysema noted in the left chest wall (chevron head) and bullet fragment (white arrow)

lung injury, which can be used by radiologists to clearly and effectively communicate the severity of lung injuries to the treating surgeon [33]. Table 5.2 the AAST scoring scale takes into account the severity of pulmonary contusions as well as the presence of pulmonary lacerations or injury to the pulmonary vasculature [12].

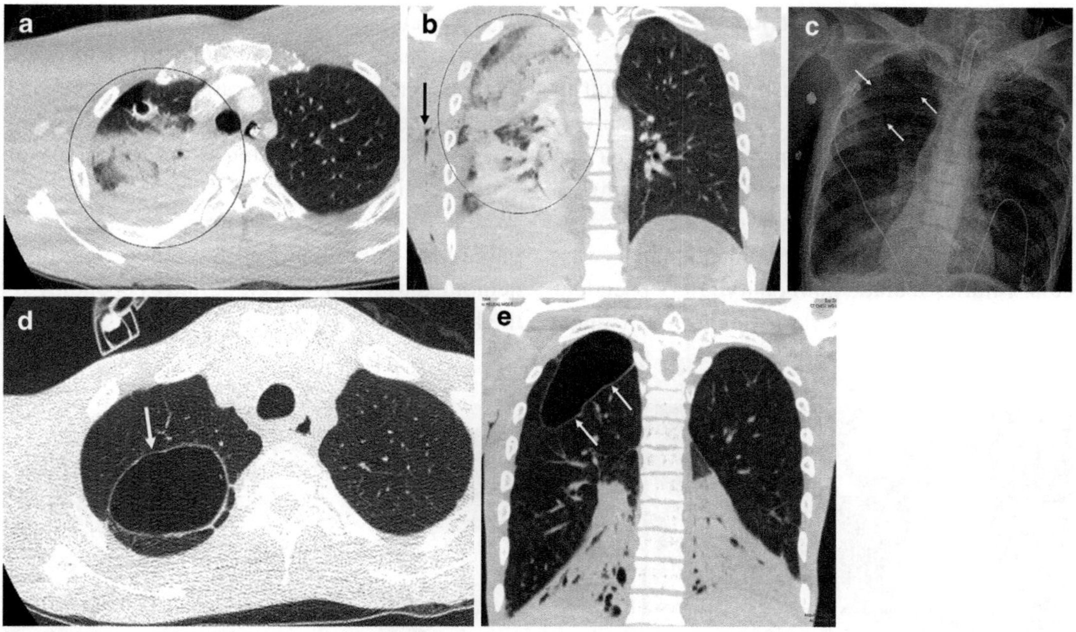

Fig. 5.17 Axial and coronal CT (**a**, **b**), chest X-ray (**c**), axial and coronal (**d** and **e**): 30-year-old male presented with multiple GSW's and cervical spinal cord injury sustained approximately 3 months prior to presentation. Initial Chest CT demonstrates near complete white out of the right hemithorax likely a combination of aspiration and pulmonary contusion (black circle). Subcutaneous emphysema noted in the right lateral chest wall (black arrow). Follow up CXR and CT, 3 months after the initial presentation shows an air-filled cyst at the right lung apex (white arrows) compatible with a pneumatocele

Table 5.2 AAST organ injury scale for lung injury

Grade	Injury type	Description of injury
I	Contusion	Unilateral contusion, segmental or subsegmental involvement
II	Contusion Laceration	Unilateral contusion, lobar involvement Peripheral laceration, with or without simple pneumothorax
III	Contusion Laceration Hematoma	Unilateral contusion with more than single lobe involvement or bilateral contusions Persistent laceration (>72 h); injury to distal airways, with or without air leak Intraparenchymal hematoma (nonexpanding)
IV	Laceration Hematoma Vascular injury	Major laceration (segmental or lobar) with imaging findings suggestive of air leak Expanding intraparenchymal hematoma (expanding over consecutive imaging examinations or with active contrast material extravasation) Primary branch intrapulmonary vessel disruption
V	Vascular injury	Hilar vascular injury (contained, without active contrast material extravasation)
VI	Vascular injury	Transection of pulmonary hilum or hilar vessel injury with uncontained bleeding (active contrast material extravasation)

Pulmonary Vascular Injuries

Both penetrating and blunt trauma can result in pulmonary vascular injury. As discussed previously, injury to the pulmonary parenchyma can damage the pulmonary vasculature, leading to pulmonary contusions, hematomas, hematoceles, and hemothoraces. Less common pulmonary vascular injuries include pulmonary artery pseudoaneurysms and arteriovenous fistulae. Pseudoaneurysms are seen as outpouchings of the pulmonary arteries which opacify at the same rate as the pulmonary arteries (Fig. 5.18). Arteriovenous fistulae are typically identified by early filling of the pulmonary veins [12]. Rare vascular injuries include pulmonary artery transection, rupture, and dissection [34]. Injury to the pulmonary artery can lead to hemopericardium, hemomediastinum, or hemothorax depending on the location of the injury.

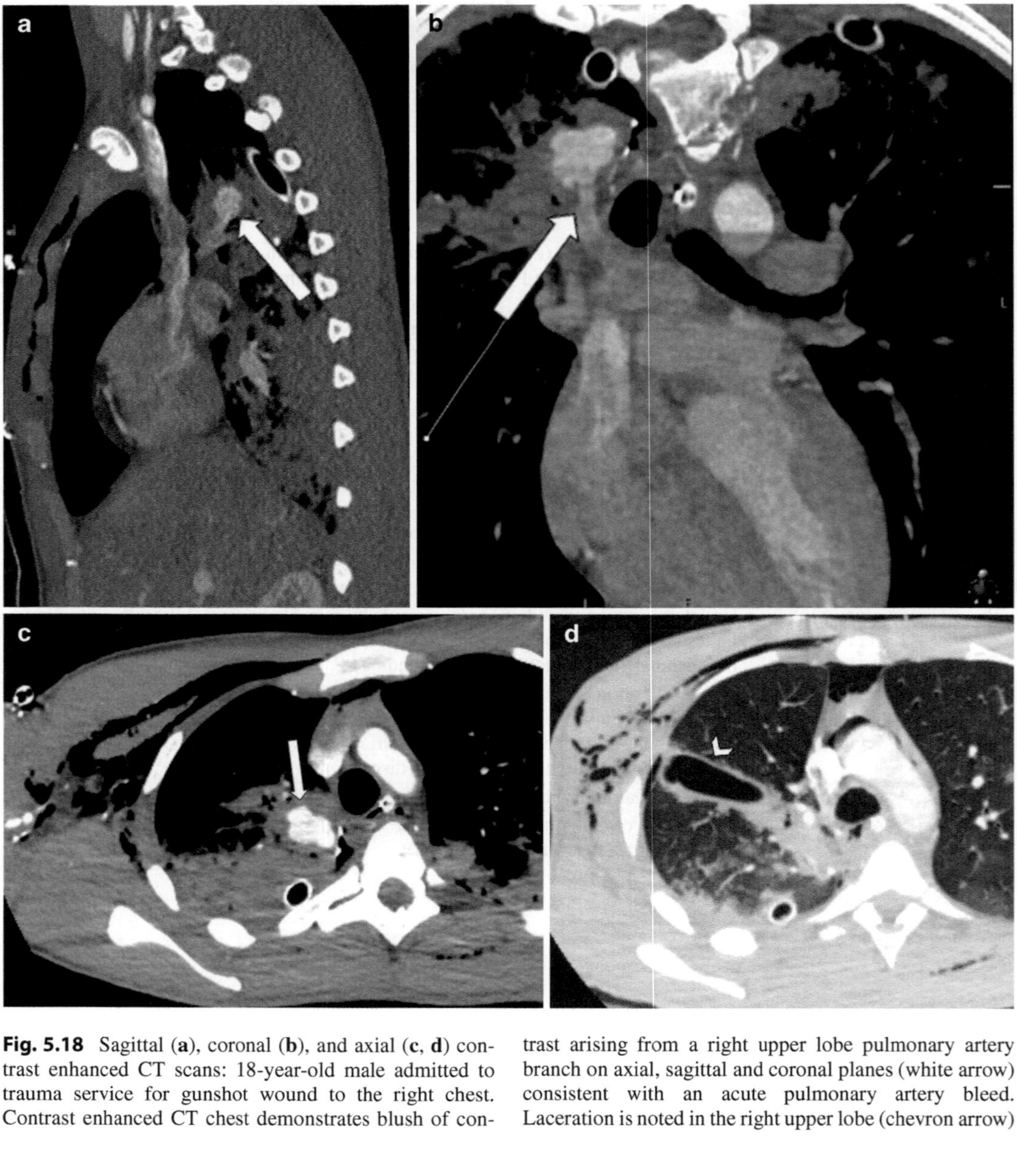

Fig. 5.18 Sagittal (**a**), coronal (**b**), and axial (**c**, **d**) contrast enhanced CT scans: 18-year-old male admitted to trauma service for gunshot wound to the right chest. Contrast enhanced CT chest demonstrates blush of contrast arising from a right upper lobe pulmonary artery branch on axial, sagittal and coronal planes (white arrow) consistent with an acute pulmonary artery bleed. Laceration is noted in the right upper lobe (chevron arrow)

Another potential complication of trauma involving the pulmonary vasculature is fat embolism. While most skeletal fractures will lead to fat droplets being released into the circulatory system and some level of fat embolism, the clinical entity known as fat embolism syndrome (FES) is rare, typically requiring a long bone fracture. FES is a clinical syndrome classically presenting with hypoxia, confusion, and petechial rash [35]. In patients with FES, chest radiographs will generally demonstrate non-specific, patchy opacities. CT is generally more useful in supporting the diagnosis. The most common CT pattern in ground glass opacities and interlobular septal thickening is a "crazy paving" pattern.

Esophageal Injuries

Esophageal injuries are most frequently encountered in the setting of iatrogenic trauma, forceful retching, and foreign body or caustic ingestion; however, they can also be encountered in the setting of both blunt and penetrating trauma. In one series, esophageal injuries were diagnosed in 0.14% of patients presenting with penetrating trauma and 0.06% of patients presenting with blunt trauma [36]. While rare, these injuries are important to identify, as esophageal perforation can rapidly lead to mediastinitis and carries a mortality rate of 10–20% factoring in all causes [37]. The spectrum of traumatic esophageal injuries includes contusions/intramural hematomas, partial thickness lacerations, full thickness lacerations, and segmental loss or devascularization [38]. Full thickness lacerations involving >50% of the esophageal circumference increase the risk of post-operative complications.

Blunt trauma to the esophagus is rare due to the deep location of the esophagus and the protection afforded by surrounding structures [22] and are most often seen in the cervical and abdominal portions of the esophagus. In the neck, the esophagus is more superficially located and relatively less protected. In the abdomen, the risk of esophageal injury is increased by the connection of the esophagus to the stomach as well as the transiting of the esophagus through the diaphragmatic crura, which both create potential for increased stresses and shear forces [39].

Penetrating trauma can lead to injury to any portion of the esophagus depending on the trajectory of the projectile. Overall, gunshot wounds (GSW) account for approximately 75% of penetrating esophageal injuries while stab wounds account for the remaining 15% [39]. Stab injuries to the esophagus are more common in the neck secondary to the more superficial location of the esophagus in this region as compared to the chest and abdomen. In the case of GSW, the path of the projectile does not need to directly traverse the esophagus to cause esophageal injury. Blast injury can lead to esophageal contusions or intramural hematomas as well as tissue necrosis, which can lead to delayed esophageal perforation.

Chest radiographs are neither sensitive nor specific for esophageal injury in the setting of blunt or penetrating trauma. The most common plain film findings of esophageal perforation are left-sided pleural effusion and cervical or mediastinal gas [40]. Pneumothorax, hemothorax, and mediastinal widening can all be seen, but are non-specific in the setting of trauma. The most specific finding of esophageal injury on chest radiographs is displacement of the nasogastric/orogastric tube outside of the expected esophageal lumen, but this is not often encountered.

Standard trauma protocol CTs are more sensitive for esophageal injury (53% sensitivity) [41, 42], but specificity remains low. Contrast enhanced CT findings that can suggest esophageal injury include esophageal wall thickening, pneumomediastinum, and fluid in the mediastinum. Esophageal mural hematoma or intramural air within the esophagus can occasionally be identified and are more specific findings for esophageal injury. If esophageal injury is suspected on the initial CECT, fluoroscopic esophagram or CT esophagram can be used for further evaluation (Fig. 5.19).

Traditionally, fluoroscopy has been the test of choice for evaluating esophageal injuries. The primary purpose of the fluoroscopic esophagram in the setting of suspected traumatic esophageal injury is to evaluate for esophageal perforation as

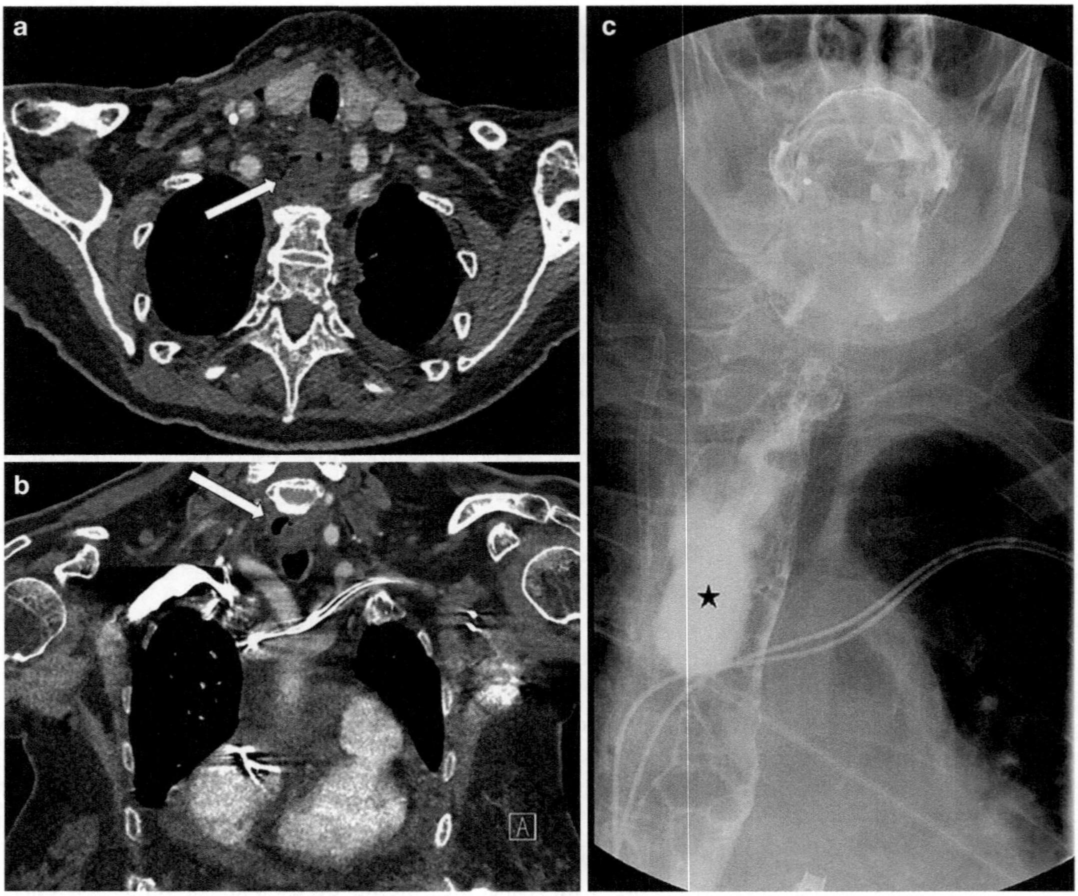

Fig. 5.19 Axial (**a**) and coronal (**b**) contrast enhanced CT scan and esophagogram (**c**): 70-year-old female presented to an outside hospital ED after possible seizure events. She was intubated for airway protection, with iatrogenic esophageal perforation. CT chest with IV contrast demonstrates extensive eccentric wall thickening of the upper esophagus with indistinct stranding and density of the adjacent mediastinal fat planes, with gas outside of the lumen suspicious for esophageal perforation (white arrows). Flouroscopy confirmed a moderate size right posterolateral cervical esophageal leak at the approximate level of C7 (black star)

evidenced by extravasation of contrast from the esophageal lumen. Less severe esophageal injuries such as mural hematomas and partial thickness lacerations are often occult on single contrast fluoroscopic esophagography. While fluoroscopic esophagography is more sensitive for esophageal injury than CECT, the procedure carries a false negative rate of 10–38% [37]. The sensitivity of the procedure can be improved by administering barium contrast if water soluble contrast fails to demonstrate a leak.

More recently, many departments have adopted CT esophagography as a replacement for fluoroscopic esophagography in the evaluation of suspected esophageal injury. Typical protocols include imaging before and after the administration of water soluble oral contrast in the supine position. Modifications such as prone imaging and the administration of effervescent granules vary by institution and clinical situation [37]. The sensitivity of CT esophagography for esophageal perforation is reported to be between 59 and 100% with specificity between 80 and 100%. Benefits over fluoroscopy include decreased time of examination and increased availability as well as the fact that the procedure does not need to be directly supervised by the radiologist. If esophageal injury is suspected on the initial trauma CT,

CT esophagography can be performed while the patient is still on the table, further decreasing time to diagnosis. Additionally, CT esophagography allows for better evaluation of periesophageal collection and non-transmural tears as compared to fluoroscopy [37, 43], but evaluation of mucosal details remains poorer. While CT esophagography holds many advantages over traditional fluoroscopy, endoscopic esophagoscopy remains the gold standard for diagnosing esophageal injuries.

Conclusion

Thoracic injuries are significant causes of morbidity and mortality in trauma patients. Imaging plays an important role in the diagnosis and management of chest trauma. Conventional radiography and multidetector computed tomography can quickly and accurately help diagnose a wide variety of injuries in trauma patients.

References

1. McCollough CH, Bruesewitz MR, Kofler JM. CT dose reduction and dose management tools: overview of available options. Radiographics. 2006;26:503–12. https://doi.org/10.1148/rg.262055138.
2. Dogrul BN, Kiliccalan I, Asci ES, Peker SC. Blunt trauma related chest wall and pulmonary injuries: an overview. Chin J Traumatol. 2020;23(3):125–38.
3. Oikonomou A, Prassopoulos P. CT imaging of blunt chest trauma. Insights Imaging. 2011;2(3):281–95.
4. Adam A, Dixon AK, Gillard JH, Schaefer-Prokop C. Grainger & Allison's diagnostic radiology: a textbook of medical imaging. 6th ed. Edinburgh: Churchill Livingstone/Elsevier; 2015. 2 volumes (xix, 2214, 176 pages) p. 184–207.
5. Sabri YY, Hafez MAF, Kamel KM, Abbas DA. Evaluating the role of ultrasound in chest trauma: common complications and computed tomography comparative evaluation. Egypt J Radiol Nucl Med. 2018;49:986–92.
6. Ho ML, Gutierrez FR. Chest radiography in thoracic polytrauma. AJR Am J Roentgenol. 2009;192(3):599–612.
7. Porhomayon J, Doerr R. Pneumothorax and subcutaneous emphysema secondary to blunt chest injury. Int J Emerg Med. 2011;4:10.
8. Leturia Etxeberria M, Biurrun Mancisidor MC, Ugarte Nuño A, Arenaza Choperena G, Mendoza Alonso M, Esnaola Albizu M, et al. Imaging assessment of ectopic gas collections. Radiographics. 2020;40(5):1318–38.
9. Panda A, Kumar A, Gamanagatti S, Patil A, Kumar S, Gupta A. Traumatic diaphragmatic injury: a review of CT signs and the difference between blunt and penetrating injury. Diagn Interv Radiol. 2014;20(2):121–8.
10. Ufuk F. Intercostal lung hernia. Radiology. 2021;299(2):277.
11. Lee CM, Jeon CH, Lee R, Kwon H, Kim CW, Kim JH, et al. Traumatic hemothorax caused by thoracic wall and intrathoracic injuries: clinical outcomes of transcatheter systemic artery embolization. Taehan Yongsang Uihakhoe Chi. 2021;82(4):923–35.
12. Lewis BT, Herr KD, Hamlin SA, Henry T, Little BP, Naeger DM, et al. Imaging manifestations of chest trauma. Radiographics. 2021;41(5):1321–34.
13. Tran J, Haussner W, Shah K. Traumatic pneumothorax: a review of current diagnostic practices and evolving management. J Emerg Med. 2021;61(5):517–28.
14. Omar HR, Abdelmalak H, Mangar D, Rashad R, Helal E, Camporesi EM. Occult pneumothorax, revisited. J Trauma Manag Outcomes. 2010;4:12.
15. Husain LF, Hagopian L, Wayman D, Baker WE, Carmody KA. Sonographic diagnosis of pneumothorax. J Emerg Trauma Shock. 2012;5(1):76–81.
16. Brant WE, Helms CA. Fundamentals of diagnostic radiology, vol. xix. 3rd ed. Philadelphia, PA: Lippincott, Williams & Wilkins; 2007. p. 1559.
17. Kattea MO, Lababede O. Differentiating pneumothorax from the common radiographic skinfold artifact. Ann Am Thorac Soc. 2015;12(6):928–31.
18. Ball CG, Kirkpatrick AW, Laupland KB, Fox DL, Litvinchuk S, Dyer DM, et al. Factors related to the failure of radiographic recognition of occult posttraumatic pneumothoraces. Am J Surg. 2005;189(5):541–6; discussion 6.
19. Blaivas M, Lyon M, Duggal S. A prospective comparison of supine chest radiography and bedside ultrasound for the diagnosis of traumatic pneumothorax. Acad Emerg Med. 2005;12(9):844–9.
20. Alrajab S, Youssef AM, Akkus NI, Caldito G. Pleural ultrasonography versus chest radiography for the diagnosis of pneumothorax: review of the literature and meta-analysis. Crit Care. 2013;17(5):R208.
21. Dennis BM, Bellister SA, Guillamondegui OD. Thoracic trauma. Surg Clin North Am. 2017;97(5):1047–64.
22. Kaewlai R, Avery LL, Asrani AV, Novelline RA. Multidetector CT of blunt thoracic trauma. Radiographics. 2008;28(6):1555–70.
23. Moy MP, Levsky JM, Berko NS, Godelman A, Jain VR, Haramati LB. A new, simple method for estimating pleural effusion size on CT scans. Chest. 2013;143(4):1054–9. https://doi.org/10.1378/chest.12-1292. PMID: 23632863; PMCID: PMC3616681.
24. Prakash PS, Moore SA, Rezende-Neto JB, Trpcic S, Dunn JA, Smoot B, Jenkins DH, Cardenas T, Mukherjee K, Farnsworth J, Wild J, Young K,

Schroeppel TJ, Coimbra R, Lee J, Skarupa DJ, Sabra MJ, Carrick MM, Moore FO, Ward J, Geng T, Lapham D, Piccinini A, Inaba K, Dodgion C, Gooley B, Schwartz T, Shraga S, Haan JM, Lightwine K, Burris J, Agrawal V, Seamon MJ, Cannon JW. Predictors of retained hemothorax in trauma: results of an Eastern Association for the Surgery of trauma multi-institutional trial. J Trauma Acute Care Surg. 2020;89(4):679–85. https://doi.org/10.1097/TA.0000000000002881.
25. Moser JB, Stefanidis K, Vlahos I. Imaging evaluation of tracheobronchial injuries. Radiographics. 2020;40(2):515–28.
26. Prokakis C, Koletsis EN, Dedeilias P, Fligou F, Filos K, Dougenis D. Airway trauma: a review on epidemiology, mechanisms of injury, diagnosis and treatment. J Cardiothorac Surg. 2014;9:117.
27. Tanrivermis Sayit A, Elmali M, Saglam D, Celenk C. The diseases of airway-tracheal diverticulum: a review of the literature. J Thorac Dis. 2016;8(10):E1163–7. https://doi.org/10.21037/jtd.2016.10.92. PMID: 27867581; PMCID: PMC5107528.
28. Sakai M, Murayama S, Gibo M, Akamine T, Nagata O. Frequent cause of the macklin effect in spontaneous pneumomediastinum: demonstration by multidetector-row computed tomography. J Comput Assist Tomogr. 2006;30:92–4.
29. Tack D, Defrance P, Delcour C, Gevenois PA. The CT fallen-lung sign. Eur Radiol. 2000;10(5):719–21.
30. Grewal HS, Dangayach NS, Ahmad U, Ghosh S, Gildea T, Mehta AC. Treatment of tracheobronchial injuries: a contemporary review. Chest. 2019;155(3):595–604.
31. Wagner RB, Crawford WO, Schimpf PP. Classification of parenchymal injuries of the lung. Radiology. 1988;167(1):77–82.
32. Barbick B, Cothren CC, Zimmerman MA, Moore EE. Posttraumatic pneumatocele. J Am Coll Surg. 2005;200(2):306–7.
33. Moore EE, Malangoni MA, Cogbill TH, Shackford SR, Champion HR, Jurkovich GJ, et al. Organ injury scaling. IV: thoracic vascular, lung, cardiac, and diaphragm. J Trauma. 1994;36(3):299–300.
34. Abbas AE. Traumatic injury of the pulmonary artery: transection, rupture, pseudoaneurysm, or dissection? Sometimes semantics do matter. J Thorac Cardiovasc Surg. 2016;152(5):1437–8.
35. Newbigin K, Souza CA, Torres C, Marchiori E, Gupta A, Inacio J, et al. Fat embolism syndrome: state-of-the-art review focused on pulmonary imaging findings. Respir Med. 2016;113:93–100.
36. Biffl WL, Moore EE, Feliciano DV, Albrecht RA, Croce M, Karmy-Jones R, et al. Western trauma association critical decisions in trauma: diagnosis and management of esophageal injuries. J Trauma Acute Care Surg. 2015;79(6):1089–95.
37. Norton-Gregory AA, Kulkarni NM, O'Connor SD, Budovec JJ, Zorn AP, Desouches SL. CT esophagography for evaluation of esophageal perforation. Radiographics. 2021;41(2):447–61.
38. Moore EE, Jurkovich GJ, Knudson MM, Cogbill TH, Malangoni MA, Champion HR, et al. Organ injury scaling. VI: extrahepatic biliary, esophagus, stomach, vulva, vagina, uterus (nonpregnant), uterus (pregnant), fallopian tube, and ovary. J Trauma. 1995;39(6):1069–70.
39. Mubang RN, Sigmon DF, Stawicki SP. Esophageal trauma. In: StatPearls. Treasure Island (FL): StatPearls Publishing; 2022. [Updated 2022 Jul 26]. https://www.ncbi.nlm.nih.gov/books/NBK470161/.
40. Gunn ML, Clark RT, Sadro CT, Linnau KF, Sandstrom CK. Current concepts in imaging evaluation of penetrating transmediastinal injury. Radiographics. 2014;34(7):1824–41.
41. Bruns BR. Trachea, bronchus, and esophagus injuries: techniques. In: Scalea TM, editor. The shock trauma manual of operative techniques. Cham: Springer; 2021. https://doi.org/10.1007/978-3-030-27596-9_8.
42. Young CA, Menias CO, Bhalla S, Prasad SR. CT features of esophageal emergencies. Radiographics. 2008;28(6):1541–53.
43. Masarapu V, Xia E, Son H. Esophageal emergencies: another important cause of acute chest pain. Insights Imaging. 2020;11(1):109. https://doi.org/10.1186/s13244-020-00915-1.

Heart and Great Vessels

6

Laura De León Benedetti, Raisa Amiruddin, and Abass M. Noor

Introduction

The management of cardiac trauma has improved significantly due to advances in medical transportation, use of emergency thoracotomy, advancements in cardiovascular surgery techniques, and application of diagnostic imaging. Mechanisms of trauma to the heart and great vessels may be categorized as blunt or penetrating. The most common cause of substantial blunt chest trauma is motor vehicle collision, and the most common cause of penetrating chest trauma are gunshot and stab wounds [1]. The American Association for the Surgery of Trauma (AAST) has developed a classification system based on severity of injury to the heart and vasculature [2].

Cardiac Trauma

Cardiac trauma remains associated with out-of-hospital mortality as high as 94% and low in-hospital survival [3]. Although cardiac trauma may occur in isolation, it often occurs concomitantly with other significant injuries [4–9]. Outcomes of blunt cardiac trauma range from arrhythmias, myocardial contusion, and myocardial rupture leading to hemopericardium—rarely blunt cardiac trauma may cause pericardial tamponade. Penetrating thoracic trauma may result in cardiac laceration and hemopericardium which may lead to pericardial tamponade and possibly exsanguination.

An anatomic understanding of the position of the heart within the thoracic cavity will reveal answers as to why certain cardiac structures are more frequently injured than others (Fig. 6.1). The right ventricle is the most anterior cardiac chamber and the most frequently injured in an anterior approach penetrating injury. The left atrium is the most posterior cardiac chamber and the least likely to be injured in an anterior approach penetrating injury. Campbell et al. in a review of 1198 cases of penetrating cardiac trauma found the most commonly injured cardiac chamber to be the right ventricle, followed by the left ventricle and right atrium [3] (Fig. 6.2).

They also found that the least commonly injured cardiac chamber to be the left atrium.

Lustenberger et al. similarly showed that pediatric penetrating cardiac injuries most frequently involved the right ventricle (46.9%), left ventricle (43.8%), and right atrium (18.8%) [10]. Most patients who survive blunt or penetrating cardiac trauma at the scene to arrive at a hospital often have less severe injuries—therefore, imaging

L. D. L. Benedetti · R. Amiruddin
Department of Radiology, Children's Hospital of Philadelphia, Philadelphia, PA, USA
e-mail: deleonbenl@chop.edu

A. M. Noor (✉)
Department of Radiology, Hospital of the University of Pennsylvania, Philadelphia, PA, USA
e-mail: abass.noor@pennmedicine.upenn.edu

F. Knollmann (ed.), *Trauma Computed Tomography*, https://doi.org/10.1007/978-3-031-45746-3_6

findings tend toward hemopericardium (Fig. 6.3) rather than cardiac herniation. Although a significant number of patients may present with electrical disturbances, computed tomography (CT) is crucial in evaluating structural cardiac injuries.

Initial evaluation of blunt and penetrating cardiac trauma should adhere to Advanced Trauma Life Support (ATLS) protocols [11]. Subsequently, imaging in the form of chest radiography and Focused Assessment of Sonography in Trauma (FAST) exam may be performed. A multicenter prospective cohort study evaluating discrepancies between chest radiography and chest CT found that 24.6% (1454/5912) of patients had radiographically occult injuries identified on chest CT, an example underscoring the superior diagnostic accuracy of chest CT as compared to radiography in characterizing thoracic injuries [12]. Brink et al. also showed improved diagnostic accuracy with routine chest CT evaluation in blunt chest trauma, where CT revealed radiographically occult injuries in 43% of patients (201/464) [13]. Thus, if a patient is clinically stable, further focused imaging such as CT angiography (CTA) of the chest may be pursued but should not delay definitive surgical management in unstable patients. Non-gated CTA of the chest in the arterial phase may be performed to identify the extent of injuries and for surgical planning in thoracic injury [14]—however, some shown that when injury to the heart and great vessels are suspected, ECG-gated CTA of the chest or heart provides important diagnostic information that may not be well characterized on non-gated exams [15, 16].

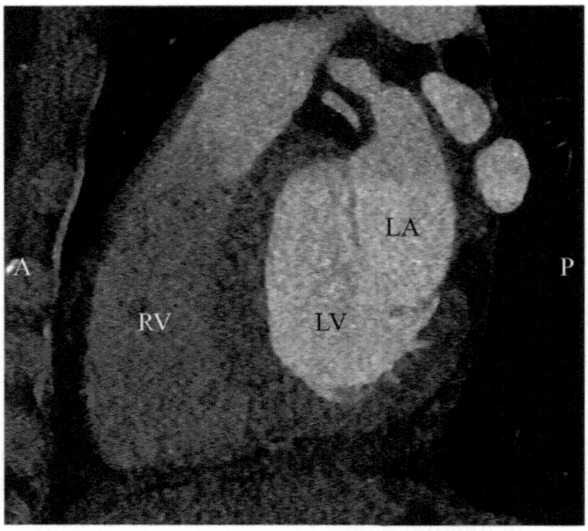

Fig. 6.1 Normal anatomy of the heart. Cardiac CTA demonstrates positioning of the cardiac chambers in the sagittal plane. Anterior (A) and posterior (P) orientation of the cardiac chambers may be appreciated, with the right ventricle being the most anterior chamber and left atrium being the most posterior

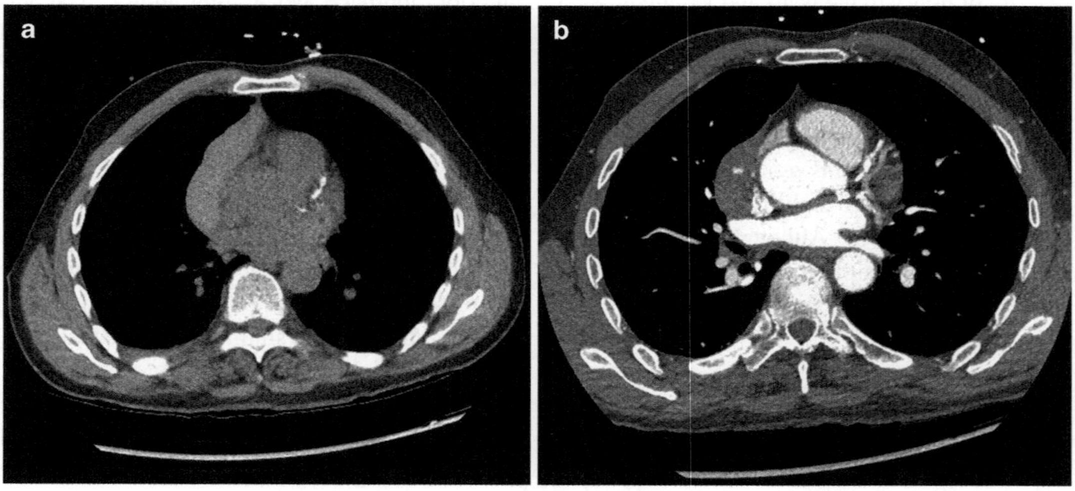

Fig. 6.2 Blunt cardiac trauma, right atrial injury. 66-year-old male who presented following blunt thoracic trauma, bicyclist versus motor vehicle. Noncontrast CT of the chest (**a**) reveals a hyperdense peri-atrial collection along the right atrium suggestive of acute hematoma. Subsequent ECG-gated CT of the heart with contrast (**b**) shows contrast extravasation within the hematoma, consistent with active bleeding from the right atrium

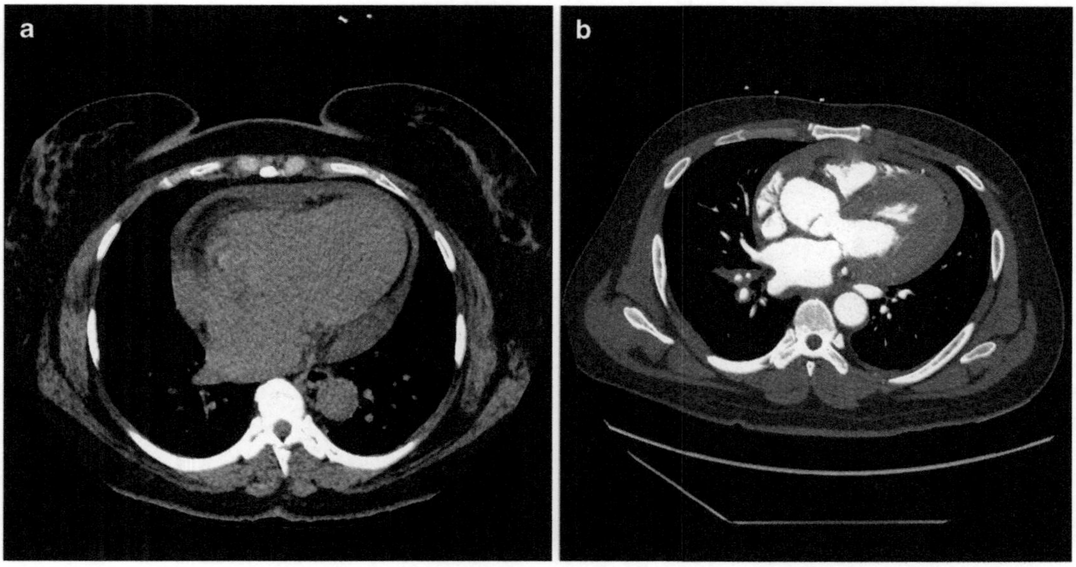

Fig. 6.3 Blunt cardiac trauma, hemopericardium. (**a**) 66-year-old female presenting after being struck by a motor vehicle while walking. Non-contrast CT of the chest showed a hyperdense pericardial effusion which represents hemopericardium. (**b**) 31-year-old male presenting with chest pain after blunt thoracic trauma. CT angiogram of the chest showed a hyperdense pericardial effusion which represents hemopericardium

Blunt Cardiac Trauma

Mechanisms of blunt cardiac trauma are thought to be threefold; transfer of energy resulting in sternal or rib fractures which may injure subjacent structures, rapid deceleration resulting in traction or torsion of the heart, and sudden rise of intrathoracic pressure due to compression of the heart between the sternum and vertebral bodies or secondary to increased abdominal pressure [17, 18]. Myocardial contusion commonly occurs following blunt cardiac trauma and may cause arrhythmia and acute heart failure; however, myocardial contusion is not usually resolved on CTA of the chest and is generally seen on surgical exploration or autopsy. However, studies have shown that myocardial hypoenhancment on CT may indicate myocardial contusion, although with low specificity [19]. Blunt cardiac trauma may, in severe cases, result in rupture of the cardiac chambers, coronary arteries, and great vessels as well as valve injury. Clinical series have shown the most commonly injured cardiac cavities in blunt injury to be the right atrium and ventricle. Coronary artery rupture and valve injury, however, are discussed rarely in case reports. Although CT can evaluate for papillary muscle rupture, echocardiography is the main method of evaluating traumatic valvular disorders. Kan et al. reported that the most commonly injured heart valve is the aortic valve, followed by the mitral and tricuspid valves [20]. CT is essential in revealing subclinical hemorrhage due to blunt trauma (Fig. 6.4).

Penetrating Cardiac Trauma

Similar to blunt cardiac trauma, non-gated or ECG-gated CT angiography of the chest in the arterial phase is the recommended initial evaluation. Penetrating cardiac trauma is uncommon and lethal with most injuries resulting in out-of-hospital death, and the vast majority of those afflicted being men. Asensio et al., in a query of the National Trauma Database, found that penetrating cardiac injury accounts for 0.16% of all trauma admissions–the vast majority representing gunshot and stab wounds (63% and 36%, respectively) (Fig. 6.5) and an overall mortality of 33% with survival skewed in favor of those with stab wounds (76%) as compared to gunshot

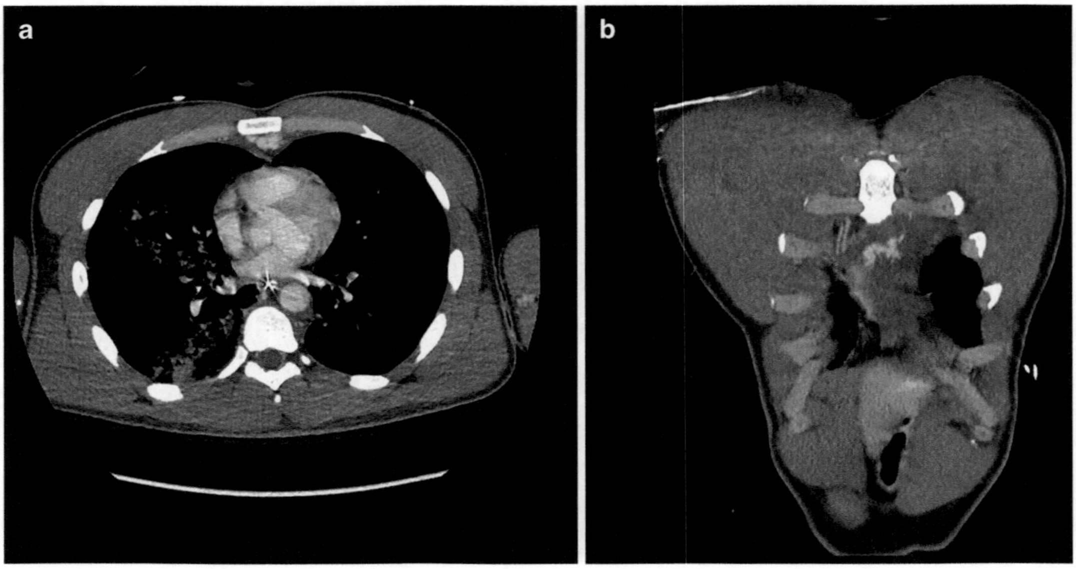

Fig. 6.4 Blunt trauma, active retrosternal hemorrhage. 35-year-old male presenting following motor vehicle collision with chest pain. (**a**) Axial post-contrast CT shows retrosternal pooling contrast. (**b**) Coronal reconstruction in the same patient shows pooling contrast within hyperdense retrosternal fluid. Findings represent active bleeding

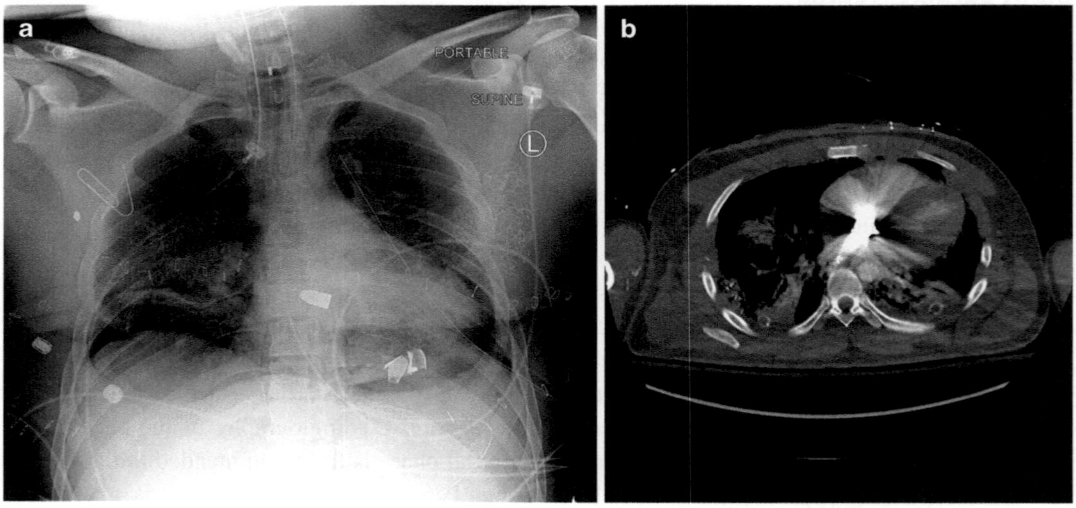

Fig. 6.5 Penetrating cardiac trauma. 34-year-old male presenting following ballistic trauma. (**a**) Post-operative radiograph notable for retained bullet projecting over the heart. (**b**) CT confirms the location of the retained bullet to be within the heart, near the interatrial septum

wounds (10%) [21]. Isaza-Restrepo et al., in an analysis of 240 cases showed the overall mortality of penetrating cardiac trauma to be 14.6%—with gunshot wounds having a much higher mortality than stab wounds (41.2% and 11.7%, respectively). Of those presenting with penetrating cardiac injuries, 67% had pericardial tamponade [22].

Although cardiac tamponade commonly occurs following cardiac trauma, it is rare to

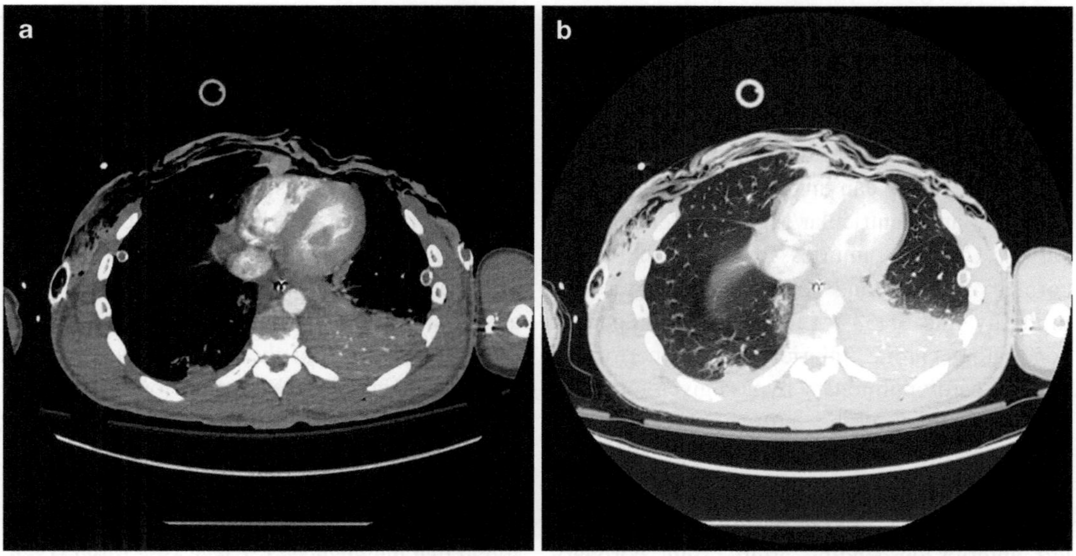

Fig. 6.6 Penetrating cardiac injury, clamshell thoracotomy. Post-contrast axial CT chest in soft tissue (**a**) and lung (**b**) windows showing a patient who underwent thoracotomy for cardiac tamponade secondary to stab wound. Surgical exploration revealed AAST Grade IV right ventricular penetrating cardiac injury with tamponade

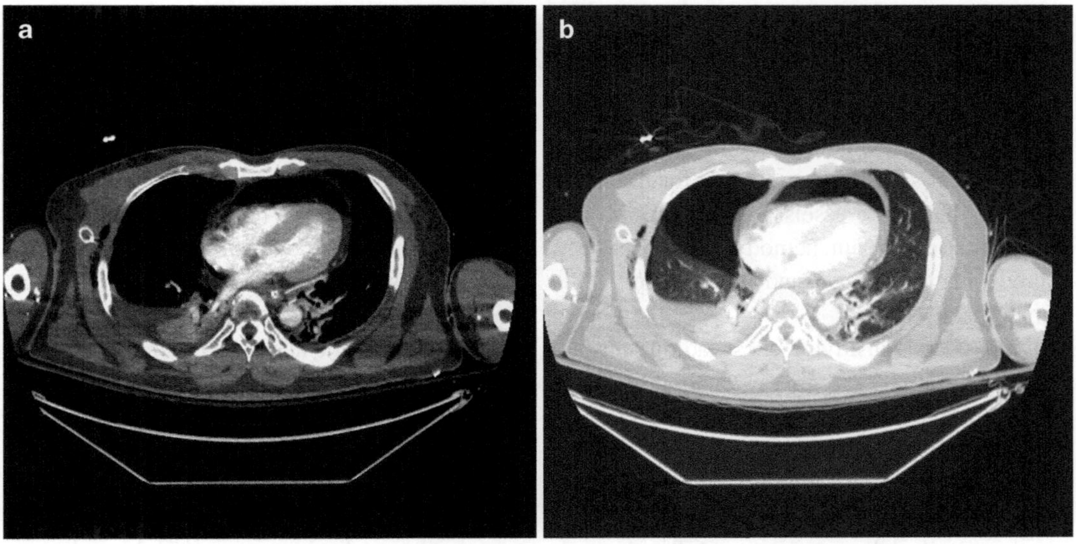

Fig. 6.7 Pneumopericardium. Post-contrast axial CT chest in soft tissue (**a**) and lung (**b**) windows showing a patient with clinical findings of pericardial tamponade and pneumopericardium. A right pneumothorax is also present

image pericardial tamponade as patients often undergo procedures such as subxiphoid window or thoracotomy prior to CT imaging (Fig. 6.6). Pericardial tamponade may also be due to pneumopericardium in addition to hemopericardium (Fig. 6.7). The discrepancy in mortality between gunshot and stab wounds may be explained by multi-chamber and multi-cavitary injuries having a higher association with ballistic trauma as compared to stab wounds [23].

Pediatric penetrating cardiac trauma appears more likely to involve stab wounds and a much higher mortality than in adult populations. In a study on pediatric trauma, Lustenberger et al.

found only 0.7% of those admitted sustained penetrating cardiac injuries, with the majority presenting with stab wounds (81.2%), and an overall in-hospital mortality of 71.9% [10].

In addition to the cardiac chambers, penetrating cardiac injury can involve the coronary arteries, atrial and ventricular septa, as well as heart valves. Complex injuries involving the septa, coronary arteries, and heart valves carry a high mortality rate of 53% [24]. Although repair of penetrating cardiac injuries may be performed without cardiopulmonary bypass given the time-sensitive nature of the injuries [25], proximal lesions of the coronary arteries may require a coronary artery bypass. The frequency of coronary artery injury from most to least common is: left anterior descending artery, right coronary artery, and left circumflex artery [24].

Great Vessels

The great vessels are the large arteries and veins which directly connect to the heart; these vessels are the inferior vena cava, superior vena cava, pulmonary arteries, pulmonary veins, and aortic root. Clinical signs and symptoms for traumatic injury to the great vessels are non-specific and may include chest pain, hemodynamic instability, altered mental status, and other nonspecific symptoms.

Despite low sensitivity, chest radiographs are used as the initial screening evaluation. A FAST examination is usually insufficient in clearing great vessel injuries but is important in identifying associated findings, such as hemopericardium. Advancements in imaging technology have greatly improved the sensitivity of CT in the evaluation of the great vessels [26]. CT angiography is now the gold standard, replacing conventional angiography as the primary diagnostic modality. In 2016, the National Institute for Health and Care Excellence in the United Kingdom commissioned a report that detailed a meta-analysis compiling data from seven studies comprising 3741 patients that assessed the use of CT in aortic injury in adults [27]. They found a pooled sensitivity of 95% and a pooled specificity of 94% for the detection of aortic injury.

As with most medical procedures and imaging techniques, there are limitations to the use of CT. It is important to remember and consider that there may be situations where CT angiography is not appropriate or that results may be inconclusive and additional intervention may be needed to arrive at a diagnosis [28]. There may be limited additional diagnostic information garnered from an ECG-gated CT of the heart or chest [29], as compared to a non-gated exam. However, if there is suspicion for great vessel or thoracic aortic injury, an ECG-gated non-contrast CT of the chest followed by an ECG-gated CTA of the chest is recommended. For example, Lovy et al. found that unenhanced CT was 89% (40/45) sensitive and 100% (45/45) specific for acute aortic syndrome [30]. In combination with breath-hold, ECG-gating allows for complete evaluation of the great vessels by limiting cardiopulmonary motion artifacts which are known to mimic or obscure vessel injury [31]. An unenhanced CT of the chest will allow for evaluation of hemothorax, hemopericardium, or intramural hematoma. Additionally, if a multiphase acquisition is needed, hyperdensities (e.g., shrapnel or suture material) can be cross referenced between non-contrast and post-contrast images to confirm extravasation of contrast. Early recognition, diagnosis, and appropriately timed management are essential to provide adequate treatment [32].

Vena Cava

Lesions to the vena cava are rare and often lethal even before medical attention [33]. Mortality can be elevated due to their location in the retroperitoneum, as they are usually present in polytraumatized patients. As the vena cava location is retroperitoneal, they are mainly caused by penetrating injuries, either gunshot wounds or stabbing, with blunt injuries rare [34].

The union of the brachiocephalic veins defines the origin of the superior vena cava (SVC) and the inferior margin is the superior cavo-atrial junction. More common than blunt or penetrating trauma, SVC injury is often iatrogenic and may, for example, be caused by central venous catheter placement [35]. Management depends on the hemodynamic stability of the patient; a small portion of patients can be treated conservatively.

The inferior vena cava (IVC) is divided into infrarenal, juxtarenal, suprarenal/intrahepatic, and retrohepatic and suprahepatic portions. Traumatic injury to the inferior vena cava (IVC) is rare; however, it is the most common traumatic abdominal vascular injury and is associated with high mortality—reported up to 70%, with the worst survival involving the retrohepatic and suprahepatic IVC [36]. Ramos and et al. described their experience with 36 polytrauma patients with vena cava injuries where they found 100% mortality for retrohepatic IVC injuries and poor prognosis for patients presenting with hemodynamic instability [34]. The most common mechanism of IVC injury is penetrating trauma. Due to its location in the abdominal cavity, penetrating trauma to the IVC is highly likely to affect other organs, thus having a higher chance of hemodynamic instability [34].

Diagnosis can, on occasion, be made promptly through FAST; however, there are limitations in detection of retroperitoneal hemorrhage on ultrasound. CT is the main imaging modality for evaluating IVC trauma, specifically non-gated contrast-enhanced CT of the chest in the venous phase. Imaging findings include direct signs such as abnormalities of vessel contour, extravasation of contrast medium, pseudoaneurysms, and thrombus [37]. Indirect signs include pericaval hematoma and hepatic laceration that extends to the IVC [35, 37]. Tsai et al. conducted a study with 12 patients to evaluate CT findings of IVC injury due to penetrating or blunt trauma. They reported equal distribution between both mechanisms. However, mortality was only associated with blunt IVC injury and injury in the retrohepatic portion of the IVC [38]. Management of these patients depends on their hemodynamic stability and the severity of injuries.

Pulmonary Trunk

Pulmonary artery injury can be classified as transection, rupture, perforation, or laceration [39]. Traumatic injury to the pulmonary trunk is often associated with other severe injuries and has a reported survival rate of less than 30% [40]. Non-gated or ECG-gated CT angiography of the pulmonary arteries with single phase reconstruction is the best initial imaging technique to evaluate injury to the pulmonary trunk [41].

Imaging findings for pulmonary trunk injuries include widened mediastinum, first rib fractures, or pleural capping on plain film [40].

Pulmonary Veins

Although traumatic injury to the pulmonary veins is rare, it may occur in penetrating or blunt trauma. There are case reports of isolated pulmonary venous injury following blunt chest trauma—thought to be caused by rapid deceleration [42–46]. Rib fractures due to blunt chest trauma may result in penetrating injuries and pulmonary vein laceration [44]. Given the relatively low mean left atrial pressure of 5–8 mmHg, hemothorax due to an isolated avulsion of a pulmonary vein may not be as evident hemodynamically—and this may explain the comparatively good prognosis of patients presenting with this type of injury [45].

Aorta and Proximal Arch Vessels

The aortic annulus is a fibrous ring that demarcates the transition between the left ventricular outflow tract and aortic valve. The aortic root is a complex anatomic structure which supports the aortic valve and the orifices of the coronary arteries—the superior margin of which is the sinotubular junction. The ascending aorta is the portion of the thoracic aorta that is between the sinotubular junction and aortic arch. The aortic arch commonly gives rise to the arch vessels which are, in order, the brachiocephalic, left common carotid, and left subclavian arteries—although, anatomic variants are common [47]. Regarding reporting standards for thoracic endovascular aortic repair, the thoracic aorta may be divided into six landing zones (Fig. 6.8) [48].

Although aortic injuries are rare, the prevalence of blunt traumatic thoracic aortic injury increased by 196% in the decade leading up to 2013 [47]. Despite imaging and management advances, the morbidity and mortality associated with traumatic aortic injury continue to be substantial. The reported mortality rate of traumatic aortic injury ranges from 33 to 85% [48, 49]. Most thoracic aortic injuries are due to blunt trauma from motor vehicle collision and, similar to cardiac trauma, the vast majority are instantly fatal and penetrating injuries are also most commonly due to stabbing or gunshot wounds [50, 51].

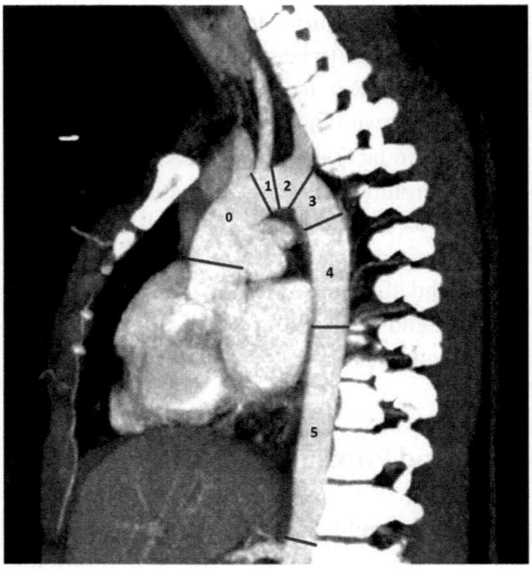

Fig. 6.8 Landing zones of the ascending aorta, aortic arch, and proximal descending aorta. *Zone 0* begins at the sinotubular junction and extends to the posterior wall of the brachiocephalic artery. *Zone 1* is demarcated by the origin of the left common carotid artery. *Zone 2* is demarcated by the origin of the left subclavian artery. *Zone 3* can be summarized as the aortic isthmus. *Zone 4* is the proximal descending aorta to the level of the T4 vertebral body. *Zone 5* is the mid-descending thoracic aorta to the origin of the celiac artery. *Zone 6–11*, not imaged, are the various segments of the abdominal aorta and the proximal common iliac arteries

Aortic root and ascending aortic injuries which may be observed on CT angiography include intraluminal filling defect, abnormal vessel contour, pseudoaneurysm, or extravasation of contrast (Fig. 6.9). In a 5-year retrospective study on motor vehicle fatalities, Williams et al. found the incidence of aortic injuries to be 17% (90/530), with majority, 66%, seen in the proximal descending aorta [52]. The most frequent location of thoracic aortic injury in blunt trauma is the aortic isthmus—although care should be taken to differentiate traumatic pseudoaneurysm of the aortic isthmus from a ductus diverticulum (Fig. 6.10). There are several potential causes of aortic injury in blunt trauma with acceleration and deceleration type injury favored to be the most common mechanism. Other described mechanisms are shearing forces, water-hammer phenomenon, or osseous pinch [53]. Traumatic aortic injury likely results from one or more of these combined factors.

Separately, acute aortic syndromes are entities which require emergent evaluation and possible surgical intervention—these include intramural hematoma, limited intimal tear, aortic dissection, and penetrating atherosclerotic ulcer. Although limited intimal tear, aortic dissection and intramural hematoma can be due to trauma, it is more likely that penetrating atherosclerotic ulcers are due to a chronic inflammatory process. Each, however, have characteristic appearances on CTA. In consideration of the three layers of the aortic wall (tunica intima, media, and adventitia), intimal tear refers to the disruption of the tunica intima which may be isolated or allow for blood to accumulate within the tunica media and result in dissection. Intramural hematoma, on the other hand, is caused by low pressure accumulation of blood within the tunica media without identifiable disruption of the tunica intima.

There are several different classification systems for blunt traumatic aortic injury [47–50, 54–57]. Azizzadeh et al. described four grades of injury: intimal tear, intramural hematoma, pseudoaneurysm, and rupture (Figs. 6.11, 6.12, 6.13, and 6.14) [56]. Starnes et al. maintained the classification system; however, they proposed that grade 2 describe a large intimal flap, intimal

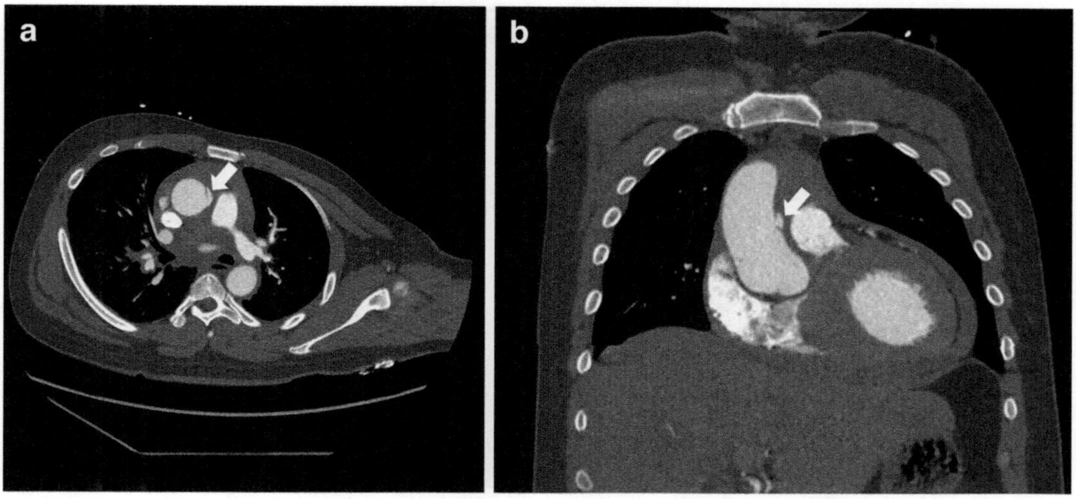

Fig. 6.9 Blunt trauma, ascending aortic injury. 42-year-old male presenting following motor vehicle collision. Axial (**a**) and coronal multiplanar reformation (**b**) of post-contrast CT chest in soft tissue window showing an intimal tear of the ascending aorta with pseudoaneurysm (white arrow), intramural hematoma, and hemopericardium in a patient presenting with chest pain following motor vehicle collision

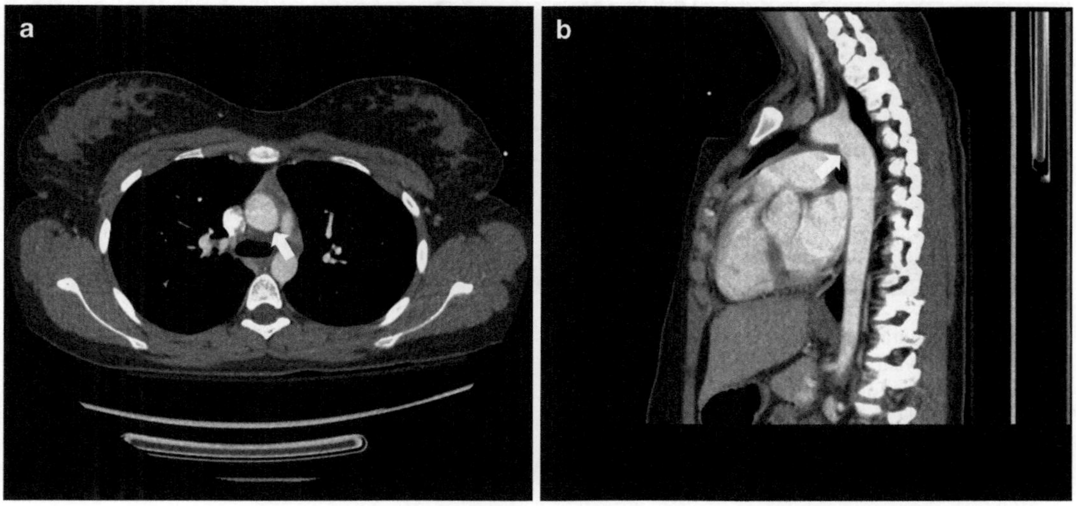

Fig. 6.10 Ductus diverticulum. 21-year-old female presenting following motor vehicle collision. Axial (**a**) and (**b**) sagittal maximal intensity projection of post-contrast CT chest in soft tissue window showing a ductus diverticulum (white arrow) at the anteromedial aortic isthmus

defect, or thrombus (>10 mm of length or width) instead of intramural hematoma [57]. The reported prevalence of intramural hematoma is 5–25% [58]. Although they are not aortic dissections, they are classified using the Stanford Classification for aortic dissection, where Stanford A involves the ascending aorta and Stanford type B may involve the aortic arch, descending aorta, and abdominal aorta. Pseudoaneurysm refers to a disruption in the tunica intima and media which results in focal hemorrhage contained by adventitia and may lead to rupture.

Diagnosis of intramural hematoma and definition of the diameter of the aorta and thickness of the hematoma can help determine prognosis and management [58]. In a 2013 review, Kruse et al. described high-risk features of CT for intramural

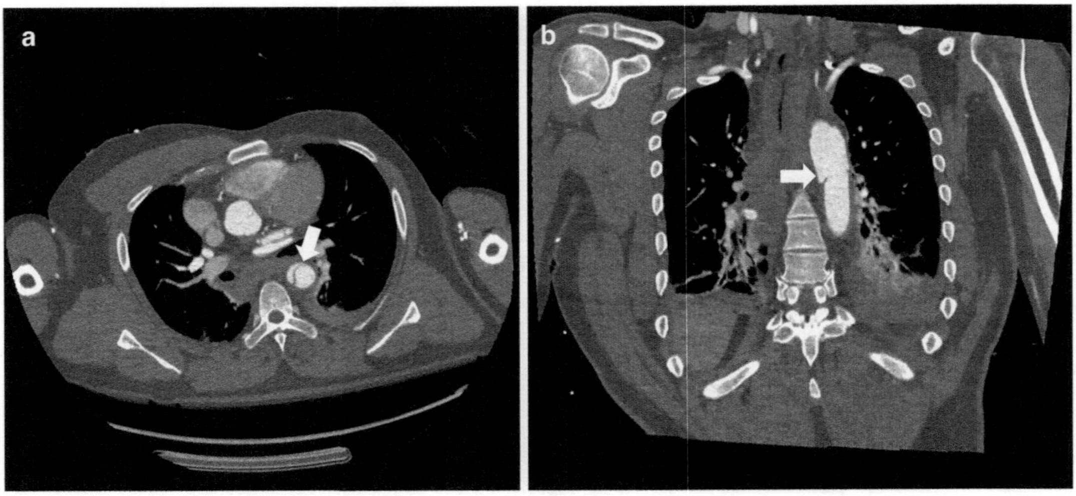

Fig. 6.11 Intimal tear. 39-year-old male presenting following motor vehicle collision. Axial (**a**) CTA of the chest and coronal multiplanar reformation (**b**) demonstrate a curvilinear hypodensity within the lumen of the descending aorta (white arrow), consistent with an intimal tear

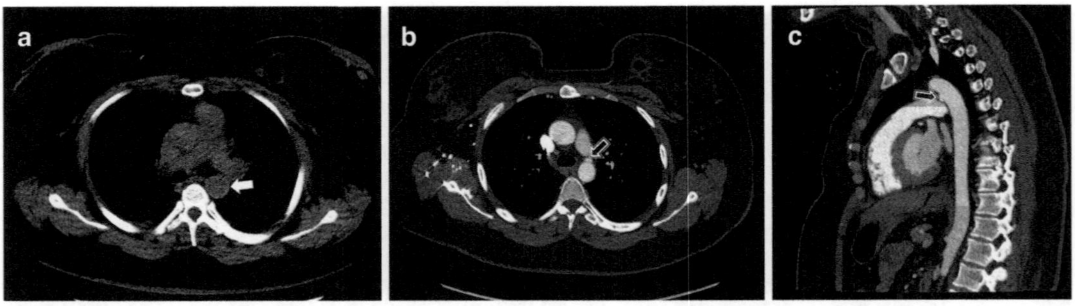

Fig. 6.12 Intramural hematoma of the descending aorta and pseudoaneurysm of the aortic isthmus. 29-year-old female presenting following motor vehicle collision. Axial unenhanced CT of the chest (**a**) demonstrates curvilinear hyperdensity within the aortic wall (white arrow); although subtle, this finding represents an intramural hematoma. Proximally, Axial (**b**) CTA of the chest with sagittal multiplanar reformation (**c**) show a focal outpouching of the anteromedial aspect of the very proximal descending aorta, consistent with a pseudoaneurysm of the aortic isthmus (yellow arrow)

hematoma—these include an enlarged diameter of the aorta, hematoma thickness, and classification as Stanford A [59]. CT can effectively diagnose minor aortic injuries and differentiate them from more severe injuries which require immediate treatment. The definition of minimal aortic injuries varies according to the referenced classification. Generally, it includes those involving only the intima of the vessel wall, including pseudoaneurysms which may depend on size [26].

Traumatic injuries to the aortic arch vessels are uncommon; however, these injuries have increased mortality and should be diagnosed promptly for adequate management. Radiographic screening for supra-aortic vessel injuries is not useful except in penetrating trauma [29].

Previously, conventional angiography was considered the gold standard for diagnosis; however, CTA has become the main imaging technique to evaluate the arch vessels [60, 61]. Still, there may be instances where CTA is inconclusive and patients may proceed to conventional angiography (Fig. 6.15).

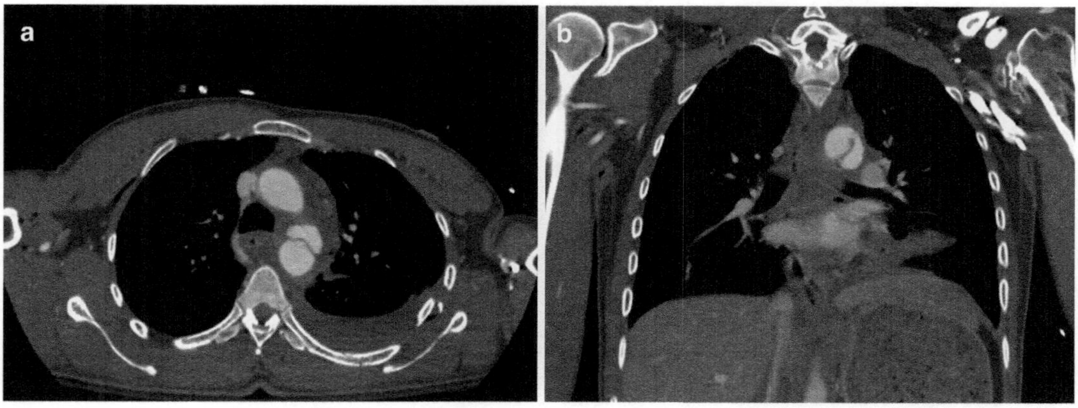

Fig. 6.13 Transection at the aortic isthmus. 45-year-old male presenting following motor vehicle collision. Axial (**a**) CTA of the chest with coronal multiplanar reformation (**b**) shows transection of the aortic isthmus with mediastinal hematoma

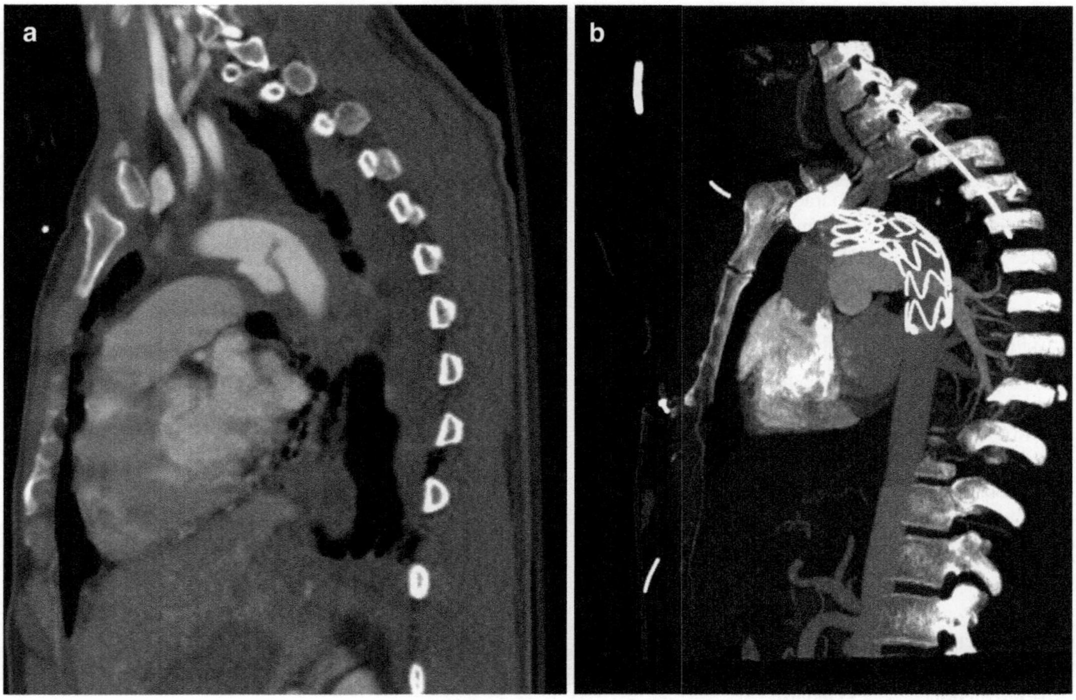

Fig. 6.14 Transection at the aortic isthmus status-post thoracic endovascular aortic repair. 45-year-old male presenting following motor vehicle collision. Sagittal (**a**) CTA of the chest again shows the transection of the aortic isthmus (same patient as Fig. 6.13) and sagittal maximum intensity projection (**b**) after successful transcatheter endovascular aortic repair

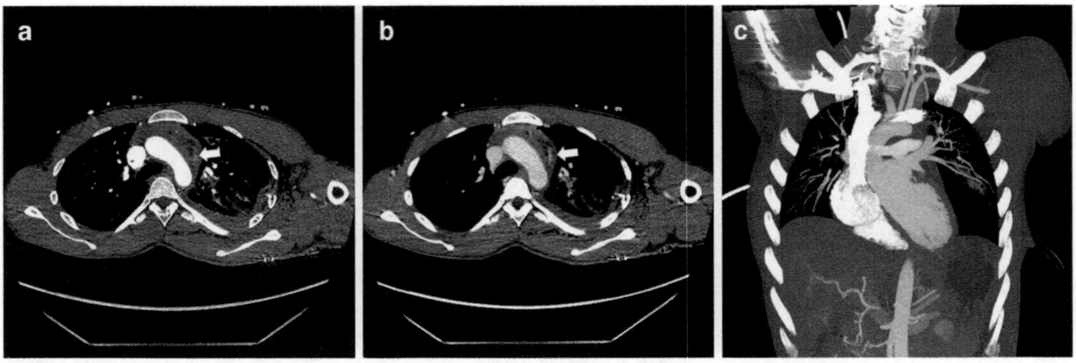

Fig. 6.15 Gunshot trauma with bullet adjacent to the aortic arch. (**a**) Coronal maximum intensity projection of CTA of the chest demonstrating a bullet adjacent to the aortic arch. Arterial phase (**b**) axial images just below the level of the bullet shows a prevascular mediastinal hematoma with increasing density on delayed phase (**c**) concerning for contrast extravasation secondary to arch vessel injury (white arrow). Patient subsequently underwent evaluation with conventional angiogram which showed normal contour of the aortic arch and arch vessels without contrast extravasation

CT Protocol

Protocol name	Thoracic trauma
Indication	Heart and great vessels
Patient preparation	Arms to be elevated
Anatomical coverage	Thoracic inlet to upper abdomen
Series	Unenhanced CT of the chest (non-gated)
Oral contrast	N/A
ECG/gating	OFF
Tube settings	
• kV	120
• mA	Automatic exposure control: mA 150–650
Tube rotation time (s)	0.5 s
Table speed (mm/s)	226.79 mm/s
Pitch	0.992
Slice width	1.25 mm
Reconstructed slice thickness	5 mm
Reconstruction kernel	Standard
Breath hold	Inspiration
Window settings	400/40
Series	CT angiography of the chest, arterial phase (ECG-gated)
Oral contrast	N/A
IV contrast (mL, mL/s)	100 mL at 3.5–5.0 mL/s
Saline flush	30 mL at 3.5–5.0 mL/s
ECG/gating	RR 65–70%, 150 mA

Protocol name	Thoracic trauma
Tube settings	
• kV	120
• mA	Automatic exposure control: mA 120–550
Tube rotation time (s)	0.5 s
Table speed (mm/s)	158.75 mm/s
Pitch	0.992
Slice width	0.625 mm
Reconstructed slice thickness	5 mm
Reconstruction kernel	Standard
Breath hold	Inspiration
Window settings	400/40
Post processing	Axial 1 mm standard kernel Axial 1 mm lung kernel Axial 3 mm standard and Lung kernel Sagittal and Coronal reconstruction 2 mm standard kernel

References

1. Gosavi S, Tyroch AH, Mukherjee D. Cardiac trauma. Angiology. 2016;67(10):896–901.
2. Moore EE, Malangoni MA, Cogbill TH, Shackford SR, Champion HR, Jurkovich GJ, et al. Organ injury scaling. IV: thoracic vascular, lung, cardiac, and diaphragm. J Trauma. 1994;36(3):299–300.

3. Campbell NC, Thomson SR, Muckart DJ, Meumann CM, Van Middelkoop I, Botha JB. Review of 1198 cases of penetrating cardiac trauma. Br J Surg. 1997;84(12):1737–40.
4. Teixeira PGR, Inaba K, Barmparas G, Georgiou C, Toms C, Noguchi TT, et al. Blunt thoracic aortic injuries: an autopsy study. J Trauma. 2011;70(1):197–202.
5. Turan AA, Karayel FA, Akyildiz E, Pakis I, Uzun I, Gurpinar K, et al. Cardiac injuries caused by blunt trauma: an autopsy based assessment of the injury pattern. J Forensic Sci. 2010;55(1):82–4.
6. Kaptein YE, Talving P, Konstantinidis A, Lam L, Inaba K, Plurad D, et al. Epidemiology of pediatric cardiac injuries: a National Trauma Data Bank analysis. J Pediatr Surg. 2011;46(8):1564–71.
7. Shackelford S, Nguyen L, Noguchi T, Sathyavagiswaran L, Inaba K, Demetriades D. Fatalities of the 2008 Los Angeles train crash: autopsy findings. Am J Disaster Med. 2011;6(2):127–31.
8. Turk EE, Tsang Y-W, Champaneri A, Pueschel K, Byard RW. Cardiac injuries in car occupants in fatal motor vehicle collisions–an autopsy-based study. J Forensic Legal Med. 2010;17(6):339–43.
9. Teixeira PGR, Georgiou C, Inaba K, Dubose J, Plurad D, Chan LS, et al. Blunt cardiac trauma: lessons learned from the medical examiner. J Trauma. 2009;67(6):1259–64.
10. Lustenberger T, Talving P, Lam L, Inaba K, Mohseni S, Smith JA, et al. Penetrating cardiac trauma in adolescents: a rare injury with excessive mortality. J Pediatr Surg. 2013;48(4):745–9.
11. Bakshi A, Wall MJ, Ghanta RK. Trauma to the heart and great vessels. In: Raja SG, editor. Cardiac surgery: a complete guide. Cham: Springer; 2020. p. 697–702.
12. Langdorf MI, Medak AJ, Hendey GW, Nishijima DK, Mower WR, Raja AS, et al. Prevalence and clinical import of thoracic injury identified by chest computed tomography but not chest radiography in blunt trauma: multicenter prospective cohort study. Ann Emerg Med. 2015;66(6):589–600.
13. Brink M, Deunk J, Dekker HM, Kool DR, Edwards MJR, van Vugt AB, et al. Added value of routine chest MDCT after blunt trauma: evaluation of additional findings and impact on patient management. AJR Am J Roentgenol. 2008;190(6):1591–8.
14. Branco BC, Musonza T, Long MA, Chung J, Todd SR, Wall MJ, et al. Survival trends after inferior vena cava and aortic injuries in the United States. J Vasc Surg. 2018;68(6):1880–8.
15. Giambuzzi M, Seitun S, Salsano A, Passerone G, Ferro C, Santini F. Nongated vs electrocardiography-gated CT imaging of blunt aortic root rupture in a trauma patient. J Cardiovasc Comput Tomogr. 2015;9(2):146–8.
16. Schertler T, Glücker T, Wildermuth S, Jungius K-P, Marincek B, Boehm T. Comparison of retrospectively ECG-gated and nongated MDCT of the chest in an emergency setting regarding workflow, image quality, and diagnostic certainty. Emerg Radiol. 2005;12(1–2):19–29.
17. Orliaguet G, Ferjani M, Riou B. The heart in blunt trauma. Anesthesiology. 2001;95(2):544–8.
18. Prêtre R, Chilcott M. Blunt trauma to the heart and great vessels. N Engl J Med. 1997;336(9):626–32.
19. Hammer MM, Raptis DA, Cummings KW, Mellnick VM, Bhalla S, Schuerer DJ, et al. Imaging in blunt cardiac injury: computed tomographic findings in cardiac contusion and associated injuries. Injury. 2016;47(5):1025–30.
20. Kan CD, Yang YJ. Traumatic aortic and mitral valve injury following blunt chest injury with a variable clinical course. Heart. 2005;91(5):568–70.
21. Asensio JA, Ogun OA, Petrone P, Perez-Alonso AJ, Wagner M, Bertellotti R, et al. Penetrating cardiac injuries: predictive model for outcomes based on 2016 patients from the National Trauma Data Bank. Eur J Trauma Emerg Surg. 2018;44(6):835–41.
22. Isaza-Restrepo A, Bolívar-Sáenz DJ, Tarazona-Lara M, Tovar JR. Penetrating cardiac trauma: analysis of 240 cases from a hospital in Bogota, Colombia. World J Emerg Surg. 2017;12:26.
23. Morse BC, Mina MJ, Carr JS, Jhunjhunwala R, Dente CJ, Zink JU, et al. Penetrating cardiac injuries: a 36-year perspective at an urban, level I trauma center. J Trauma Acute Care Surg. 2016;81(4):623–31.
24. Wall MJ, Mattox KL, Chen CD, Baldwin JC. Acute management of complex cardiac injuries. J Trauma. 1997;42(5):905–12.
25. Stranch EW, Zarzaur BL, Savage SA. Thinking outside the box: re-evaluating the approach to penetrating cardiac injuries. Eur J Trauma Emerg Surg. 2017;43(5):617–22.
26. Forman MJ, Mirvis SE, Hollander DS. Blunt thoracic aortic injuries: CT characterisation and treatment outcomes of minor injury. Eur Radiol. 2013;23(11):2988–95.
27. National Clinical Guideline Centre. Major trauma: assessment and initial management [Internet]. 2016 [cited 2023 Apr 12]. Available at https://www.ncbi.nlm.nih.gov/books/NBK344252/.
28. Gunn ML. Imaging of aortic and branch vessel trauma. Radiol Clin N Am. 2012;50(1):85–103.
29. Ketai L, Primack SL. Thoracic trauma. In: Hodler J, Kubik-Huch RA, von Schulthess GK, editors. Diseases of the chest, breast, heart and vessels 2019-2022: diagnostic and interventional imaging. Cham: Springer; 2019.
30. Lovy AJ, Rosenblum JK, Levsky JM, Godelman A, Zalta B, Jain VR, et al. Acute aortic syndromes: a second look at dual-phase CT. AJR Am J Roentgenol. 2013;200(4):805–11.
31. Bennett JM, Sileshi B. Incorrect diagnosis of type A aortic dissection attributed to motion artifact during computed tomographic angiography: a case report. Case Rep Dermatol. 2017;9(9):254–7.
32. Brinkman WT, Szeto WY, Bavaria JE. Overview of great vessel trauma. Thorac Surg Clin. 2007;17(1):95–108.
33. Bourricaudy NM, García AIP, Junco NM, Toledo OG. Lesión traumática de la vena cava superior,

parénquima e hilio pulmonar. Rev Cubana Med Mil. 2008;37:1.
34. Ramos Perkis JP, Ottolino Lavarte PR, Zinco Acosta A, Muñoz Alarcon CA, Diaz Fernandez A. Trauma de vena cava en pacientes politraumatizados: experiencia en el hospital Dr. Sótero del Río Rev Cir. 2020;72:1.
35. Sonavane SK, Milner DM, Singh SP, Abdel Aal AK, Shahir KS, Chaturvedi A. Comprehensive imaging review of the superior vena cava. Radiographics. 2015;35(7):1873–92.
36. Balachandran G, Bharathy KG, Sikora SS. Penetrating injuries of the inferior vena cava. Injury. 2020;51(11):2379–89.
37. Eleti S, Roshen M, Griffiths M, Cross S. Imaging in traumatic injury to the inferior vena cava. Clin Radiol. 2021;76(10):787.e15–25.
38. Tsai R, Raptis C, Schuerer DJ, Mellnick VM. CT appearance of traumatic inferior vena cava injury. AJR Am J Roentgenol. 2016;207(4):705–11.
39. Yanagawa Y, Ishikawa K, Nagasawa H, Takeuchi I, Jitsuiki K, Ohsaka H, et al. Traumatic pulmonary artery injury: a review of the recent literature. VP J. 2018;2(1):1.
40. Qamar SR, Wu Y, Nicolaou S, Murray N. State of the art imaging review of blunt and penetrating cardiac trauma. Can Assoc Radiol J. 2020;71(3):301–12.
41. Lin Y-Y, Tiu C-M, Chen J-D, Chou Y-H, Hsueh H-C, Tseng T-K, et al. Segmental pulmonary artery transection after blunt trauma. J Chin Med Assoc. 2014;77(7):389–92.
42. Le Guyader A, Bertin F, Laskar M, Cornu E. Blunt chest trauma: a right pulmonary vein rupture. Eur J Cardiothorac Surg. 2001;20(5):1054–6.
43. Fang R, Miller OL, Cai T, Kupferschmid JP, Stewart RM. Blunt avulsion of the right inferior pulmonary vein. J Trauma. 2004;56(1):191–3.
44. Nwaejike N, Mosca R, Hooper TL, Soon SY. Surgical repair of pulmonary vein injury from blunt trauma. Ann R Coll Surg Engl. 2015;97(3):e34–6.
45. Ishay SY, Raichel L, Tabo LY, Semyonov M, Barsky G, Acker A, et al. Penetrating pulmonary vein laceration following blunt chest trauma. Trauma Case Rep. 2022;37:100596.
46. Varghese D, Patel H, Cameron EW, Robson M. Repair of pulmonary vein rupture after deceleration injury. Ann Thorac Surg. 2000;70(2):656–8.
47. Isselbacher EM, Preventza O, Hamilton Black J, Augoustides JG, Beck AW, Bolen MA, et al. 2022 ACC/AHA guideline for the diagnosis and management of aortic disease: a report of the American heart association/American College of Cardiology Joint Committee on clinical practice guidelines. Circulation. 2022;146(24):e334–482.
48. Fillinger MF, Greenberg RK, McKinsey JF, Chaikof EL, Society for Vascular Surgery Ad Hoc Committee on TEVAR Reporting Standards. Reporting standards for thoracic endovascular aortic repair (TEVAR). J Vasc Surg. 2010;52(4):1022–33.
49. Bruckner BA, DiBardino DJ, Cumbie TC, Trinh C, Blackmon SH, Fisher RG, et al. Critical evaluation of chest computed tomography scans for blunt descending thoracic aortic injury. Ann Thorac Surg. 2006;81(4):1339–46.
50. Estrera AL, Miller CC, Guajardo-Salinas G, Coogan S, Charlton-Ouw K, Safi HJ, et al. Update on blunt thoracic aortic injury: fifteen-year single-institution experience. J Thorac Cardiovasc Surg. 2013;145(3):154–8.
51. Aghaei Afshar M, Mangeli F, Nakhaei A. Evaluation of injuries caused by penetrating chest traumas in patients referred to the emergency room. Indian J Surg. 2015;77(3):191–4.
52. Williams JS, Graff JA, Uku JM, Steinig JP. Aortic injury in vehicular trauma. Ann Thorac Surg. 1994;57(3):726–30.
53. Cullen EL, Lantz EJ, Johnson CM, Young PM. Traumatic aortic injury: CT findings, mimics, and therapeutic options. Cardiovasc Diagn Ther. 2014;4(3):238–44.
54. Prijon T, Ermenc B. Classification of blunt aortic injuries a new systematic overview of aortic trauma. Forensic Sci Int. 2010;195(1–3):6–9.
55. Duhaylongsod FG, Glower DD, Wolfe WG. Acute traumatic aortic aneurysm: the Duke experience from 1970 to 1990. J Vasc Surg. 1992;15(2):331–42; discussion 342.
56. Azizzadeh A, Keyhani K, Miller CC, Coogan SM, Safi HJ, Estrera AL. Blunt traumatic aortic injury: initial experience with endovascular repair. J Vasc Surg. 2009;49(6):1403–8.
57. Starnes BW, Lundgren RS, Gunn M, Quade S, Hatsukami TS, Tran NT, et al. A new classification scheme for treating blunt aortic injury. J Vasc Surg. 2012;55(1):47–54.
58. Spanos K, Kölbel T, Giannoukas AD. Current trends in aortic intramural hematoma management-a shift from conservative to a more aggressive treatment. Ann Cardiothorac Surg. 2019;8(4):497–9.
59. Kruse MJ, Johnson PT, Fishman EK, Zimmerman SL. Aortic intramural hematoma: review of high-risk imaging features. J Cardiovasc Comput Tomogr. 2013;7(4):267–72.
60. Waller CJ, Cogbill TH, Kallies KJ, Ramirez LD, Cardenas JM, Todd SR, et al. Contemporary management of subclavian and axillary artery injuries-A Western Trauma Association multicenter review. J Trauma Acute Care Surg. 2017;83(6):1023–31.
61. Jacks R, Degiannis E. Endovascular therapy and controversies in the management of vascular trauma. Scand J Surg. 2014;103(2):149–55.

Imaging of Gastrointestinal Trauma

7

Joanie Garratt, Paul Hill, and Mathew Hensley

Gastrointestinal Trauma

Abdominal and pelvic injuries, which involve both the gastrointestinal and genitourinary systems, are common in trauma patients, particularly in the setting of high-energy injuries such as falls from height, motor vehicle collisions, explosive trauma, and crush injuries [1]. The incidence of abdominal and pelvic injury in trauma patients varies with the population, diagnostic criteria, and grade of injury. Overall, abdominal and pelvic injuries occur in approximately 15–20% of all trauma patients [1, 2].

In abdominal trauma, injuries are most common in the spleen and liver [3]. In pelvic trauma, the bones, bladder, and urethra are the most commonly injured structures. Treatment for abdominal and pelvic injury varies with injury severity and may include conservative management, interventional radiology procedures, or surgery. Prompt recognition and treatment of these injuries are critical to avoid life-threatening complications such as bleeding and organ dysfunction.

J. Garratt (✉) · M. Hensley
Department of Radiology, University of Pennsylvania, Philadelphia, PA, USA
e-mail: joanie.garratt@pennmedicine.upenn.edu; mathew.hensley@pennmedicine.upenn.edu

P. Hill
Department of Radiology, Winchester Radiologists, Winchester, VA, USA

Blunt Trauma

Blunt injury accounts for approximately 70 percent of traumatic medical evaluations and includes motor vehicle collisions, falls, sports-related activities, and physical assaults [2, 4]. While there is an increased risk of trauma with higher velocity injuries, significant injury can occur from a seemingly minor impact, such as a ground-level fall; this is particularly true in the setting of underlying medical conditions and comorbidities. For example, underlying splenomegaly is associated with an increased risk of splenic injury. Likewise, there is an increased risk of bleeding complications, including from low-impact injuries, in the setting of anticoagulation therapy.

Penetrating Trauma

Although less common than blunt trauma, penetrating trauma causes significant morbidity and mortality. Penetrating trauma includes both non-ballistic (knife or puncture injury) and ballistic (gunshot wound) mechanisms, the latter accounting for the majority of mortality. Between 2013 and 2017, firearms were associated with 182,000 deaths and 500,000 cases of non-fatal injury in America. During the same period, there were 13,000 deaths from non-ballistic penetrating trauma [4].

F. Knollmann (ed.), *Trauma Computed Tomography*, https://doi.org/10.1007/978-3-031-45746-3_7

Injuries from ballistic trauma are secondary to direct injury from the projectile itself. In higher velocity ballistic injuries, there is an associated wound cavity produced by the displacement of tissue along the path of the projectile; therefore, it is important to evaluate for injury to structures adjacent to, in addition to along, the ballistic path. Of note, shotguns may use multiple pellets that can injure a patient; additionally, the cartridge wadding from a shotgun can become a projectile, embed within the soft tissues, and act as a nidus for infection. Suspicion for retained cartridge wadding should be high for all close-range shotgun injuries, as these are often radiolucent and may be more challenging to localize.

Imaging of Gastrointestinal Trauma

Imaging is critically important in the evaluation for gastrointestinal injuries in trauma patients. CT is the imaging modality of choice due to the speed of imaging acquisition, broad anatomical coverage, and accuracy in identifying clinically important injuries [5]. CT scanning can detect the extent and severity of injuries to the gastrointestinal system, including the liver, spleen, pancreas, bowel, and mesentery. Radiologists play a crucial role in identifying actionable gastrointestinal injuries that may quickly be treated by interventional radiology or surgeons to reduce morbidity and mortality of GI trauma. Some specific roles of CT in the evaluation of gastrointestinal trauma include:

- **Rapid and accurate diagnosis**: CT allows rapid identification of injuries to gastrointestinal structures, including lacerations, contusions, perforations, and hematomas. This information is important for making timely management decisions, particularly as some injuries may be clinically occult.
- **Non-invasive**: CT is a non-invasive imaging modality, which may be particularly beneficial in unstable trauma patients.
- **Identification of free fluid or air in the peritoneum**: CT allows detection of free air, fluid, or hemorrhage within the abdominal cavity.
- **Detection of specific injuries**: CT permits detailed identification of injuries to the abdominal organs and gastrointestinal tract, such as liver or splenic laceration, bowel wall thickening, mesenteric injury, or the presence of foreign bodies.
- **Assessment of the severity of injury**: CT provides information on the severity of gastrointestinal injury, including degree of organ involvement, presence of associated injuries, and extent of hemorrhage or inflammation.
- **Detection of associated injuries**: CT can also detect injuries to adjacent organs, including the adrenal glands and kidneys, which may affect management decisions.
- **Planning of surgical intervention**: CT can help guide the surgical approach to gastrointestinal injury, including the selection of the optimal surgical technique and the determination of the extent of resection or repair needed.
- **Follow-up**: CT can also be used to monitor the progression of healing in gastrointestinal injuries and to assess for any complications that may arise.

Management decisions in trauma patients are in part determined by imaging findings. For example, CT scanning can help determine whether surgery is necessary, or whether nonsurgical management such as observation or interventional radiology procedures is appropriate. CT scanning can also help determine the need for admission to the intensive care unit, blood transfusions, or other interventions.

In summary, CT is a valuable tool in the evaluation of gastrointestinal injury in trauma patients, as it can provide detailed information on the presence and extent of injury, guide treatment decisions, and help to optimize patient outcomes.

CT Protocol

To expertly evaluate for gastrointestinal trauma, the method of diagnostic imaging acquisition must be tailored to each patient, including consideration of clinical and functional status. Contrast-enhanced CT imaging is considered the gold standard diagnostic choice to evaluate of injuries to the gastrointestinal system because of its high sensitivity and specificity [6–8]; however, this relies on factors such as a readily available CT scanner and a hemodynamically stable patient. For contrast-enhanced CT of the abdomen and pelvis, images can be obtained at one or more phases of the contrast enhancement cycle. Common phases of contrast acquisition include

- **Unenhanced phase**: Prior to administration of intravenous contrast. Unenhanced, or non-enhanced, images are useful in the detection of hematomas, including intraparenchymal hematomas, and renal calculi.
- **Early arterial phase** (15–20 seconds after intravenous contrast or immediately after bolus-tracking): Contrast is located within arteries (angiographic phase), but has not reached abdominopelvic organs. This phase is useful for assessing vascular injuries.
- **Late arterial phase** (35–40 s after intravenous contrast administration or 20 s after bolus-tracking): This phase is also known as late hepatic arterial phase because some contrast is seen in the portal vein. There is optimal enhancement of hypervascular liver lesions, pancreatic parenchyma, and spleen during this phase. This phase is useful for detecting active bleeding from solid organs, including the liver and kidneys (Fig. 7.1).
- **Corticomedullary phase** (40–70 s after intravenous contrast): There is optimal enhancement of the renal cortex during this phase, which is distinct from the hypoenhancing renal medulla. This phase is helpful in evaluation for enhancing urothelial lesions.
- **Portovenous phase** (70–80 s after intravenous contrast administration or 50–60 s after bolus-tracking): This phase is also known as the hepatic phase because there is optimal enhancement of hepatic parenchyma, which receives most of its blood supply from the portal vein. Contrast should be seen in the portal and hepatic veins during this phase of contrast. This phase is useful for assessing parenchymal injuries to solid organs, including the liver (Fig. 7.1).
- **Nephrographic phase** (100 s after intravenous contrast administration or 80 s after bolus-tracking): There is homogenous enhancement of the renal parenchyma, including both the cortex and medulla. This phase of contrast allows detection of small renal lesions and has limited use in the trauma setting.
- **Delayed phase** (5–10 min after intravenous contrast administration or bolus-tracking): This phase is also known as the washout or equilibrium phase as contrast has washed out of all abdominal structures.
- **Excretory phase** (5–15 min after intravenous contrast or bolus-tracking): This phase is useful in evaluation for filling defects, strictures, or extravasation of contrast involving the collecting systems, ureters or urinary bladder.

The specific trauma CT protocol varies by institution and may include single, multiple or combined phases of contrast. Many institutions utilize a version of the "pan scan," in which rapid whole-body CT is performed [1].

- **Single phase imaging:** A single set of images during one phase of contrast is acquired. Typically, the portal venous phase is preferred as this phase of contrast is both sensitive and specific for solid organ injury [1]; however, repeat imaging in the arterial phase is often necessary if there is concern for active bleeding or pseudoaneurysm on the portal venous phase, requiring additional intravenous contrast. Alternatively, acquisition of delayed-phased images may help differentiate a contained hematoma from an active bleed or underlying vascular injury; if performed in a timely manner, additional intravenous contrast may not be necessary [9]. Visualization of active contrast extravasation is a positive sign of active hemorrhage, and the presence of an underlying vascular injury closely correlates with an elevated injury grade [10].
- **Multiphase imaging**: Multiple sets of images are obtained concurrently at different phases of contrast (Fig. 7.1). For instance, multiphase imaging with both arterial and portal venous phases (also known as dual phase imaging)

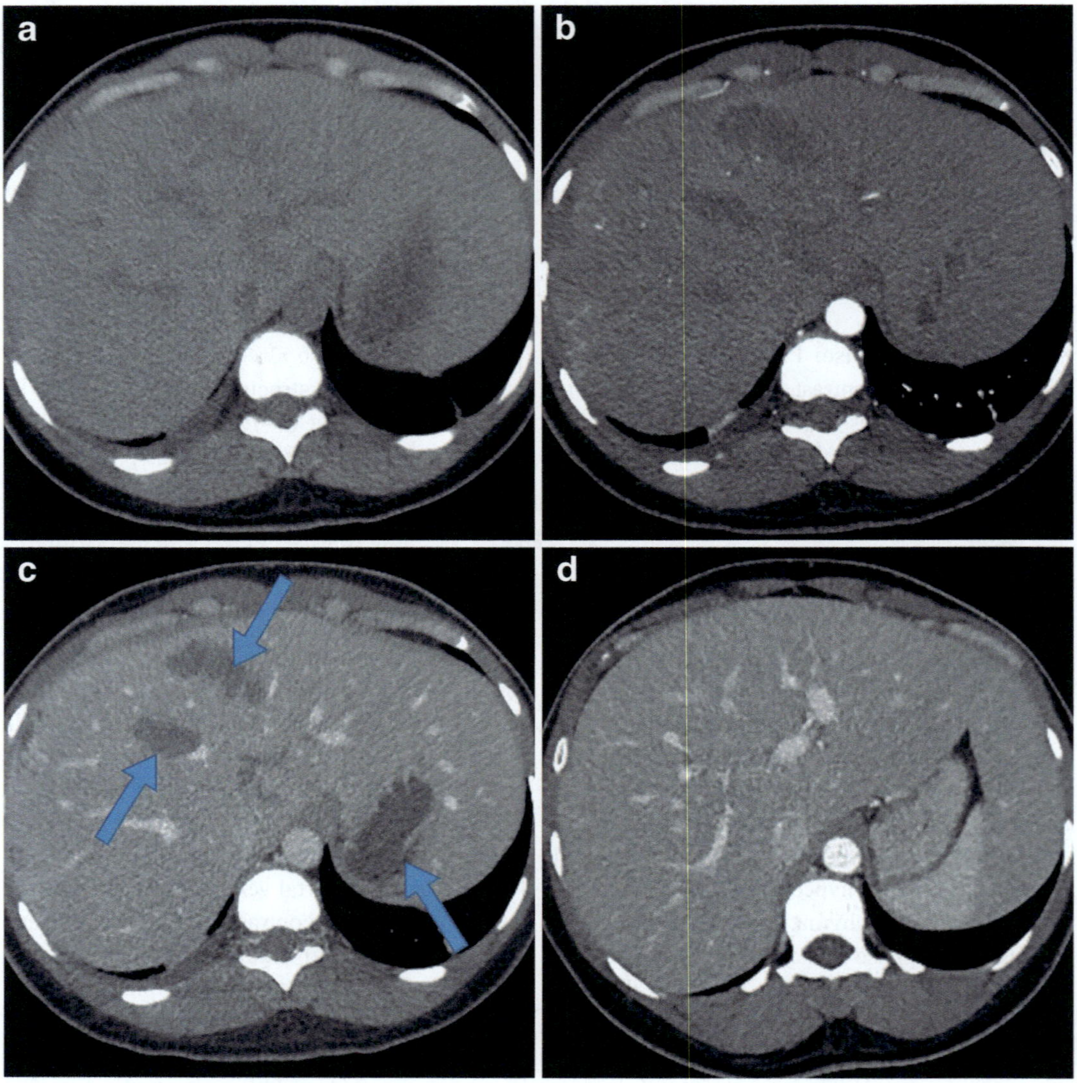

Fig. 7.1 Axial CT images of the liver on unenhanced (**a**), late hepatic arterial (**b**), and portal venous (**c**) phases of contrast in a 29-year-old patient with a history of motor vehicle collision. The arterial phase of contrast (**b**) best delineates vascular injury, noting that there is no vascular injury in this patient. The portal venous phase (**c**) provides better evaluation of the hepatic parenchyma, including parenchymal injury. Several areas of linear hypoattenuation are seen within the liver (arrows), in keeping with lacerations. This patient was managed conservatively without surgery. Follow-up axial CT performed 1 year later (**d**) shows interval healing of those lacerations. AAST grade III/IV liver injury

provides a thorough evaluation of the abdomen and pelvis as vascular injury is best evaluated on the arterial phase and parenchymal injury is best evaluated on the portal venous phase.

- **Combined arterial and portal venous phase imaging**: Intravenous contrast is administered in two boluses. A single set of images is then obtained, which has contrast in both the arterial and portal venous phases of enhancement (Fig. 7.2) [11]. This technique requires a larger contrast volume but reduces the radiation dose compared to multiphase imaging; it also prevents repeat imaging in patients with

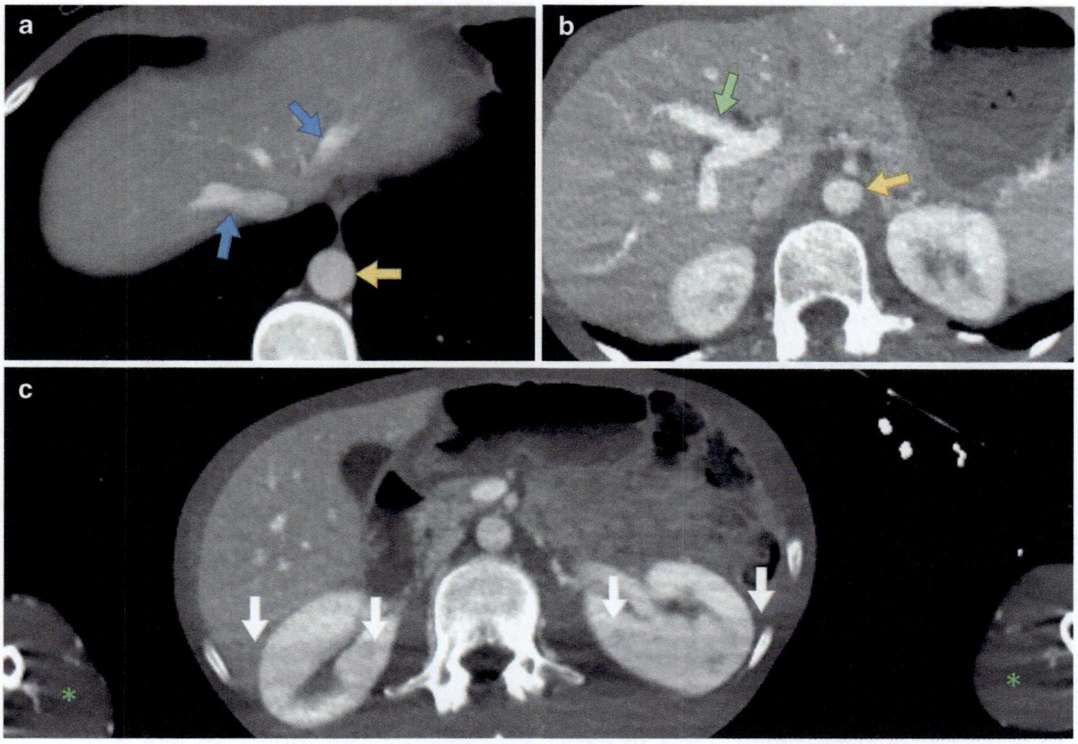

Fig. 7.2 Axial (**a**, **b**) CT images show contrast opacification of the aorta (yellow arrows), portal veins (green arrow), and hepatic veins (blue arrows) in the setting of combined arterial and portal venous phase imaging. Intravenous contrast was administered in two boluses; a single set of images was then obtained, which has contrast in both the arterial (as demonstrated by contrast in the aorta) and portal venous phases of enhancement (as demonstrated by contrast in the portal and hepatic veins). Axial (**c**) CT image at the level of the kidneys shows artifact (white arrows) from arms (green asterisks) overlying the upper abdomen, mimicking renal parenchymal injury

suspected active bleeding on single phase portal venous phase imaging. Combined arterial and portal venous phase images allow detection of vascular injuries and active bleeding as well as parenchymal injuries on the same set of images (Fig. 7.3). An example protocol is given in Table 7.1.

Other considerations in developing a trauma CT protocol are as follows:

- Dual energy CT imaging, when available, utilizes two different photon energies during the image acquisition, typically a high energy of 140 kVp and a low energy of 80–100 kVp. There are several benefits to using dual energy CT, including the ability to create virtual unenhanced images, monoenergetic images, and iodine maps. Monoenergetic images improve detection of subtle solid organ injuries by increasing the contrast to noise ratio. Iodine maps also improve visualization of subtle injuries by accentuating differences in contrast [12].
- Another described technique is a "triple-contrast" CT protocol, which includes oral, rectal, and intravenous without additional contrast. This protocol particularly useful in the setting of penetrating trauma as it demonstrates high sensitivity and specificity in identifying visceral injury and peritoneal violation [13].
- Patient positioning is important. Elevation of the arms above the head is particularly important because the beam hardening artifact that results from arms overlying the upper abdomen mimics organ injury (Fig. 7.2).

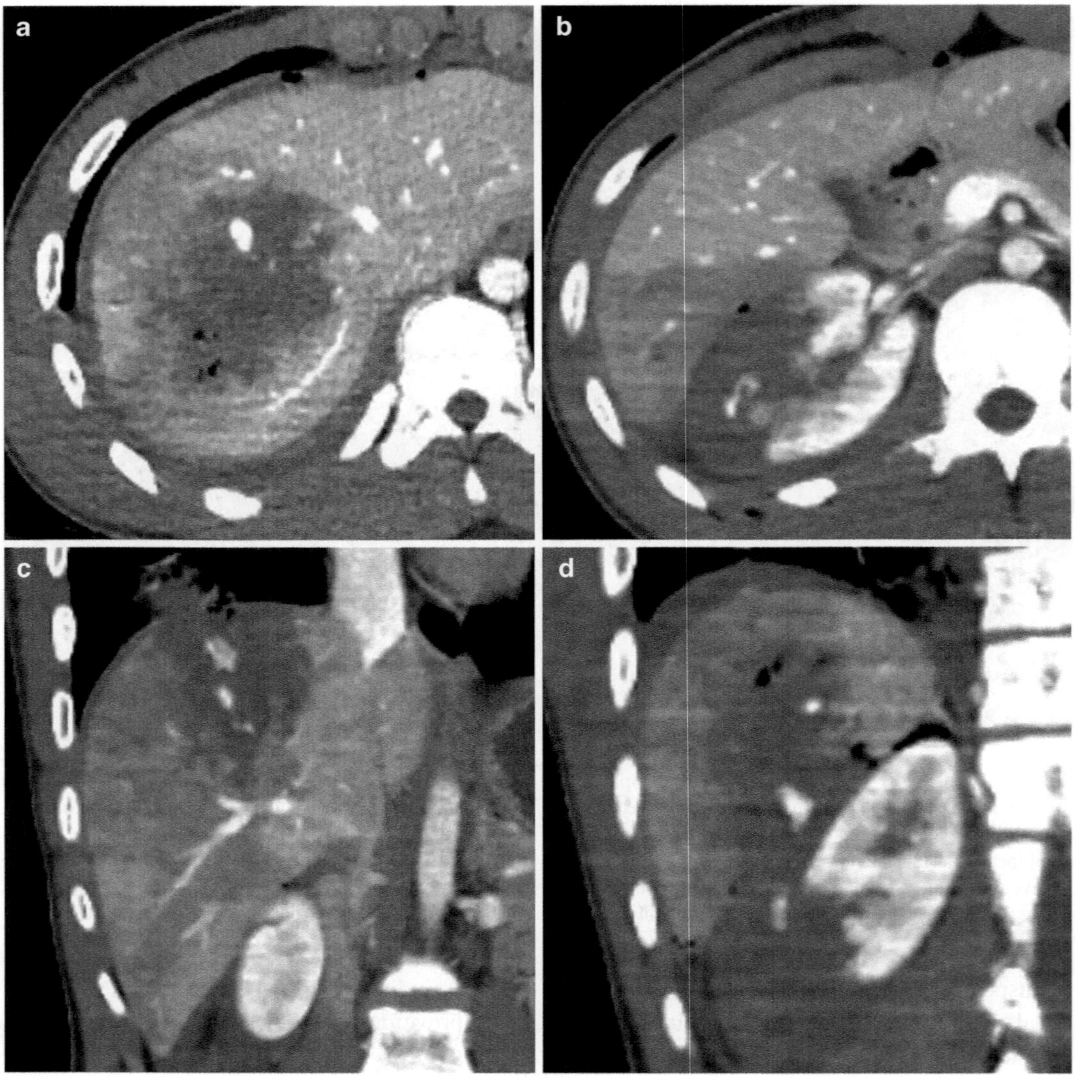

Fig. 7.3 A 30-year-old patient presents with penetrating trauma. Axial (**a**, **b**) and coronal (**c**, **d**) CT images from combined arterial and venous phase scan demonstrate active bleeding (blue arrows) from both the liver (**a**, **c**, **d**) and kidney (**b**). This combined phase technique allows concurrent evaluation of the hepatic and renal parenchyma, noting a hepatic laceration and right renal segmental infarction in this patient

It is essential to optimize the CT technique and protocols used in the evaluation of trauma patients. There are many factors to consider, including contrast material as well as the number and timing of phases.

Table 7.1 Example CT protocol to evaluate for gastrointestinal trauma

CT trauma chest, abdomen and pelvis protocol (one run): combined arterial and portal venous phase imaging			
Clinical indication		Severe, life threatening head and or body trauma. To be requested by the trauma surgeon	
Age		Adult	
Dose range		38.64–60.41 mGy	
Body habitus		mA modulation and automated kV selection are utilized to account for different patient body habitus	
Prep		18 or 20 gauge IV	
Contrast administration		125 mL Isovue 370	
Scan parameters	kV	120	
	mA	Smart mA	
	mA Min/Max	100–550	
	Noise Index	12.23	
	Scan Type	Helical	
	SFOV	Large body	
	DFOV	36.0	
	Detector coverage (mm)	80	
	Pitch	0.992:1	
	Coverage speed (mm/s)	65.62	
	Rotation time (s)	0.80	
	Slice collimation (mm)	0.625	
	Thickness (mm)	5	
	Scan interval (mm)	5	
	ASIR	50%	
	WW/WL	40/40	
	Algorithm (Recon type)	Standard; 2 mm and 5 mm	
Scan procedure		Every attempt should be made to raise the arms above head	
		Lung apices through lesser trochanters	
		Start scan and injector simultaneously	
IV injection	Notes	Dual syringe, 325 psi (PICC or power port- 300 psi)	
		SPLIT injection: 70 mL @ 3 mL/s, 55 mL @ 2 mL/s	
		Injection delay: 65 seconds	
	Solution	**Rate**	**Amount**
	Saline	3 mL/s	20 mL
	Contrast	3 mL/s	70 mL
	Contrast	2 mL/s	55 mL
	Saline	2 mL/s	20 mL

Injury Assessment and Grading

The Organ Injury Scale (OIS) created by the American Association for the Surgery of Trauma (AAST) is a classification system that standardizes the assessment and severity of traumatic organ injury and guides management. OIS grades injuries from minor (grade I or II) to severe or life-threatening (grade V or VI). This grading system accounts for location, size, and depth of injury, including vascular injury such as arteriovenous fistulae or pseudoaneurysm. The most recent update in 2018 includes imaging findings, acknowledging the importance of imaging evaluation of trauma patients since its first use in the 1980s [1, 12, 14–19]. In fact, the accuracy of CT imaging in evaluating injuries in trauma patients has allowed nonsurgical management to become the standard of care in hemodynamically stable patients. The imaging findings for the AAST OIS are detailed in this text; there are separate criteria for operative and pathologic findings. Overall, the most common injuries are grade II [12].

The AAST OIS are the most widely accepted classification systems and are most commonly used in the evaluation of solid viscera injuries, including traumatic injuries of the liver, spleen, and pancreas. A grading system helps clinicians to better understand the extent of the injury and to guide further management, such as whether surgical intervention is required. In addition, a classification system can help to standardize communication among healthcare professionals, facilitating accurate and consistent reporting of injuries in trauma patients.

Hepatic Trauma

Although the reported prevalence and incidence varies, hepatic injury is common in abdominal trauma, particularly in the setting of high-energy blunt abdominal trauma such as falls from height and motor vehicle collisions [3, 5, 12]. Hepatic injury is less common in the setting of penetrating trauma, such as stab or gunshot wounds. Complications from hepatic injury range from minor contusions to life-threatening lacerations or ruptures.

Anatomy

About the size of a football, the liver is the largest and one of the most commonly injured internal organs. The liver is comprised of two lobes, noting that the caudate lobe is considered part of the left hepatic lobe [1]. The liver has a dual blood supply from the portal vein, formed by the convergence of the splenic and superior mesenteric veins, and the common hepatic artery, one of the three branches from the celiac axis [1]. Blood is returned from the liver into circulation via the hepatic veins, which converge at the hepatic dome and drain into the inferior vena cava.

Anatomically, the liver is divided into eight functional segments using the Couinaud system, which separates the liver vertically by the portal veins and horizontally by the hepatic veins [12]:

- **Caudate lobe**: Segment I
- **Left hepatic lobe**: Segments II, III, Iva, and IVb
- **Right hepatic lobe**: Segments V, VI, VII, and VIII

Except for the bare area of the liver along the posterior aspect of segment VII, which communicates with the retroperitoneal space, the liver is covered by visceral peritoneum [12].

In blunt trauma, injuries typically occur at the segmental divisions, likely because of the strength of the portal triad covering. In vascular injury of the liver, the hepatic veins are more often injured because of the absence of this fibrous covering. Penetrating trauma, however, can transect any structure [1].

The liver is located in the right upper quadrant inferior to the right hemidiaphragm. The right adrenal gland and right kidney are located along the medial aspect of the liver, adjacent to the bare area. The hepatic flexure of the colon, stomach, duodenum, pancreas, and gallbladder are located inferior to the liver.

Imaging and Grading

CT is the modality of choice for imaging evaluation of traumatic hepatic injury because of its ability to determine the severity and extent of the injury. Some specific CT findings of liver injury include:

- **Hematoma**: Collection of blood within the liver, which typically appears as an area of hypoattenuation (decreased density) relative to the parenchyma on CT images. However, if the blood is acute or hyperacute, it may appear hyper- or isoattenuating (increased or similar density).
  - Subcapsular hematomas are peripherally located collections that are confined by the

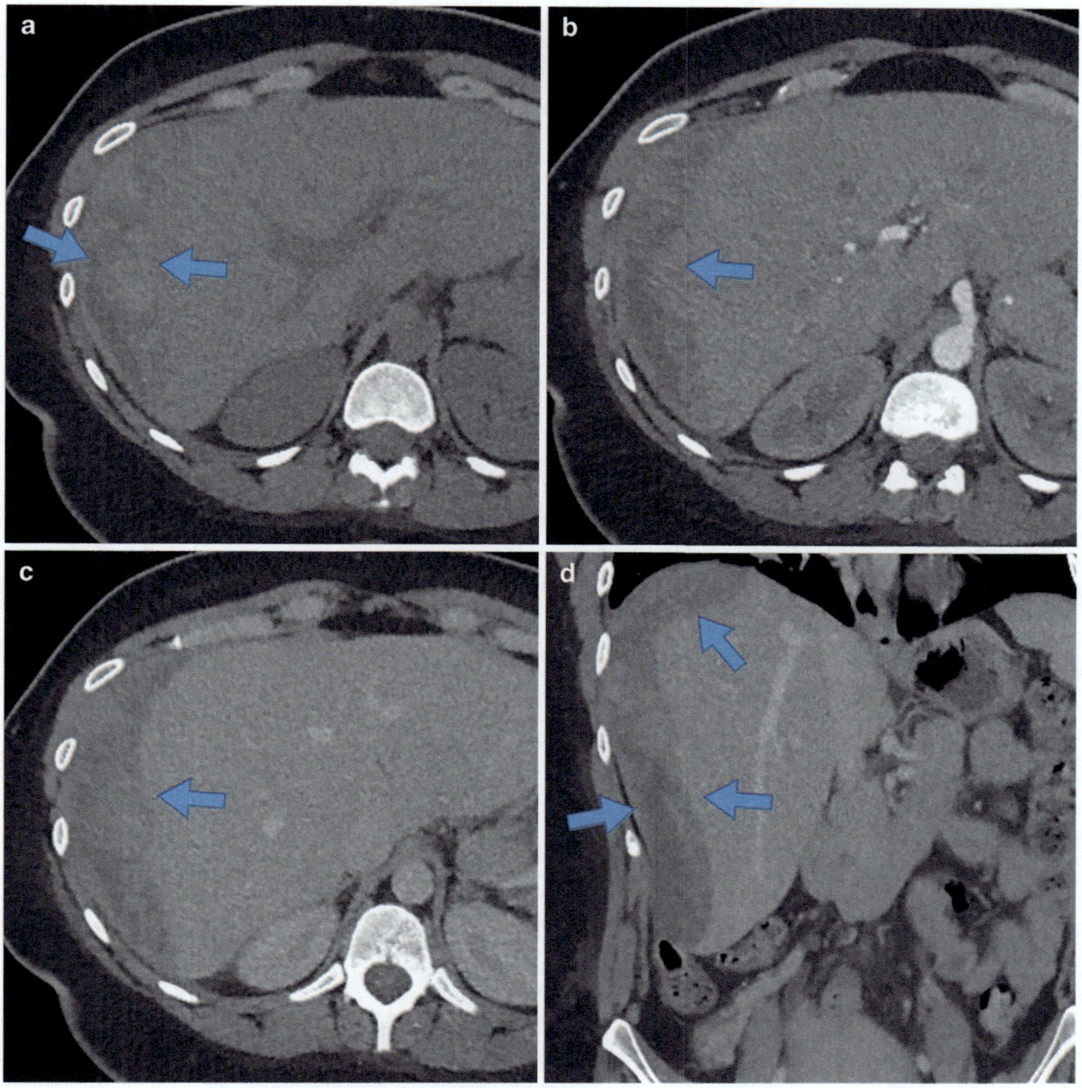

Fig. 7.4 CT images of the liver, including axial unenhanced (**a**), axial late hepatic arterial (**b**), and axial (**c**) and coronal (**d**) portal venous phases, in a 30-year-old patient show a large, crescent-shaped area of heterogeneity along the periphery of the right hepatic lobe. This collection conforms to the expected contour of the liver with mass effect of the underlying parenchyma. Findings are in keeping with a subcapsular hematoma of the liver. No associated foci of contrast extravasation on the arterial phase to suggest active bleeding. AAST grade III liver injury

liver capsule; often crescent-shaped and exert mass effect upon the underlying parenchyma (Fig. 7.4).
  - Intraparenchymal hematomas are located within the parenchyma, are often oval or rounded, and also exert mass effect upon the parenchyma (Fig. 7.5) [12].
- **Laceration**: Tear in the liver tissue, which most often appears as linear or branching area of hypoattenuation within the liver parenchyma (Figs. 7.1 and 7.6). If a laceration extends to the bare area, there may be an associated retroperitoneal hematoma. Lacerations are the most common hepatic injury [12]. Hypoattenuation along the falciform ligament related to focal fatty infiltration or a perfusional variant may mimic a hepatic laceration (Fig. 7.7)

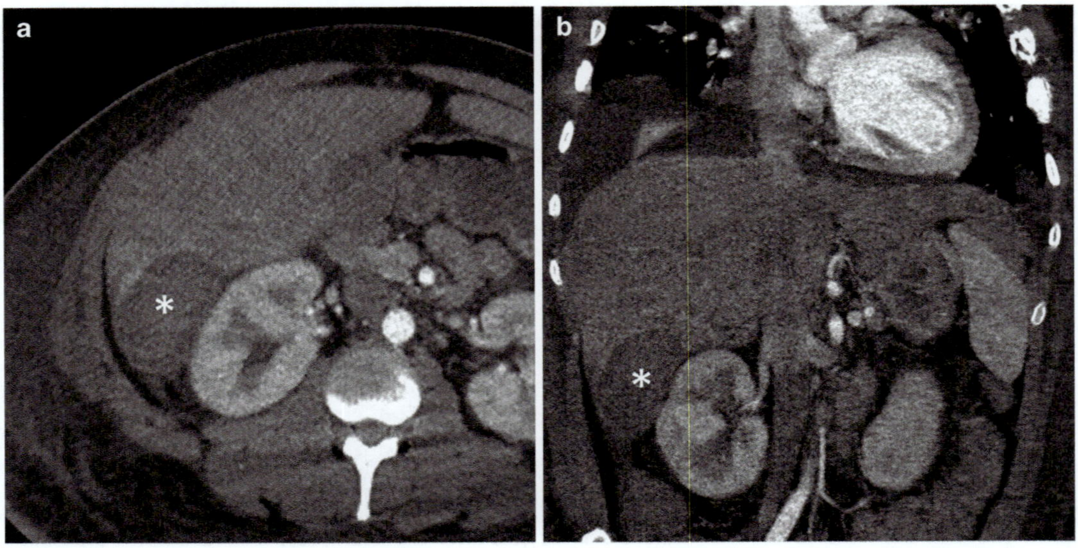

Fig. 7.5 Axial (**a**) and coronal (**b**) contrast-enhanced images of a 28 year old show an intraparenchymal hematoma (asterisk) in segment 5/6 of the liver. AAST grade II/III liver injury

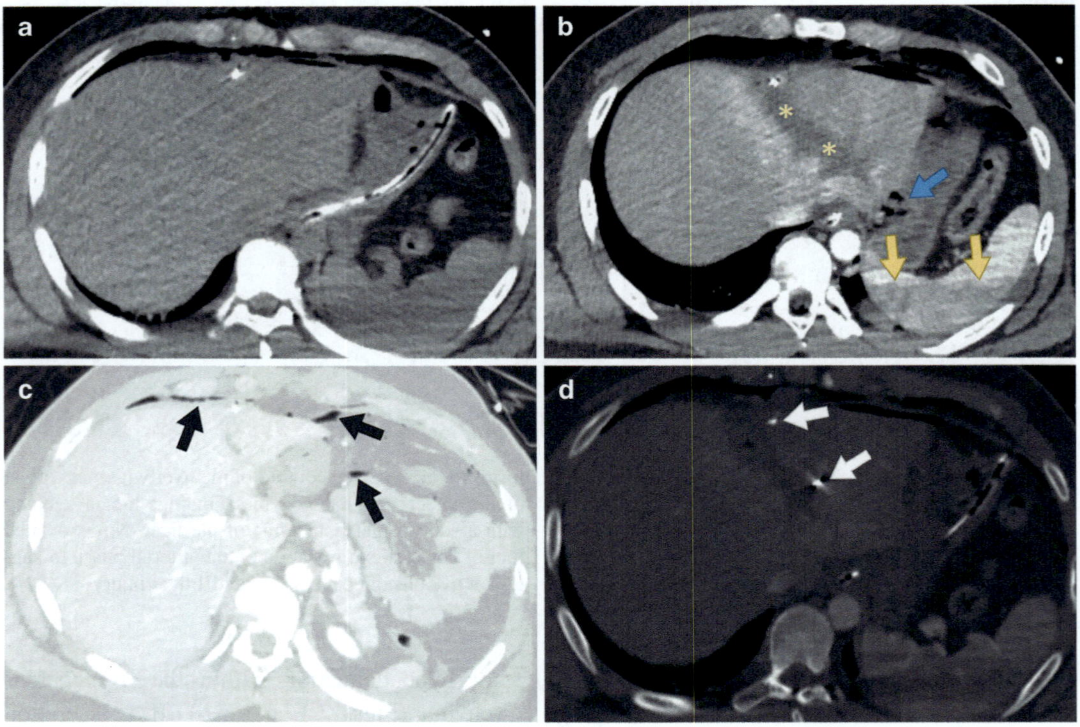

Fig. 7.6 CT images of the upper abdomen in a 25-year-old trauma patient presenting with gunshot wounds. Hepatic injury is inconspicuous on the axial unenhanced image (**a**), demonstrating the importance of intravenous contrast in trauma patients. Linear area of hypoattenuation (asterisks) in the left hepatic lobe on axial portal venous phase image (**b**), in keeping with a liver laceration; adjacent hyperattenuating band likely reflects component of hematoma. Linear band of hypoattenuation in the spleen (yellow arrows) is related to beam hardening artifact from the patient's overlying arms, which is a mimic of trauma. Foci of extraluminal air abutting the lesser curvature of the stomach (blue arrow) suggests gastric wall injury, located along the ballistic trajectory. Foci of extraluminal air (pneumoperitoneum) within the upper abdomen (black arrows) are more conspicuous on axial image with lung window (**c**). Metallic ballistic fragments within the liver (white arrows) are more conspicuous on axial image with bone window (**d**). AAST grade III liver injury

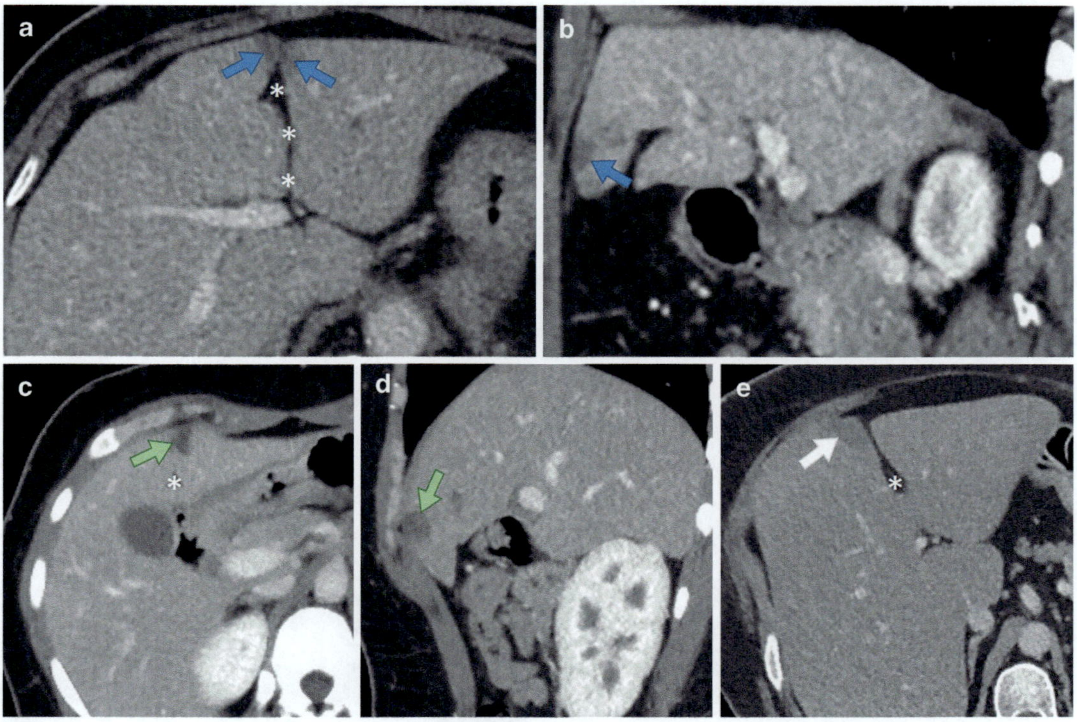

Fig. 7.7 CT images of the upper abdomen in a 26-year-old trauma patient presenting with gunshot wounds. Axial arterial phase images (**a**, **b**) show hyperattenuating foci (similar attenuation to intravenous contrast) that represent areas of active bleeding, including within the liver (blue arrows), from the left gastric artery (green arrow) and into the stomach (white arrow). Extraluminal air along the stomach (yellow arrow) is more conspicuous on lung window (**c**) and indicates full-thickness mural injury/laceration. The ballistic trajectory (yellow asterisks) through the liver and stomach in the upper abdomen is best seen on coronal imaging (**d**). Axial (**e**) and coronal (**f**) portal venous images show extensive hepatic parenchymal injury (white asterisks) that extends to the porta hepatis. Hyperattenuating contrast in the stomach on portal venous phase is related to blood products from active bleeding (black asterisk). Patient was taken directly to the operating room from the CT scanner. AAST grade V liver injury and grade II gastric injury

- **Active bleeding**: Contrast extravasation, which is leakage of contrast material from the blood vessels within the liver, may indicate active bleeding. This appears as an area of hyperattenuating contrast material (similar in attenuation to that within the vessels) outside the blood vessels on CT images (Fig. 7.8). The area of hemorrhage enlarges on the slightly later portal venous phase of contrast. Patients with active bleeding usually require management with surgery or interventional radiology [12].
- **Pseudoaneurysm**: Localized outpouchings of an artery, most often the hepatic artery, secondary to injury of a vessel with contained hematoma. Pseudoaneurysms appear as well-circumscribed, contrast-enhancing structures on CT images. Although asymptomatic, pseudoaneurysms are at risk of rupturing and causing fatal hemorrhage [12].
- **Arteriovenous fistula** (AVF): Rare abnormal communication between the hepatic artery and a vein, either a portal vein or a suprahepatic vein, that usually results from penetrating trauma. On imaging, an AVF should be suspected if there is enhancement of a structure during both arterial and venous phases [5].
- **Major venous injury**: Injury to at least one major vein, including portal veins, hepatic veins, and the inferior venous cava. On imaging, this should be suspected if there is a lac-

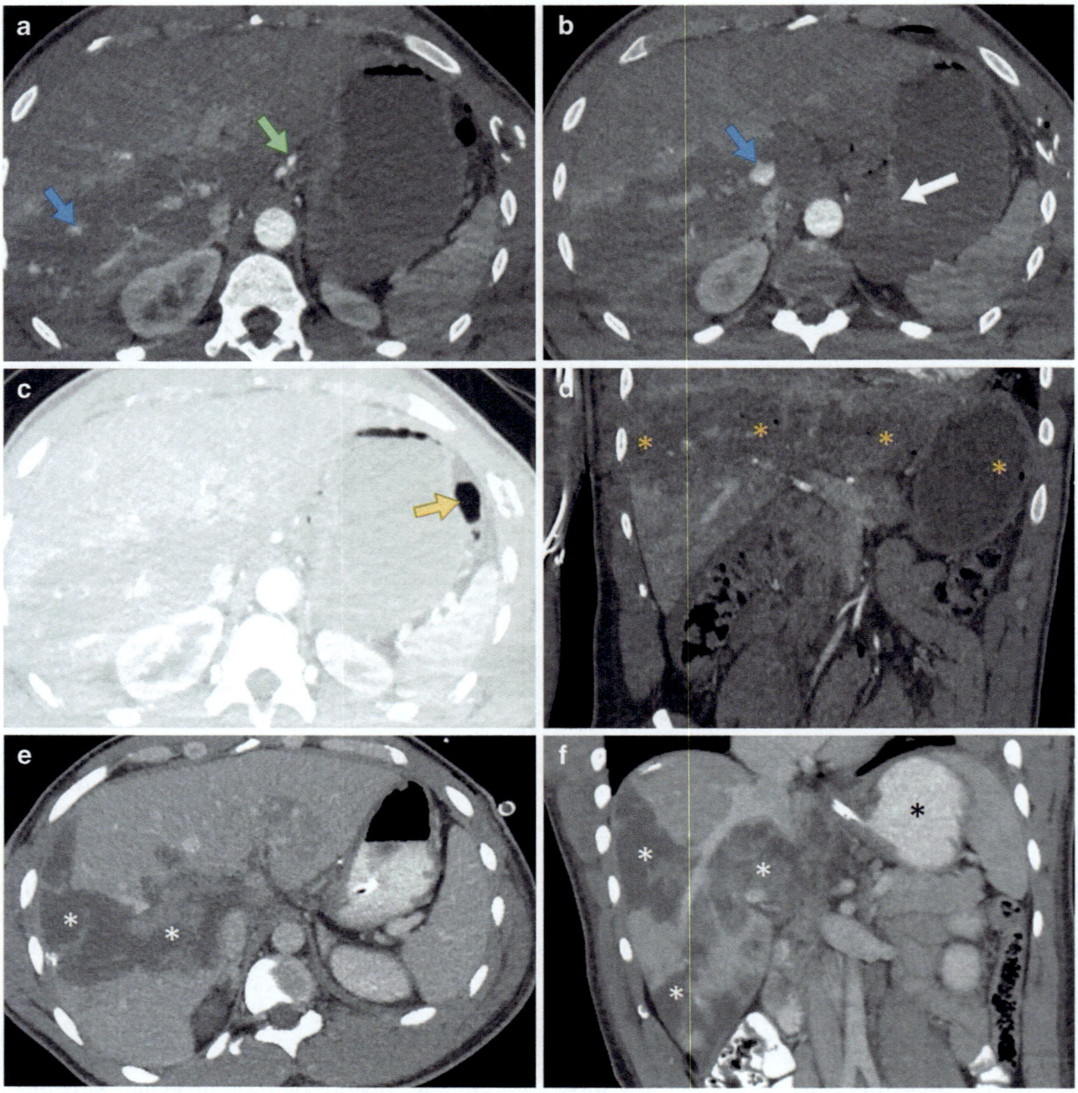

Fig. 7.8 Axial (**a**) and sagittal (**b**) portal venous images in a patient show an area of hypoattenuation (blue arrows) along the falciform ligament (white asterisks on **a**). This finding is a common variant seen on imaging, which is secondary to focal fatty infiltration or a perfusional variant. However, it mimics a hepatic parenchymal injury. Axial (**c**, **e**) and sagittal (**d**) portal venous phase images in two additional patients show similar findings of hepatic pseudolesions/pseudoinjuries (green and white arrows) along the falciform ligament (white asterisks on **c**, **e**)

eration that extends to a major vein (Fig. 7.8). Typically in the setting of severe injury, mortality from major venous injuries has been reported as high as 70 percent [12].

The AAST OIS is the most commonly used scale to assess liver injury and the CT findings are detailed in Table 7.2.

Management and Complications

Liver injury grading can help guide management decisions for trauma patients, as management depends on the severity of the injury, associated injuries, and whether or not the patient is hemodynamically stable. Controlling bleeding, preventing further injury, and promoting liver tissue

Table 7.2 AAST liver injury scale [14, 19]

AAST grade[b]	Hematoma	Laceration	Vascular injury
I	Subcapsular, <10% surface area	Capsular tear, <1 cm Parenchymal depth	
II	Subcapsular, 10% to 50% surface area	Capsular tear 1–3 cm parenchymal depth, <10 cm in length	
	Intraparenchymal <10 cm in diameter		
III	Subcapsular, >50% surface area of ruptured subcapsular or parenchymal hematoma	>3 cm parenchymal depth	Any injury in the presence of a liver vascular injury[a] (pseudoaneurysm or arteriovenous fistula) or active bleeding contained within liver parenchyma
	Intraparenchymal hematoma >10 cm or expanding		
IV		Parenchymal disruption involving 25% to 75% hepatic lobe or 1–3 Couinaud's segments	Active bleeding[c] extending beyond the liver parenchyma into the peritoneum
V		Parenchymal disruption involving >75% of hepatic lobe or > 3 Couinaud's segments within a single lobe	Juxtahepatic venous injuries; i.e., retrohepatic vena cava/central major hepatic veins
VI			Hepatic avulsion

[a]Vascular injuries are defined as a pseudoaneurysm or arteriovenous fistula
[b]Advance one grade for multiple liver injuries up to grade III
[c]Active bleeding should increase in size or attenuation on delayed phases

healing are the primary clinical goals of care. Management strategies for liver injury in trauma patients includes the following:

- **Conservative management**: Hemodynamically stable patients are treated without surgery, including high grade injuries, as the liver has a rich reparative capacity (Fig. 7.1) [5]. Measures include blood transfusions, supportive care, and close monitoring of vital signs and laboratory values.
- **Interventional radiology procedures**: In some cases, arterial or venous embolization may be performed to stop active bleeding from a damaged vessel. Interventional radiologists use minimally invasive endovascular angiographic techniques utilizing embolizing particles or metal coils [5].
- **Surgical interventions**: Surgery is necessary in hemodynamically unstable patients and more severe liver injuries, such as those that involve large vessels or associated injuries to other organs (grades IV and V). Surgery may involve techniques such as liver resection and packing of the liver with gauze [5].
- **Liver transplantation**: In rare cases, liver transplantation may be necessary if the liver injury is too severe to be managed with other interventions.

A multidisciplinary approach, involving trauma surgeons, interventional radiologists, and critical care specialists, is necessary to ensure optimal management of liver injury in trauma patients. Because non-operative management of liver injuries has become the standard of care in many patients, there has also been an increase in delayed complications, with a reported prevalence of up to 23 percent [12]. Delayed complications may be seen on imaging weeks to months after the trauma and include:

- **Delayed hemorrhage**: Occurs in up to 6% of patients with liver trauma and may be secondary to worsening injury or ruptured pseudoaneurysm [12]. Active arterial bleeding is usually

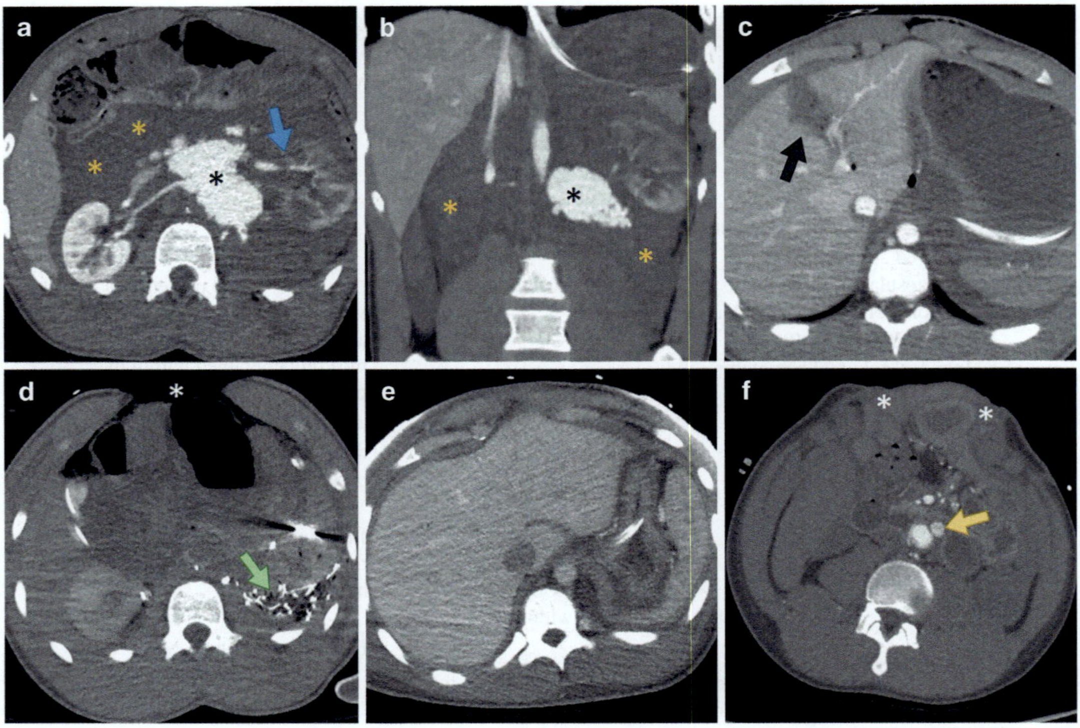

Fig. 7.9 CT images of the upper abdomen in a 16-year-old trauma patient with presenting with gunshot wounds. Axial (**a**) and coronal (**b**) arterial phase images show large extravasation of intravenous contrast, in keeping with active bleeding (black asterisk). There is associated devascularization of the left kidney because of involvement of the left renal artery (blue arrow). Hypoattenuation throughout the retroperitoneum is in keeping with extensive blood products (hemoretroperitoneum) (yellow asterisks). Axial portal venous phase image (**c**) shows hepatic laceration (black arrow). Following surgical intervention, axial arterial image shows an open abdomen (white asterisk), (**d**) surgical sponge (green arrow) in the left nephrectomy bed, and surgical drains. Graft repair of the abdominal aorta was also performed (not shown). A 6-month follow-up axial contrast-enhanced image (**e**) shows interval healing of the liver laceration. A 12-month follow-up axial arterial phase image (**f**) shows persistent ventral abdominal wound (white asterisks) and pseudoaneurysm arising from the abdominal aorta at site or prior repair (yellow arrow). The patient passed following the last exam secondary to ruptured aortic pseudoaneurysm. AAST grade III liver injury

treated with embolization by interventional radiology, while active venous bleeding is usually treated surgically [5].

- **Abscess**: Organized, superinfected collection, most often at site of prior hematoma or infarction. On imaging, an abscess has a thick, enhancing organized wall with central hypoattenuation, potentially with surrounding edema or hyperemia. There may be central foci of gas, which can also be seen in necrotic tissue. Abscesses are rare and associated with higher grades of liver injury [5].
- **Pseudoaneurysm**: Delayed formation can occur (Fig. 7.9), such as in the setting of a biloma [12]. Hemobilia, which appears as hyperattenuation of the biliary tract, may be seen on imaging if a pseudoaneurysm ruptures into a bile duct; of note, hemobilia may manifest as gastrointestinal bleeding [1, 5].

Recognition of these complications on imaging is essential for early treatment and low morbidity and mortality [12].

Biliary Tract Trauma

Occurring in only 2–3 percent of trauma patients, injury to the biliary tract is rare because of the inherent protection from the liver. Of the biliary tract, the gallbladder is most commonly injured, followed by the common bile duct. In most cases, biliary tract injury is associated with polytrauma, most commonly with hepatic injuries, or penetrating trauma [1, 12].

Anatomy

The biliary tract is comprised of intrahepatic and extrahepatic bile ducts and the gallbladder. Branching ducts collect bile from the liver and deliver it to the duodenum. There are many variants of the biliary tree anatomy. Left and right hepatic ducts converge to form the common hepatic duct, which then units with the cystic duct (from the gallbladder) and forms the common bile duct. The common bile duct drains into the duodenum at the ampulla of Vater. The gallbladder is located along the liver undersurface.

The common bile duct travels with the portal vein and hepatic artery, which are the three components of the portal triad. Throughout the liver, the biliary tree parallels branches of the portal vein and hepatic artery; these structures are protected by a fibrous covering [1].

Imaging and Grading

CT is the modality of choice for imaging evaluation for a traumatic biliary tract injury. Some specific CT findings of biliary tract injury include:

- **Contusion/hematoma**: Intramural hematoma, which manifests as focal wall thickening.
- **Laceration/perforation**: Full-thickness mural injury with extravasation of bile, which manifests as nonspecific intrahepatic or perihepatic free fluid that may be mistaken for ascites or postoperative fluid on CT (Fig. 7.7). Clues to the diagnosis of gallbladder laceration/perforation include poorly defined gallbladder wall, gallbladder wall thickening, collapsed gallbladder, discontinuous mural enhancement of the gallbladder wall, and hepatic injury that extends to the gallbladder fossa [12].
- **Avulsion injury**: Avulsion of the gallbladder from the liver bed may be associated with injury to the cystic duct and artery, potentially leading to significant hemorrhage.

In some cases, further evaluation with nuclear medicine hepatobiliary scan, which is a type of imaging that uses radiotracers to evaluate the liver and biliary tree, may be needed to confirm a bile leak. Endoscopic retrograde cholangiopancreatography (ERCP), performed by gastroenterology, or MR with Egotist contrast (gadolinium contrast that is excreted into the biliary tree) could also be used to evaluate for bile leak [12].

The AAST OIS is the most commonly used scale to assess extrahepatic biliary tree injury and is detailed in Table 7.3. Intrahepatic biliary tree injury is treated based on hepatic injury.

Table 7.3 AAST extrahepatic biliary tree injury scale [17]

AAST grade[a]	Description of injury
I	Gallbladder contusion/hematoma
	Portal triad contusion
II	Partial gallbladder avulsion from liver bed; cystic duct intact
	Laceration or perforation of the gallbladder
III	Complete gallbladder avulsion from liver bed
	Cystic duct laceration
IV	Partial or complete right hepatic duct laceration
	Partial or complete left hepatic duct laceration
	Partial common hepatic duct laceration (<50%)
	Partial common bile duct laceration (<50%)
V	>50% transection of common hepatic duct
	>50% transection of common bile duct
	Combined right and left hepatic duct injuries
	Intraduodenal or intrapancreatic bile duct injuries

[a]Advance one grade for multiple injuries up to grade III

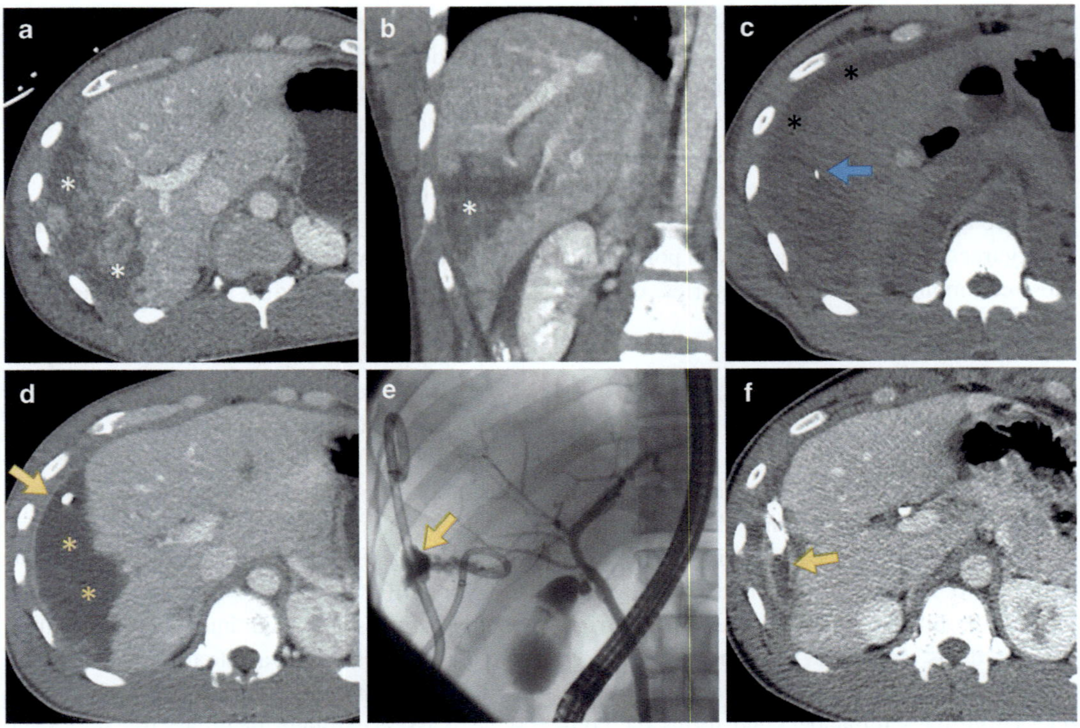

Fig. 7.10 Images of a 16-year-old trauma patient. Axial (**a**) and coronal (**b**) CT images of the liver show a large area of hypoattenuation in the periphery of the right hepatic lobe (white asterisks), in keeping with a liver laceration. Axial unenhanced image (**c**) obtained after surgical intervention shows a clip (blue arrow) at the site of a bile duct injury that was discovered and treated during surgery. Small amount of perihepatic fluid is also present (black asterisks). Axial portal venous image (**d**) from a follow-up CT a few weeks later shows an organizing, thick-walled perihepatic collection abutting the parenchymal laceration (yellow asterisks and arrow), which was favored to reflect a biloma; a drain is partially seen. Fluoroscopic image from follow-up ERCP (**e**) shows normal retrograde contrast opacification of the biliary tree and gallbladder; however, there is extravasation of contrast near the drain, confirming persistent bile leak (yellow arrow). Axial portal venous phase CT image (**f**) performed a few months later shows persistent, but decreased size of the perihepatic biloma (yellow arrow), which contains a drain. There was interim healing of the liver laceration (now shown). AAST grade IV liver injury

Management and Complications

Similar to hepatic injury, biliary tract injury grading can help guide management decisions for trauma patients. However, additional injuries must be taken into account when determining management of the patient. A multidisciplinary approach is necessary to ensure optimal management of injury in trauma patients. Management strategies for biliary tract injury in trauma patients include the following:

- **Conservative management**: Patients with gallbladder contusion/hematoma are managed conservatively [5].
- **Interventional minimally invasive procedures**: ERCP may be necessary to confirm a diagnosis of biliary leak and perform treatment with stenting (Fig. 7.10) [1]. Arterial embolization may be performed by interventional radiology to stop active bleeding from a damaged vessel [5].
- **Surgical intervention**: Surgical cholecystectomy is required for gallbladder lacerations and perforations as these are full-thickness injuries [12]. Gallbladder avulsion usually requires surgical management due to the high risk for cystic artery massive hemorrhage. If there is injury to the right hepatic artery or cystic duct, cholecystectomy is necessary

because of the risk of gallbladder ischemia and infarction. If there is severe injury to the distal common bile duct, pancreaticoduodenectomy may be required [1].

The management of biliary tract injuries often involves a multidisciplinary approach, including trauma surgeons, interventional radiologists, and gastroenterologists. Although often self-limiting, biliary complications are common and may be seen on imaging weeks to months later. Most biliary complications are related to bile leakage and include:

- **Biloma**: Intrahepatic or intraperitoneal collection of leaked bile that is often secondary to hepatic laceration (Fig. 7.10). A biloma that measures less than 3 cm can often be treated conservatively [5].
- **Biliary fistula**: Abnormal communication of the biliary tract, usually with an artery (arteriobiliary fistula) [5]. Pleurobiliary fistula is rare and typically associated with penetrating trauma [1].
- **Bile peritonitis** (coleperitoneum): Bile leakage collecting in the peritoneum.
- Cholecystitis: Blood within the gallbladder lumen can cause cystic duct obstruction and acute cholecystitis [1].

Unfortunately, there is often a delay in diagnosis for biliary complications because bile is water density on CT and mimics ascites or postoperative fluid. Therefore, a high degree of suspicion is needed for timely diagnosis of a bile leak [5].

Splenic Trauma

Splenic injury is the one of the most frequently injured solid abdominal organs in trauma patients, with a reported incidence of up to 49 percent in patients with a history of blunt trauma [5]. Splenic injury is less common in patients with penetrating abdominal trauma, such as stab or gunshot wounds. Splenic injury ranges from minor contusions to life-threatening ruptures. Splenic injuries can be fatal from initial presentation as well as from delayed pseudoaneurysm or expanding subcapsular hematoma rupture.

Anatomy

Anatomically, the spleen is approximately the size of a clenched fist. Except for the entry and exit sites of the splenic artery and vein, respectively, the splenic surface is covered with visceral peritoneum and a fibroelastic capsule. The spleen is composed of red pulp, which filters old red blood cells, and white pulp, which is primarily composed of lymphocytes [1].

The spleen is posteriorly located in the left upper quadrant of the abdomen. The left kidney abuts the inferomedial surface of the spleen, which is referred to as the renal impression. The posterolateral surface of the spleen, or diaphragmatic surface, has impressions from the adjacent left hemidiaphragm as well as from the left 9th through 11th ribs. Therefore, careful evaluation of the spleen should be undertaken when the aforementioned ribs are injured, as well as careful evaluation of the integrity of the left hemidiaphragm when the posterolateral aspect of the spleen is injured. The anterior aspect of the spleen is impressed upon by the splenic flexure of the colon.

Imaging and Grading

Imaging plays an essential role in the clinical management of splenic trauma by providing detailed information about the extent of the injury. CT is the modality of choice, with sensitivity and specificity of diagnosing splenic injuries near 96–100% [5]. The imaging findings of splenic injury on CT of trauma patients include:

- **Hematoma**: Collection of blood within the spleen, which typically appears as an area of hypoattenuation (decreased density) relative to the parenchyma on CT images. However, if the blood is acute or hyperacute, it may appear hyper- or isoattenuating (increased or similar density).

 - Subcapsular hematomas are peripherally located collections that are confined by the splenic capsule, are often crescent-shaped and exert mass effect upon the underlying parenchyma.
 - Intraparenchymal hematomas are located within the parenchyma, are often oval or rounded, and also exert mass effect upon the parenchyma.
- **Laceration**: Tear of the splenic tissue, which most often appears as linear or branching area of hypoattenuation within the parenchyma (Figs. 7.11, 7.12, 7.13, and 7.14). Lacerations can range from a small, superficial tears to a shattered spleen, in which there is severe disruption.
- **Active bleeding**: Contrast extravasation, which is leakage of contrast material from the blood vessels within the spleen, may indicate active bleeding. Bleeding may collect within the spleen or into the peritoneal cavity. This appears as an area of hyperattenuating contrast material (similar in attenuation to that within the vessels) outside the blood vessels on CT images. The area of hemorrhage enlarges on the slightly later portal venous phase of contrast. Patients with active bleeding usually require management with surgery or interventional radiology.

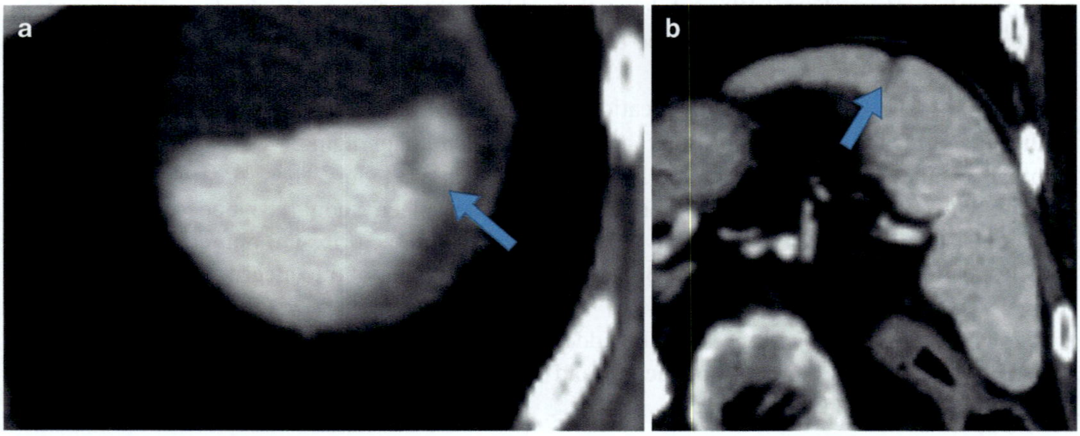

Fig. 7.11 Axial (**a**) and coronal (**b**) CT images of the spleen in the portal venous phase show a linear area of hypoattenuation in the lateral, superior aspect of the spleen (arrow), which measures less than 1 cm in length and is in keeping with a laceration. The patient was treated conservatively. AAST grade I injury

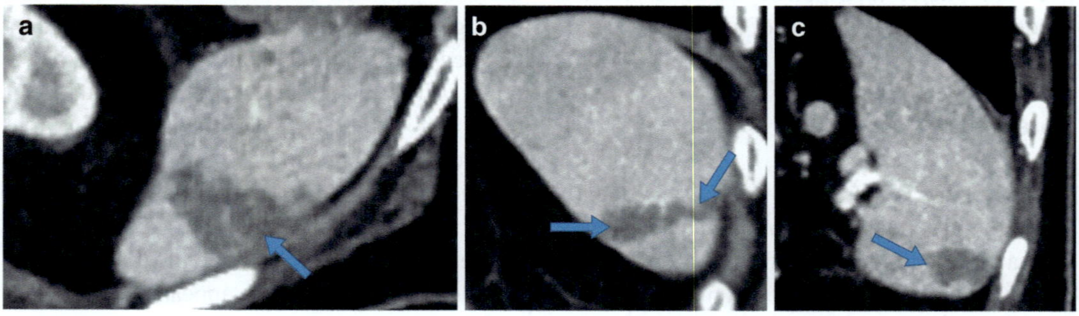

Fig. 7.12 Axial (**a**), coronal (**b**), and sagittal (**c**) CT images of the spleen in the portal venous phase show background heterogeneity of the spleen. There is a 4 cm linear area of hypoattenuation in the posterior, inferior aspect of the spleen (arrow), which measures less than 4 cm in length and is in keeping with a laceration. The hilar vessels (not shown) are intact. AAST grade III injury

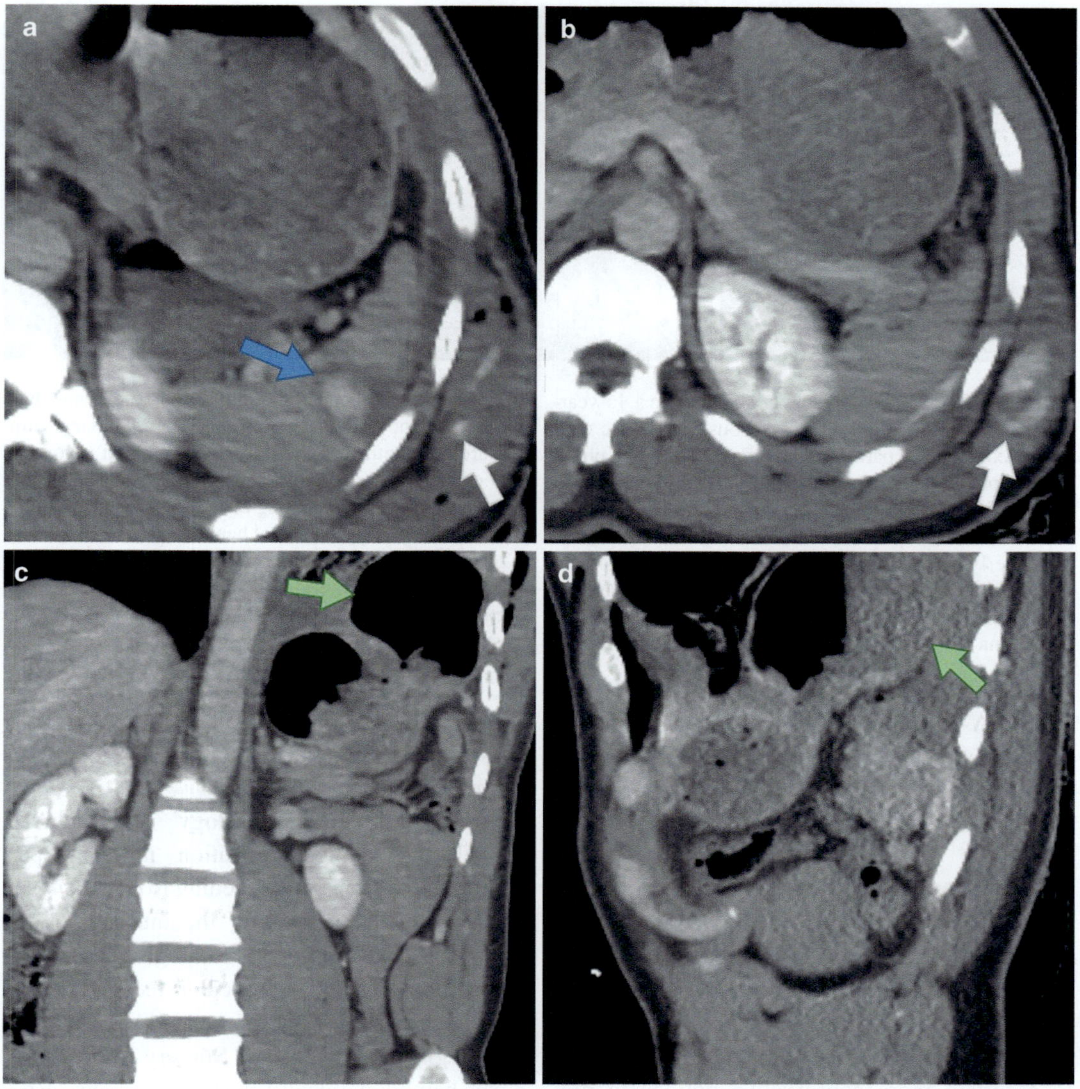

Fig. 7.13 CT images of the upper abdomen in a 28-year-old trauma patient presenting with multiple stab wounds. Axial portal venous phase images through the spleen (**a**, **b**) show a laceration involving between 25% and 50% of the parenchyma with active extravasation into the spleen (blue arrow), around the splenic capsule and into the chest wall (white arrows). Coronal (**c**) and (**d**) sagittal images demonstrate herniation of the gastric body into the left chest (green arrows) through a posttraumatic diaphragmatic laceration. Left lateral thoracoabdominal wall subcutaneous emphysema and lacerations are also noted. AAST grade III splenic injury

- **Pseudoaneurysm**: Localized outpouchings of an artery secondary to injury of a vessel with contained hematoma. Pseudoaneurysms appear as well-circumscribed, contrast-enhancing structures on CT images. Although asymptomatic, pseudoaneurysms are at risk of rupturing and causing fatal hemorrhage.
- **Arteriovenous fistula** (AVF): Rare abnormal communication between an artery and vein that usually results from penetrating trauma. On imaging, an AVF should be suspected if there is enhancement of a structure during both arterial and venous phases.
- **Hilar vascular injury**: Injury to at least one hilar vessel, often resulting in life-threatening bleeding. On imaging, this should be suspected if there is a laceration that extends to the splenic hilum (Figs. 7.15 and 7.16).

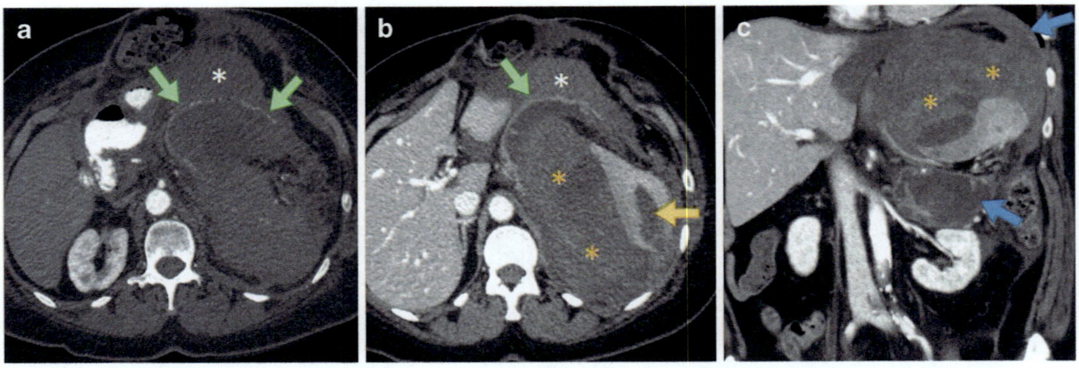

Fig. 7.14 CT images of the upper abdomen in a 46-year-old patient, performed with intravenous and enteric contrast. Axial late hepatic arterial phase (**a**), axial portal venous phase (**b**), and coronal portal venous phase (**c**) images show a large, heterogenous collection along the superior medial aspect of the spleen with mass effect on the underlying parenchyma, in keeping with a large subcapsular hematoma (yellow asterisks). There is an associated small splenic laceration or intraparenchymal hematoma (yellow arrow). There is associated rupture of the subcapsular hematoma into the peritoneum (blue arrows), but no findings of active bleeding. Thin, curvilinear area of contrast in the left upper quadrant represents the enhancing mucosa of a collapsed stomach (green arrow). Focal wall thickening of the anterior aspect of the distal stomach suggests mural hemotoma (white asterisk). No findings of extraluminal enteric contrast to suggest gastric perforation, noting that enteric contrast is seen in the duodenum. AAST grade III splenic injury and grade I gastric injury

The AAST OIS is the most commonly used scale to assess splenic injury and the CT findings are detailed in Table 7.4.

Management and Complications

The mainstay of treatment of splenic injuries in the past, or currently in developing nations, was splenectomy. As knowledge of the immunological function of the spleen grew, so did the desire to ascertain more conservative options to preserve the spleen and avert the immunological deterioration that accompanies a splenectomy. The treatment of splenic injury is determined by injury grading, the clinical status of the patient, and other factors, such as the presence of associated injuries. Management strategies that may be used for splenic injury in trauma patients are as follows:

- **Conservative management**: Non-operative management is generally the first-line approach for low-grade splenic injuries (Fig. 7.8), and may include observation, blood transfusions, and supportive care. This typically involves close monitoring of the patient's vital signs, regular blood tests to assess for signs of ongoing bleeding, and a period of bed rest.
- **Interventional radiology procedures**: Selective angioembolization may be performed to stop active bleeding from a damaged vessel while preserving the integrity of the spleen. Interventional radiologists use minimally invasive endovascular technique with angiography and particles or metal coils [5].
- **Surgical intervention**: Surgery is necessary in hemodynamically unstable patients, especially in the setting of polytrauma; these patients may proceed emergently to surgery without obtaining CT imaging, depending upon the bedside assessment with radiographs and ultrasound [5]. Surgery may also be necessary in hemodynamically stable patients with severe splenic injuries (grades IV and V) (Figs. 7.15 and 7.16).
- The management of pancreatic injury often involves a multidisciplinary approach, including trauma surgeons, interventional radiologists, and gastroenterologists.

The management of splenic injury often involves a multidisciplinary approach, including

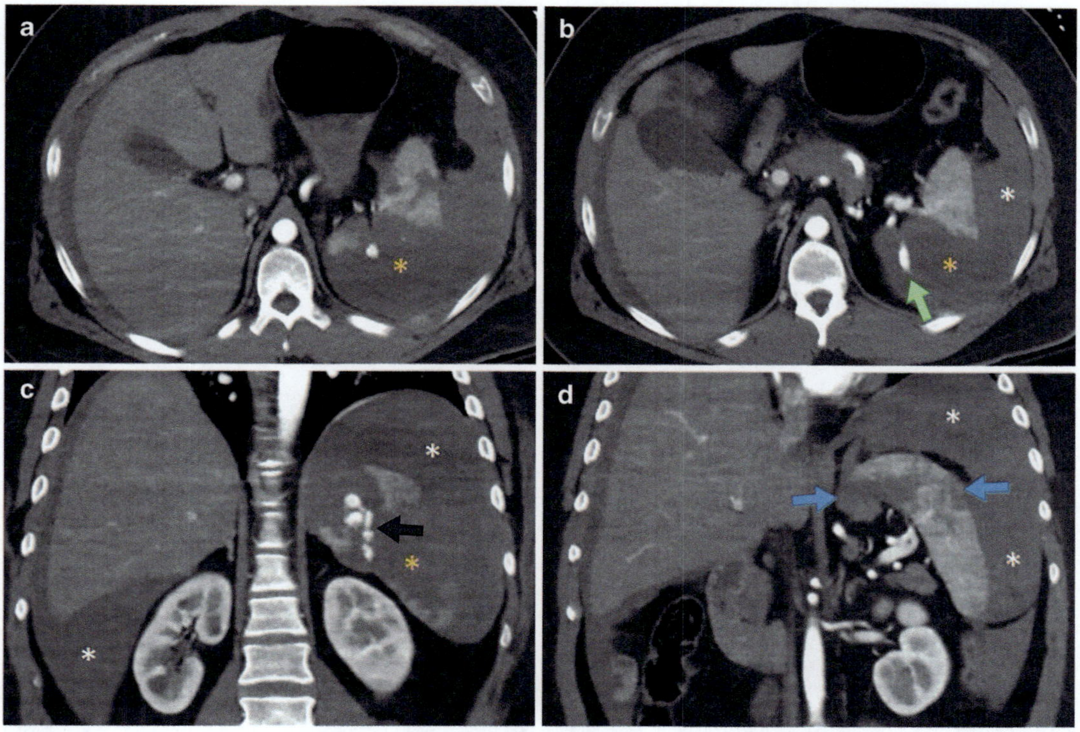

Fig. 7.15 CT images of the upper abdomen in a 35-year-old trauma patient presenting after a fall from 5 feet. Axial (**a**, **b**), coronal (**c**, **d**) late hepatic arterial phase images show a 5 cm laceration extending from the posterior splenic capsule toward the hilum (blue arrows). The spleen is devascularized, as characterized by diffuse hypoenhancement (greater than 50%) (yellow asterisks). A blush of active contrast extravasation from a branch of the splenic artery (green arrow), consistent with active bleeding. Presumed pseudoaneurysms along the expected course of a splenic artery branch (black arrow). Associated large volume hemoperitoneum (white asterisks). AAST grade V splenic injury

trauma surgeons, interventional radiologists, and gastroenterologists. Potential complications in the management of patients with splenic trauma include:

- **Bleeding**: Non-operative management of splenic trauma is most often complicated by persistent or delayed bleeding, which often required surgical intervention. Operative management may also be complicated by bleeding [1].
- **Associated intra-abdominal injury**: When splenic trauma is managed without surgery, there is a risk of missing an occult associated intra-abdominal injury that should be managed with surgery. For instance, a small bowel injury with subtle or nonspecific CT findings may be missed on imaging and will go undetected with non-operative management, although it would have been detected at the time of surgery. Also, there is a risk of injury to adjacent organs, such as the pancreas, during surgery [1].
- **Arteriovenous fistula**: Although rare, fistula formation between the ligated vessels at the splenic hilum has been reported following splenectomy.
- **Gastric necrosis**: Necrosis of the greater curvature of the stomach may result if a portion of the gastric wall is included in the ligation ties for the short gastric vessels during splenectomy. With necrosis, gastric leak results and is associated peritonitis and abscesses [1].
- **Postsplenectomy thrombocytosis**: Splenectomy is associated with increased long-term risk of thrombotic events,

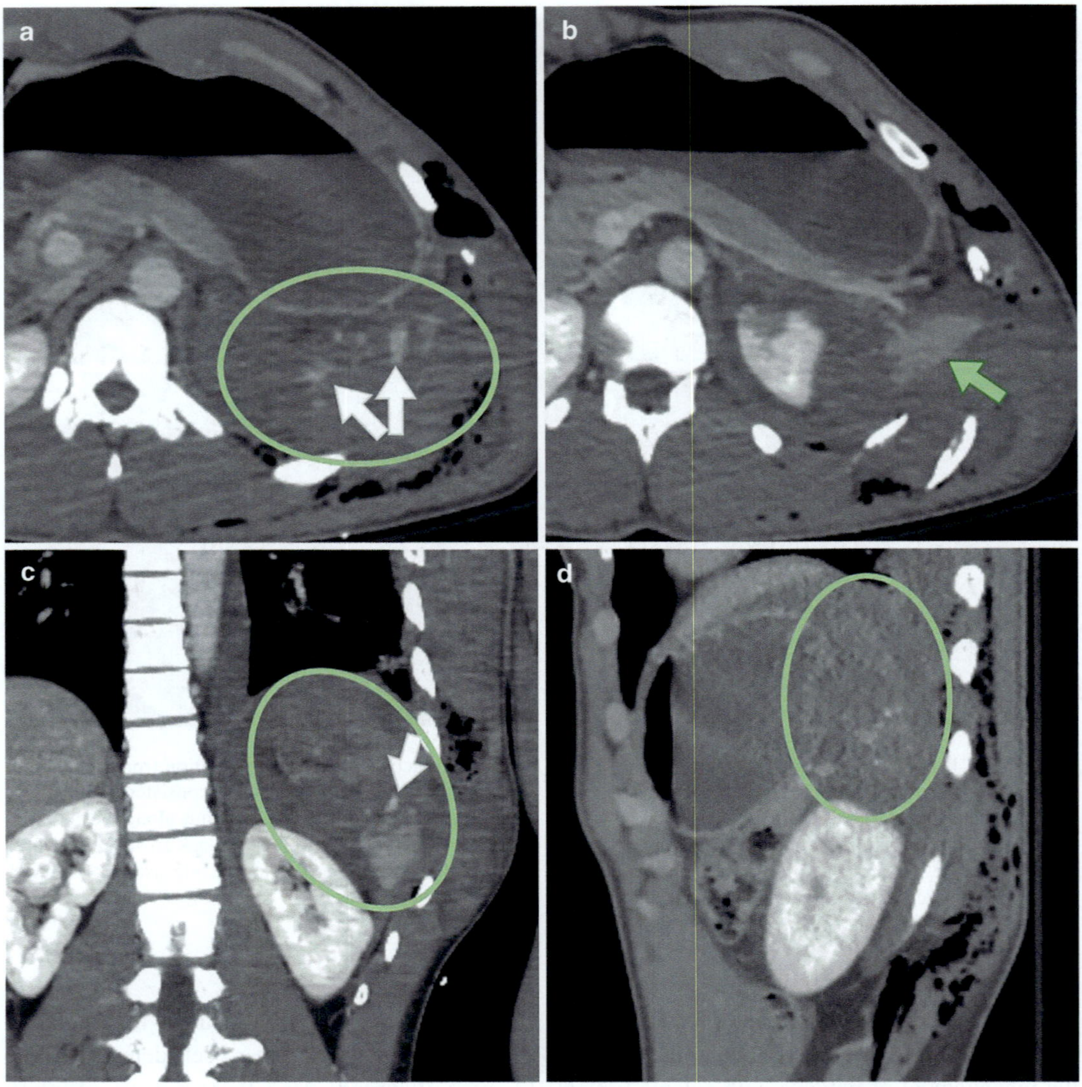

Fig. 7.16 CT images of the upper abdomen in a 28-year-old trauma patient presenting after a motorcycle accident. Axial (**a**, **b**), coronal (**c**), and sagittal (**d**) contrast-enhanced images show diffuse hypoenhancement of the spleen (green ellipse), in keeping with devascularization. There is a small area of enhancing parenchyma at the splenic tip (green arrow). Foci of hyperattenuation suggest active bleeding (white arrows). Extensive subcutaneous emphysema and numerous rib fractures are also shown. AAST grade V splenic injury

although less common in trauma patients than patients post splenectomy for other reasons [1].

- **Infection**: Asplenic state is associated with a very low risk of life-threatening infection. Infections with encapsulated organisms are most are common in asplenia, such as pneumococcus; therefore, these patients should be vaccinated against these organisms following splenectomy [1].

Recognition of these complications on imaging is essential for early treatment and decreasing morbidity and mortality.

Table 7.4 AAST spleen injury scale [14, 19]

AAST grade[b]	Hematoma	Laceration	Vascular injury
I	Subcapsular, <10% surface area	Capsular tear, <1 cm parenchymal depth	
II	Subcapsular, 10%–50% surface area	Capsular tear, 1–3 cm parenchymal depth that does not involve a trabecular vessel	
	Intraparenchymal, <5 cm in diameter		
III	Subcapsular, >50% surface area or expanding	>3 cm parenchymal depth or involving trabecular vessels	
	Ruptured subcapsular or parenchymal hematoma		
	Intraparenchymal hematoma >5 cm or expanding		
IV		Laceration involving segmental or hilar vessels producing major devascularization (>25% of spleen)	Any injury in the presence of a splenic vascular injury[a] (pseudoaneurysm or arteriovenous fistula) or active bleeding[c] confined within splenic capsule
V		Completely shattered spleen	Hilar vascular injury with devascularized spleen

[a]Vascular injuries are defined as a pseudoaneurysm or arteriovenous fistula
[b]Advance one grade for multiple injuries up to grade III
[c]Active bleeding should increase in size or attenuation on delayed phases

Pancreatic and Duodenal Trauma

Although rare, pancreatic and duodenal injury is a potentially life-threatening complication of abdominal trauma. Overall, pancreatic or duodenal injury is estimated to occur in less than 5% of all trauma patients [1]. However, there is an increased incidence of pancreatic injury with blunt trauma or polytrauma, particularly from high-energy trauma from falls from height or motor vehicle collisions. Pancreatic injury is less common in patients with penetrating abdominal trauma, such as stab or gunshot wounds.

Anatomy

The pancreas is located in the retroperitoneum; except for the first few centimeters that are intraperitoneal, the remainder of the duodenum is retroperitoneal. The retroperitoneal location of these structures is protective, accounting for the rare incidence of injury. The duodenum is a hollow C-shaped structure, which begins as the duodenal bulb at the pylorus, sweeps around the pancreatic head, crosses midline anterior to the spine, and transitions to jejunum distal to the ligament of Treitz. Approximately 30 cm in length, the duodenum is divided into four segments, known as D1 (superior), D2 (descending), D3 (transverse), and D4 (ascending) [1]. In the right upper quadrant, the pancreatic head is located in the duodenal C-loop, encases the distal common bile duct and abuts the superior mesenteric vein. The pancreas crosses midline and courses superiorly toward the spleen. The pancreatic tail is attached to the spleen in the left upper quadrant. Branches of the pancreaticoduodenal arteries supply both the C-loop of the duodenum and the pancreas; therefore, if there is severe injury to this region, combined resection of both structures is required [1].

Imaging and Grading

Pancreatic injury is often a difficult diagnosis, as symptoms may be delayed and physical examination findings may be subtle. CT is the gold standard in the evaluation of pancreatic injury in trauma patients. The CT findings of pancreatic injury in trauma patients include:

- **Contusion**: A focal area of pancreatic parenchymal edema without visible disruption of the pancreatic duct or parenchyma (Fig. 7.17).
- **Laceration**: A visible disruption of the pancreatic duct or parenchyma with or without associated hematoma (Fig. 7.18).
- **Hematoma**: A collection of blood within or adjacent to the pancreas.

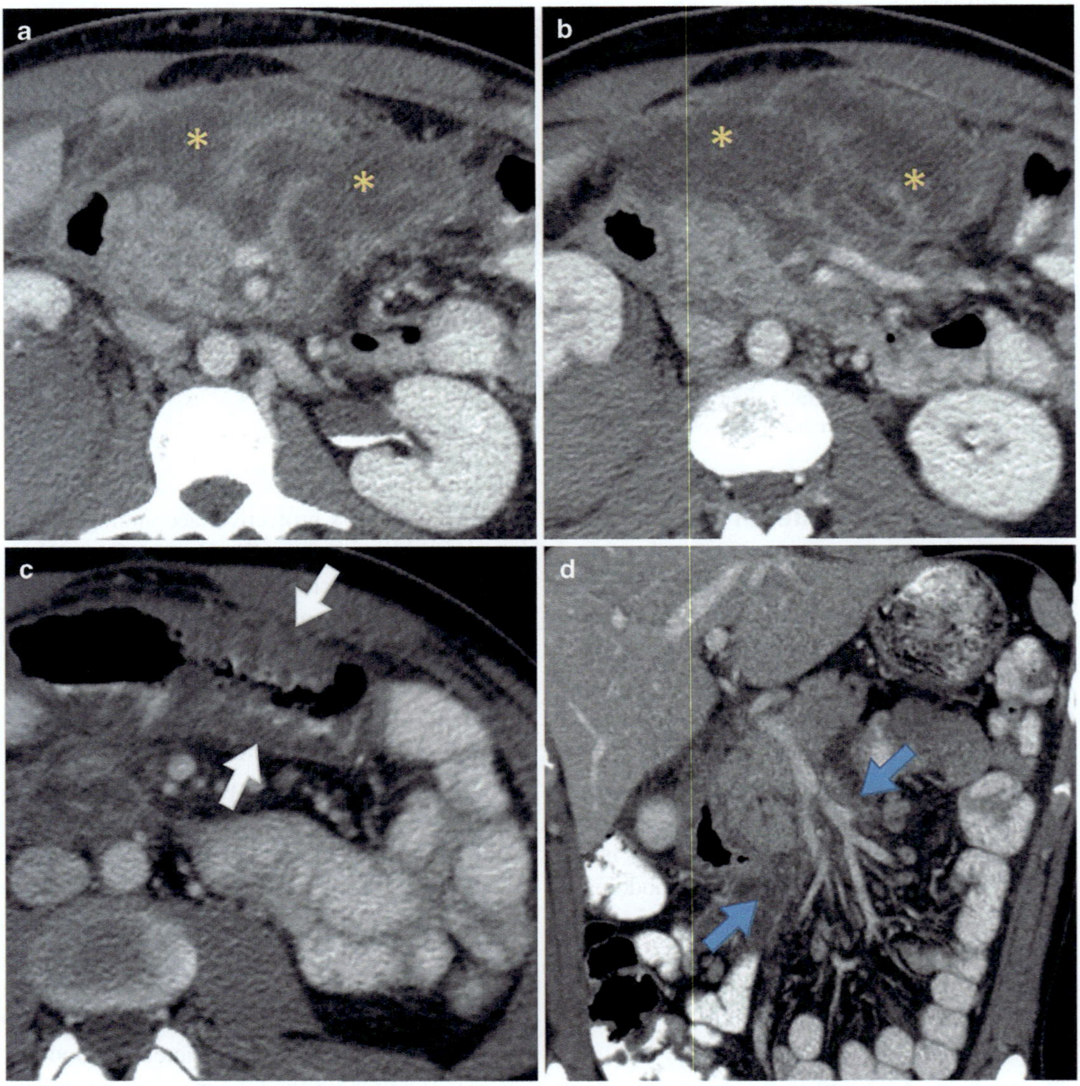

Fig. 7.17 CT images of the upper abdomen in a 26-year-old trauma patient. Axial (**a**–**c**) and coronal (**d**) portal venous phase images show a complex, multiloculated collection of fluid and phlegmon in the peripancreatic region (yellow asterisks) that extends into the omentum and mesentery (blue arrows on **d**), suggestive of pancreatic injury. No focal pancreatic parenchyma defect to suggest laceration. Associated thickening of the adjacent transverse colon (white arrows on **c**) is likely reactive. AAST grade II pancreatic injury

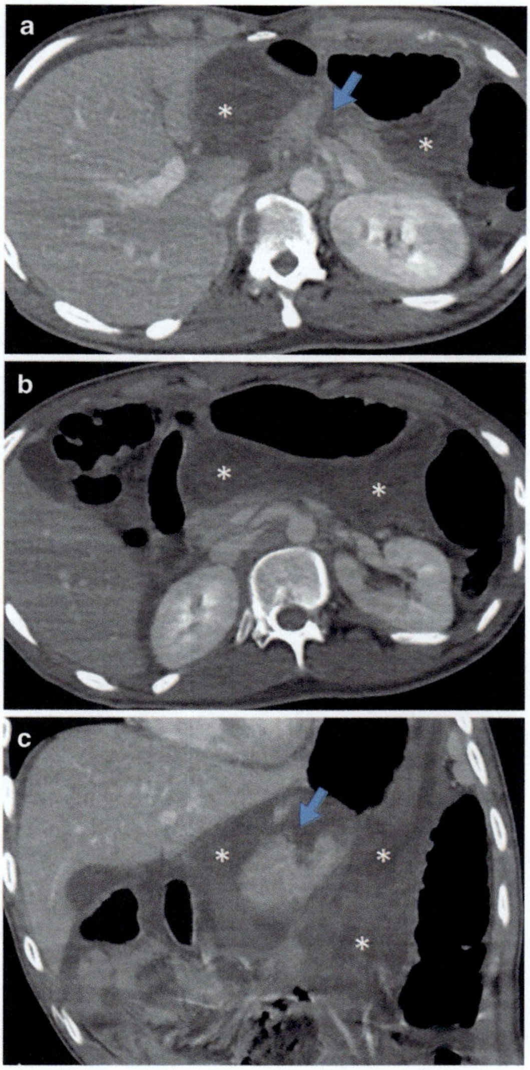

Fig. 7.18 CT images of the upper abdomen in a trauma patient with unknown age and history. Axial (**a**, **b**) and coronal (**c**) images in the portal venous phase show a focal parenchymal defect of the anterior, superior aspect of the pancreatic body (blue arrow) with large surrounding complex fluid collection (white asterisks). There is normal enhancement of both the proximal and distal portions of the pancreas. The fluid collection extends throughout the lesser sac, from the left infradiaphragmatic space and inferiorly into the mid abdomen. AAST grade III pancreatic injury

- **Duct injury**: A visible disruption of the main pancreatic duct, which can lead to pancreatic ductal leakage and pancreatic fistula formation.

Table 7.5 AAST pancreas injury scale [15]

AAST grade[b]	Hematoma	Laceration
I	Minor contusion without duct injury	Superficial laceration without duct injury
II	Major contusion without duct injury or tissue loss	Major laceration without duct injury or tissue loss
III		Distal transection or parenchymal injury with duct injury
IV		Proximal[a] transection or parenchymal injury involving ampulla
V		Massive disruption of pancreatic head

[a]Proximal pancreas is to the patients' right of the superior mesenteric vein
[b]Advance one grade for multiple injuries up to grade III

The most commonly used grading system is the AAST OIS, which is detailed in Tables 7.5 and 7.6 for the pancreas and duodenum, respectively.

Management and Complications

The clinical management depends on the severity of the pancreatic or duodenal injury and the hemodynamic status of the patient. Management strategies for pancreatic or duodenal traumatic injury include the following:

- **Conservative management**: For low-grade injuries, conservative management may be appropriate.
- **Endoscopic retrograde cholangiopancreatography** (ERCP): In cases of suspected pancreatic duct injury or pancreatic fistula, ERCP (Figure 7.10e) may be used to diagnose and treat the condition if there are no other abdominal injuries that require surgery. This procedure involves the insertion of a flexible tube through the mouth and into the small intestine to visualize the pancreatic duct and bile ducts. If a ductal injury is identified, stenting or sphincterotomy may be performed to promote healing and prevent further complications [1].

Table 7.6 AAST duodenum injury scale [15]

AAST grade[a]	Hematoma	Laceration	Vascular injury
I	Involving single portion of duodenum	Partial thickness, no perforation	
II	Involving more than one portion	Disruption <50% of circumference	
III		Disruption 50–75% of circumference of D2	
		Disruption 50–100% of circumference of D1,D3,D4	
IV		Disruption >75% of circumference of D2	
		Involving ampulla or distal common bile duct	
V		Massive disruption of duodenopancreatic complex	Devascularization of duodenum

(D1-first position of duodenum; D2-second portion of duodenum; D3-third portion of duodenum; D4-fourth portion of duodenum)
[a]Advance one grade for multiple injuries up to grade III

- **Surgical intervention**: For more severe pancreatic injuries, surgical intervention may be necessary. This may involve either closure of duodenal injury, partial resection or pancreatoduodenectomy, depending on the extent of the injury. In cases of massive bleeding or suspected pancreatic ductal injury, emergency surgery may be required to control the bleeding and stabilize the patient.

The management of pancreatic or duodenal injury often involves a multidisciplinary approach, including trauma surgeons, interventional radiologists, and gastroenterologists. Potential complications in the management of patients with pancreatic or duodenal trauma include:

- **Duodenal leak/fistula**: Following repair of duodenal injury, a small portion of patients will develop a leak or fistula. The risk is higher in the setting of penetrating trauma. If there is an associated fluid collection, these patients are typically treated with percutaneous drainage. Postoperative fistulae take weeks to heal and occasionally require surgical management [1].
- **Pancreatic leak/fistula:** Usually self-limiting, although a high output fistula is associated with a poor prognosis. If intervention is necessary, ERCP with stent placement is sufficient in most cases. If there is an associated fluid collection, it is typically treated with percutaneous drainage [1].
- **Abscess**: Organized, superinfected collection, most often at a site of prior hematoma or parenchymal infarction. On imaging, an abscess has a thick, enhancing wall with central hypoattenuation, potentially with surrounding edema or hyperemia. There may be central foci of gas, which can also be seen in necrotic tissue. Abscesses are typically managed with percutaneous drainage [1].

As previously stated, recognition of these complications on imaging is essential for early treatment and decreased morbidity and mortality.

Gastric and Intestinal Trauma

Traumatic injury to the thick-walled stomach is rare; gastric injury is more common in the setting of gastric distention or penetrating trauma. Similarly, injuries to the hollow viscus are rare, occurring in 1–3% of trauma patients. The small bowel accounts for 70–90% of hollow viscus injuries; the colon is the second most commonly injured intestinal structure [1, 5]. Hollow viscus injuries are more common in blunt trauma, particularly seat belt injuries [1]. Injury to the bowel and mesentery is also associated with concomitant injuries to other solid abdominal organs or osseous structures. Rectal trauma, for instance, is much more in patients with pelvic fractures; of note, the presence of blood on a digital rectum exam is suspicious for rectal injury. The incidence for gastric and intestinal injuries may be underestimated, as these injuries can be difficult to diagnose clinically and may be missed on initial imaging studies.

Anatomy

The stomach is located superiorly within the left upper quadrant of the abdomen and is partially protected by the lower chest wall; when the stomach is distended or the patient is erect, the stomach may extend into the lower abdomen. The greater omentum loosely joins the stomach with the transverse colon; the gastrosplenic ligament joins the stomach with the spleen. The stomach is thick-walled and has a rich blood supply.

About 5–6 m in length, the small bowel (or intestine) begins after the duodenum and includes the jejunum, which begins distal to the ligament of Treitz in the left upper quadrant, and the ileum, which extends to the ileocecal valve in the right lower quadrant. Small bowel injuries are most common near the ligament of Treitz and the ileocecal valve as these portions are less mobile. The small bowel is vulnerable to injury as it occupies a large portion of the abdominal cavity and is only protected by the abdominal wall musculature. The small bowel is attached to the retroperitoneum by the mesentery and has a rich blood supply [1].

The colon, known as the large bowel or intestine, is approximately 1.5 m in length. It is a hollow viscus that is composed of the cecum, ascending colon, transverse colon, descending colon, and sigmoid colon. The cecum, transverse colon and sigmoid colon are intraperitoneal and mobile. The ascending colon and descending colon are partially retroperitoneal, located in the lateral aspects of the right and left abdomen respectively; these portions of the colon are fixed and more vulnerable to trauma [5]. The cecum is located in the right lower quadrant, communicates with the ileum through the ileocecal valve and is the structure from which the appendix arises. The transverse colon is located in the anterior upper abdomen. The sigmoid colon is located in the left lower quadrant and pelvis.

Approximately 15 cm in length, the rectum joints the sigmoid colon with the anus. The proximal and midportion of the rectum is intraperitoneal, while the distal rectum is extraperitoneal.

Imaging and Grading

Traumatic injury to the stomach and intestines can range from minor contusions to life-threatening perforations. A high index of suspicion and comprehensive imaging evaluation is necessary, as clinical findings are often unreliable [5]. CT is the modality of choice for the assessment of these traumatic injuries, which can help determine the severity of the injury and guide treatment decisions. The imaging findings of gastric and intestinal injuries on CT of trauma patients include:

- **Wall discontinuity**: Focal discontinuity of the gastric or bowel wall that is most conspicuous on the portal venous phase but is an uncommon CT finding because the discontinuities are typically quite small. When visualized, this finding is 100 percent specific for injury. Multiplanar evaluation is essential to evaluate the superior and inferior walls.
- **Extraluminal air or contrast**: Free, extraluminal air within the peritoneum (pneumoperitoneum), retroperitoneum or extraperitoneum (seen with distal rectal injury) is best visualized on lung window (wide window setting) (Figs. 7.7, 7.8, 7.19, 7.20, and 7.21). Bowel perforation accounts for the majority of extraluminal air, but there are other potential sources, such as intraperitoneal bladder rupture and pneumothorax with diaphragmatic injury [5]. Free air within the retroperitoneum suggests injury to a retroperitoneal structure.

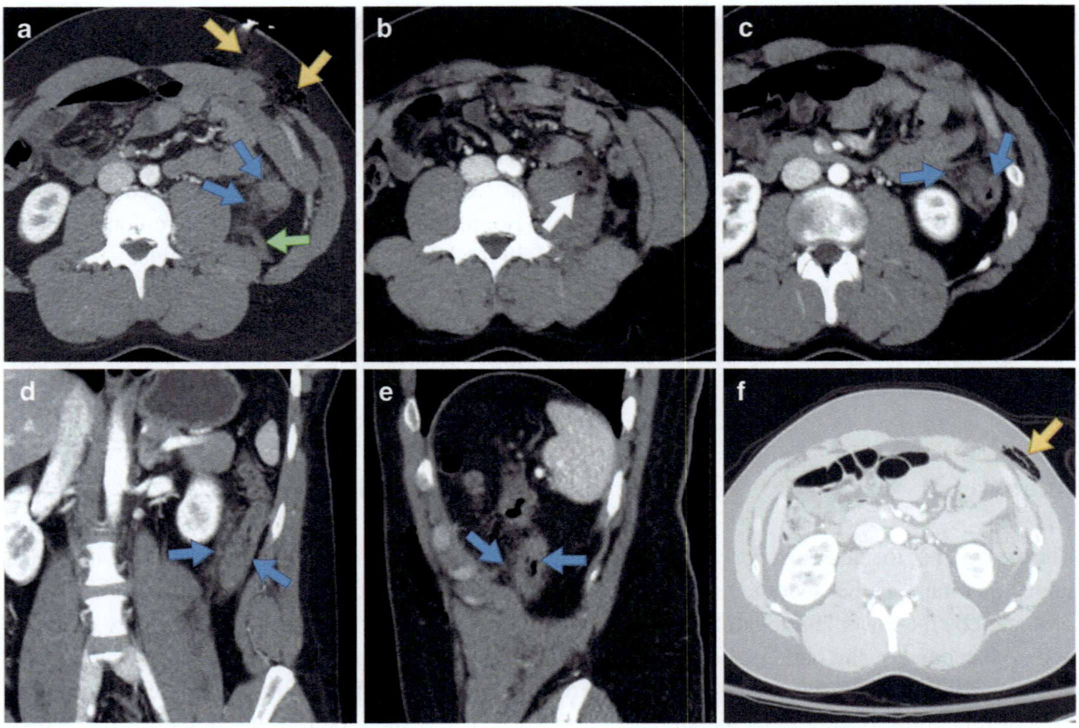

Fig. 7.19 CT images of the upper abdomen in a 32-year-old trauma patient presenting with gunshot wounds. Axial (**a–c**), coronal (**d**), and sagittal (**e**) portal venous phase images show wall thickening and surrounding edema of the descending colon (blue arrows) with fluid layering the left interfascial plane (green arrow). Associated subcutaneous emphysema and fat stranding (yellow arrows); the air within the soft tissues is best appreciated on axial image with lung window (**f**). AAST grade II bowel injury

Although enteric contrast is rarely used in the setting of trauma, extraluminal contrast is specific, but not sensitive, for bowel injury [1].

- **Intramural air**: Foci of air within the wall of a hollow viscus, best seen on lung window (wide window setting). This finding raises concern for full-thickness injury in trauma patients [5].
- **Wall thickening**: Focal (Fig. 7.14) or diffuse wall thickening is sensitive, but not specific, for stomach or bowel injury. If adequately distended, small bowel wall should measure less than 3 mm in thickness and the colon should measure less than 5 mm. Mural thickening may reflect intramural hematoma, partial thickness injury or full-thickness injury a trauma patient [5].
- **Active bleeding**: Contrast extravasation, which is leakage of contrast material from the blood vessels within the liver, may indicate active bleeding (Fig. 7.22). This appears as an area of hyperattenuating contrast material (similar in attenuation to that within the vessels) outside the blood vessels on CT images (Fig. 7.7). The area of hemorrhage enlarges on the slightly later portal venous phase of contrast. Patients with active bleeding usually require management with surgery or interventional radiology.
- **Abnormal enhancement**: Subjective finding of hyper- (Fig. 7.23) or hypoenhancement of a bowel segment compared to the enhancement of the remainder of the bowel; hyperenhancement (increased enhancement) suggests

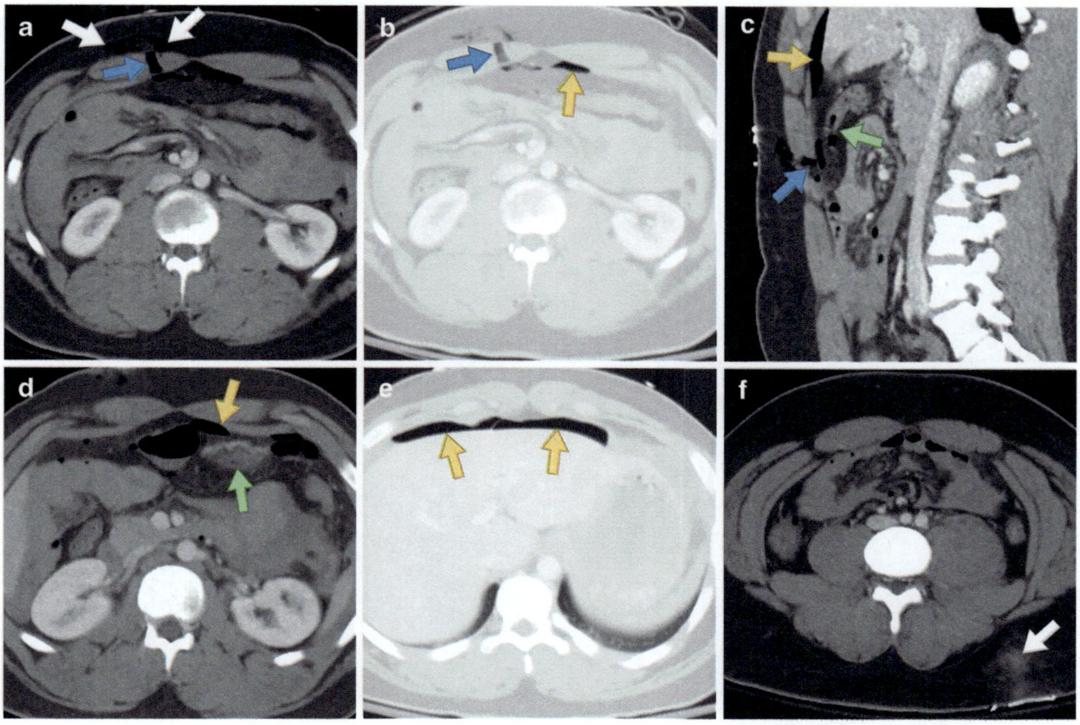

Fig. 7.20 CT images of the upper abdomen in a 19-year-old trauma patient presenting with stab wounds. Axial (**a**, **d**, **f**) and coronal (**c**) portal venous phase images show several areas of subcutaneous fat stranding and emphysema from soft tissue wounds (white arrows) with an associated linear defect of the right rectus abdominus muscle (blue arrow). There is associated free air (yellow arrows), best appreciated on axial images with lung window (**b**, **e**). Several of these foci of free air closely about the transverse colon and there is focal edema within the mesentery (green arrow). On the sagittal image (c), the proximity of the transverse colon (green arrow) to the overlying soft tissue injury is seen. Findings are in keeping with perforation of the transverse colon from penetrating trauma. AAST grade II injury

bowel injury with vascular involvement, while hypoenhancement (decreased enhancement) suggests bowel ischemia. Diffuse hyperenhancement of the small bowel has been described in the setting of hypovolemic shock [5].

- **Intraperitoneal or Retroperitoneal Fluid**: In the absence of solid organ injury, intraperitoneal or retroperitoneal free fluid suggests an underlying bowel or mesenteric injury, particularly interloop fluid (Figs. 7.19, 7.20, 7.23). Conversely, the absence of free fluid is reassuring that there is no underlying bowel or mesenteric injury. The location of the fluid may hint at a nearby injury. Of note, hypoattenuating fluid could also represent urine from bladder injury [5].

The AAST OIS is the most commonly used grading system to assess traumatic injury to the stomach and intestines, which is detailed in Tables 7.7, 7.8, 7.9, and 7.10 for the stomach, small bowel, colon, and rectum. Higher-grade injuries are associated with a higher risk of complications such as infection, abscess formation, and perforation, and may require more aggressive surgical intervention. However, it is important to note that the severity of the injury on

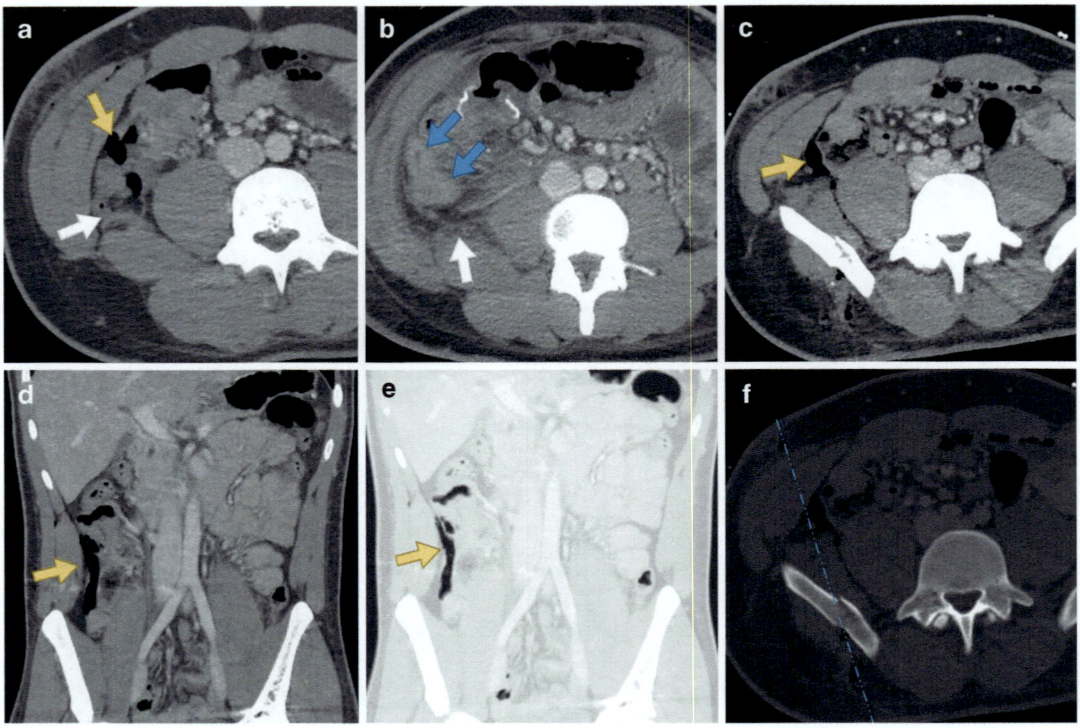

Fig. 7.21 CT images of the abdomen in a 22-year-old trauma patient presenting with gunshot wounds. Axial (**a**–**c**) and coronal (**d**) portal venous phase images show wall thickening of the ascending colon (blues arrow on **b**) with surrounding fat stranding and fluid (white arrows). An anteroposterior ballistic trajectory is seen in the right lower quadrant (dashed line on **f**), through the region of the ascending colon. There is associated free air along the ascending colon (yellow arrows), best appreciated on coronal image with lung window (**e**). Findings are in keeping with colonic perforation. Axial image with bone window demonstrates comminuted right iliac fracture along the ballistic trajectory (**f**). There is subcutaneous emphysema and fat stranding as well as muscular thickening (**f**). AAST grade IV grade II/III colonic injury

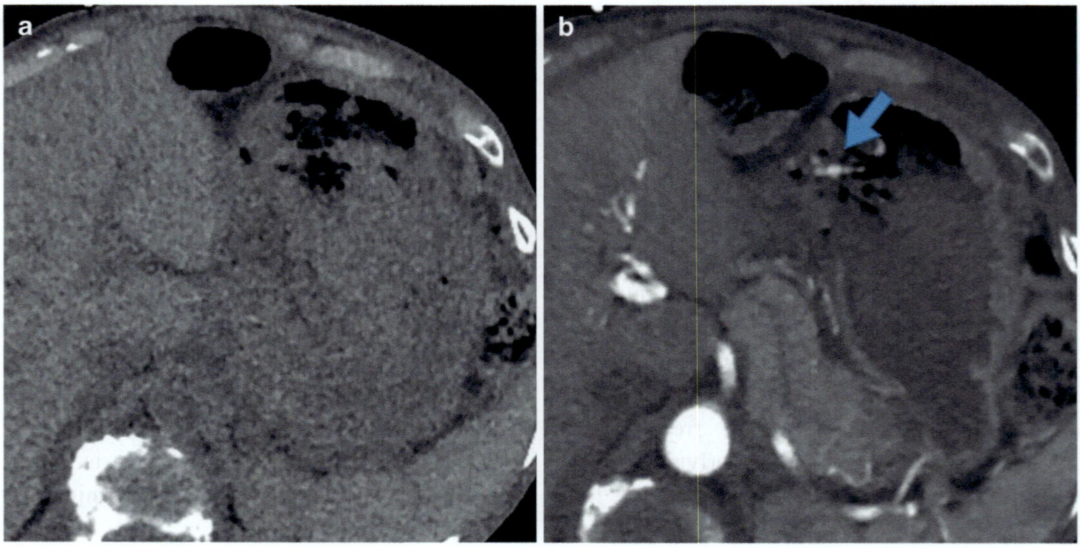

Fig. 7.22 CT images of the upper abdomen in a 56-year-old patient. Axial unenhanced (**a**) and arterial (**b**) phase images show extravasation of contrast into the gastric lumen (blue arrow), in keeping with active bleeding

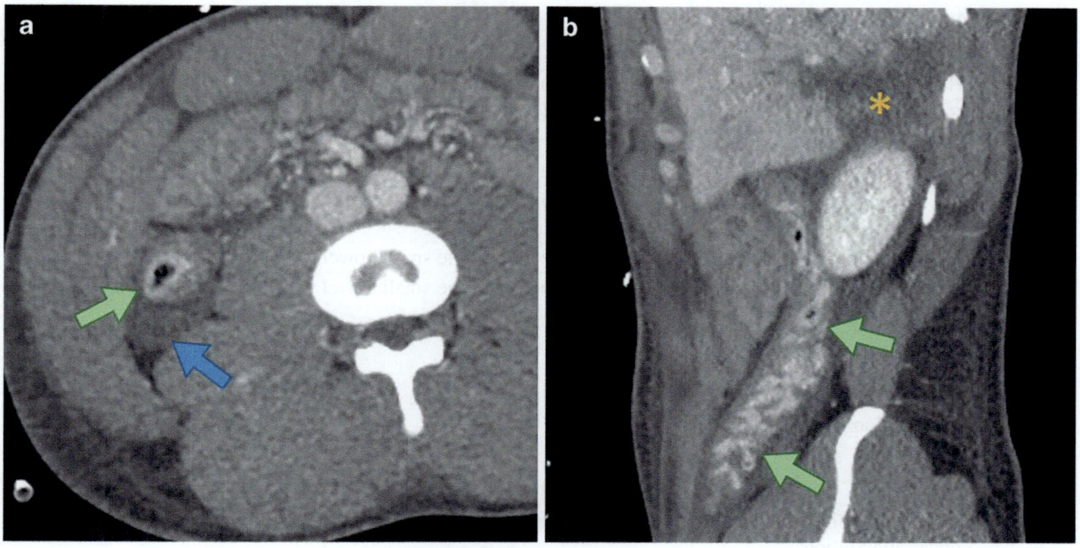

Fig. 7.23 CT images of the abdomen in a 16-year-old trauma patient. Axial (**a**) and sagittal (**b**) images show mucosal hyperenhancement (green arrows) and wall thickening of the ascending colon. Fluid closely abuts he colon (blue arrow), which may be in part related to a liver laceration (yellow asterisk). There are no findings of free air. The remainder of the small and large bowel appeared normal (not shown). Findings are suggestive of bowel injury. AAST grade I bowel injury

Table 7.7 AAST stomach injury scale [17]

AAST grade[a]	Description of injury
I	Contusion/hematoma
	Partial thickness laceration
II	Laceration <2 cm in GE junction or pylorus
	<5 cm in proximal 1/3 stomach
	<10 cm in distal 2/3 stomach
III	Laceration >2 cm in GE junction or pylorus
	>5 cm in proximal 1/3 stomach
	>10 cm in distal 2/3 stomach
IV	Tissue loss or devascularization <2/3 stomach
V	Tissue loss or devascularization >2/3 stomach

[a]Advance one grade for multiple injuries up to grade III

imaging does not always correlate with the patient's clinical condition, and the management of traumatic bowel injuries must be individualized based on the patient's overall clinical status and the presence of associated injuries.

Management and Complications

The management of gastric and intestinal injuries in trauma patients depends on the severity of the injury, the patient's clinical condition, and the presence of associated injuries. Management strategies that may be used for gastric and intestinal injury in trauma patients include:

- **Conservative management**: Patients with less severe injuries, such as Grade I or II injuries, may be managed conservatively with close monitoring and serial imaging to ensure healing and resolution of the injury. However, even patients with seemingly minor injuries may require close monitoring because of the risk of complications.
- **Surgical intervention**: Patients with gastric or intestinal injuries often require prompt surgical evaluation and intervention, as these injuries can be life-threatening and have a high risk of complications. Treatment options may include repair, resection with anastomo-

Table 7.8 AAST small bowel injury scale [15]

AAST grade[a]	Hematoma	Laceration	Vascular injury
I	Contusion or hematoma without devascularization	Partial thickness, no perforation	
II		Laceration <50% of circumference	
III		Laceration >50% of circumference without transection	
IV		Transection of the small bowel	
V		Transection of the small bowel with segmental tissue loss	Devascularized segment

[a]Advance one grade for multiple injuries up to grade III

Table 7.9 AAST colon injury scale [15]

AAST grade[a]	Hematoma	Laceration	Vascular injury
I	Contusion or hematoma without devascularization	Partial thickness, no perforation	
II		Laceration <50% of circumference	
III		Laceration >50% of circumference without transection	
IV		Transection of the colon	
V		Transection of the colon with segmental tissue loss	Devascularized segment

[a]Advance one grade for multiple injuries up to grade III

Table 7.10 AAST rectum injury scale [15]

AAST Grade[a]	Hematoma	Laceration	Vascular Injury
I	Contusion or hematoma without devascularization	Partial thickness laceration	
II		Laceration <50% of circumference	
III		Laceration >50% of circumference	
IV		Full-thickness laceration with extension into the perineum	
V			Devascularized segment

[a]Advance one grade for multiple injuries up to grade III

sis (Fig. 7.24), or diversion procedures such as gastrostomy or jejunostomy tubes, ileostomy or colostomy. For the surgeons, it is critical to preserve as much small bowel as possible.

- Repair of the distal rectum is difficult because of the extraperitoneal location; these injuries are more likely to require diversion. The intraperitoneal portion of the rectum has the same management as the remainder of the colon. In the setting of perineal injury or pelvic fractures, colostomy is the procedure of choice. [1].

The management of gastric or intestinal injury often involves a multidisciplinary approach, including trauma surgeons, interventional radiologists, and gastroenterologists. Although rare, potential complications in the management of patients with gastric and intestinal trauma include:

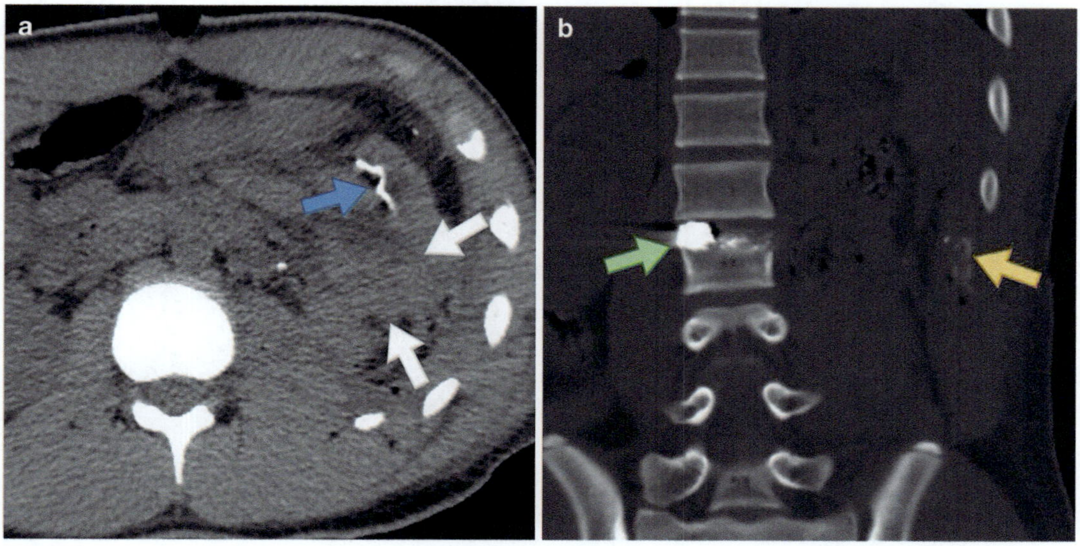

Fig. 7.24 CT images of the upper abdomen in a 15-year-old trauma patient presenting with gunshot wounds. The patient was hemodynamically unstable and proceeded directly to surgery without imaging. Axial unenhanced image (**a**) from follow-up CT shows suture material (blue arrow) along the descending colon, in keeping with colonic anastomosis. Associated retroperitoneal fluid and blood products are seen (white arrows). Coronal image with bone window (**b**) shows ballistic fragment lodged in the L1-L2 intervertebral disc space (green arrow) with associated fracture of the L2 superior endplate. Acute comminuted fracture of distal tip of left 11th rib is partially imaged (yellow arrow)

- **Bleeding**: Bleeding may occur into the bowel lumen or peritoneal cavity. Vascular injury to the short gastric vessels or tearing of the splenic capsule can present as gastric bleeding. Another potential source of bleeding is gastric or intestinal anastomoses [1].
- **Infection**: Normal gastric fluid is acidic and typically free of bacteria; similarly, small bowel contents are relatively sterile. However, the stomach and small bowel often contain ingested material, which acts as a potential source of infection following perforation. Peritoneal fecal contamination from the colon or rectum, which is related to either the initial trauma or anastomotic dehiscence, is associated with infection and sepsis [1].
- **Anastomotic disruption**: This complication may present as peritonitis, abscess or fistula and is associated with increased morbidity and mortality. Leaks from colonic anastomoses are more common in the left colon and transverse colon [1]. Anastomotic leaks should be treated with reoperation.
- **Small bowel obstruction**: Mechanical blockage of the small bowel that is a potential complication following any abdominal operation (Fig. 7.25).
- **Short gut**: Extensive resection of small bowel can lead to malabsorption.

As previously stated, recognition of these complications on imaging is essential for early treatment and decreasing morbidity and mortality.

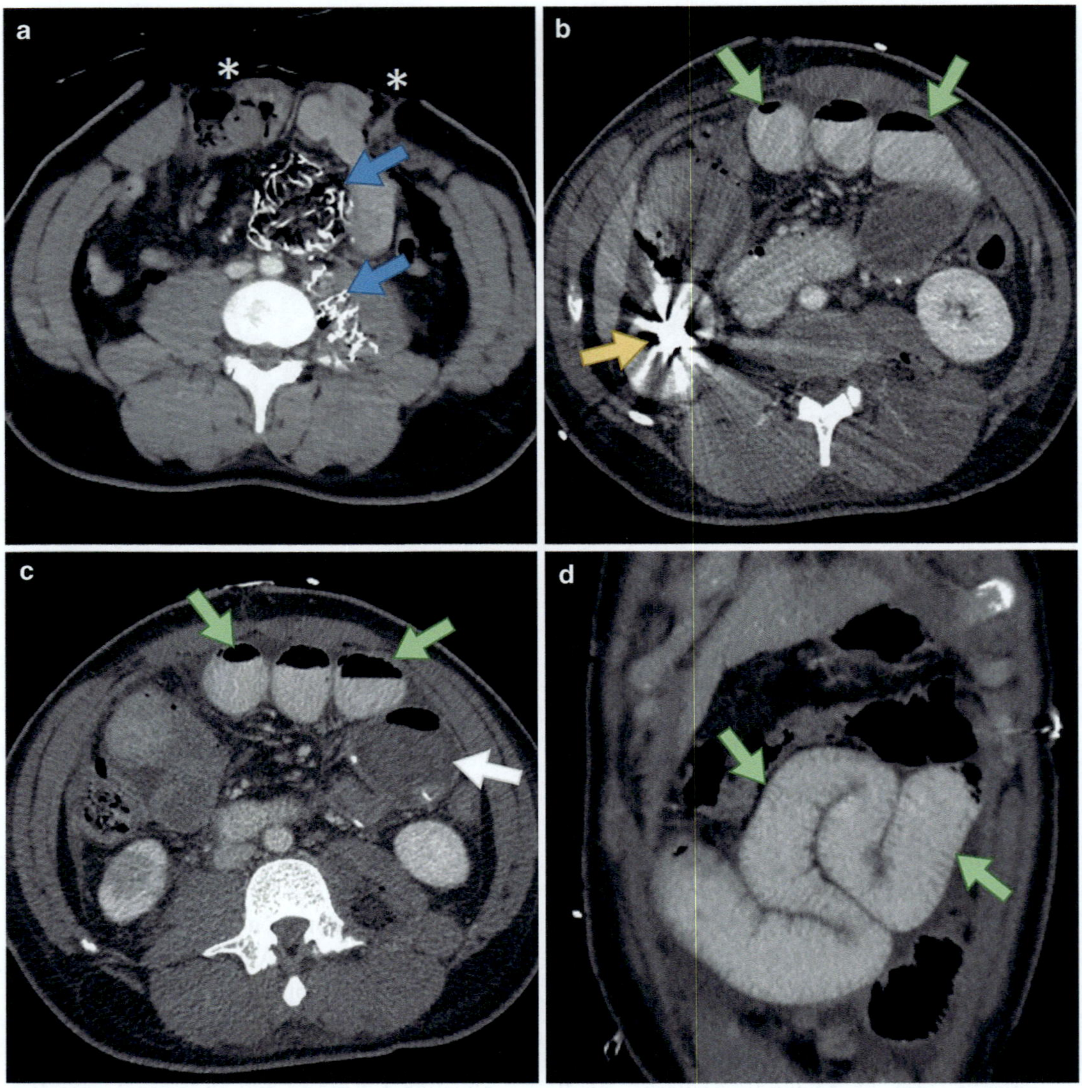

Fig. 7.25 CT images of the upper abdomen in a 25-year-old trauma patient presenting with gunshot wounds. The patient was hemodynamically unstable and proceeded directly to surgery without imaging. Axial unenhanced image after surgery (**a**) shows an open abdomen (white asterisks) and packing with surgical sponges (blue arrows). Axial (**b**, **c**) and coronal (**d**) portal venous phase images from CT performed several weeks after abdominal closure show a ballistic fragment in the right kidney (yellow arrow). There are several disproportionately dilated small bowel segments in the anterior central abdomen with air-contrast levels (green arrows), with transition point in the pelvis, distal to a patent enteroenteric anastomosis in the left midabdomen (white arrow). Findings are in keeping with small bowel obstruction, likely related to adhesions

Mesenteric Trauma

Mesenteric injury is relatively uncommon in trauma patients, but it can be a serious complication when it occurs. The incidence of mesenteric injury in trauma patients has been reported to range from 0.2% to 2.7% depending on the population studied and the severity of the trauma. Mesenteric injury is more common in patients with high-energy blunt trauma, such as those involved in motor vehicle collisions, falls from height, or industrial accidents. It is also more common in patients with associated injuries to the abdomen, such as injuries to the liver, spleen, or bowel.

Imaging and Grading

CT is the modality of choice for the detection and characterization of mesenteric traumatic injury. On CT, mesenteric injury may be indicated by the following findings:

- **Hematoma:** Collection within the mesentery that is well-defined. Attenuation varies with the age of the blood products, but is typically hyperattenuating. The area of highest attenuation usually indicates a "sentinel clot sign" near the site of bleeding [5]. When large, can exert mass effect on adjacent structures, including vessels.
- **Active bleeding**: Extravasation of intravenous contrast is suggestive of active bleeding and indicates high grade injury that requires urgent surgery [5]. Bleeding at the mesenteric root raises concern for injury to the superior mesenteric artery or vein.
- **Beading/termination of mesenteric vessels**: Focal variation in the size of a mesenteric vessel, which is isoattenuating to arteries, is known as beading. Discontinuity or absence of tapering of mesenteric vessels suggests abrupt termination. These findings are specific for high grade injury and may be better visualized on coronal or sagittal planes.
- **Bowel ischemia**: Segmental bowel ischemia, such as intramural air and hypoenhancement, may be indicative of an underlying mesenteric injury in this region.
- **Stranding in the mesentery**: Haziness of the mesenteric fat is sensitive but not specific for mesenteric injury (Fig. 7.26). This finding may also reflect underlying bowel injury, particularly if there is adjacent bowel wall thickening (Fig. 7.27). Alternatively, pre-existing mesenteric panniculitis also manifests as mesenteric haziness on imaging.
- **Intraperitoneal or Retroperitoneal Fluid**: In the absence of solid organ injury, intraperitoneal or retroperitoneal free fluid suggests an underlying bowel or mesenteric injury, particularly interloop fluid. Conversely, the absence of free fluid is reassuring that there is no

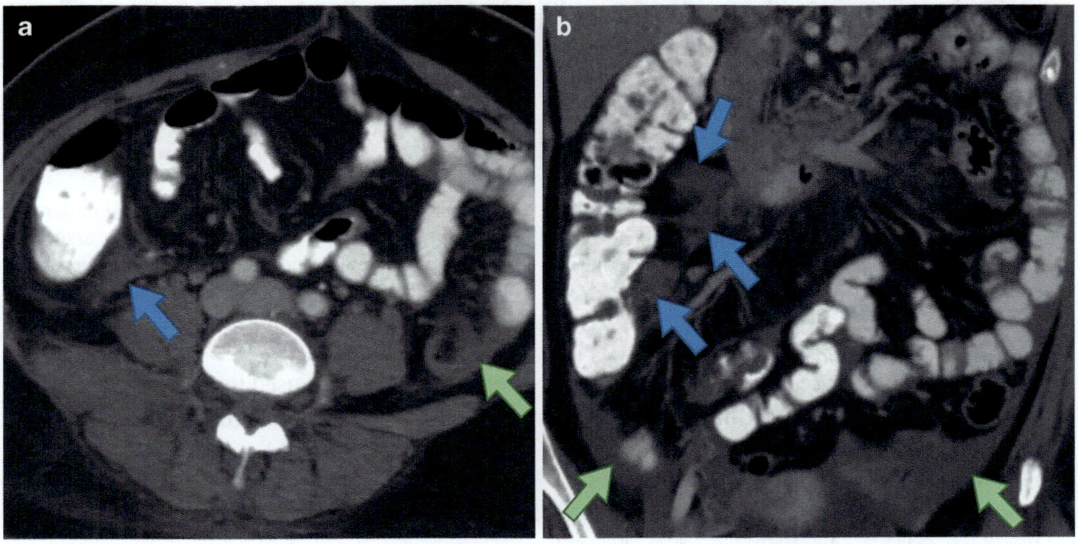

Fig. 7.26 CT images of the upper abdomen in a 35-year-old trauma patient presenting after motor vehicle collision. Axial (**a**) and coronal (**b**) images show multiple areas of mesenteric edema (blue arrows) and small volume hemoperitoneum (42 Hounsfield units) (green arrows). No findings of associated bowel injury. Findings are in keeping with mesenteric injury. BIPS grade 1 injury

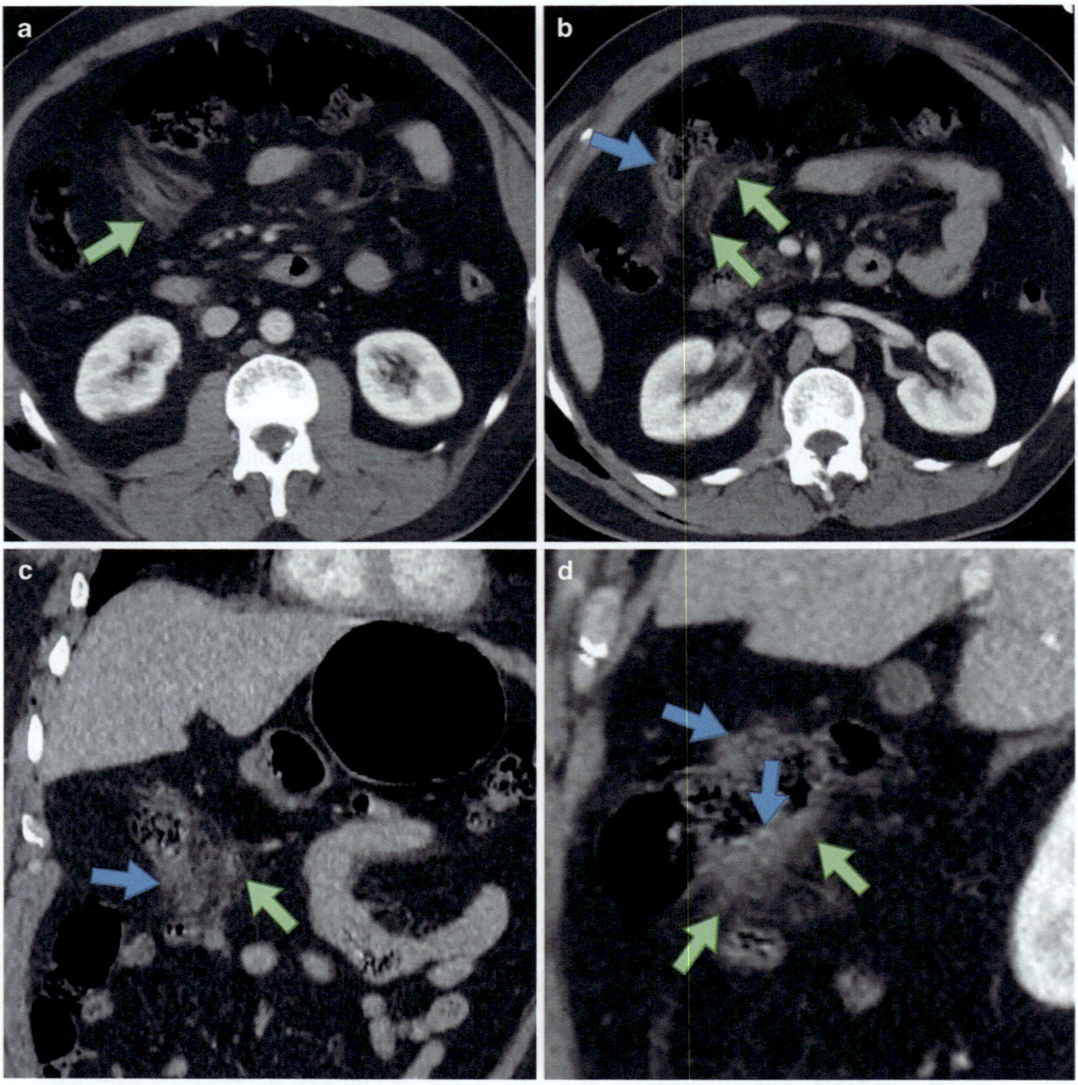

Fig. 7.27 CT images of the upper abdomen in a 33-year-old trauma patient presenting after motor vehicle collision. Axial (**a**, **b**) and coronal (**c**, **d**) portal venous phase images show short segment wall thickening of the proximal transverse colon (blue arrows) with focal mesenteric stranding and edema (green arrows). The associated bowel wall thickening increases the grade of mesenteric injury. BIPS grade 4 injury

underlying bowel or mesenteric injury. The location of the fluid may hint at a nearby injury. Of note, hypoattenuating fluid could also represent urine from bladder injury [5].

A commonly used grading system for CT findings of mesenteric injury or bowel injury is the Blunt Injury Prediction Score (BIPS), which is detailed in Table 7.11. The Mesenteric Injury Score (MIS) may be used to assess intraoperative findings of mesenteric and bowel injury [20].

Management and Complications

The clinical management of mesenteric injury depends on the severity and extent of the injury. In general, more severe injuries require surgical

Table 7.11 Blunt injury prediction score (BIPS) [20, 21]

BIPS grade	Description of Injury
1	Isolated mesenteric contusion without associated bowel wall thickening or adjacent interloop fluid collection
2	Mesenteric hematoma <5 cm without associated bowel wall thickening or adjacent interloop fluid collection
3	Mesenteric hematoma >5 cm without associated bowel wall thickening or adjacent interloop fluid collection
4	Mesenteric contusion or hematoma (any size) with associated bowel wall thickening or adjacent interloop fluid collection
5	Active vascular or oral contrast extravasation, bowel transection or pneumoperitoneum

intervention, while less severe injuries may be managed conservatively. Management strategies that may be used for mesenteric injury in trauma patients include:

- **Conservative management**: Less severe injuries, including grade 1 and 2 injuries, may be managed conservatively.
- **Surgical Intervention**: More severe injuries may require surgical intervention, which may involve resection of devitalized bowel and repair or ligation of damaged vessels.

Potential complications in the management of patients with mesenteric trauma include:

- **Bleeding**: Bleeding may be inconspicuous on initial imaging and can unfortunately continue in patients managed conservatively. Additionally, mesenteric injuries may not be detected during surgery, particularly in polytrauma patients, leading to continued bleeding [1].

Conclusion

CT imaging is an essential tool in the evaluation of gastrointestinal injuries in trauma patients. It is the preferred imaging modality because it is widely available, rapid, and accurate in detecting both the presence and the extent of injury.

References

1. Mattox KL, Moore EE, Feliciano DV. Trauma. 9th ed. New York: McGraw-Hill Medical; 2021.
2. Simel DL. Does this adult patient have a blunt intra-abdominal injury? JAMA. 2012;307(14):1517.
3. Isenhour JL, Marx J. Advances in abdominal trauma. Emerg Med Clin North Am. 2007;25(3):713–33.
4. Durso AM, Paes FM, Caban K, Danton G, Braga TA, Sanchez A, et al. Evaluation of penetrating abdominal and pelvic trauma. Eur J Radiol. 2020;130:109187.
5. Miele V, Trinci M, editors. Diagnostic imaging in polytrauma patients. Cham: Springer; 2018.
6. Carr JA, Roiter C, Alzuhaili A. Correlation of operative and pathological injury grade with computed tomographic grade in the failed nonoperative management of blunt splenic trauma. Eur J Trauma Emerg Surg. 2012;38(4):433–8.
7. Bee TK, Croce MA, Miller PR, Pritchard FE, Fabian TC. Failures of splenic nonoperative management: is the glass half empty or half full? J Trauma Inj Infect Crit Care. 2001;50(2):230–6.
8. Clark TJ, Cardoza S, Kanth N. Splenic trauma: pictorial review of contrast-enhanced CT findings. Emerg Radiol. 2011;18(3):227–34.
9. Anderson SW, Varghese JC, Lucey BC, Burke PA, Hirsch EF, Soto JA. Blunt splenic trauma: delayed-phase CT for differentiation of active hemorrhage from contained vascular injury in patients. Radiology. 2007;243(1):88–95.
10. Marmery H, Shanmuganathan K, Mirvis SE, Richard H, Sliker C, Miller LA, et al. Correlation of multidetector CT findings with splenic arteriography and surgery: prospective study in 392 patients. J Am Coll Surg. 2008;206(4):685–93.
11. Wirth S, Hebebrand J, Basilico R, Berger FH, Blanco A, Calli C, et al. European Society of Emergency Radiology: guideline on radiological polytrauma imaging and service (short version). Insights Imaging. 2020;11(1):135.
12. Stephens J, Yu HS, Uyeda JW. Hepatobiliary trauma imaging update. Radiol Clin N Am. 2022;60(5):745–54.
13. Shanmuganathan K, Mirvis SE, Chiu WC, Killeen KL, Hogan GJF, Scalea TM. Penetrating torso trauma: triple-contrast helical CT in peritoneal violation and organ injury—a prospective study in 200 patients. Radiology. 2004;231(3):775–84.
14. Moore EE, Shackford SR, Pachter HL, McAninch JW, Browner BD, Champion HR, et al. Organ injury scaling: spleen, liver, and kidney. J Trauma. 1989;29(12):1664–6.
15. Moore EE, Cogbill TH, Malangoni MA, Jurkovich GJ, Champion HR, Gennarelli TA, et al. Organ injury scaling, II: pancreas, duodenum, small bowel, colon, and rectum. J Trauma. 1990;30(11):1427–9.
16. Moore EE, Cogbill TH, Jurkovich GJ, McAninch JW, Champion HR, Gennarelli TA, et al. Organ

injury scaling. III: chest wall, abdominal vascular, ureter, bladder, and urethra. J Trauma. 1992;33(3):337–9.

17. Moore EE, Jurkovich GJ, Knudson MM, Cogbill TH, Malangoni MA, Champion HR, et al. Organ injury scaling. VI: extrahepatic biliary, esophagus, stomach, vulva, vagina, uterus (nonpregnant), uterus (pregnant), fallopian tube, and ovary. J Trauma. 1995;39(6):1069–70.
18. Moore EE, Malangoni MA, Cogbill TH, Peterson NE, Champion HR, Jurkovich GJ, et al. Organ injury scaling VII: cervical vascular, peripheral vascular, adrenal, penis, testis, and scrotum. J Trauma. 1996;41(3):523–4.
19. Kozar RA, Crandall M, Shanmuganathan K, Zarzaur BL, Coburn M, Cribari C, et al. Organ injury scaling 2018 update: spleen, liver, and kidney. J Trauma Acute Care Surg. 2018;85(6):1119–22.
20. Bekker W, Hernandez MC, Zielinski MD, Kong VY, Laing GL, Bruce JL, et al. Defining an intraoperative blunt mesenteric injury grading system and its use as a tool for surgical-decision making. Injury. 2019;50(1):27–32.
21. Wandling M, Cuschieri J, Kozar R, O'Meara L, Celii A, Starr W, et al. Multi-center validation of the bowel injury predictive score (BIPS) for the early identification of need to operate in blunt bowel and mesenteric injuries. Injury. 2022;53(1):122–8.

Imaging of Genitourinary Trauma

8

Joanie Garratt, Jay Im, Akshya Gupta, Paul Hill, and Kalpana Suresh

Genitourinary Trauma

Abdominal and pelvic injuries occur in approximately 15–20% of all trauma patients. In abdominal and pelvic trauma, the kidneys, urinary bladder, and urethra are commonly injured organs. Significant genitourinary injuries result from either blunt or penetrating trauma. More than 90 percent of closed traumatic injuries are secondary to wide-impact blunt trauma, such as motor vehicle collisions. Renal and urinary bladder traumatic injuries frequently occur in motor vehicle collisions, with an incidence of 43 percent and 16 percent, respectively [1]. Male genitalia, typically testes, and kidneys are the most commonly injured genitourinary organs in the setting of two-wheeled motorized vehicle collisions, occurring in 64% and 28% of cases, respectively [1]. Genitourinary injury, particularly renal injury, is also common in penetrating trauma. Unfortunately, traumatic injuries are often more severe in the setting of penetrating trauma. Additional details regarding blunt and penetrating trauma are discussed in Chap. 7. CT plays an essential role in the diagnosing and guiding management of genitourinary injury in trauma patients.

Imaging of Genitourinary Trauma

Imaging is critically important in the evaluation for genitourinary injuries in trauma patients. CT is the imaging modality of choice because of the speed of imaging acquisition, broad anatomical coverage, and accuracy in identifying clinically important injuries. The benefits of CT in the evaluation of genitourinary trauma overlap those discussed in Chap. 7 for the evaluation of gastrointestinal trauma, including:

- Rapid and accurate diagnosis
- Non-invasive
- Identification of free fluid or air in the peritoneum
- Detection of specific injuries
- Assessment of the severity of injury
- Detection of associated injuries
- Planning of surgical intervention
- Follow-up.

Management decisions in trauma patients are in part determined by imaging findings. For example, CT can help determine whether surgery is necessary or whether nonsurgical manage-

J. Garratt (✉) · K. Suresh
Department of Radiology, University of Pennsylvania, Philadelphia, PA, USA
e-mail: joanie.garratt@pennmedicine.upenn.edu; kalpana.suresh@pennmedicine.upenn.edu

J. Im · A. Gupta
Department of Radiology, University of Rochester, Rochester, NY, USA

P. Hill
Department of Radiology, Winchester Radiologists, Winchester, VA, USA

F. Knollmann (ed.), *Trauma Computed Tomography*, https://doi.org/10.1007/978-3-031-45746-3_8

ment, such as observation or interventional radiology procedures, is appropriate. CT can also help determine the need for additional imaging, admission to the intensive care unit, blood transfusions, or other interventions.

In summary, CT is a valuable tool in the evaluation of genitourinary injury in trauma patients, as it can provide detailed information on the presence and extent of injury, guide treatment decisions, and help to optimize patient outcomes.

CT Protocol

Contrast-enhanced CT imaging plays a significant role in the evaluation of injury to the genitourinary system, particularly in the evaluation of the upper and lower urinary tract [1].

In addition to standard CT trauma protocols for the abdomen and pelvis (discussed in Chap. 7; an example protocol is provided in Table 8.1), GU-specific CT protocols are also beneficial.

Table 8.1 Example protocol to evaluate for genitourinary trauma

CT trauma chest, abdomen and pelvis protocol (one run): combined arterial and portal venous phase imaging			
Clinical indication		Severe, Life threatening Head and or Body Trauma. To be requested by the Trauma Surgeon	
Age		Adult	
Dose range		38.64–60.41 mGy	
Body habitus		mA modulation and automated kV selection are utilized to account for different patient body habitus	
Prep		18 or 20 gauge IV	
Contrast administration		125 mL Isovue 370	
Scan parameters	kV	120	
	mA	Smart mA	
	mA Min/Max	100–550	
	Noise Index	12.23	
	Scan Type	Helical	
	SFOV	Large Body	
	DFOV	36.0	
	Detector Coverage (mm)	80	
	Pitch	0.992:1	
	Coverage speed (mm/s)	65.62	
	Rotation time (s)	0.80	
	Slice collimation (mm)	0.625	
	Thickness (mm)	5	
	Scan interval (mm)	5	
	ASIR	50%	
	WW/WL	40/40	
	Algorithm (Recon Type)	Standard; 2 mm and 5 mm	
Scan procedure		Every attempt should be made to raise the arms above head	
		Lung apices through lesser trochanters	
		Start scan and injector simultaneously	
IV injection	Notes	Dual syringe, 325 psi (PICC or power port- 300 psi)	
		SPLIT injection: 70 mL @ 3 mL/s, 55 mL @ 2 mL/s	
		Injection delay: 65 s	
	Solution	**Rate**	**Amount**
	Saline	3 mL/s	20 mL
	Contrast	3 mL/s	70 mL
	Contrast	2 mL/s	55 mL
	Saline	2 mL/s	20 mL

Excretory phase imaging, for instance, should be obtained to evaluate the collecting systems and ureters in patients with suspected injury of these structures. The excretory phase is timed to allow the kidneys to excrete contrast into and opacify the urine. A CT urography protocol typically includes a three-phase set of images through the abdomen and pelvis [2], including:

- **Unenhanced phase**: Useful in the evaluation for renal calculi, intraparenchymal hematoma, and acute bleeding.
- **Corticomedullary phase** (40–70 s after intravenous contrast): Useful in evaluation for enhancing urothelial lesions.
- **Excretory phase** (5–15 min after intravenous contrast): Useful in evaluation for filling defects, strictures, or extravasation of contrast involving the collecting systems, ureters or urinary bladder.

While CT urography is most often performed to evaluate microscopic hematuria, the most salient phase of contrast for suspected traumatic injury of a collecting system or ureter is the excretory phase. Also, most trauma patients are initially evaluated with a standard contrast-enhanced CT of the abdomen and pelvis, either single phase or multi-phase. The solution is to perform delayed imaging in the excretory phase in patients who have already received intravenous contrast; these patients can return to the scanner as the excretory phase can last hours after intravenous contrast administration. Therefore, if there is suspected collecting system or ureteral injury based on the initial CT abdomen and pelvis, the patient should return to the CT scanner for additional images. In a busy trauma center, it is not ideal to keep every trauma patient on the CT scanner for more than 10 min to obtain excretory phase imaging. An example CT urogram protocol is provided in Table 8.2.

Cystography is essential in patients with suspected urinary bladder injury and CT cystography can be performed as an alternative to traditional fluoroscopic cystography. Passive filling of the urinary bladder during excretory phase imaging from intravenous contrast does not sufficiently distend the urinary bladder to evaluate for injury [1, 3]. A cystogram involves instilling contrast (350 mL of 3–5% iodinated contra) via a Foley catheter to achieve distention of the urinary bladder. CT cystography includes images of the pelvis before and after instillation of contrast into the urinary bladder; although not required with CT cystography, some protocols include images after the urinary bladder is emptied to potentially improve sensitivity for injury [4]. Postvoid imaging is necessary with conventional cystography to improve visualization anterior and posterior to the urinary bladder [5]. An example CT cystogram protocol is provided in Table 8.3.

CT may provide clues to the diagnosis of urethral or genitalia injury, although additional imaging is often necessary. In evaluation of the urethra, fluoroscopic urethrography remains the

Table 8.2 Example CT urogram (CTU) protocol

CT urogram protocol	
Clinical indication	Hematuria, detection or follow-up of urothelial or renal malignancy, evaluation for congenital or posttraumatic abnormalities of the urinary tract
Age	Adult
Dose range	8.970–48.54 mGy
Body habitus	mA modulation and automated kV selection are utilized to account for different patient body habitus
Prep	18 or 20 gauge IV
Contrast administration	120 mL Isovue 370

(continued)

Table 8.2 (continued)

CT urogram protocol					
Scan parameters		**Unenhanced phase**	**Corticomedullary phase**	**Excretory phase**	**Prone (if needed)**
	kV	120			
	mA	Smart mA			
	mA Min/Max	100–550			
	Noise index	18.0	25.0	18.0	18.0
	Scan type	Helical			
	SFOV	Large body			
	Detector coverage (mm)	80			
	Pitch	0.992:1	0.991:1	0.992:1	0.992:1
	coverage speed (mm/s)	283.48	283.48	158.75	158.75
	Rotation time (s)	0.28	0.28	0.50	0.50
	Thickness (mm)	5.0	2.5	1.25	1.25
	Scan interval	5.0	1.25	1.25	1.25
	ASIR	30%	30%	50%	50%
	WW/WL	400/40	400/40	350/50	350/50
	Algorithm (Recon type)	Standard; 2 mm and 5 mm			
	Scan coverage	Abdomen and Pelvis			A&P Prone
	Scan delay	–	Smart Prep +12 s	15 min	Immediate
Scan procedure		Every attempt should be made to raise the arms above head			
		Scout: Abdomen and Pelvis from above diaphragm through pubic symphysis			
		Unenhanced phase: Above kidneys to bladder			
		Pre-monitoring/monitoring: ROI on aorta @ level of celiac			
		Corticomedullary phase: Diaphragm to pubic symphysis			
		Pause: 15 minute delay			
		Excretory phase: Diaphragm to pubic symphysis			
		Scroll through excretory phase images; if ureters are not enhanced through the bladder, have the patient lie prone on the table. Take one prone scout image and scan an unenhanced prone abdomen and pelvis			
IV injection	Notes	Dual syringe, 325 psi (PICC or power port- 300 psi)			
	Smart prep	120 mL contrast			
		ROI: Aorta @ level of celiac			
		130 HU trigger			
		Peak +10 s			
	Solution	**Rate**	**Amount**		
	Saline test	4 mL/s	20 mL		
	Contrast	4 mL/s	120 mL		
	Saline flush	4 mL/s	140 mL		

Table 8.3 Example CT cystogram protocol

CT cystogram protocol			
Clinical indication		Bladder leak, post op bladder surgery, TRAUMA, bladder perforation, possible fistula	
Age		Adult	
Dose range		5.88–28.85 mGy	
Body habitus		mA modulation and automated kV selection are utilized to account for different patient body habitus	
Prep		Foley catheter placement	
Contrast administration		15 mL Isovue 370 with 500 mL saline	
Scan parameters		Unenhanced Pelvis and Filled Bladder phases	
	kV	120	
	mAs	160	
	Slide collimation (mm)	32 × 1.2	
	Slice width (mm)	2	
	Pitch	0.8	
	Rotation time (s)	0.5	
Scan procedure		Every attempt should be made to raise the arms above head; feet first into scanner	
		Scout: Pelvis from above iliac crest through greater trochanters	
		Unenhanced phase: Scan full pelvis unenhanced before contrast is administered into bladder	
		Mix 15 mL of Isovue 370 into a 500 mL saline bag via syringe and blunt tip needle. IV drip tubing is inserted into 500 mL bag of saline. Clamp Foley tubing with hemostats below the site of IV drip connection (preferably use gauze in between hemostat and Foley tubing to avoid puncturing the tubing).	
		Instill 300 mL of the contrast into the urinary bladder under gravity. If the patient is experiencing extreme discomfort, stop the contrast and scan the pelvis. The amount of contrast instilled into the bladder depends on the patient and depends on the physician's discretion how much the patient can tolerate due to their specific injury/clinical indication. In the setting of trauma, approximately 200 mL is often needed to fully distend the bladder to evaluate for leak	
		Filled bladder phase: Scan the pelvis with contrast-filled bladder	
		Reconnect Foley catheter to drainage bag and drop below table to empty bladder.	
		Scan postvoid bladder if needed or requested.	
IV injection	Notes	Dual syringe, 325 psi (PICC or power port- 300 psi)	
		SPLIT injection: 70 mL @ 3 mL/s, 55 mL @ 2 mL/s	
		Injection delay: 65 s	
	Solution	**Rate**	**Amount**
	Saline	3 mL/s	20 mL
	Contrast	3 mL/s	70 mL
	Contrast	2 mL/s	55 mL
	Saline	2 mL/s	20 mL

gold standard [1]. However, CT is performed in nearly every trauma patient and it is important to detect subtle findings that may suggest further investigation of the urethra or genitalia is needed.

It is essential to optimize the CT technique and protocols used in the evaluation of trauma patients. There are many factors to consider, including contrast material as well as the number and timing of phases. Additional details regarding the CT protocol for imaging of the abdomen and pelvic in trauma patients are discussed in Chap. 7: Imaging of Gastrointestinal Trauma.

Injury Assessment and Grading

The Organ Injury Scale (OIS) created by the American Association for the Surgery of Trauma (AAST) is a classification system that standardizes the assessment and severity of traumatic organ injury and guides management. This injury scale grades injuries from minor (grade I or II) to severe or life threatening (grade V or VI). This grading system accounts for location, size, and depth of injury, including vascular injury such as arteriovenous fistulae or pseudoaneurysm. The most recent update in 2018 includes imaging findings, acknowledging the importance of imaging evaluation of trauma patients since its first use in the 1980s [1, 5–7]. In fact, the accuracy of CT imaging in evaluating injuries in trauma patients has allowed nonsurgical management to become the standard of care in hemodynamically stable patients [1]. The imaging findings for the AAST OIS are detailed in this text; there are separate criteria for operative and pathologic findings.

The AAST OIS are the most widely accepted classification systems and are most commonly used in the evaluation of solid viscera injuries, including renal trauma. A grading system helps clinicians to better understand the extent of the injury and to guide further management, such as whether surgical intervention is required. In addition, a classification system can help to standardize communication among healthcare professionals, facilitating accurate and consistent reporting of injuries in trauma patients. Although there are AAST organ injury scales for all genitourinary organs, there is no consensus regarding their use and, except for renal injury, they are less commonly used for genitourinary injuries. However, knowledge of the classification systems does provide insight into the information that should be included on a radiologist's report for imaging of trauma patients.

Adrenal Trauma

With an incidence of less than 4% in blunt trauma patients, adrenal gland traumatic injury is uncommon and is most often associated with massive trauma. In the absence of substantial trauma, an adrenal abnormality is unlikely to represent a traumatic adrenal injury. Patients with underlying adrenal disorders may be predisposed to adrenal gland injury, even in minor trauma [1]; prior imaging is indispensable in the evaluation for underlying adrenal lesions. Unilateral right adrenal gland injury is most common, while isolated left adrenal injury is uncommon and bilateral injury is rare [1]. The mechanisms of adrenal gland injury include direct trauma and decreased blood supply.

Hyperenhancement of both adrenal glands on CT has also been suggested as an indicator of hypoperfusion complex (Fig. 8.1). The differential diagnosis for this finding is bilateral acute adrenal hemorrhage; the presence of normal adreniform shape and absence of surrounding inflammation, such as periadrenal fat stranding, favors shock adrenals [8].

Anatomy

The adrenal glands are two V- or Y-shaped structures that are located superior to each kidney in the retroperitoneum. These glands are responsible for producing hormones, such as cortisol, that regulate a variety of bodily functions [1]. The

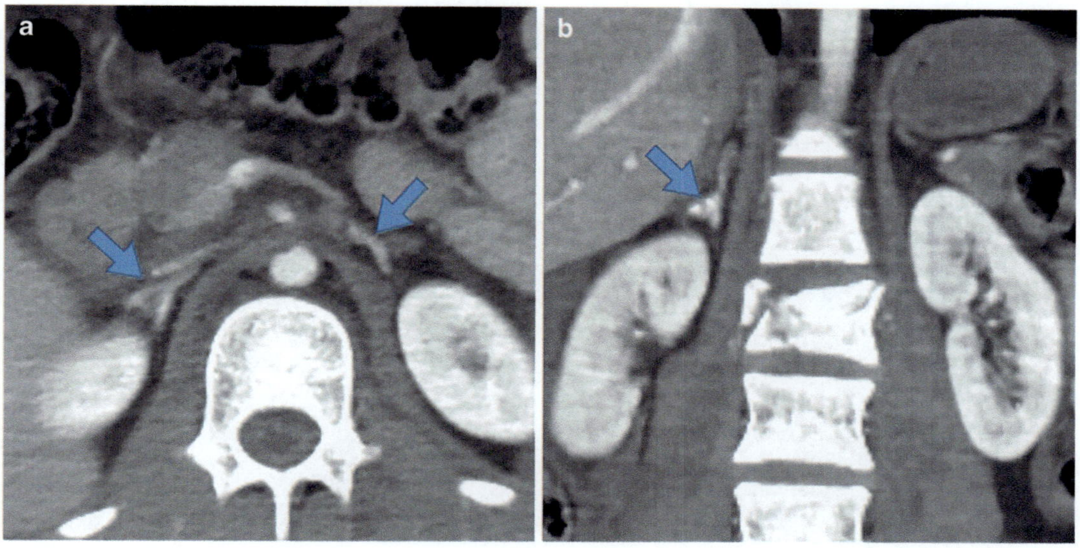

Fig. 8.1 CT images of the upper abdomen in a 21-year-old trauma patient presenting with extensive injuries (not shown) after jumping from a second story window. Axial (**a**) and coronal (**b**) portal venous phase images of the adrenals show hyperenhancement of the adrenal glands (blue arrows), which have a normal adreniform shape. Findings favor shock adrenal changes in the setting of hypoperfusion complex

right adrenal gland is located between the liver and the spine, making it susceptible to compression during blunt trauma. Additionally, the right adrenal vein drains directly into the IVC; because of the increased intra-abdominal pressure with blunt trauma, the short course of the adrenal vein predisposes the right adrenal gland to injury from increased venous pressure [1, 9]. The left adrenal gland is located superior and slightly anterior to the left kidney.

Imaging and Grading

CT is important in the evaluation of adrenal gland injury in trauma patients. Some specific CT findings of adrenal injury include:

- **Contusion/hematoma**: Typically a well-defined, round or oval, hyperattenuating (> 50 HU) nodule or mass that expands the adrenal gland (Figs. 8.2 and 8.3) [1, 9]. A centrally located hematoma may splay the limbs of the adrenal gland. Less often, a contusion or hematoma appears as diffuse swelling/edema with indistinct margins or complete obliteration of the gland [9].
- **Laceration**: Tear in the tissue, which most often appears as linear or irregularly-shaped area of hypoattenuation. There may be an associated perinephric hematoma.
- **Active bleeding**: Contrast extravasation, which is leakage of contrast material from the blood vessels within the adrenal gland, may indicate active bleeding; active bleeding is best appreciated on arterial phase imaging. Associated hemorrhage in the retroperitoneum will be present.
- **Fat stranding**: Periadrenal fat stranding is often related to blood products from adrenal injury (Fig. 8.3).
- **Fluid accumulation**: Accumulation of fluid or blood products in the retroperitoneum may indicate adrenal injury. Associated hemorrhage is most common in the posterior pararenal space, layering along the diaphragmatic crus, but may extend to any portion of the retroperitoneum [9]. In the presence of a large retroperitoneal hemorrhage, consider adrenal gland rupture.

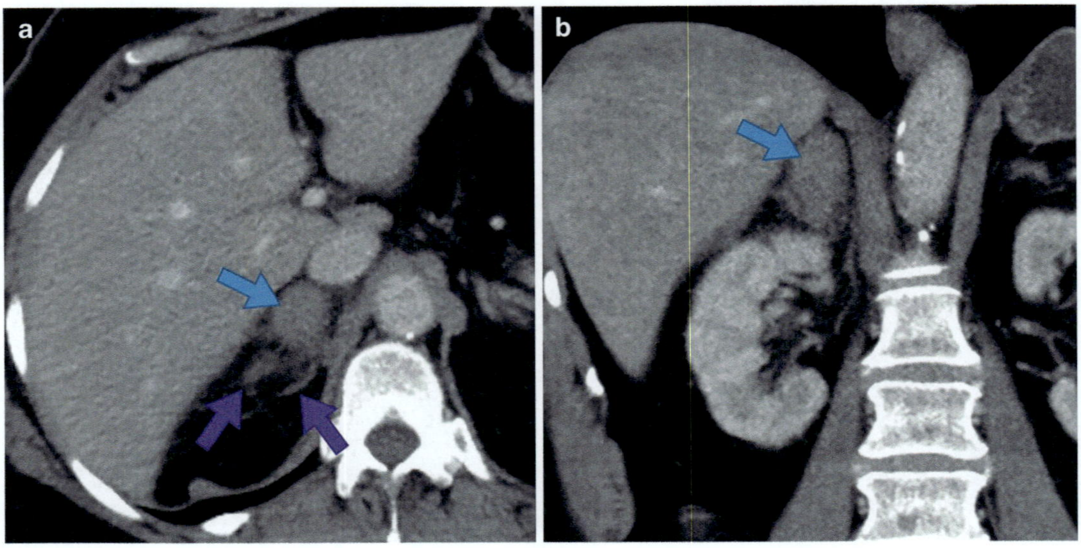

Fig. 8.2 CT images of the upper abdomen in a 63-year-old trauma patient presenting after a fall down a flight of stairs. Axial (**a**) and coronal (**b**) portal venous phase images show enlargement of the right adrenal gland (blue arrows) with surrounding fat stranding. The posterior limbs of the adrenal gland may be preserved, but splayed (purple arrows). Findings are in keeping with intraparenchymal hemorrhage. AAST grade IV adrenal injury

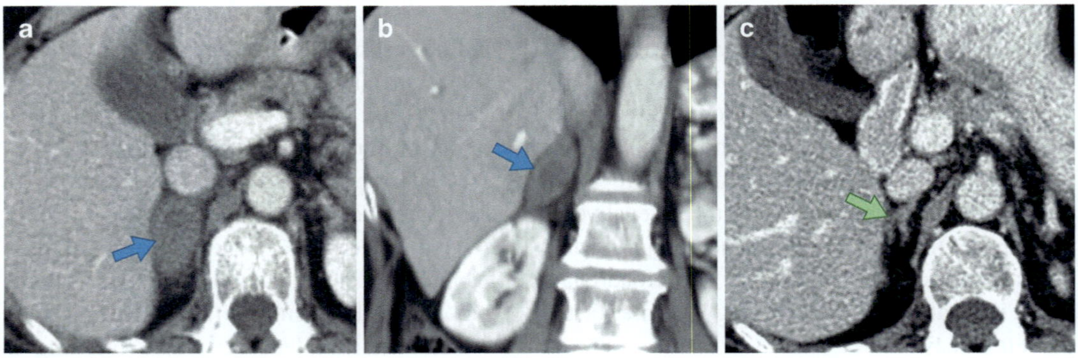

Fig. 8.3 CT images of the right upper abdomen in a 71-year-old trauma patient presenting after a fall. Axial (**a**) and coronal (**b**) portal venous phase images show heterogeneous enlargement of the right adrenal gland (blue arrows) with subtle surrounding fat stranding, new from recent CT with normal appearance of the adrenal gland (**c**). Findings are in keeping with intraparenchymal hemorrhage and associated loss of the normal adrenal architecture. AAST grade V adrenal injury

The AAST OIS is the most commonly used scale to assess adrenal injury and is detailed in Table 8.4.

Management and Complications

Unilateral adrenal injury has little, if any, clinical significance. Because adrenal injuries often occur in the setting of multiorgan injury, management, including the need for surgical intervention, is guided by the associated traumatic injuries [1]. Rarely, endocrine abnormalities, such as post-traumatic pheochromocytoma-like syndrome or adrenal insufficiency, occur following bilateral adrenal injury. On follow-up imaging, adrenal hematomas should decrease in size or resolve; if an adrenal abnormality does not resolve within 3 months, it may be unrelated to the patient's trauma [1].

Table 8.4 AAST adrenal injury scale [10]

AAST grade[a]	Description of injury
I	Contusion
II	Laceration involving only cortex (<2 cm)
III	Laceration extending into medulla (>2 cm)
IV	>50% parenchymal destruction
V	Total parenchymal destruction (including massive intraparenchymal hemorrhage)
	Avulsion from blood supply

[a]Advance one grade for bilateral lesions up to grade V

Renal Trauma

In the U.S., traumatic injuries account for over 150,000 deaths in addition to over three million non-fatal injuries per year. Of those, renal trauma and injury to the genitourinary tract are involved in roughly 10% [11]. Injuries may result in renovascular compromise, urinary tract leakage, and parenchymal damage. Blunt trauma is by far the more common mechanism of injury involving approximately 71–95% of renal trauma [5]. Typical scenarios involve motor vehicle collisions, falls, sports injuries, and pedestrian struck injuries in order of descending frequency [10]. Direct blows to an organ can cause a crush injury from surrounding musculature or cause a deceleration injury resulting in shearing or avulsion of the collecting system and vasculature. Ureteropelvic junction injuries are most commonly sudden deceleration injuries causing shearing of the renal pedicle causing either avulsion or laceration [12]. Penetrating trauma typically results from gunshots or stab wounds [13].

Independent of the mechanism of injury, multiorgan injury is common with renal traumatic injuries, occurring in 80–95% of trauma patients [1]. Flank ecchymosis or palpable abnormalities in the flank, abdomen, or back can raise suspicion for renal trauma [14]. Rib fractures should also raise concern for adjacent organ injury. Hematuria raises suspicion but may not be present [14].

Anatomy

The kidneys lie within the retroperitoneal space in the abdomen, generally at the level of the T12 through L3 vertebral bodies. The oblique orientation positions the superior pole more medially relative to the lower pole. They are well protected by the rib cage, paraspinal musculature, and surrounding perirenal fat. One or more renal arteries, with a draining renal vein, supply the kidneys. Urine produced by the kidney drains into the renal collecting system. Calyces drain into the renal pelvis and subsequently the ureter. The renal parenchyma itself consists of the cortex and medulla, while the renal sinus contains the renal pelvis, vascular supply/hilum, lymphatics, and renal sinus fat.

The perirenal space immediately surrounding the kidney contains fat and is separated by the anterior pararenal space of the retroperitoneum by the anterior renal fascia, known as Gerota fascia. The perirenal space is separated from the posterior pararenal space of the retroperitoneum by the posterior renal fascia, known as Zuckerkandl fascia. For the purposes of injury scoring, both the anterior and posterior renal fascia are referred to as Gerota fascia.

Imaging and Grading

Grading of renal injury, evaluation and recognition of concomitant injuries, and communication to providers in a prompt manner for management intervention are imperative for affecting morbidity and mortality [11]. CT with IV iodinated contrast is the gold standard for evaluation and management of renal injury allowing for detection of active hemorrhage, urinary leakage, and concomitant injuries. It is also imperative to assess the contralateral kidney and to recognize any pre-existing renal abnormalities, which may put patients at higher risk even from low-grade trauma (Fig. 8.4).

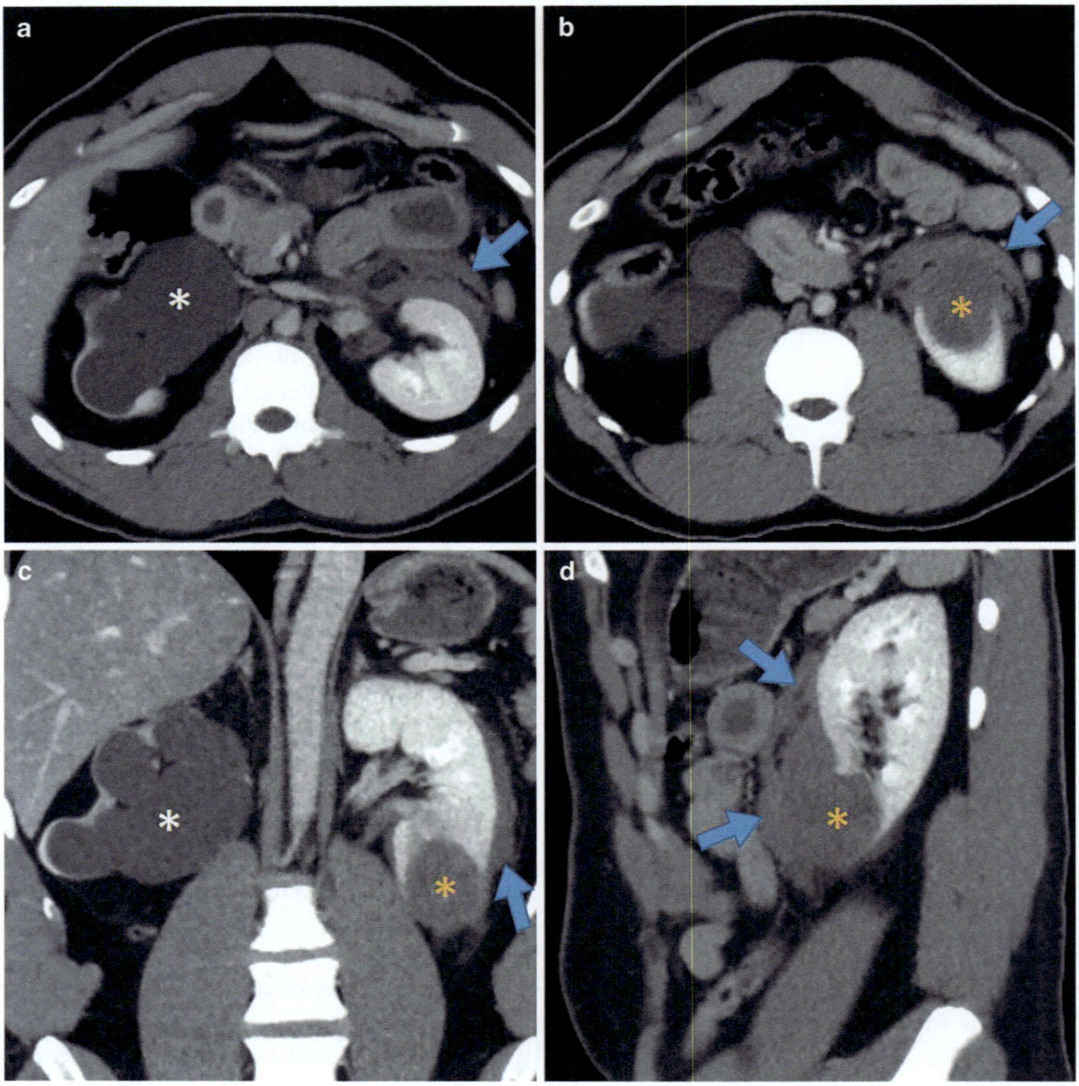

Fig. 8.4 CT images of the upper abdomen in a 28-year-old trauma patient presenting with pain after a fall. Axial (**a**, **b**), coronal (**c**), and sagittal (**d**) portal venous phase images show small left perirenal hematoma (blue arrows). There is a 4 cm ovoid lesion in the left lower renal pole that is heterogeneous and mildly hyperattenuating (yellow asterisks), favored to reflect hemorrhage within a renal cyst. There is wall thickening of the duodenum and proximal jejunum (green arrow), which may be reactive or related to traumatic injury. Right pelvocaliectasis (white asterisks) with associated parenchymal atrophy is related to known congenital UPJ obstruction. AAST grade II renal injury

CT is a valuable imaging tool for evaluating renal trauma, as it can provide detailed information about the extent and severity of the injury. The CT findings in renal trauma can vary depending on the severity and extent of the injury. Some common CT findings in renal trauma may include:

- **Contusion/hematoma**: Focal area of edema or hemorrhage within the kidney tissue, which may appear as ill-defined, round, or striated areas of hypoattenuation with possible retention of contrast material on delayed nephrogram (Fig. 8.5) [12].

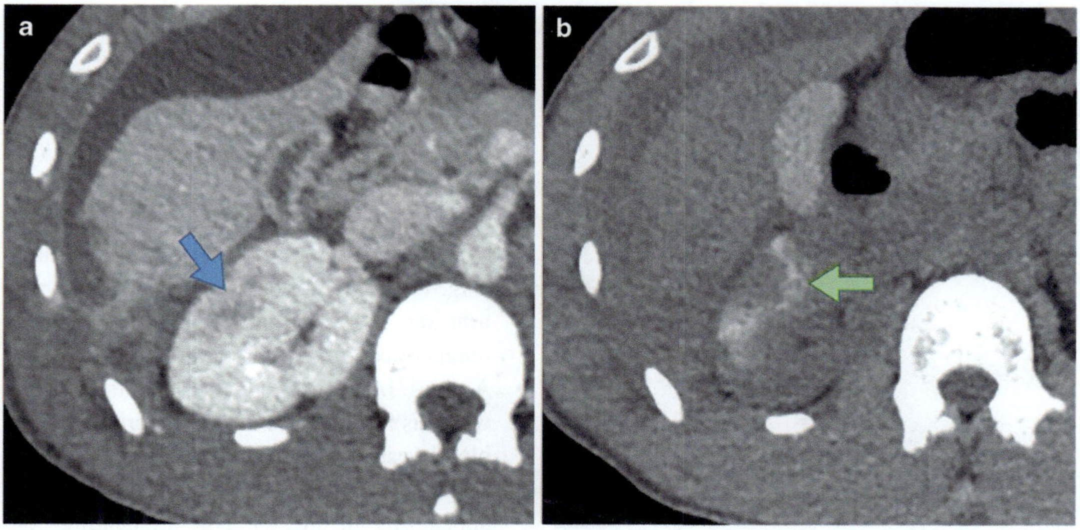

Fig. 8.5 CT images of the right kidney in a 32-year-old trauma patient. Axial image in the portal venous phase (**a**) shows small area of heterogeneity of the right renal parenchyma (blue arrow); the background renal parenchyma homogeneously enhances. Liver injury is also partially imaged. Axial unenhanced axial CT image (**b**) from a follow-up exam a few days later shows retained contrast within the injured renal parenchyma. Findings are in keeping with renal contusion. AAST grade I renal injury

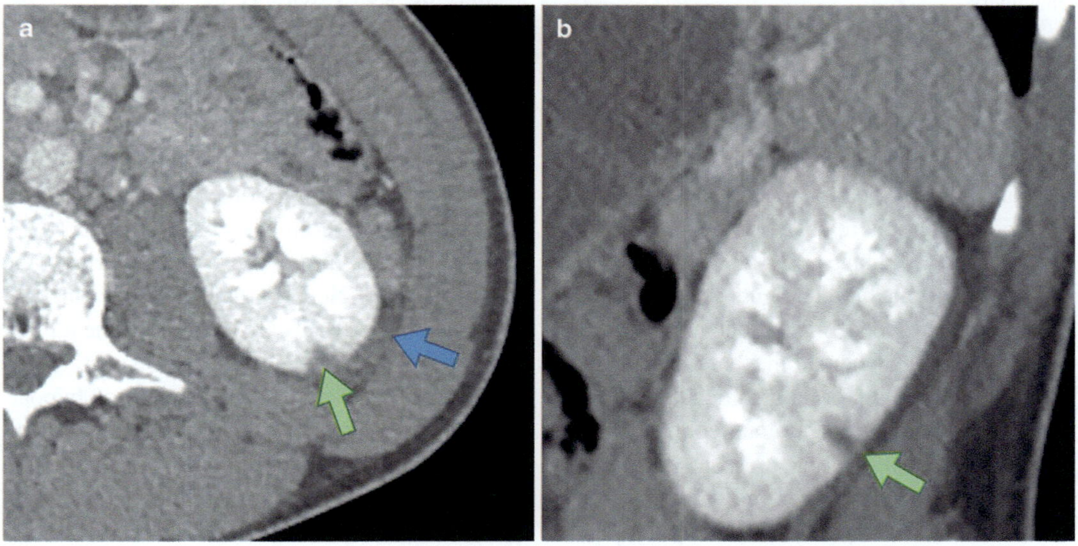

Fig. 8.6 CT images of the left kidney in a 63-year-old trauma patient. Axial (**a**) and sagittal (**b**) portal venous phase images show a linear focus of hypoattenuation (green arrows) in the posterior aspect of the left lower renal pole, in keeping with a laceration. There is an associated small left retroperitoneal hemorrhage (blue arrow). AAST grade II renal injury

- **Laceration**: Focal cut or disruption in the kidney tissue, which may extend to the collecting system or vascular pedicle (main renal artery or vein). Typically appears as a linear or irregular hypoattenuating defects along the periphery of the parenchyma, with possible hematoma extending through the capsule and confined to the perirenal fascia (Figs. 8.6, 8.7 and 8.8) [12].

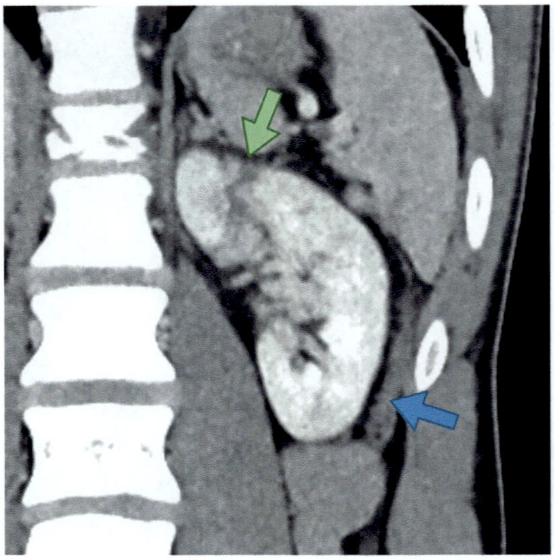

Fig. 8.7 CT image of the left kidney in a 19-year-old patient presenting with a history of blunt trauma. Coronal portal venous phase image shows a linear focus of hypoattenuation (green arrow) in the left upper renal pole, in keeping with a laceration. There is an associated small left retroperitoneal hemorrhage (blue arrow). AAST grade III renal injury

- **Perinephric hemorrhage/hematoma**: Bleeding around the kidney, either confined by the caspule or extending into the perinrenal space, that typically appears as an area of hypoattenuation relative to the renal parenchyma on CT images (Figs. 8.8, 8.9 and 8.10). However, if the blood is acute or hyperacute, it may appear hyper- or isoattenuating.
  - Subcapsular hematomas are peripherally located round or ellipsoid collections of blood that are deep to and confined by the renal capsule; often crescent-shaped collections with convex margins that exert mass effect upon the underlying parenchyma, characterized by flattening or indentation of the renal parenchyma (Fig. 8.10) [11, 15].
  - Perirenal hematomas are collections that are located around the kidney, which are located outside of the renal capsule; often contained by Gerota fascia (Fig. 8.4) but may extend further into the retroperitoneum.
- **Urinoma**: This refers to the accumulation of urine outside the kidney due to a tear or rupture of the collecting system. Urinomas may appear as a fluid-filled collection with a thin wall on CT. If imaging or clinical findings are concerning for a collecting system injury, a delayed excretory phase after 5–15 min is necessary to assess for urinary extravasation (Fig. 8.9). The absence of urinary extravasation on excretory phase imaging excludes renal collecting system violation [11].
- **Active bleeding**: Contrast extravasation, which is leakage of contrast material from the blood vessels within the kidney, should raise suspicion for vascular injury [11]. This appears as an area of hyperattenuating contrast material (similar in attenuation to that within the vessels) outside the blood vessels on CT images (Figs. 8.8 and 8.9). The area of hemorrhage enlarges on the slightly later portal venous phase of contrast. Active bleeding may be seen extending beyond the perirenal fascia into the retroperitoneum. Patients with active bleeding usually require management with surgery or interventional radiology.
- **Renal artery dissection/occlusion**: Focal injury to the renal artery resulting in infarction or devascularization of the kidney (Fig. 8.11). Renal artery thrombosis is often caused by deceleration injury stretching/tearing the intima [12]. Nephrogram will show lack of distal renal arterial enhancement of the injured kidney.
- **Infarction**: Wedge-shaped defect of hypoattenuating or non-enhancing parenchyma with sharply demarcated margins (Figs. 8.8 and 8.12). Segmental or complete parenchymal infarct is evidence of arterial injury, usually secondary to renal vessel thrombosis without active bleeding.
- **Shattered kidney**: Multiple severe lacerations with one or more devitalized fragments; possible concomitant arterial extravasation and ureteropelvic junction disruption (Fig. 8.9). A fragment is deemed devitalized if there is loss of identifiable parenchymal renal anatomy [11]. It is important to differentiate

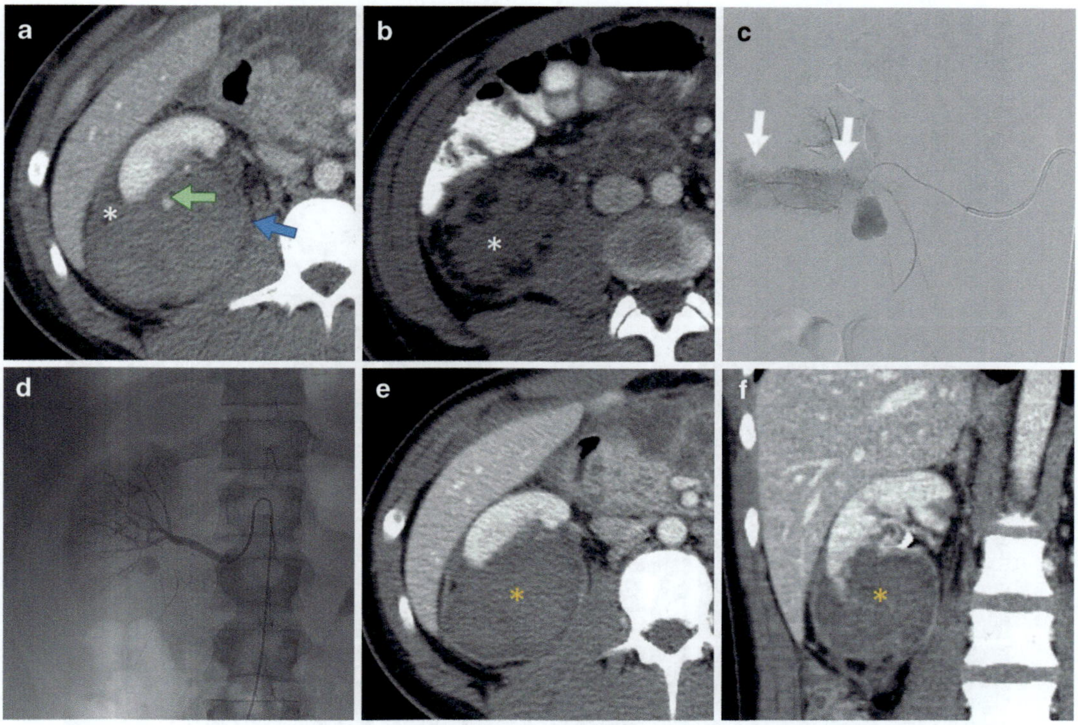

Fig. 8.8 Imaging of the left kidney in a 26-year-old trauma patient. Axial portal venous phase images (**a**, **b**) show a renal laceration, subcapsular hematoma (blue arrow), and perirenal hemorrhage (white asterisks). A small focus of hyperenhancement (green arrow) is favored to represent active bleeding. Fluoroscopic image from subsequent interventional radiology procedure (**c**) shows contrast extravasation from a renal artery branch (white arrows). There is no contrast extravasation on a fluoroscopic image following embolization (**d**). Axial (**e**) and coronal (**f**) portal venous phase images from follow-up CT show evolution of right renal subcapsular hematoma (yellow asterisks) following embolization. A small trauma-related right upper renal pole infarct is also seen (yellow arrow). AAST grade IV renal injury

foci of active arterial extravasation from islands of enhancing renal parenchyma.

- **Pseudoaneurysm**: Localized outpouchings of an artery, most often the hepatic artery, secondary to injury of a vessel with contained hematoma. Pseudoaneurysms appear as well-circumscribed, contrast-enhancing structures on CT images. Although asymptomatic, pseudoaneurysms are at risk of rupturing and causing fatal hemorrhage.
- **Arteriovenous fistula** (AVF): Rare abnormal communication between a renal artery and vein, often resulting from penetrating trauma. On imaging, an AVF should be suspected if there is enhancement of a structure during both arterial and venous phases.
- **Avulsion**: Complete transection of the vascular pedicle/hilum (main renal artery or vein).

The AAST OIS is the most commonly used scale to assess renal injury and the CT findings are detailed in Table 8.5 and Fig. 8.13. Grade I injuries are the most common type of renal injury accounting for approximately 75–85% of cases [11]. The hallmark of both grade II and III injuries is sparing of the urinary collecting system and vascular structures [15]. Injuries involving the collecting system with urinary extravasation are grade IV or V. Vascular injuries, including pseudoaneurysms and arteriovenous fistulae, are uncommon but associated with a higher rate of failure of nonsurgical management. If the pattern

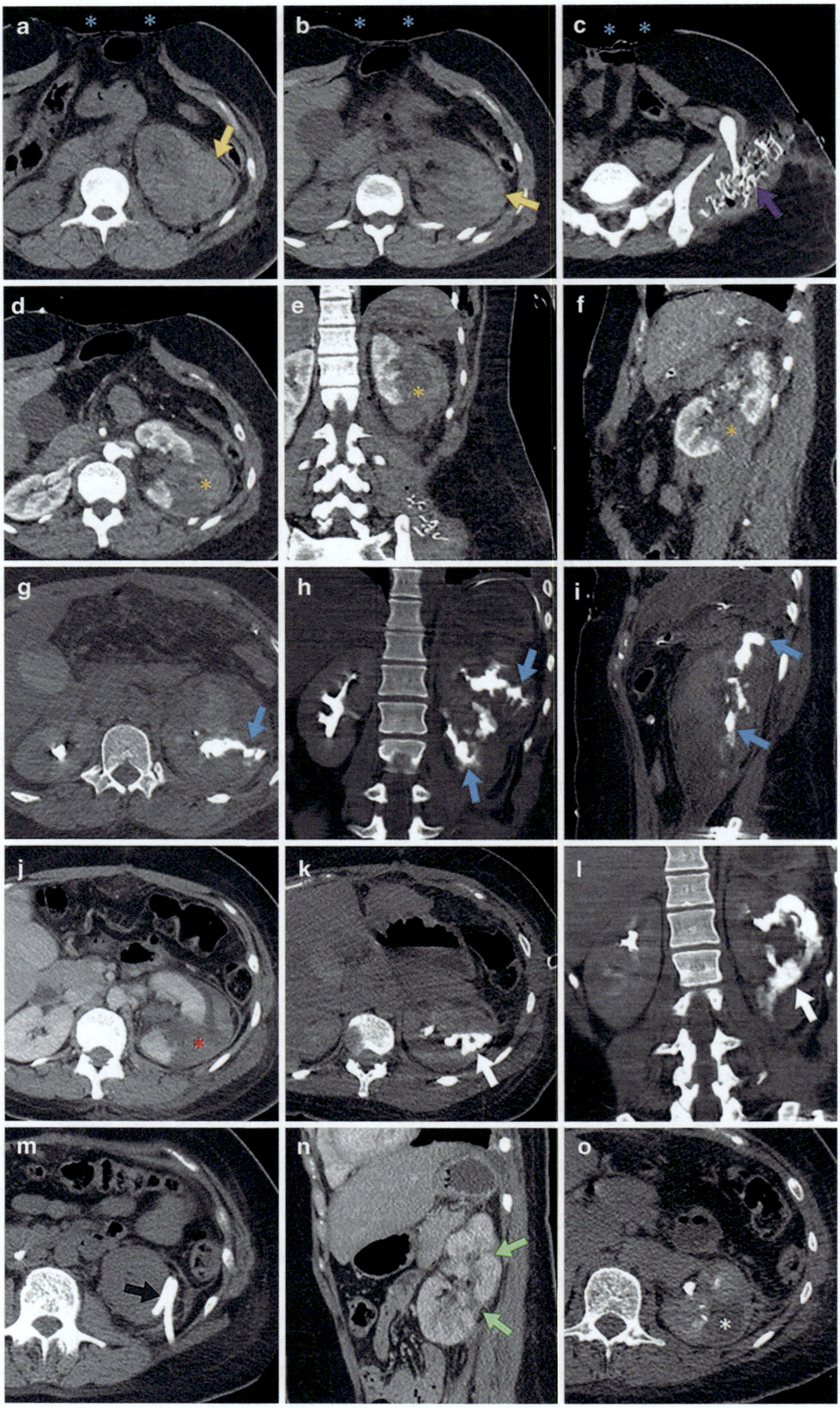
a
b
c
d
e
f
g
h
i
j
k
l
m
n
o

Fig. 8.9 Imaging of the left kidney in a 26-year-old trauma patient presenting with history of pedestrian versus auto. Axial unenhanced images (**a–c**) show left perirenal hyperattenuation (yellow arrows). The patient has an open abdomen (blue asterisks) from exploratory laparotomy and splenectomy. A comminuted left iliac wing fracture, surgical packing material in the left gluteal region (purple arrow), subcutaneous emphysema and subcutaneous fat stranding are also seen. Axial (**d**), coronal (**e**), and sagittal (**f**) portal venous phase images demonstrate a shattered left kidney with perirenal hematoma (yellow asterisks) that extends into the left retroperitoneum. Axial (**g**), coronal (**h**) and sagittal (**i**) excretory phase images (obtained 15 min after intravenous contrast administration) show contrast extravasation from the left renal collecting system (blue arrows), in keeping with collecting system injuries, urine extravasation and urinoma. Following 1 week of conservative management, CT urogram was performed. Similar findings of shattered kidney with perirenal hematoma and urinoma (red asterisk) are seen on axial portal venous phase image (**j**). Persistent urinary extravasation from collecting system injuries (white arrows) are shown on axial (**k**) and coronal (**l**) excretory phase images. A percutaneous drain (black arrow) was subsequently placed into the perirenal hematoma/urinoma by interventional radiology, as shown on axial unenhanced image (**m**) from follow-up CT urogram performed 1 month later. On this 1 month follow-up study, sagittal portal venous phase image (**n**) shows interval healing of the left kidney with areas of parenchymal scarring (green arrows). Axial excretory phase image (**o**) shows no findings of contrast extravasation, in keeping with healing of the collecting system injuries. Evolution and decreased size of the perinephric hematoma/urinoma are seen (white asterisk). AAST grade V renal injury

of traumatic injury falls under multiple grades, the highest grade should be reported. Other imaging modalities such as ultrasound and magnetic resonance imaging (MRI) may also be used depending on the clinical situation.

The anatomic differences in renal transplants, including the absence of Gerota fascia and other retroperitoneal anatomical structures, requires conceptual modification of the AAST criteria by the interpreting radiologist for injuries to transplant kidneys (Fig. 8.14).

Management and Complications

Kidney injury grading can help guide management decisions for trauma patients, as management depends on the severity of the injury, associated injuries, and whether or not the patient is hemodynamically stable. Controlling bleeding, preventing further injury, and promoting parenchymal tissue healing are the primary clinical goals of care. Management strategies for renal injury in trauma patients includes the following:

- **Conservative management**: The standard of care for hemodynamically stable patients is nonsurgical management [1]. Supportive measures include blood transfusions, supportive care, and close monitoring of vital signs and laboratory values.
- **Interventional radiology procedures**: In some cases, arterial or venous embolization may be performed to stop active bleeding from a damaged vessel. Interventional radiologists use minimally invasive endovascular angiographic techniques utilizing embolizing particles or metal coils.
- **Surgical intervention**: Surgical exploration is necessary in hemodynamically unstable patients and more severe renal injuries, such as those that involve large vessels or associated injuries to other organs (grades IV and V). Surgery may involve techniques such as nephrectomy (Fig. 8.15).

A multidisciplinary approach, involving trauma surgeons, interventional radiologists, and critical care specialists, is necessary to ensure optimal management of renal injury in trauma patients. Because nonoperative management of renal injuries has become the standard of care in many patients, there has also been an increase in delayed complications. Delayed complications may be seen on imaging weeks to months after the trauma and include:

- **Bleeding**: Delayed bleeding can occur from blood vessels that were damaged during the initial trauma, which can cause further kidney damage and lead to hemorrhage.
- **Hypertension**: The injured kidney may release excess renin, a hormone that can raise

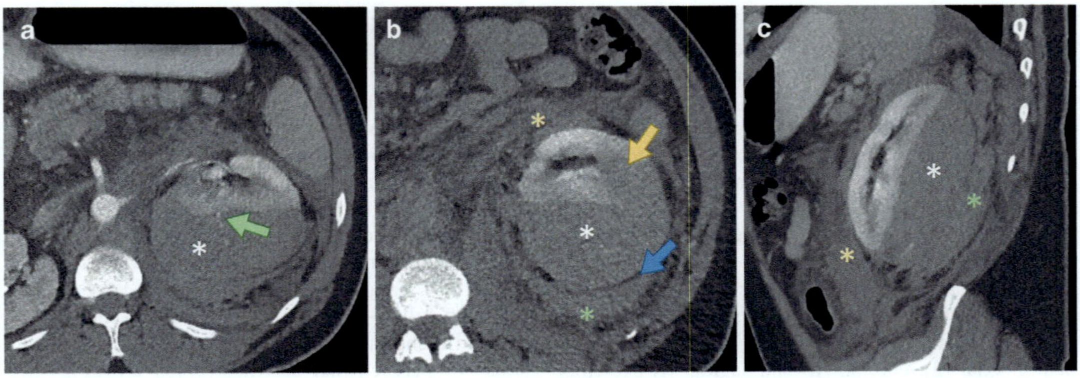

Fig. 8.10 CT images of the upper abdomen in a 38-year-old trauma patient. Axial (**a**, **b**) and sagittal (**c**) late hepatic arterial phase images show a large subcapsular hematoma (white asterisks) with associated mass effect on the underlying parenchyma. There is a focus of contrast extravasation, in keeping with active bleeding (green arrow) from a renal artery branch. Hemorrhage extends into perinephric and retroperitoneal spaces, including the anterior (yellow asterisk) and posterior (green asterisk) pararenal spaces; a portion of Zuckerkandl's fascia (blue arrow) is seen, which separates the perinephric space from the posterior pararenal space. An ill-defined area of hypoattenuation of the lateral left renal parenchyma may represent a small contusion (yellow arrow). AAST grade IV renal injury

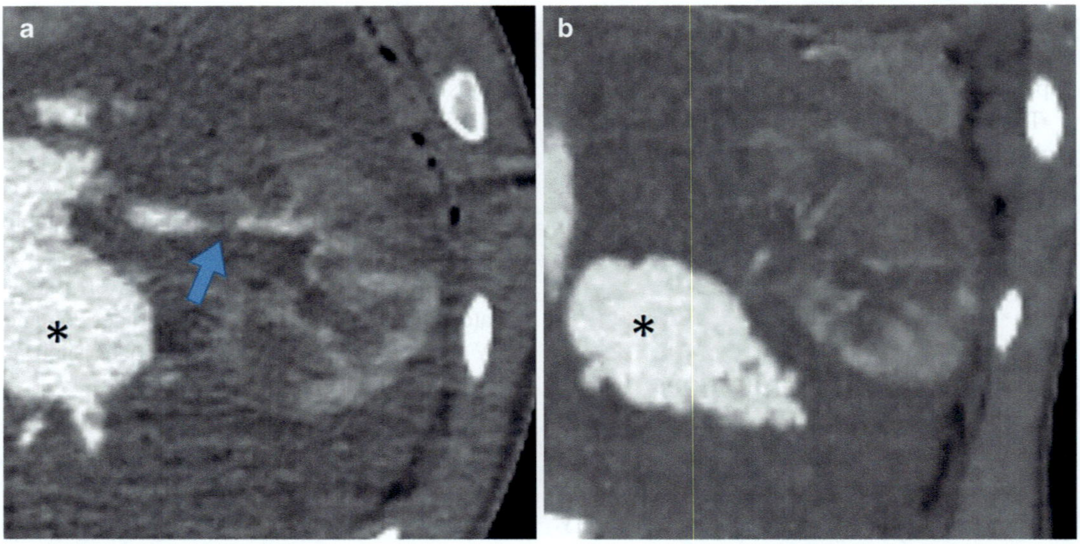

Fig. 8.11 CT images of the left kidney in a 16-year-old trauma patient with presenting with gun shot wounds. Axial (**a**, **b**) arterial phase images show large extravasation of intravenous contrast, in keeping with active bleeding (black asterisk). There is associated devascularization of the left kidney because of involvement of the left renal artery (blue arrow). Additional findings related to this patient are shown in Fig. 7.6. AAST grade V renal injury

Fig. 8.12 CT images of the upper abdomen in a 57-year-old patient (**a**–**d**). Axial corticomedullary (**a**) and axial (**b**), coronal (**c**), and sagittal (**d**) nephrographic phase images of the left kidney show a sharply demarcated, wedge-shaped area of hypoattenuation in the posterior upper pole of the left kidney, in keeping with a segmental infraction. This infarction is more conspicuous on the later nephrographic phase (**b**) in comparison to the corticomedullary phase (**a**). Additional coronal nephrographic phase image (**e**) of both kidneys in a different patient shows numerous bilateral wedge-shaped areas of hypoattenuation/hypoenhancement, in keeping with multiple small infarcts

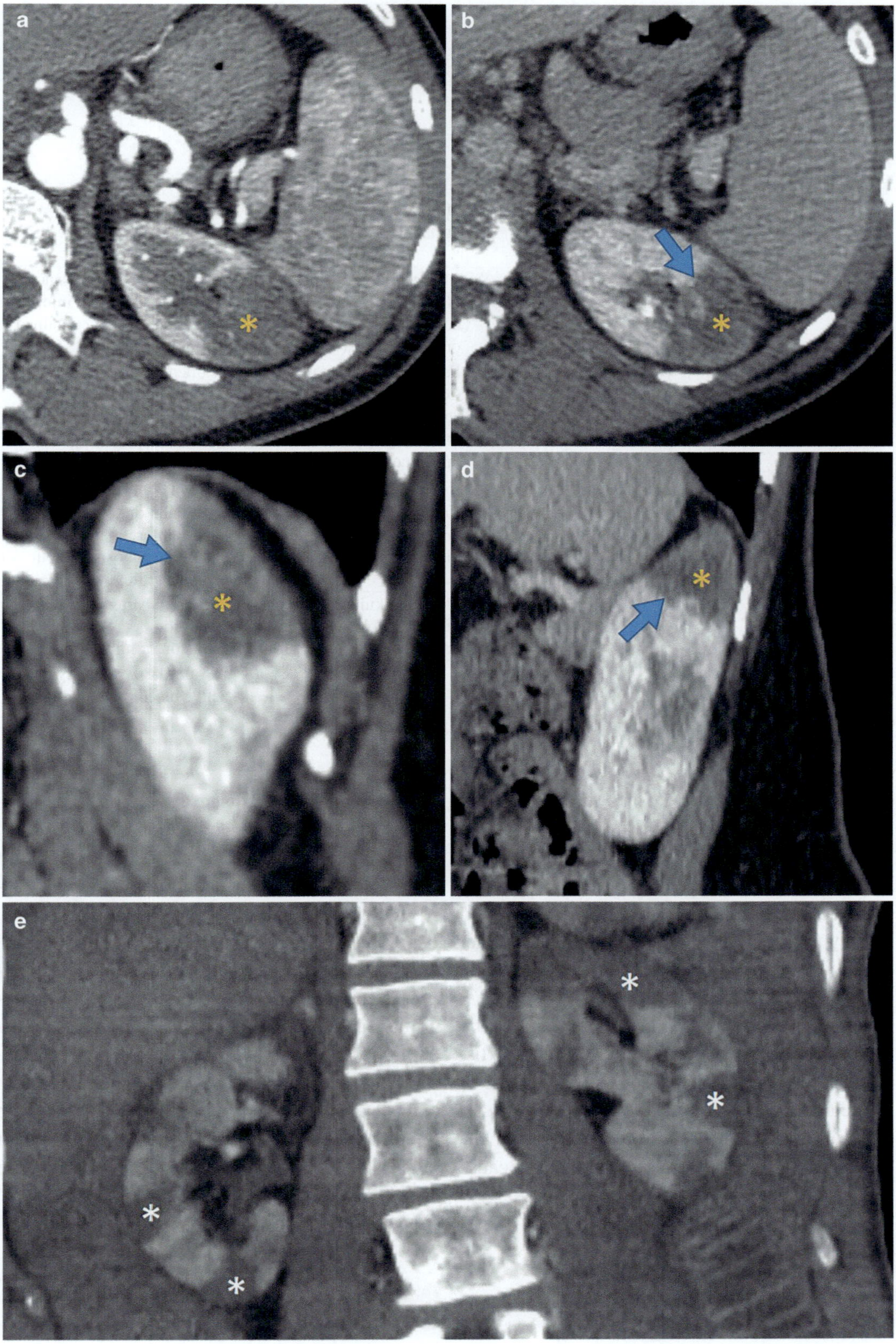
a
b
c
d
e

Table 8.5 AAST kidney injury scale [6, 7]

AAST grade[a]	Contusion	Hematoma	Laceration	Vascular injury
I	Microscopic or gross hematuria, urologic studies normal	Subcapsular, nonexpanding without parenchymal laceration		
II		Nonexpanding perirenal hematoma confirmed to renal retroperitoneum	<1.0 cm parenchymal depth of renal cortex without urinary extravasation	
III			>1.0 cm parenchymal depth of renal cortex without collecting system rupture or urinary extravasation	Any injury in the presence of a kidney vascular injury or active bleeding contained within Gerota fascia
IV			Parenchymal laceration extending through renal cortex, medulla, and collecting system with urinary extravasation	Segmental renal vein or artery injury
				Active bleeding beyond Gerota fascia into the retroperitoneum or peritoneum
			Renal pelvis laceration and/or complete ureteropelvic disruption	Segmental or complete kidney infarction(s) due to vessel thrombosis without active bleeding
V			Shattered kidney with loss of identifiable Parenchymal renal anatomy	Main renal artery or vein laceration or Avulsion of hilum
				Devascularized kidney with active bleeding

[a]Advance one grade for bilateral up to grade III

blood pressure. Hypertension in the setting of external compression, most often from a subcapsular hematoma, is known as a Page kidney or Page phenomenon [16].

- **Infection**: Trauma can increase the risk of urinary tract infections, which can cause further damage to the affected kidney and potentially spread to other parts of the body.
- **Urinary fistula**: Abnormal communication between the kidney and other organs or tissues, which can cause urine to leak outside of the urinary tract.
- **Urinary tract obstruction**: Blockage of the flow of urine from the affected kidney because of blood clots or scar tissue formation.
- **Chronic kidney disease**: Higher grade injuries can cause parenchymal scarring (Fig. 8.9). The damage caused by the trauma can result in reduced kidney function, which can progress to chronic kidney disease over time [1, 5].

Recognition of these complications on imaging is essential for early treatment and low morbidity and mortality. Management of renal trauma is highly individualized and may depend on factors such as the patient's overall health, the extent and severity of the injury, and the expertise of the medical team. Therefore, the specific management approach may vary even within each grade of the AAST renal injury scale.

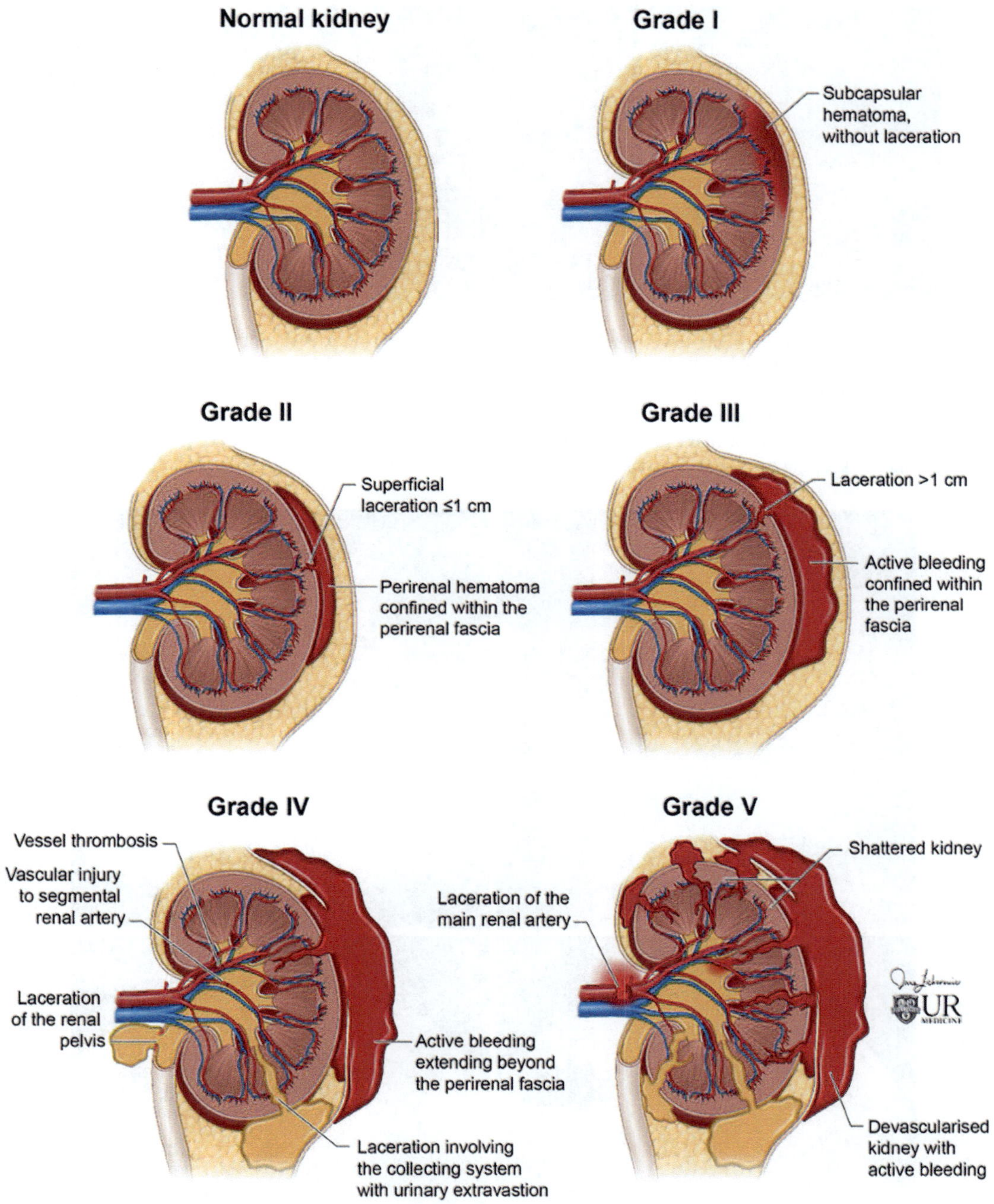

Fig. 8.13 Pictorial depiction of renal injury grading by the AAST OIS, courtesy of University of Rochester Department of Radiology

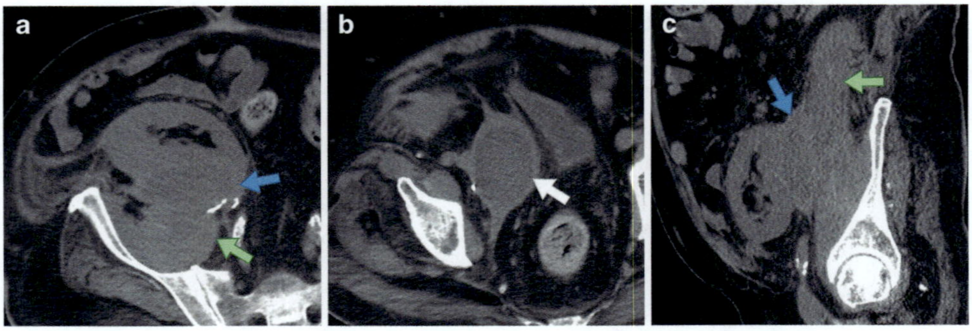

Fig. 8.14 CT images of a right lower quadrant renal transplant in a 63-year-old patient. Axial (**a**, **b**) and sagittal (**c**) unenhanced images show a hypoattenuating fluid collection along the posterior aspect of the renal transplant (blue arrows), with associated mass effect on the renal parenchyma, in keeping with a subcapsular hematoma. There is inferior extension of this hematoma into the pelvis (white arrow), which displaces the urinary bladder (yellow asterisk). This hematoma also extends into the right iliopsoas muscle (green arrows). When accommodating for the anatomical differences of a renal transplant, findings are most consistent with AAST grade II renal injury

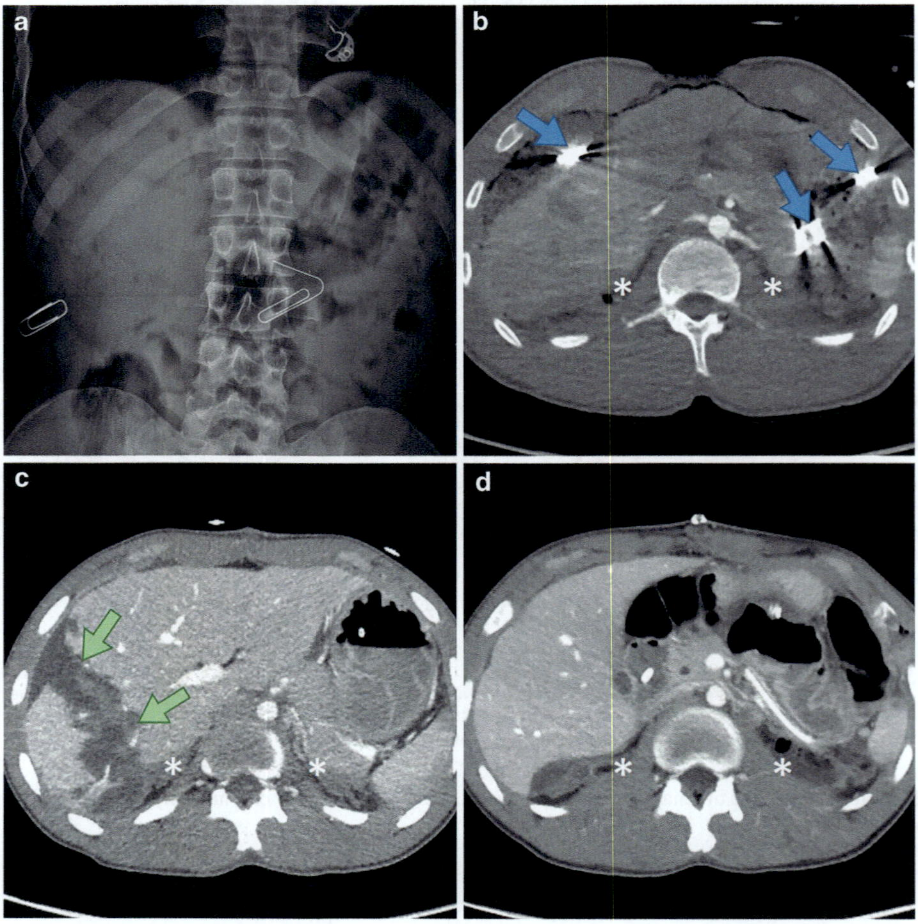

Fig. 8.15 Images of the abdomen in a 21-year-old trauma patient presenting with gunshot wounds. Frontal radiograph (**a**) shows open and closed paperclips overlying the left paramidline and right midabdomen, denoting the entry and exit sites from ballistic injury. A few punctate metallic ballistic fragments are seen near the open paperclip. Small foci of air overly the liver shadow, likely pneumoperitoneum. The patient proceeded directly to surgery without CT imaging. Postoperative axial arterial phase CT image (**b**) of the upper abdomen shows an open abdomen packed with surgical sponges (blue arrows). Following bilateral nephrectomies, the renal fossae (white asterisks) are empty (**c** and **d**). Liver laceration is also noted (green arrows) (**c**)

Ureteral Trauma

Well protected in the retroperitoneum, the ureters are rarely injured in trauma patients. Serious complications can result from ureteral injury, such as urinary leakage, infection, or sepsis. Ureteral injury occurs in approximately 4% of patients with penetrating trauma and less than 1% of blunt trauma cases [5]. Because the majority of traumatic ureteral injury is related to penetrating trauma, it is accompanied by additional injuries; the distal ureter is most commonly injured. In the setting of blunt trauma, ureteral injury is most often associated with rapid deceleration injury and involves the ureteropelvic junction (UPJ) [1]. Hematuria is present in only half of patients with ureteral injury, requiring a high degree of clinical suspicion [5]. Unfortunately, ureteral injury is also one of the most commonly missed injuries during exploratory laparotomy [5].

Anatomy

The ureters are muscular tubes that carry urine from the ureteropelvic junction (UPJ) of each kidney to the ureterovesical junctions (UVJ) at the urinary bladder. Each ureter is approximately 25 cm in length and overlies the psoas muscle before crossing the iliac vessels into the pelvis. The ureter is near multiple other abdominopelvic structures along its course from the kidney to the bladder.

Imaging and Grading

CT can help to identify and localize ureteral injury by providing detailed images of the urinary tract and surrounding structures. However, it should be noted that excretory phase CT imaging, intraluminal endoscopic view, or surgical exploration is usually needed to make the diagnosis (Fig. 8.16). Some common CT/CTU findings in ureteral trauma include:

- **Contrast extravasation**: Contrast material that has been excreted into the urinary tract should remain within the urinary system; if there is an injury to the ureter, the contrast material may leak into the surrounding tissues, indicating an extravasation. With complete transection, the ureter distal to the injury will not be opacified (Fig. 8.16).
- **Perinephric or retroperitoneal fluid**: Ureteral injury may cause accumulation of fluid in the perinephric or retroperitoneal space, which can be detected on CT scan. Excretory phase imaging is necessary to differentiate a urinoma from a hematoma.
- **Ureteral obstruction or dilation**: Ureteral injury may cause obstruction or dilation of the ureter, which can be visualized on CT scan. Partial thickness laceration involves less than 50% of the ureteral wall thickness.
- **Direct visualization of ureteral injury**: In some cases, the ureteral injury may be directly visualized on CT scan as a focal discontinuity or interruption in the ureter.

  - Full-thickness laceration without ureteropelvic disruption refers to a laceration that involves the full thickness of the ureteral wall, but does not result in any disruption of the ureteropelvic junction (Fig. 8.16).
  - Ureteropelvic disruption or avulsion refers to a severe injury that results in complete disruption of the ureteropelvic junction or avulsion of the ureter from the kidney.

Once a ureteral injury is identified on CT scan, further imaging or invasive procedures may be necessary to confirm the diagnosis and guide treatment. In addition, CT can also help to identify other injuries that may be present in trauma patients, which can help guide overall management and treatment decisions.

The AAST OIS can assist in guiding management decisions and treatment planning; however, the AAST OIS is not widely accepted for CT reporting as it is often difficult to distinguish between grades on imaging, such as the degree of

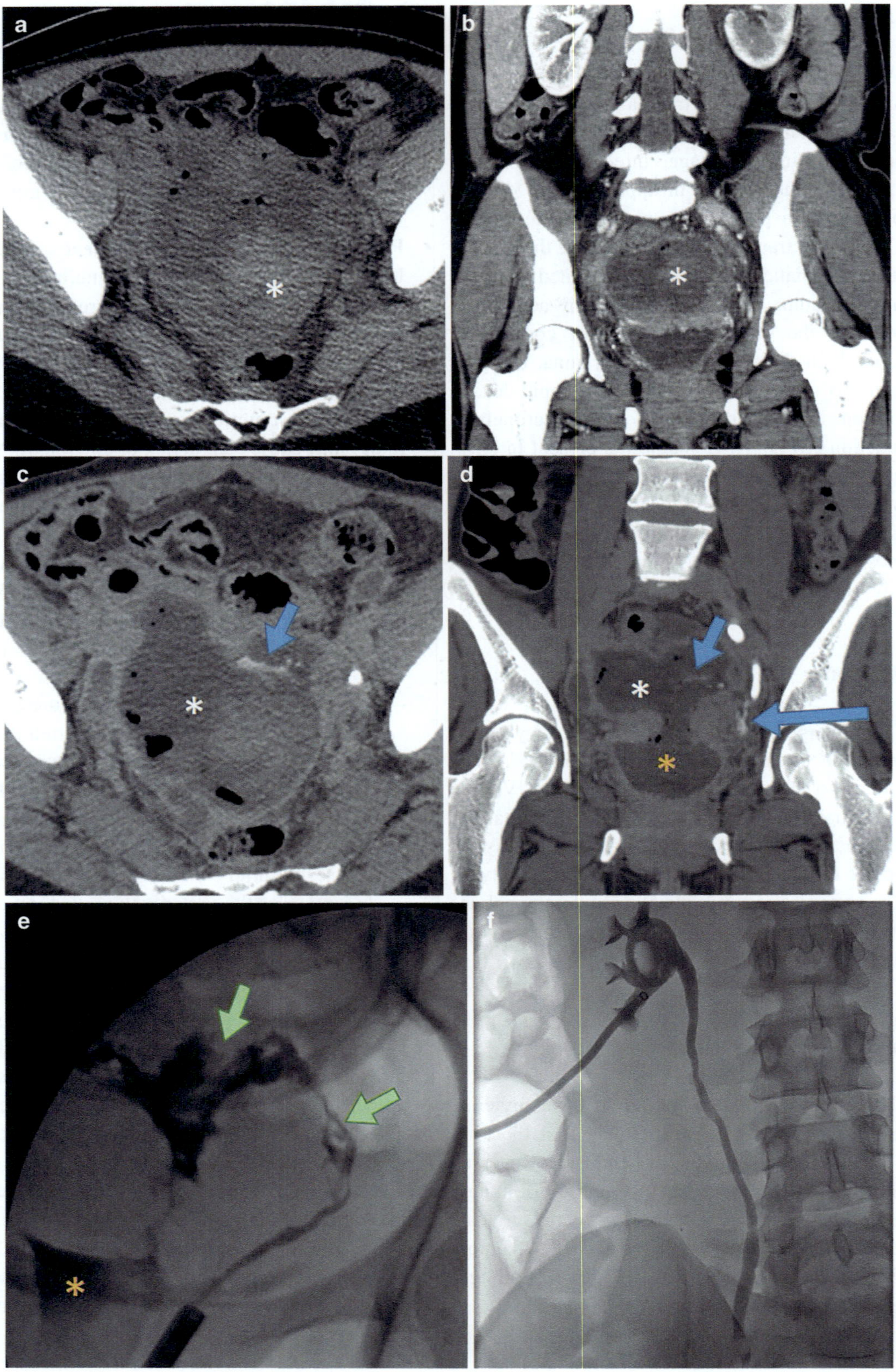
a
b
c
d
e
f

Fig. 8.16 Images in a 47-year-old patient. Axial unenhanced image (**a**) and coronal portal venous image (**b**) shows a heterogeneous collection within the pelvis (white asterisks), including fluid, foci of gas, and areas of hyperattenuation that are favored to reflect blood products. Axial (**c**) and coronal (**d**) excretory phase images show abrupt termination of the left pelvis ureter (yellow arrow) and associated contrast extravasation (blue arrows). There is communication between the pelvic collection (likely a combination of hematoma and urinoma) and the vagina (orange asterisk) secondary to dehiscence of the vaginal cuff in this female post hysterectomy. Fluoroscopic image (**e**) from intraoperative retrograde ureterogram shows contrast extravasation from the left distal left ureter (green arrows), in keeping with complete transection. Contrast is also seen within the vagina (yellow asterisk). Because the diagnosis was delayed, the patient was treated with percutaneous nephrostomy and later surgical repair. Fluoroscopic image from antegrade pyeloureterogram (**f**) through the percutaneous nephrostomy shows healing of the left ureter several months later. AAST grade IV ureteral injury

Table 8.6 AAST ureter injury scale [17]

AAST grade[a]	Hematoma	Laceration
I	Contusion or hematoma without devascularization	
II		<50% transection
III		>50% transection
IV		Complete transection with <2 cm devascularization
V		Avulsion with >2 cm of devascularization

[a]Advance one grade for bilateral up to grade III

ureteral transection; these findings are more readily detected surgically, particularly ureteral contusions and partial thickness lacerations. However, knowing the injury grading allows the radiologist to provide appropriate imaging details to guide management; for instance, ureteral injury with nonvisualization of the distal ureter on excretory phase suggests complete transection, which is essential information for the multidisciplinary team. The AAST ureter injury scale is detailed in Table 8.6.

Management and Complications

The treatment of ureteral injury in trauma patients depends on the severity and location of the injury, as well as the patient's overall clinical status. Generally, the goals of treatment are to control bleeding, prevent infection, and restore normal urinary function. Management strategies for ureteral injury in trauma patients includes the following:

- **Conservative management**: Minor contusions and partial thickness lacerations may be treated with conservative management, including observation, pain management, and antibiotics. However, conservative management is not possible for most ureteral injuries [5].
- **Endoscopic or interventional radiology procedures**: Endoscopic placement of a ureteral stent or percutaneous nephrostomy tube diversion by interventional radiology is necessary in many cases of ureteral injury, particularly full-thickness injuries. Because of inflammation, edema and friability caused by urinomas, the preferred management in cases of delayed diagnosis includes stenting or diversion with percutaneous nephrostomy tube, followed by delayed operative reconstruction [5]. Urinomas typically require percutaneous drainage by interventional radiology [1].
- **Surgical intervention**: Primary anastomosis or autotransplantation may be required for full-thickness lacerations, particularly those involving the ureteropelvic junction and midureter. Injury of the distal ureter is treated with ureteroneocystectomy with or without vesico-psoas hitch, as primary anastomosis of the distal ureter is difficult [1]. Injuries involving the ureteropelvic disruption or avulsion must be treated urgently to restore normal urinary flow and prevent further complications.

Overall, the treatment of ureteral injury in trauma patients is individualized and based on the severity of the injury and the patient's overall clinical status. A multidisciplinary approach involving urologists, trauma surgeons, and critical care specialists is often necessary to optimize patient outcomes. With any trauma patient, there is always a risk of delayed complications; this is particularly true for cases in which there is a delayed diagnosis of ureteral injury, in which the complication rate is about 40% [5]. Delayed complications of ureteral injury may be seen on imaging weeks to months after the trauma and include:

- **Urinary leakage or delayed perforation**: With nonoperative management of ureteral contusions (typically diagnosed operatively) and other injuries, there is a risk of delayed perforation; ureteral stenting reduces this risk [5]. In the setting of partial or complete transection of the ureter, urine can leak and accumulate, forming a urinoma.
- **Urinary tract obstruction or stricture**: There is a relatively high risk of ureteral stricture following management with stenting or percutaneous nephrostomy diversion, occurring in up to 50 percent of cases. Delayed diagnosis and treatment of ureteral injury is also associated with an increased risk of stricture. Patients may be further managed with endourologic management, but a large proportion of patients will require delayed surgical reconstruction [5]. Ureteral obstruction can lead to hydronephrosis and impaired renal function.
- **Infection**: Urinomas can lead to infection or abscess [5].
- **Ureterovaginal fistula**: Rarely, ureteral injury can lead to an abnormal communication between the ureter and the vagina, called a ureterovaginal fistula (Fig. 8.16). These fistulae are associated with chronic urinary tract infections [18].

Recognition of these complications on imaging is essential for early treatment and low morbidity and mortality.

Bladder Trauma

Injuries to the bladder are rare as the urinary bladder is well protected by the bony pelvis. Bladder injuries are most common in the setting of pelvic trauma, particularly in motor vehicle collisions and falls where there is sudden compression of the bladder [4]; injury is more likely in a distended bladder, in comparison to a decompressed bladder. Pelvic fractures are associated with 60–90% of bladder injuries; nearly 30% of patients with pelvic fractures will also have a bladder injury [1]. A high degree of suspicion is needed because delayed diagnosis of bladder injury increases morbidity and mortality [4]. Present in 95% of cases, gross hematuria is an indication for further evaluation of the bladder; by comparison, microhematuria is only present in five percent of cases of urinary bladder injury [5]. Additional relative indications for further evaluation of the bladder include suprapubic pain or ecchymosis, perineal ecchymosis, inability to void and renal dysfunction. The severity of a bladder injury may not correlate with the severity of symptoms or the need for intervention.

Anatomy

The urinary bladder located deep in the pelvic cavity, posterior to the pubic symphysis and inferior aspect of the rectus abdominis. In male patients, the rectum is located posterior to the urinary bladder, while in female patients, the uterus and vagina are seen posteriorly. The paired ureters drain from the kidneys into the bladder, inserting along the posterosuperior aspect of the bladder. The urinary bladder is composed of inner and outer longitudinal muscles surrounding a middle circular muscle. The dome is the weakest portion of the urinary bladder; this portion of the bladder is covered by peritoneum and injury to the dome causes intraperitoneal extravasation [1].

Imaging and Grading

Although bladder injury cannot be diagnosed on standard CT imaging performed in trauma patients, secondary signs of bladder injury can be detected, including pelvic free fluid, pelvic hematoma, and irregular contour of the urinary bladder. Associated injuries, including pelvic fractures and injury to adjacent organs, can also be identified on CT, providing clues that should prompt further evaluation of the urinary bladder [5].

Traumatic injury of the urinary bladder can be categorized into extraperitoneal, intraperitoneal or mixed-type. Extraperitoneal bladder injuries can be further divided into simple and complex. Nearly 60 percent of injuries are extraperitoneal, while intraperitoneal injuries account for 35 percent and mixed-type account for the remaining 5% [1, 5].

- **Extraperitoneal**: Does not extend to the peritoneal space. These injuries are associated with pelvic fractures, possibly related to direct laceration by osseous fragments or tearing from ligamentous injury.
  - Simple: Confined to the extraperitoneal space.
  - Complex: Extend into adjacent structures, including perineum, penis, scrotum, and abdominal wall.
- **Intraperitoneal**: Involves the peritoneal space. These injuries are associated with direct compression of the lower abdomen in the setting of urinary bladder distention, causing rupture from the weakest portion of the urinary bladder. Pelvic fractures can be seen in 25% of intraperitoneal bladder injuries.
- **Mixed/combined**: Combined extraperitoneal and intraperitoneal injuries. Co-existing urethral injury may be confused for a mixed-type injury.

CT cystography or conventional cystography is necessary to diagnose bladder injury because the bladder must be adequately distended. Passive filling of the urinary bladder during excretory phase imaging from intravenous contrast is not adequate to evaluate for bladder injury, even if the Foley catheter is clamped and the bladder appears distended. Other than bladder contusion, which cannot be diagnosed on imaging, cystography permits diagnosis of bladder injury and differentiation between the remaining types of bladder injury. In cystography, contrast outside of the urinary bladder confirms bladder injury. Some common CT cystography findings in urinary bladder trauma include:

- **Extraperitoneal**:
  - Simple: Extraluminal opacified urine is confined to the extraperitoneal space, referred to as a molar tooth appearance given the shape of the extraperitoneal space.
  - Complex: Extraluminal contrast in the extraperitoneal space that also extends to adjacent structures, such as the abdominal wall and superficial soft tissues (Fig. 8.17). Contrast should not be seen in the peritoneum.
- **Intraperitoneal**: Extraluminal contrast extends into the peritoneal space (Fig. 8.18), outlining bowel and possibly extending to the paracolic gutters/interfascial planes. The estimated size of the bladder wall defect should be reported.
- **Mixed/combined**: Combined extraperitoneal and intraperitoneal injuries (Fig. 8.19). Co-existing urethral injury may be confused for a mixed-type injury.

Concurrent injuries of the bladder and prostatomembranous urethra can occur in up to 30% of males; if there are clinical signs of urethral injury, such as blood at the urethral meatus, retrograde urethrography should be performed prior to catheterization of the urinary bladder [1].

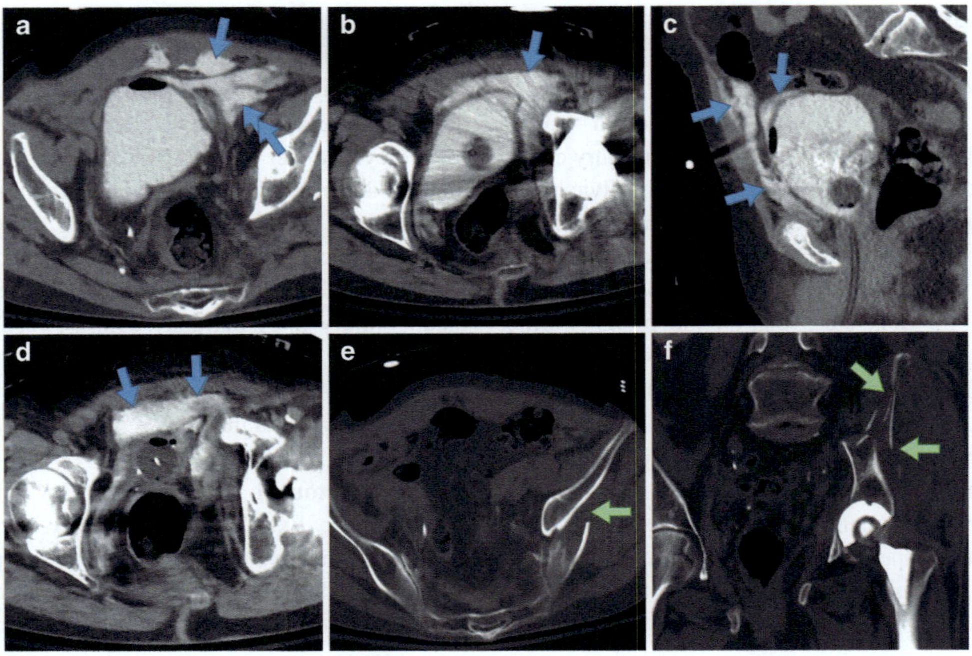

Fig. 8.17 CT images of the pelvis in an 88-year-old trauma patient. Axial (**a**–**d**) CT cystogram images show contrast extravasation from the urinary bladder (blue arrows) anteriorly into the extraperitoneal space of Retzius, which extends superiorly to the level of the umbilicus. No findings of intraperitoneal contrast. Findings are in keeping with extraperitoneal bladder rupture in the setting of pelvic trauma with multiple fractures (green arrows on **e** and **f**). AAST grade II/III bladder injury

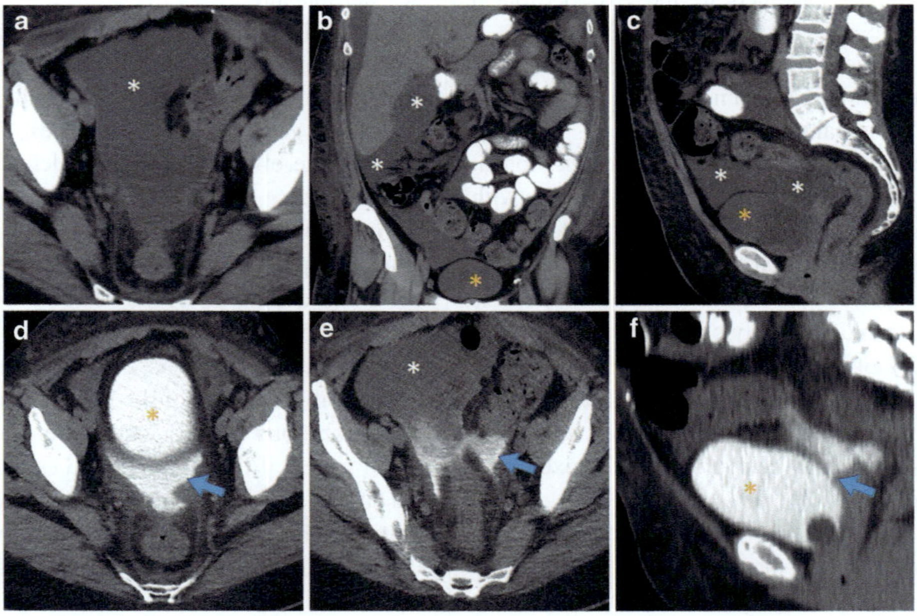

Fig. 8.18 CT images of the pelvis in a 53-year-old trauma patient. Axial (**a**, **d**, **e**), coronal (**b**), and sagittal (**c**, **f**) CT cystogram images show moderate volume ascites (white asterisks) on the unenhanced images (**a**–**c**). Following instillation of contrast into the urinary bladder (yellow asterisks) through a Foley catheter, images (**d**–**f**) show contrast extravasation (blue arrows) from the urinary bladder. The contrast extends superiorly from the bladder dome into the peritoneal cavity, abutting several bowel loops. No findings of extraperitoneal contrast. Findings are in keeping with intraperitoneal bladder rupture. AAST grade III bladder injury

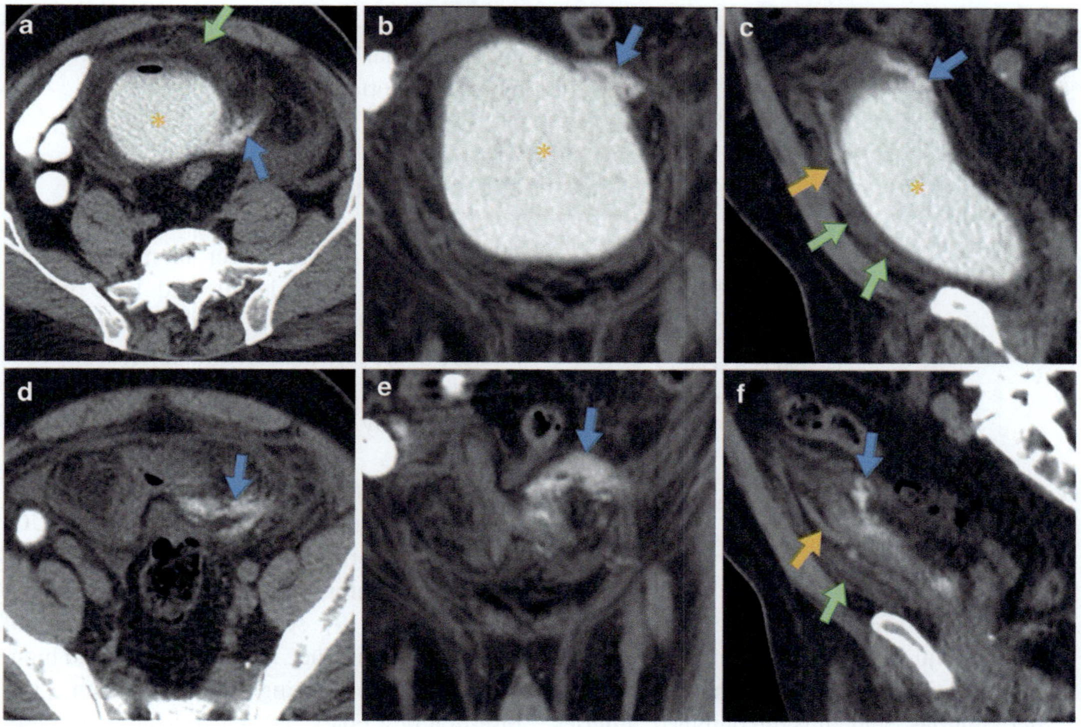

Fig. 8.19 CT images of the pelvis in a 53-year-old patient transferred from an outside hospital with provided history of bladder perforation. Following instillation of contrast into the urinary bladder (yellow asterisks) through a Foley catheter, axial (**a**), coronal (**b**), and sagittal (**c**) CT cystogram images show contrast extravasation through a defect in the left posterolateral bladder dome (blue arrows) into the peritoneal cavity. Contrast and fluid is also seen anterior to the bladder (yellow arrow) in the extraperitoneal space of Retzius (green arrows). Following drainage of the bladder, axial (**d**), coronal (**e**), and sagittal (**f**) images show retained extravasated contrast in the pelvis. Findings are in keeping with combination intraperitoneal and extraperitoneal bladder rupture. AAST grade IV bladder injury

The AAST OIS can contribute in directing management decisions and treatment planning; however, the AAST OIS is not widely accepted for CT reporting as it is often difficult to distinguish between grades on imaging, including the size of laceration; these findings are more readily detected surgically. However, knowing the injury grading allows the radiologist to provide appropriate imaging details to guide management; for instance, distinguishing extraperitoneal from intraperitoneal injury is essential information for the multidisciplinary team. The AAST bladder injury scale is detailed in Table 8.7.

It is important to note that the AAST grading system is just one tool used by healthcare providers to guide treatment decisions for bladder injuries in trauma patients. The severity of the injury, as well as the patient's overall clinical condition and comorbidities, also play a role in determining the most appropriate treatment plan.

Management and Complications

By diagnosing bladder injuries, imaging plays an essential role in guiding the management of trauma patients. The treatment of bladder injury in trauma patients depends on the severity and location of the injury, associated injuries, and the patient's overall clinical status. Management strategies for bladder injury in trauma patients includes the following:

Table 8.7 AAST bladder injury scale [17]

AAST grade[a]	Hematoma	Laceration
I	Contusion, intramural hematoma	Partial thickness
II		Extraperitoneal bladder wall laceration <2 cm
III		Extraperitoneal (>2 cm) or intraperitoneal (<2 cm) bladder wall laceration
IV		Intraperitoneal bladder wall laceration >2 cm
V		Intraperitoneal or extraperitoneal bladder wall laceration extending into the bladder neck or ureteral orifice (trigone)

[a]Advance one grade for multiple lesions up to grade III

- **Conservative management**: Extraperitoneal bladder injuries are treated conservatively.
- **Surgical intervention**: Intraperitoneal bladder injuries and mixed/combined injuries require urgent surgical repair.

A multidisciplinary approach involving urologists, trauma surgeons, and critical care specialists is often necessary to optimize patient outcomes. Complications that can arise from bladder injury in trauma patients include:

- **Infection:** Infection, peritonitis, and sepsis can occur.
- **Urinary incontinence:** Trauma may damage the muscles and nerves that control bladder function, resulting in inability to control urination.
- **Fistula formation:** Bladder injury can lead to the formation of a fistula, which is an abnormal connection between the bladder and another organ, such as the vagina or rectum. This can cause chronic urinary tract infections and other complications. Fistulae are associated with chronic urinary tract infections.
- **Chronic kidney disease**: If severe, bladder injury can affect the function of the kidneys.

Recognition of these complications on imaging is essential for early treatment and low morbidity and mortality.

Urethral Trauma

Most urethral injuries occur in male patients. Because of its short length and lack of firm attachment to the pubic bone, the female urethra is rarely injured; female urethral injuries do occur in conjunction with vaginal and rectal injuries [1]. Injury may be the result of blunt or penetrating trauma.

In male trauma patients with blood at the urethral meatus, a retrograde urethrogram (RUG) should be performed to assess for urethral injury, particularly before attempting Foley catheter placement [1, 19]. Additional clinical signs of urethral injury include inability to void and high-riding prostate on digital rectal exam [19]. Insertion of a Foley catheter into an injured urethra may cause further damage, such as converting a partial urethral tear into a complete tear [1]. Unfortunately, it is common in trauma centers for Foley catheterization prior to RUG to monitor intake and output [1, 20].

Imaging plays a pivotal role in early diagnosis of urethral injury, which is necessary to avoid increased morbidity that is associated with delayed management [19].

Anatomy

The urethra is a hollow tube that carries urine external to the body from the urinary bladder. The female urethra is approximately 5 cm in length, while the male urethra is approximately 22 cm in length [20]. The male urethra is eccentrically located toward the dorsum of the penis, surrounded by corpus spongiosum along most of its length. It is divided into anterior and posterior segments. The posterior segment begins at the bladder neck and includes the prostatic and membranous urethra, both of which are located above the urogenital diaphragm. The anterior urethra is located below the urogenital diaphragm and extends to the meatus of the penis, including the bulbar and penile urethra [1, 5, 20].

Imaging and Grading

Retrograde urethrogram (RUG) is the modality of choice for diagnosing urethral injury, which involves injecting contrast in a retrograde manner into the urethra from the fossa navicularis and taking radiographs. Although not as sensitive or specific as RUG for urethral injury, CT can be useful in the evaluation of urethral injury, especially as many patients will have a CT performed prior to RUG. CT is even more important in patients without clinical signs or symptoms of urethral injury and in the setting of severe injuries that may make RUG difficult or risky. If urethral injury is suspected on CT, further evaluation with RUG is necessary [1].

There are typically two primary types of urethral injury, depending on the cause of trauma.

- **Anterior pelvic arch fracture**: Although the reported incident varies, urethral injury occurs up to 20 percent of males with a pelvic fracture [19]. The membranous urethra (posterior urethra) or the proximalmost portion of the bulbar urethra (anterior urethra just distal to the urogenital diagpbragm) are most commonly affected [1, 19, 20]. Injury may result from direct injury by osseous spicules or tearing from puboprostatic ligamentous injury [1].
- **Straddle injury**: Crush injury to the perineum with direct compression of the corpus spongiosum and bulbar urethra (anterior urethra) against the inferior aspect of the pubic symphysis, resulting in partial or complete rupture of the bulbar urethra [1]. Typically, there is no associated fracture.

Urethral injuries can have different appearances on CT, depending on the type and severity of the injury. Some common CT findings that may be seen in urethral injury:

- **Disruption of the urethra**: In cases of complete urethral disruption, CT may show a discontinuity or separation of the urethral walls. This may appear as a gap or break in the urethral wall on axial or coronal images.
- **Deviation or kinking of the urethra**: In cases of partial urethral injury or partial obstruction, CT may show a deviation or kinking of the urethra. This may appear as a narrowing or tortuosity of the urethral lumen on axial or coronal images. In the setting of Foley catheter placement in severe injury, the Foley catheter may be eccentrically located.
- **Extravasation of urine**: In cases of urethral injury with urine extravasation, CT may show an accumulation of urine around the urethra or in adjacent soft tissues. This may appear as a low-attenuation fluid collection on CT images. If the urine is opacified with contrast, extraluminal contrast will be seen (Fig. 8.20).
- **Hematoma**: Hypoattenuating or hyperattenuating blood products in the perivesical or retropubic space (Fig. 8.20) is a clue to associated urethral injury. Intramuscular hematomas may also be seen, including in the ischiocavernosus (located along the medial aspect of the ischiopubic rami) or obturator internus (covering the inner aspect of the obturator foramen) muscles; on CT, intramuscular hematoma often presents as heterogeneous enlargement of the muscle with surrounding fat stranding or hematoma.
- **Loss of normal anatomic contours**: Obscuration of the prostatic contour, urogenital diaphragmatic fat plane, or bulbocavernosus muscle (a U-shaped muscle that wraps around the penile bulb) are additional CT findings of urethral injury [1].

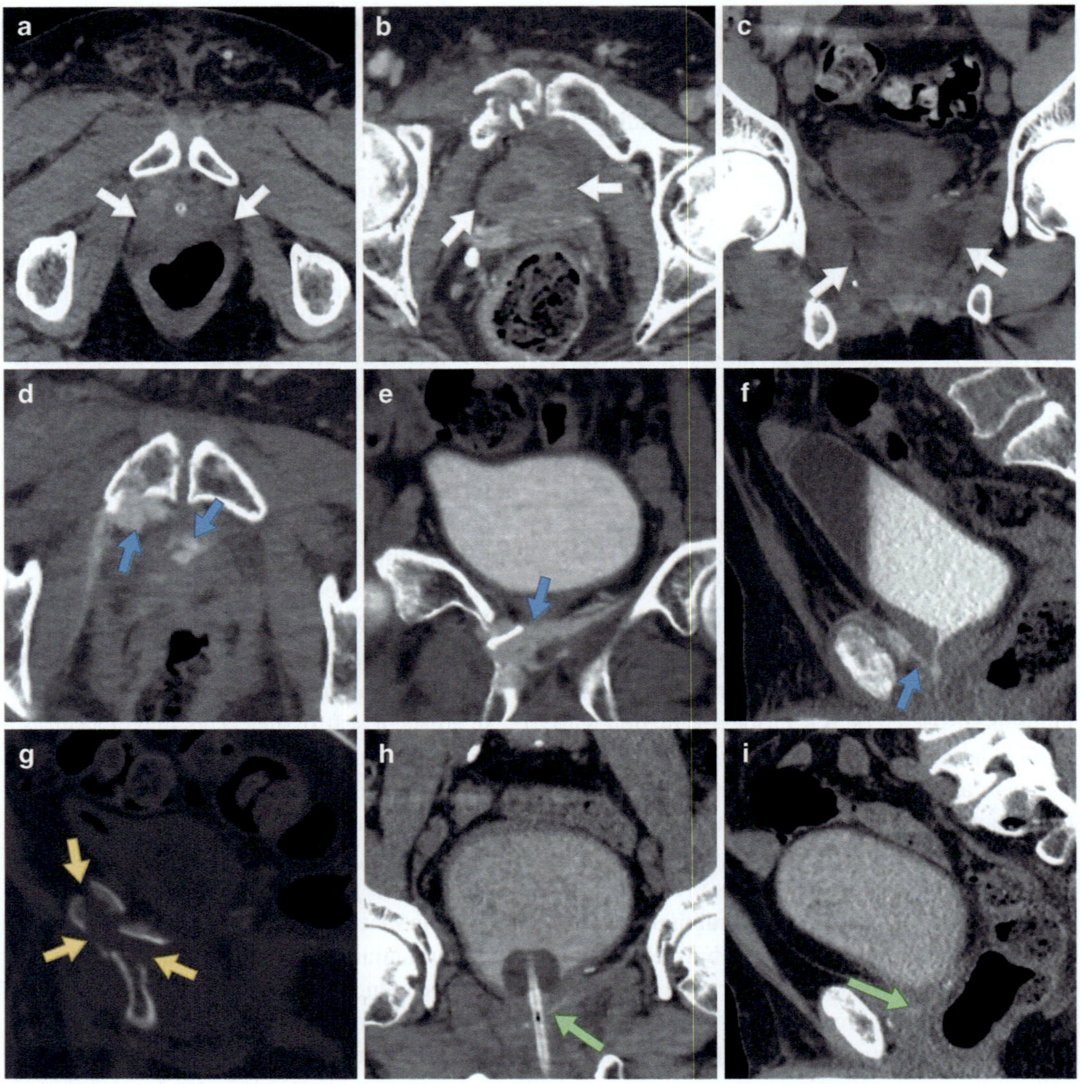

Fig. 8.20 CT images of the pelvis in a 66-year-old trauma patient presenting after a high speed motor vehicle collision (auto versus tree) with hypotension and blood at urethral meatus. The patient has an additional history of prostate cancer post-prostatectomy and vesicourethral anastomosis. Axial (**a**, **b**), coronal (**c**) show fat stranding (white arrows) surrounding the urethra, which is delineated by the Foley catheter (green arrow), and the bladder neck (**b**). Fractures involve the right pelvis (**b**). Given the history of blood at the urethral meatus and initial imaging findings, CT cystogram was obtained. Axial (**d**), coronal (**e**) and sagittal (**f**) images after Foley catheter removal show contrast extravasation (blue arrows) from the posterior urethra, just distal to the vesicourethral anastomosis; findings are in keeping with ureteral injury. The ureteral injury is at the level of pelvic fractures which are best appreciated on sagittal image with bone window (**g**). The extravasated contrast extends toward the pelvic fractures (**e**). Coronal (**h**) and sagittal (**i**) images from follow-up CT cystogram performed 10 days later shows trace residual leak (green arrows)

- **Associated injuries**: In addition to the urethral injury itself, CT may also show associated injuries in the pelvic region, such as bladder injury, pelvic fractures, or soft tissue injuries. The urethra, particularly the membranous and proximal bulbar urethra, should be closely evaluated in all patients with fractures of the anterior pelvic arch.

Table 8.8 Goldman classification of urethral injury [20]

Injury type	Injury description	Urethrographic appearance
I	Stretching or elongation of an intact posterior urethra resulting from ligament rupture	Intact but stretched urethra
II	Membranous urethral disruption above an intact urogenital diaphragm	Contrast extravasation above the urogenital diaphragm, no inferior contrast extravasation into the perineum
III	Disruption of the membranous urethra with injury of the urogenital diaphragm	Contrast extravasation above the urogenital diaphragm and below the urogenital diaphragm into the perineum
IV	Bladder neck injury extending into the proximal urethra	Extraperitoneal contrast extravasation around the bladder base
V	Isolated anterior urethral injury as from a straddle-type injury	Contrast extravasation below the urogenital diaphragm, confined to the anterior urethra

Table 8.9 AAST urethra injury scale [17]

AAST grade[a]	Injury type	Description of injury
I	Contusion	Blood at urethral meatus; retrourethography normal
II	Stretch injury	Elongation of urethra without extravasation on urethrography
III	Partial disruption	Extravasation of urethrography contrast at injury site with visualization in the bladder
IV	Complete disruption	Extravasation of urethrography contrast at injury site without visualization in the bladder; <2 cm of urethra separation
V	Complete disruption	Complete transaction with >2 cm urethral separation, or extension into the prostate or vagina

[a]Advance one grade for bilateral injuries up to grade III

It is important to note that the AAST grading system is just one tool used by healthcare providers to guide treatment decisions for urethral injuries in trauma patients.

Classification systems for grading urethral injury are primarily based on findings from retrograde urethrography [1]. However, CT findings may provide useful information regarding urethral injuries, such as whether urethral disruption is partial or complete; complete disruption will be associated with urinary leakage on imaging (Fig. 8.20). CT may also assist in distinguishing between anterior and posterior urethral injury as well as evaluating for extension to adjacent structures, including the bladder neck and rectum. And, CT provides invaluable information regarding associated injuries, which cannot be assessed on RUG and will guide treatment decisions [1].

The Goldman classification is the most frequently used system to grade urethral injury, which is based on the anatomic location of urethral injury and divides urethral injuries into five types. The Goldman classification is detailed in Table 8.8 [20].

Although less commonly used, the AAST OIS for urethral injury has been modified over time to better predict continence. The AAST urethra injury scale is detailed in Table 8.9.

Management and Complications

The treatment of patients with urethral injuries depends on the severity and location of the injury, as well as the presence of associated injuries. For instance, if the patient is undergoing immediate surgical exploration for associated injuries, surgical repair of the urethra may be performed concurrently [20]. The goal of treatment is to restore normal urinary function and prevent complications such as infection, stricture formation, and incontinence. Management strategies for urethral injury in trauma patients includes the following:

- **Conservative management**: Lower-grade injuries are often managed conservatively, including placement of a urinary catheter or urethral stent. Catheterization, either from Foley or suprapubic catheter, allows the urethra to heal.
- **Endoscopic procedures**: Endoscopic realignment of posterior urethra injuries is used in some situations [20].

- **Surgical interventions**: Surgical repair or reconstruction is typically needed for higher grade injuries, including complete urethral rupture. In complete disruption of the anterior urethra, patients are initially managed with suprapubic catheterization and delayed surgical repair [20]. Surgical exploration and debridement is typically needed in all penetrating injuries in this region [20].

A multidisciplinary approach involving urologists, trauma surgeons, and critical care specialists is often necessary to optimize patient outcomes. Complications that can arise from urethral injury in trauma patients include:

- **Infection**: Prophylactic antibiotics are often given to prevent infection, especially in cases where there is a delay in treatment or extravasation of urine.
- **Urinary incontinence**: Trauma may damage the muscles and nerves that control the internal (at the bladder neck) or external (at the urogenital diaphragm) urinary sphincter function, resulting in inability to control urination.
- **Urethral stricture**: Stricture or narrowing of the urethra is common following urethral injury, particularly in the setting of delayed diagnosis.

Recognition of these complications on imaging is essential for early treatment and low morbidity and mortality.

Female Genital Trauma

Trauma to the female genitalia includes a diverse range of injuries and multiple organs, including both external and internal female genitalia. Injuries may result from blunt or penetrating trauma, including assault and sports injuries. Overall, female genitalia injuries are uncommon in trauma patients.

Anatomy

The female genitalia includes numerous structures:

- Uterus: Muscular organ located posterior to the urinary bladder and anterior to the rectum.
- Ovaries: Paired structures that lie on each side of uterus, in the adnexa. Suspended by numerous ligaments.
- Fallopian tubes: Small tubes that connect the uterus to the adnexa, near the ovaries.
- Vagina: Fibromuscular tube that connects the uterus to the vestibule inferiorly.
- Vulva/external genitalia.
  - Vestibular bulbs.
  - Clitoris.
  - Vestibule: Cavity that contains the external urethral and vaginal orifices.
  - Labia majora and minora: Two folds of smooth muscle, adipose tissue, and fascia that extends from the mons pubis to the perineum.
  - Mons pubis: Adipose tissue located anterior to the pubic symphysis.

Imaging and Grading

Although not as sensitive or specific as ultrasound for female genitalia injury, CT can be useful in the evaluation of traumatic injury, especially as many patients will have a CT performed prior to ultrasonography. CT findings that may be seen in female genitalia injury include:

- **Soft tissue edema or hematoma**: Swelling of the vulvar soft tissues or subcutaneous hematoma are secondary signs of external female genitalia injury. Extravasation of contrast from intravenous contrast, which appears as

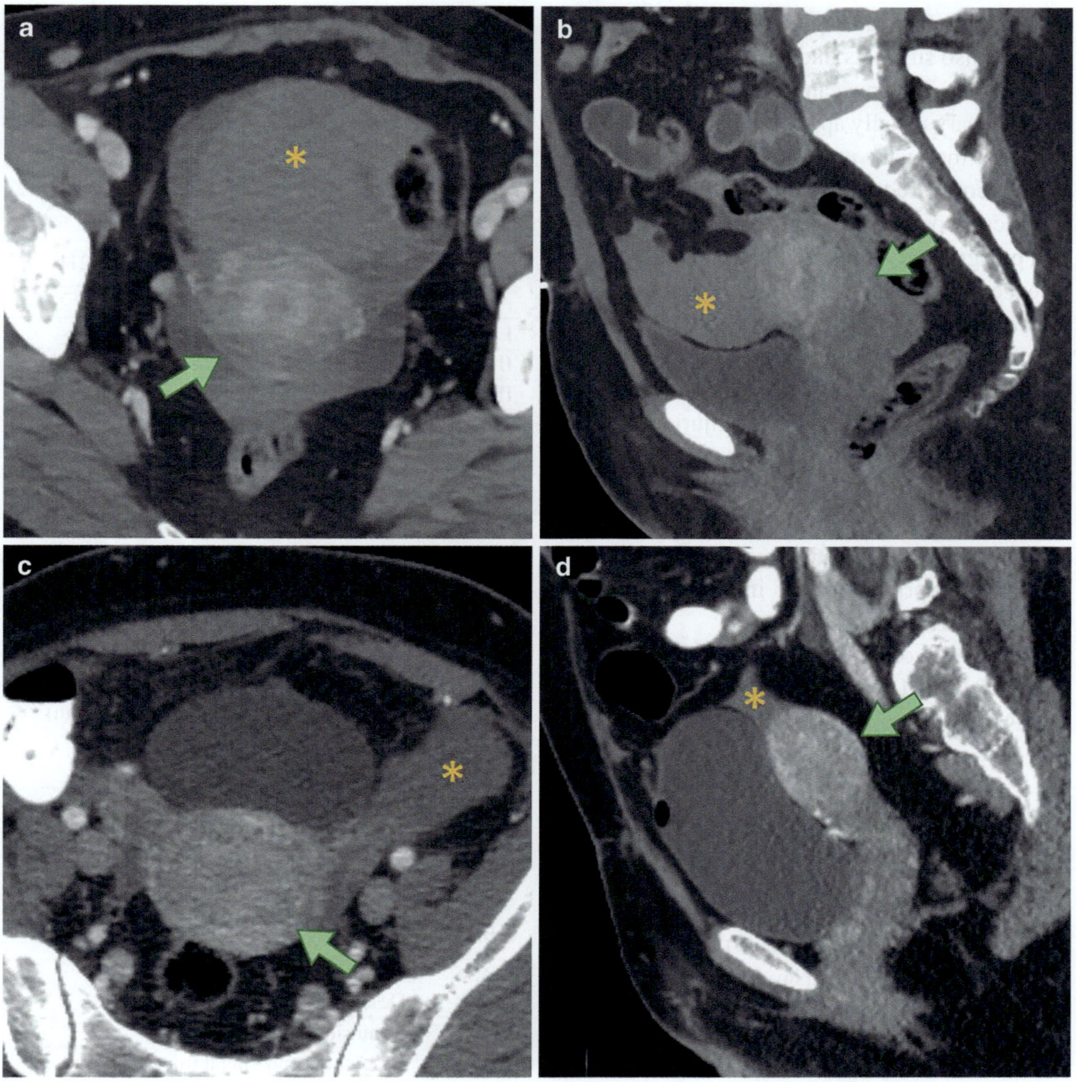

Fig. 8.21 CT images of the pelvis in a 40-year-old trauma patient presenting after a motor vehicle collision. Axial (**a**) and sagittal (**b**) images show heterogeneous enhancement of the uterus (green arrows) with small to moderate volume hemoperitoneum (orange asterisks). The densest portion of the hemoperitoneum abuts the anterior uterine body (sentinel clot sign). These findings raise concern for traumatic uterine injury. Axial (**c**) and sagittal (**d**) images on 1 week follow-up imaging show decreased hemoperitoneum and improved enhancement of the uterus

an area of hyperattenuation, may suggest active bleeding.

- **Fluid collection/hemorrhage**: Accumulation of fluid or blood (hemoperitoneum) in the pelvis is a secondary sign of internal female genitalia injury (Fig. 8.21). Extravasation of contrast from intravenous contrast, which appears as an area of hyperattenuation, may suggest active bleeding.
- **Loss of normal anatomic contours**: Obscuration of the normal anatomic contours, such as loss of the uterine contour, suggests hematoma or edema from underlying injury. Focal irregularity, disruption or distortion of a

structure, such as vaginal wall or ovarian capsule, also suggests underlying injury.

- **Torsion**: Trauma can cause ovarian torsion. The ovary usually appears enlarged and edematous; the ovary may show a change in position compared to a prior CT. A twist of the vascular pedicle is often seen.
- **Foreign body or soft tissue gas**: The presence of a foreign body within a structure of the female genitalia suggests injury. If there is a history of penetrating trauma, soft tissue gas can be seen at the site of injury.
- **Associated injuries**: Vulvar injuries are associated with pelvic fractures.

If an injury of the female genitalia is suspected on CT, further evaluation with physical exam and, if appropriate, further imaging with ultrasound or MRI is necessary.

The AAST organ injury scales are detailed in Tables 8.10, 8.11, 8.12, 8.13, 8.14, and 8.15 for uterus (nonpregnant), uterus (pregnant), fallopian tube, ovary, vagina, and vulva, respectively. It is important to note that these grading systems have not been widely adopted and there is no standardized grading system for female genitalia injuries in trauma patients.

Table 8.10 AAST uterus (nonpregnant) injury scale [21]

AAST grade[a]	Description of injury
I	Contusion/hematoma
II	Superficial laceration (<1 cm)
III	Deep laceration (>1 cm)
IV	Laceration involving uterine artery
V	Avulsion/devascularization

[a]Advance one grade for multiple injuries up to grade III

Table 8.11 AAST uterus (pregnant) injury scale [21]

AAST grade[a]	Description of injury
I	Contusion or hematoma (without placental abruption)
II	Superficial laceration (<1 cm) or partial placental abruption <25%
III	Deep laceration (>1 cm) occurring in second trimester or placental abruption >25% but <50%
	Deep laceration (>1 cm) in third trimester
	Laceration involving uterine artery
IV	Deep laceration (>1 cm) with >50% placental abruption
V	Uterine rupture, second or third trimester
	Complete placental abruption

[a]Advance one grade for multiple injuries up to grade III

Table 8.12 AAST fallopian tube injury scale [21]

AAST grade[a]	Description of injury
I	Hematoma or contusion
II	Laceration <50% circumference
III	Laceration >50% circumference
IV	Transection
V	Vascular injury; devascularized segment

[a]Advance one grade for bilateral injuries up to grade III

Table 8.13 AAST ovary injury scale [21]

AAST grade[a]	Description of injury
I	Contusion or hematoma
II	Superficial laceration (depth < 0.5 cm)
III	Deep laceration (depth > 0.5 cm)
IV	Partial disruption or blood supply
V	Avulsion or complete parenchymal destruction

[a]Advance one grade for bilateral injuries up to grade III

Table 8.14 AAST vagina injury scale [21]

AAST grade[a]	Description of injury
I	Contusion or hematoma
II	Laceration, superficial (mucosa only)
III	Laceration, deep into fat or muscle
IV	Laceration, complex, into cervix or peritoneum
V	Injury into adjacent organs (anus, rectum, urethra, bladder)

[a]Advance one grade for multiple injuries up to grade III

Table 8.15 AAST vulva injury scale [21]

AAST grade[a]	Description of injury
I	Contusion or hematoma
II	Laceration, superficial (skin only)
III	Laceration, deep into (into fat or muscle)
IV	Avulsion; skin, fat or muscle
V	Injury into adjacent organs (anus, rectum, urethra, bladder)

[a]Advance one grade for multiple injuries up to grade III

Management and Complications

The treatment of patients with female genitalia injuries depends on the severity and location of the injury, as well as the presence of associated injuries. Management strategies for female genitalia injury in trauma patients includes the following:

- **Conservative management**: Mild injuries may be treated conservatively.
- **Interventional radiology procedures:** Selective angioembolization may be performed to stop active bleeding from a damaged vessel while preserving the integrity of the uterus or ovary. Interventional radiologists use minimally invasive endovascular technique with angiography and particles or metal coils.
- **Surgical interventions**: Moderate to severe injuries require surgical management, which may include hysterectomy, salpingectomy or oophorectomy. Penetrating trauma often requires emergent surgical exploration.

A multidisciplinary approach involving gynecologists, trauma surgeons, and critical care specialists is often necessary to optimize patient outcomes.

Male Genital Trauma

Trauma to the male genitalia includes a diverse range of injuries and multiple organs, including both external and internal male genitalia. Injuries may result from blunt or penetrating trauma, including assault and sports injuries. Overall, male genitalia injuries are rare in trauma patients.

Scrotal injuries are rare and often associated with sports injuries [20]. Direct injuries to the scrotum are associated with testicular injury, such as testicular contusion, hematoma or fracture/rupture [20]. In cases of severe blunt scrotal trauma, the risk of testicular fracture/rupture is 50 percent [5].

Anatomy

The male genitalia includes numerous structures:

- Scrotum: Sac with several tissue layers that contains the vas deferens, epididymides, and testes.
- Testes: Paired organs that are suspended in the scrotum and primarily composed of seminiferous tubules. Each testis is enclosed by capsule of tunica albuginea. Outer layers protecting the testes include the tunica vaginalis.
- Penis: Erectile tissue composed of corpus spongiosum, which contains the urethra, and two corpus cavernosa. Four components include base, shaft, glans, and foreskin.
- Prostate: Gland located inferior to the bladder, surrounding the bladder neck and a portion of the posterior urethra.
- Seminal vesicles: Paired glands located posterior to the prostate, between the bladder and rectum.

Imaging and Grading

With a high sensitivity for detecting injury, ultrasonography is the preferred method of imaging for male genitalia, particularly the testes, scrotum and penis [20]. Although not as sensitive or specific as ultrasound for male genitalia injury, CT can be useful in the evaluation of traumatic injury, especially as many patients will have a CT performed prior to ultrasonography. CT findings that may be seen in male genitalia injury include:

- **Soft tissue edema or hematoma**: Swelling or hematoma of the scrotal or subcutaneous soft tissues are secondary signs of external male genitalia injury (Figs. 8.22, 8.23, and 8.24). Extravasation of contrast from intravenous contrast, which appears as an area of hyperattenuation, may suggest active bleeding (Fig. 8.24).

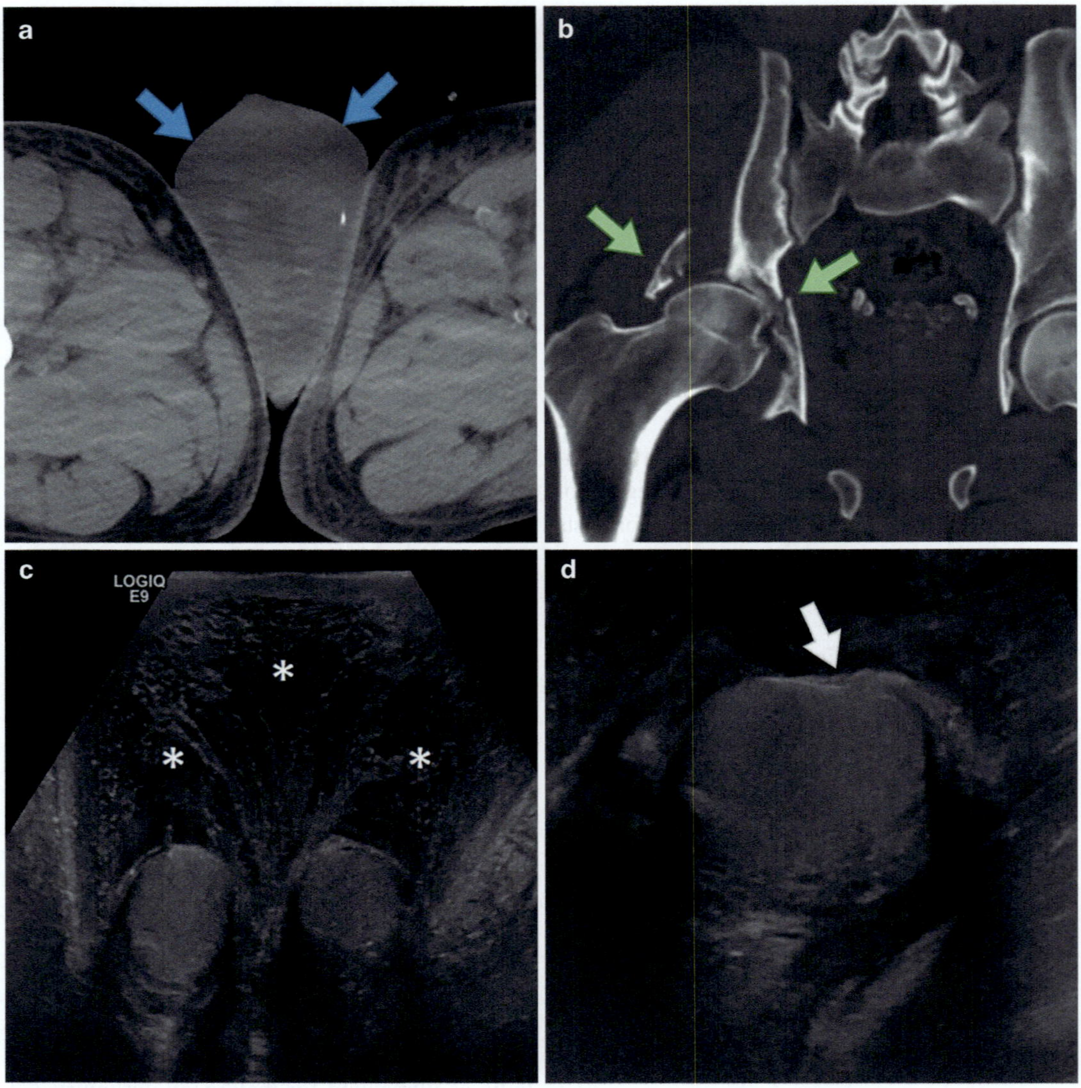

Fig. 8.22 Images of a 50-year-old trauma patient presenting after being struck by a car. Axial (**a**) unenhanced images through the scrotum show extensive scrotal edema (blue arrows). Coronal image of the pelvis with bone window (**b**) shows a comminuted right pelvic fracture (green arrows). Ultrasound images (**c**, **d**) show marked scrotal wall thickening and edema with fibrinous septations, favored to represent a large extratesticular hematoma (white asterisks). Subtle irregular contour of the tunica albuginea at the anterior lower pole of the right testicle (white arrow) suggests injury to the tunica albuginea. No testicular contusion or laceration identified

- **Fluid collection/hemorrhage**: Accumulation of fluid or blood (hemoperitoneum) in the pelvis is a secondary sign of internal male genitalia injury. Extravasation of contrast from intravenous contrast, which appears as an area of hyperattenuation, may suggest active bleeding.
- **Loss of normal anatomic contours**: Obscuration of the normal anatomic contours, such as loss of the prostatic contour or penile bulb, suggests hematoma or edema from underlying injury (Fig. 8.24). Focal irregularity, disruption or distortion of a structure, such as tunica albuginea of the testis or penis, also suggests underlying injury.
- **Torsion**: Trauma can cause testicular torsion. The testis usually appears enlarged and edematous. A twist of the vascular pedicle may be seen.

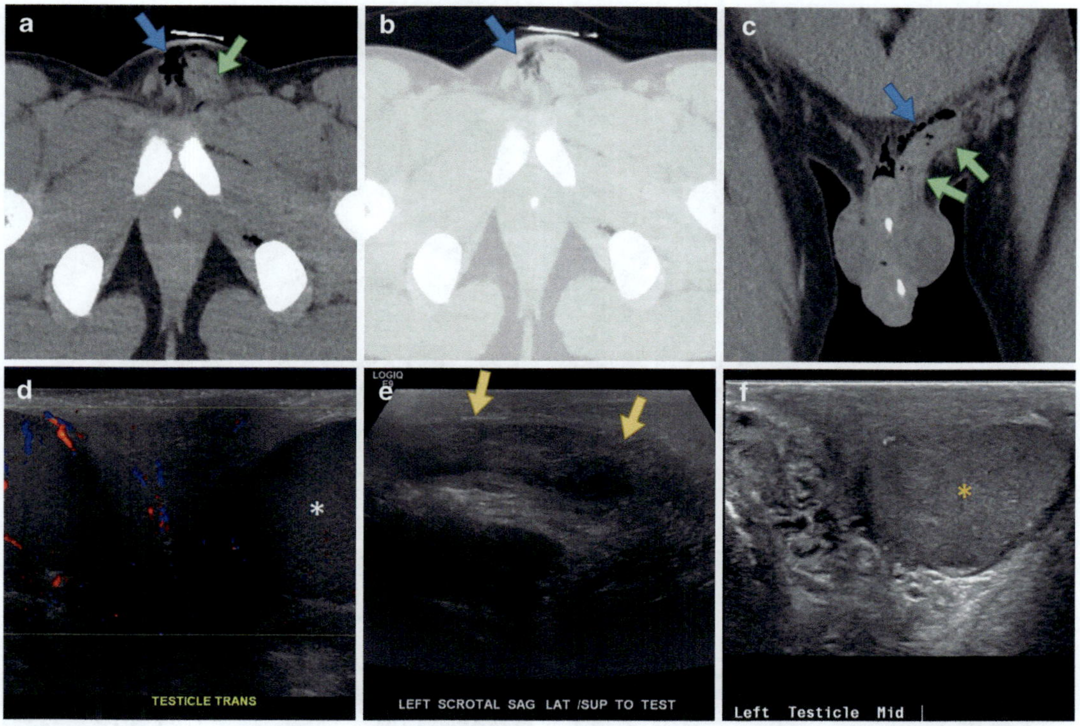

Fig. 8.23 Images of the pelvis in a 19-year-old trauma patient presenting with gunshot wounds. Axial (**a, b**) coronal (**c**) CT images through the lower pelvis show a small area of heterogeneous thickening of the left spermatic cord (green arrows), favored to represent a hematoma. Adjacent foci of subcutaneous emphysema (blue arrows) are best appreciated on lung window (**b**). Follow-up US (**d, e**) shows homogeneous echogenicity with decreased flow within the left testis (white asterisk) on color Doppler imaging (compared to the right), in keeping with ischemia. Thickening and heterogeneity of the left spermatic cord (yellow arrows) corresponds with the CT findings. Surgical intervention showed a dusky but viable left testis that was treated with orchiopexy. There was injury of the main testicular artery and multiple veins. The spermatic cord vessels were repaired and the hematoma was evacuated. A two-month follow-up ultrasound (**f**) shows a small and scarred, but viable left testis

- **Foreign body or soft tissue gas**: The presence of a foreign body within a structure of the male genitalia suggests injury. If there is a history of penetrating trauma, soft tissue gas can be seen at the site of injury (Fig. 8.23).
- **Associated injuries**: Male genitalia injuries can occurs in the setting of pelvic fractures (Fig. 8.22).

If an injury of the male genitalia is suspected on CT, further evaluation with physical exam and, if appropriate, further imaging with ultrasound or MRI is necessary.

The AAST organ injury scales are detailed in Tables 8.16, 8.17, and 8.18 for scrotum, testis, and penis, respectively. It is important to note that these grading systems have not been widely adopted and there is no standardized grading system for male genitalia injuries in trauma patients.

Management and Complications

The treatment of patients with male genitalia injuries depends on the severity and location of the injury, as well as the presence of associated injuries. Management strategies for female genitalia injury in trauma patients includes the following:

- **Conservative management**: In minor injuries, conservative management may be appropriate. For instance, patients with isolated subcutaneous tissue injury in the setting of

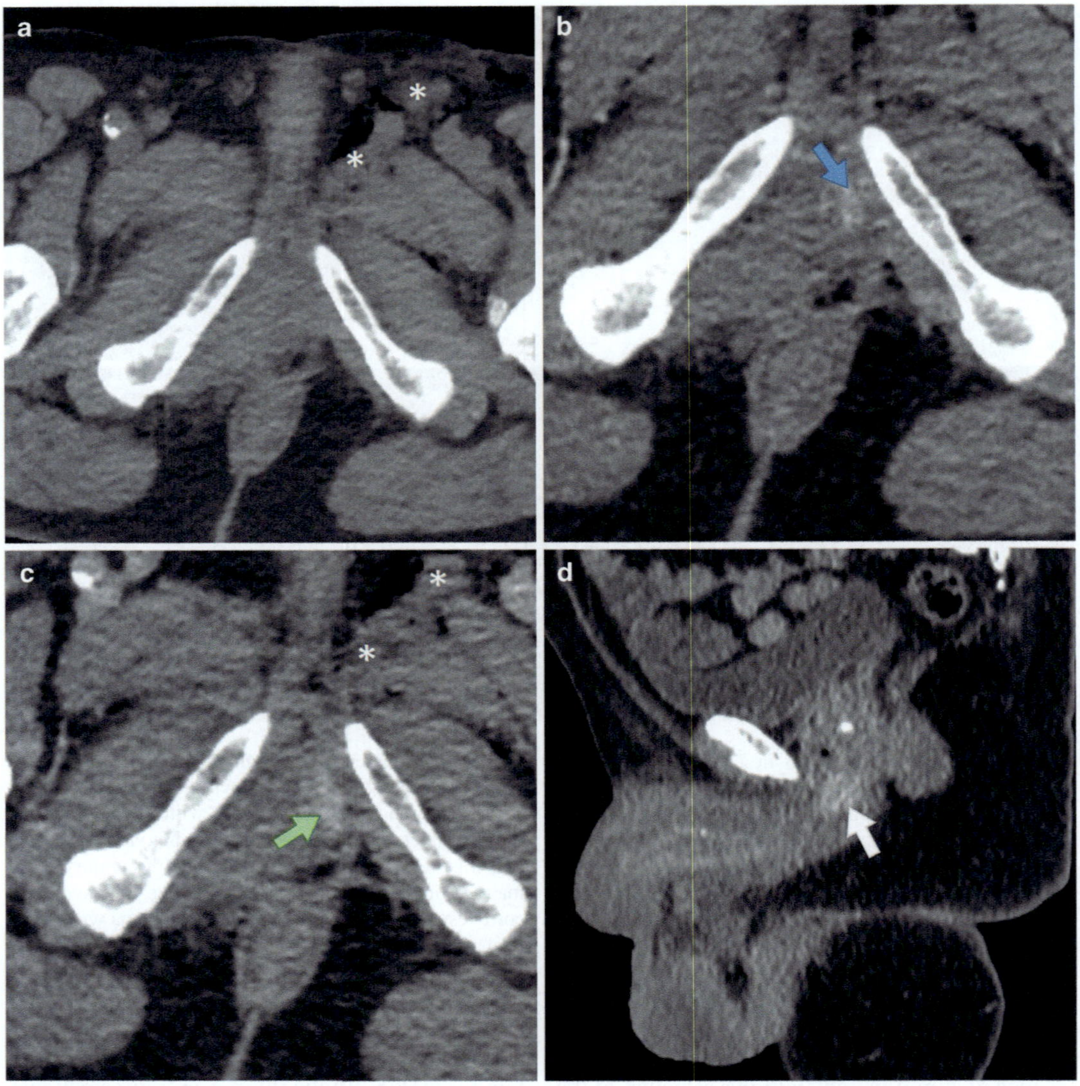

Fig. 8.24 CT images of the pelvis in a 28-year-old trauma patient presenting with gunshot wounds. Axial unenhanced (**a**), arterial phase (**b**) and portal venous phase (**c**) images as well as sagittal portal venous phase (**d**) image show subcutaneous emphysema, fat stranding and small hematomas along a ballistic path (white asterisks) in the left inguinal region. There is fat stranding along the posterior aspect of the penile bulb. There is contrast extravasation in the left penile bulb on the arterial phase (blue arrow), which enlarges on the portal venous phase (green and white arrows). Findings are in keeping with active bleeding and hemorrhage

Table 8.16 AAST scrotum injury scale

AAST grade	Description of injury
I	Contusion
II	Laceration <25% of scrotal diameter
III	Laceration of tunica albuginea with <50% parenchymal loss
IV	Avulsion <50%
V	Avulsion >50%

minor blunt trauma may be treated conservatively, including tissue debridement [5].

- **Surgical interventions**: Penetrating trauma often requires emergent surgical exploration, particularly in the setting of penile, scrotal, and testicular injuries [20]. Penile or testicular fracture/rupture also requires urgent surgery; conservative management of these injuries has been associated with poor outcomes, while

Table 8.17 AAST testis injury scale

AAST grade[a]	Description of injury
I	Contusion/hematoma
II	Subclinical laceration of tunica albuginea
III	Laceration of tunica albuginea with <50% parenchymal loss
IV	Major laceration of tunica albuginea with >50% parenchymal loss
V	Total testicular destruction or avulsion

[a]Advance one grade for bilateral lesions up to grade V

Table 8.18 AAST penis injury scale

AAST grade[a]	Description of injury
I	Cutaneous laceration/contusion
II	Buck's fascia (cavernosum) laceration without tissue loss
III	Cutaneous avulsion
	Laceration through glans/meatus
	Cavernosal or urethral defect <2 cm
IV	Partial penectomy
	Cavarnosal or urethral defect >2 cm
V	Total penectomy

[a]Advance one grade for multiple injuries up to grade III

early surgical repair has been associated with high success rates [5].

A multidisciplinary approach involving urologists, trauma surgeons, and critical care specialists is often necessary to optimize patient outcomes.

Conclusion

CT imaging is an essential tool in the evaluation of genitourinary injuries in trauma patients. It is the preferred imaging modality for renal and adrenal trauma because it is widely available, rapid, and accurate in detecting both the presence and the extent of injury. Specialized CT protocols, including CT urography and CT cystography, are invaluable for the evaluation of traumatic injury to the ureters and urinary bladder. Although not the modality of choice for evaluation of the urethra or genitalia, CT does provide useful information regarding traumatic injuries of these structures.

References

1. Ramchandani P, Buckler PM. Imaging of genitourinary trauma. Am J Roentgenol. 2009;192(6):1514–23.
2. Noorbakhsh A, Aganovic L, Vahdat N, Fazeli S, Chung R, Cassidy F. What a difference a delay makes! CT urogram: a pictorial essay. Abdom Radiol. 2019;44(12):3919–34.
3. Chan DPN, Abujudeh HH, Cushing GL, Novelline RA. CT cystography with multiplanar reformation for suspected bladder rupture: experience in 234 cases. Am J Roentgenol. 2006;187(5):1296–302.
4. Joshi G, Kim EY, Hanna TN, Siegel CL, Menias CO. CT cystography for suspicion of traumatic urinary bladder injury: indications, technique, findings, and pitfalls in diagnosis: *RadioGraphics fundamentals | online presentation.* Radiographics. 2018;38(1):92–3.
5. Mattox KL, Moore EE, Feliciano DV. Trauma. 9th ed. New York: McGraw-Hill Medical; 2021.
6. Moore EE, Shackford SR, Pachter HL, McAninch JW, Browner BD, Champion HR, et al. Organ injury scaling: spleen, liver, and kidney. J Trauma. 1989;29(12):1664–6.
7. Kozar RA, Crandall M, Shanmuganathan K, Zarzaur BL, Coburn M, Cribari C, et al. Organ injury scaling 2018 update: spleen, liver, and kidney. J Trauma Acute Care Surg. 2018;85(6):1119–22.
8. Venkatanarasimha N, Roobottom C. Intense adrenal enhancement: a feature of hypoperfusion complex. Am J Roentgenol. 2010;195(1):W82.
9. Burks DW, Mirvis SE, Shanmuganathan K. Acute adrenal injury after blunt abdominal trauma: CT findings. Am J Roentgenol. 1992;158(3):503–7.
10. Moore EE, Malangoni MA, Cogbill TH, Peterson NE, Champion HR, Jurkovich GJ, et al. Organ injury scaling VII: cervical vascular, peripheral vascular, adrenal, penis, testis, and scrotum. J Trauma. 1996;41(3):523–4.
11. Alonso RC, Nacenta SB, Martinez PD, Guerrero AS, Fuentes CG. Kidney in danger: CT findings of blunt and penetrating renal trauma. Radiographics. 2009;29(7):2033–53.
12. Kawashima A, Sandler CM, Corl FM, West OC, Tamm EP, Fishman EK, et al. Imaging of renal trauma: a comprehensive review. Radiographics. 2001;21(3):557–74.
13. Voelzke BB, Leddy L. The epidemiology of renal trauma. Transl Androl Urol. 2014;3(2):143–9.
14. Brandes SB, McAninch JW. Urban free falls and patterns of renal injury: a 20-year experience with 396 cases. J Trauma Inj Infect Crit Care. 1999;47(4):643.
15. Lee YJ, Oh SN, Rha SE, Byun JY. Renal Trauma. Radiol Clin N Am. 2007;45(3):581–92.
16. Smyth A, Collins CS, Thorsteinsdottir B, Madsen BE, Oliveira GHM, Kane G, et al. Page kidney: etiology, renal function outcomes and risk for future hypertension: page kidney. J Clin Hypertens. 2012;14(4):216–21.

17. Moore EE, Cogbill TH, Jurkovich GJ, McAninch JW, Champion HR, Gennarelli TA, et al. Organ injury scaling. III: chest wall, abdominal vascular, ureter, bladder, and urethra. J Trauma. 1992;33(3):337–9.
18. Brandes S, Coburn M, Armenakas N, McAninch J. Diagnosis and management of ureteric injury: an evidence-based analysis. BJU Int. 2004;94(3):277–89.
19. Ali M, Safriel Y, Sclafani SJA, Schulze R. CT signs of urethral injury. Radiographics. 2003;23(4):951–63.
20. Avery LL, Scheinfeld MH. Imaging of male pelvic trauma. Radiol Clin N Am. 2012;50(6):1201–17.
21. Moore EE, Jurkovich GJ, Knudson MM, Cogbill TH, Malangoni MA, Champion HR, et al. Organ injury scaling. VI: extrahepatic biliary, esophagus, stomach, vulva, vagina, uterus (nonpregnant), uterus (pregnant), fallopian tube, and ovary. J Trauma. 1995;39(6):1069–70.

A Practical Guide to Imaging Spinal Trauma

9

J. Eric Schmitt

Introduction

The incidence of traumatic spine injury has been estimated at more than 760,000 cases per year worldwide [1], with nearly 180,000 individuals experiencing injury to the spinal cord [2]. Spine injuries can be catastrophic, resulting in significant morbidity, mortality, and economic consequences. For example, there are approximately 15,000 cases of paraplegia and 5000 deaths per year in the USA owed to complications from spinal trauma [3]. Cervical spine injuries carry a particularly high risk of long-term morbidity, largely owed to an increased risk injury to the high spinal cord. Thoracic and lumbar spine injuries are often associated with severe comorbid soft tissue injures in the chest, abdomen, and pelvis. It has been estimated that of all spine injuries, about 55% involve the cervical spine, 15% the thoracic spine, 15% are at the lumbrosacral junction specifically, and about 15% are found in the lumbar spine [4].

Despite the high number of annual spine injuries, only 2–6% of trauma patients will have a significant acute spine injury [5, 6]. This is largely due to the overwhelming volume of injury-related visits to the emergency department, which approximated 35 million in the U.S. alone in 2020, or more than 10 visits per 100 people [7]. Spine imaging has therefore become a ubiquitous feature in the assessment of trauma patients, both in order to accelerate treatment for those cases with positive, time-critical findings, as well as to facilitate workflow in busy emergency rooms by rapidly clearing patients with only minor injuries.

In the modern trauma bay, multidetector CT (MDCT) has emerged as the workhorse for performing these duties [8], being able to detect serious trauma injuries quickly and with extraordinarily high sensitivity. The current chapter presents a pragmatic overview of the imaging of spine trauma, with an emphasis on providing a useful guide to CT interpretation, image-rich examples, and high-yield clinical pearls.

Overview of Basic Spine Anatomy

The spine is a miracle of evolution, simultaneously protecting the spinal cord in a rigid bony sheath, providing a scaffold to support the body, allowing for a reasonably high degree of mobility, and attenuating compressive forces along its long axis. Most individuals have 33 vertebral bodies (7 cervical, 12 thoracic, 5 lumbar, 5 sacral, 4 coccygeal). Different sections of the spine emphasize different functions (e.g., mobility in the cervical spine, protection in the thoracic

J. E. Schmitt (✉)
Departments of Radiology and Psychiatry, University of Pennsylvania, Philadelphia, PA, USA
e-mail: eric.schmitt@stanfordalumni.org

F. Knollmann (ed.), *Trauma Computed Tomography*, https://doi.org/10.1007/978-3-031-45746-3_9

spine, and the lumbar spine somewhere in between). However, all aspects of the spine share common features, and level-by-level anatomic differences largely lie along a continuum. Nearly all vertebral levels share a common segmental anatomy, with a cylindrical vertebral body providing axial support anteriorly, and a vertebral arch forming the spinal canal posteriorly [9]. The arch can be divided into two pedicles anteriorly, and two laminae posteriorly. Several elongated processes arise from the arch; the paired transverse processes at the pedicle-lamina junctions (projecting laterally), the superior and inferior articular facets which also originate near the pedicle-lamina junctions and form the facet joints, and the midline spinous process at the junction of the lamina (projecting posterio-inferiorly). These processes provide support for the paraspinal musculature and leverage to improve mechanical advantage. The foramen transversarium are unique to the cervical spine and protect the vertebral arteries for a portion of their extracranial course (the V2 segment). The anatomic features of the cervical spine are shown in Fig. 9.1, although basic features are similar in other spine regions.

Supernumerary vertebral bodies are not uncommon [9]. Other relatively common anatomic variants in the spine include cervical ribs at C7, hypoplastic ribs at T12, and transitional lumbrosacral anatomy in which either L5 resembles a sacral vertebral body (sacralization) or S1 resembles a lumbar vertebral body (lumbarization). Detailed descriptions of anatomic variants are usually not particularly important when interpreting an emergent trauma case if it is otherwise negative. However, variants may be noteworthy because precise anatomic localization of any positive findings is a critical component of spine assessment; the satisfaction of making a great

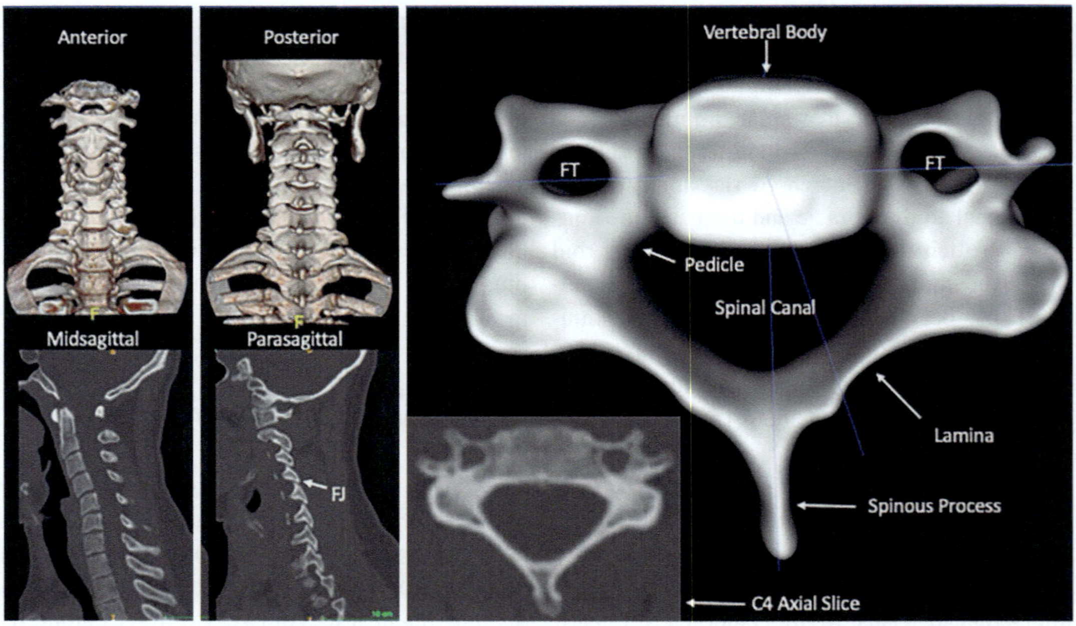

Fig. 9.1 Normal spine anatomy on high-resolution axial CT, based on data from a 28-year-old man involved in a motor vehicle collision. On top left, 3D reconstructions show the cervical spine from both anterior and posterior views. Inferiorly, both midsagittal and parasagittal CT slices are provided. The large image on the right represents 3D reconstruction of C4 modeled in ITK-SNAP [66], with important anatomical landmarks labeled. *FT* foramen transversarium, *FJ* Facet joint. A representative axial slice through C4 from the original data is also provided for reference. Most other spinal levels have a grossly similar morphology, although foramen transversarium are unique to the cervical spine

diagnosis will rapidly turn into tragedy if simple carelessness predicates a surgical intervention at the incorrect spine level.

Vertebral bodies throughout the spine are intimately associated with numerous soft tissue structures. Although detailed spine anatomy is beyond the scope of this chapter, some structures require specific mention. The intervertebral disk separates each vertebral body and allows for increased mobility as well as shock absorption [10]. The anterior longitudinal ligament (ALL) is a long band of connective tissue that extends along the anterior vertebral bodies and disks from the anterior tubercule of C1 to the sacrum. Similarly, the posterior longitudinal ligament (PLL) is a long band of fibrous tissue along the posterior margin of the vertebral bodies and disk space and runs from C2 to the sacrum. Numerous shorter bands of fibrous connective tissue are associated with the posterior elements, most importantly the intraspinous ligaments and paired ligamentum flava, which connect adjacent spinous processes and lamina, much like coupled train cars (Fig. 9.2). Although direct evidence of ligamentous injury can be difficult to appreciate on CT, it can usually be inferred indirectly—via careful assessment of spine alignment.

The Craniocervical Junction (CCJ)

The anatomy of the CCJ warrants special consideration for several reasons. First, the anatomy is substantially more complicated than the remainder of the spine. Second, it is functionally unique. For example, approximately half of head rotation occurs in this region owed to its unique anatomy. Third, fractures in the subaxial spine are common, accounting for about 65% of all cervical fractures [11]. Fourth, injuries to the CCJ can be particularly devastating, given the high likelihood of an upper spinal cord injury or traumatic vertebral artery dissection [12]. And finally, of all cervical spine injuries, those near the CCJ are the most commonly missed by interpreting radiologists [13].

Functionally, the CCJ begins at the occipital condyles (Fig. 9.2), the paired protuberances at the base of the skull [14]. The occipital condyles

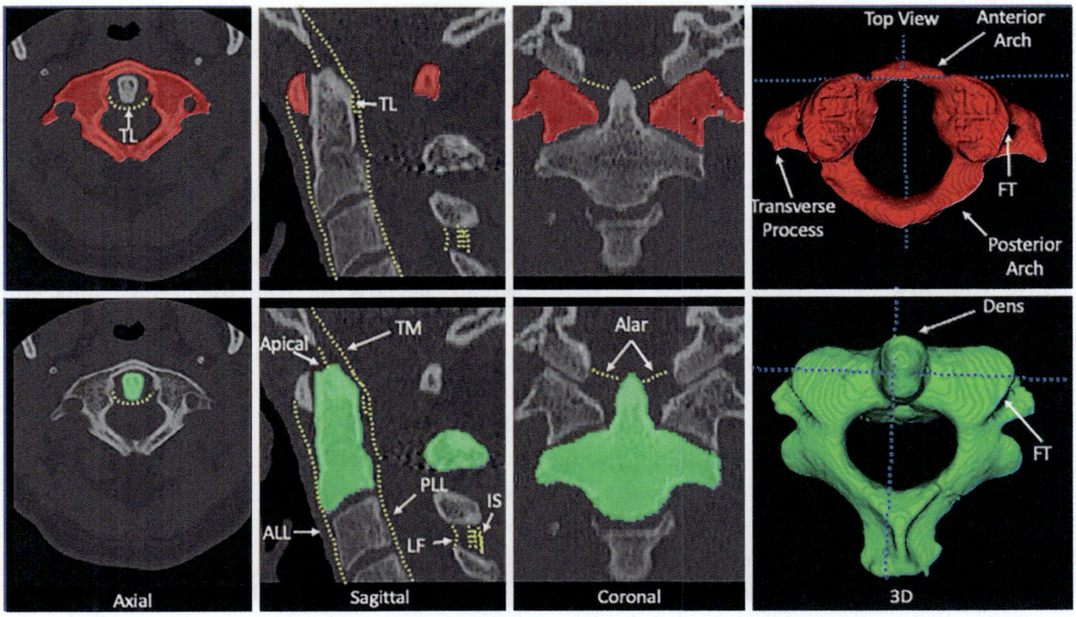

Fig. 9.2 Complex anatomy at the CCJ. Paired magnified triplanar views from MDCT highlighting either the C1 atlas (red) or C2 axis (green) via 3D segmentation [66]. Top views of 3D renders of both C1 and C2 are provided on the right. The dotted yellow lines represent the approximate locations of the most important ligaments in this region. *TL* transverse ligament, *TM* tectorial membrane, *ALL* anterior longitudinal ligament, *PLL* posterior longitudinal ligament, *LF* ligamentum flavum, *IS* intraspinous ligament, *FT* foramen transversarium

articulate with the lateral masses of the C1 ring, i.e., the *atlas*, which has neither a body nor a spinous process [15]. The C2 vertebral body, i.e., the *axis*, also has unique anatomy. A large superiorly-directly finger-like protuberance from the C2 vertebral body, i.e., the dens or odontoid process extends into the C1 ring. The dens acts as a pivot point, enabling a high degree of rotational movement at this level. The CCJ also is unique in that there are no intravertebral disks; these begin at C2/C3.

In order to maximize motion, the ligamentous anatomy of the CCJ is also significantly more complex than at lower spine levels. In the setting of trauma, the most important ligaments near the CCJ to know are: (1) the *apical* ligament which extends from the tip of the dens at midline and fans out to the anterior margin of foramen magnum [15], (2) the paired *alar* ligaments that extend from the side of the dens more laterally and insert on the lateral margins of foramen magnum, (3) the solitary *transverse ligament* which is affixed to the C1 arch but surrounds the dens, creating an osteoligamentous ring (and dividing the ring into anterior and posterior compartments) [9], and (4) the *tectorial membrane* which is a continuation of the posterior longitudinal ligament and inserts along the anterior margin of foramen magnum [8]. This complex ligamentous anatomy simultaneously allows for a large range of motion while maintaining the structural integrity of the upper cervical spine (Fig. 9.2).

Spine Stability

The function of the spine requires a balance between its roles as protector of the nervous system, scaffold for the remainder of the musculoskeletal system, and the necessities of mobility. Significant spine trauma may result in increased instability, placing the cord and other nearby soft tissue structures at risk for damage—owed to unchecked motion. It is therefore not surprising that most spinal cord injuries are associated with unstable fractures [11]. However, it is also important to remember that ligamentous integrity is the principal factor maintaining stability of the spine, and that unstable fractures seen on CT nearly always associated with ligamentous disruption [16].

Optimal classification of spine traumas into stable and unstable categories remains a matter of active debate [17]. However, for over four decades, the 3-column system of Denis has become the most widely known metric for unstable injuries [18]. Denis divides the spine in to three columns, *anterior* (ALL, anterior 2/3 of vertebral body, anterior 2/3 of disk), *middle* (PLL, posterior 1/3 of vertebral body, posterior 1/3 of disk), and *posterior* (everything else, e.g., spinal canal, posterior elements, and associated ligaments). *Any injury that results in disruption of 2 or more columns* is considered unstable with this system. It is noteworthy that some 2-column injuries may be stable if the posterior ligamentous complex is intact [19], and that in reality spine stability lies along a continuum rather than being a perfect dichotomy [20]. Regardless, the 3-column system is a useful heuristic that is predictive in most positive CT cases, and simple enough to employ routinely in a busy reading room.

Patient Triage: Who Should Get Scanned and How?

The decision of when to image trauma patients is largely beyond the control of the interpreting radiologist. In an ideal world, these decisions should be made via evidence-based protocols that emphasize a high negative predictive value (NPV, i.e., the probability that a negative study is actually negative for acute trauma). Patients with a high NPV have a low likelihood of serious trauma—and therefore should not require imaging. For the cervical spine, the most well-accepted clinical assessment tools are the Canadian cervical spine rules (CCR) and those derived from the National Emergency X-ray Utilization study (NEXUS) study [21, 22]. These clinical tools are summarized in Tables 9.1 and 9.2. NEXUS and CCR differ in specifics, but in order to consider the patient "low risk," both tools require that the patient: (1) is able to participate in their physical exam (e.g., is not intoxicated) and (2) has no localizing symptoms. If a patient is determined to be low risk by either of these tools, then there is a very low probability of significant cervical trauma (e.g., low risk of a fracture or acute ligamentous injury). While NEXUS includes only five relatively simple criteria, the CCR are somewhat more complicated, largely because they include additional risk factors (e.g., age > 65 and high risk mechanisms of injury). Both NEXUS and CCR have demonstrated a high NPV in clinical trials (>98% in most studies). The reward of the additional complexity of CCR seems to be in slightly better NPV, approaching 100% [21, 22]; however, both tools are excellent, and neither is perfect.

Table 9.1 NEXUS low risk criteria. All must be negative to be considered low risk

• No focal ***n***eurologic deficit
• No midline ***s***pine tenderness
• Normal ***a***lertness
• No ***i***ntoxication or indication of brain injury
• No painful ***d***istracting injuries
Mnemonic: **NSAID**
If low risk by NEXUS, ~99.6% NPV

Table 9.2 CCH low risk criteria

• Absence of high risk factors*	***CCH high risk factors**
• Low risk factors that allow safe assessment of range of motion	• Altered mental status
– Simple rear-end MVC	• Multiple fractures
– Sitting in ED	• Significant head or facial injury
– Ambulatory at any time	• Age > 65 years
– Delayed onset of neck pain	• Paraesthesia in extremities
– Absent midline cervical tenderness	• Rigid spine disease
• Able to rotate neck 45 degrees both sides	– Ankylosing spondylitis
	– DISH
	• Dangerous mechanisms
	– Axial load to head
	– Age > 65 years
	– Fall from >1 meter
	– High speed MVC (>60 mph)
	– MVC with large vehicle
	– MVC with rollover or ejection
	– Pedestrian or bicyclist struck by vehicle
	– Crash from motorized recreation vehicle
IF stratified to low risk using CCH, ~100% NPV	

Patients considered "high risk" by either CCR or NEXUS should undergo cervical spine CT for further evaluation. Note that although cervical radiographs have historically been used for the assessment of cervical spine trauma, they should be avoided completely in the adult population – assuming that CT is available. Numerous studies have shown that the sensitivity of radiographs is substantially lower than CT—about 50% versus 98% [23]. Radiographically subtle or occult fractures could have significant clinical implications (Fig. 9.3). Radiography in children is still considered acceptable at present, given the lower pretest probability, increased sensitivity of radiography in this population, and increased concerns about radiation exposure [24–26]. The precise role of MRI in the management of cervical spine trauma is more controversial, but it clearly plays an important role if CT or clinical findings suggest cord or ligamentous injury [26, 27]. At many institutions, MRI is routinely performed in obtunded and intubated patients with a negative CT, although this practice remains an area of active debate [28, 29].

There have been several attempts to construct similar clinical tools for triage of the thoracolumbar spine [26, 30–32], although to date they are less widely-accepted than NEXUS and CCR. The general principals of these criteria are similar to those for the cervical spine; the presence of localizing symptoms, intoxication, and high risk mechanisms of injury result in stratification of the patient into a higher risk category warranting CT. The negative predictive value of these tools is also reportedly high, approaching 100%. However, the determination of whether to image the thoracic and lumbar spine is confounded by whether to image chest and body for other reasons (e.g., concern for splenic laceration). Similar

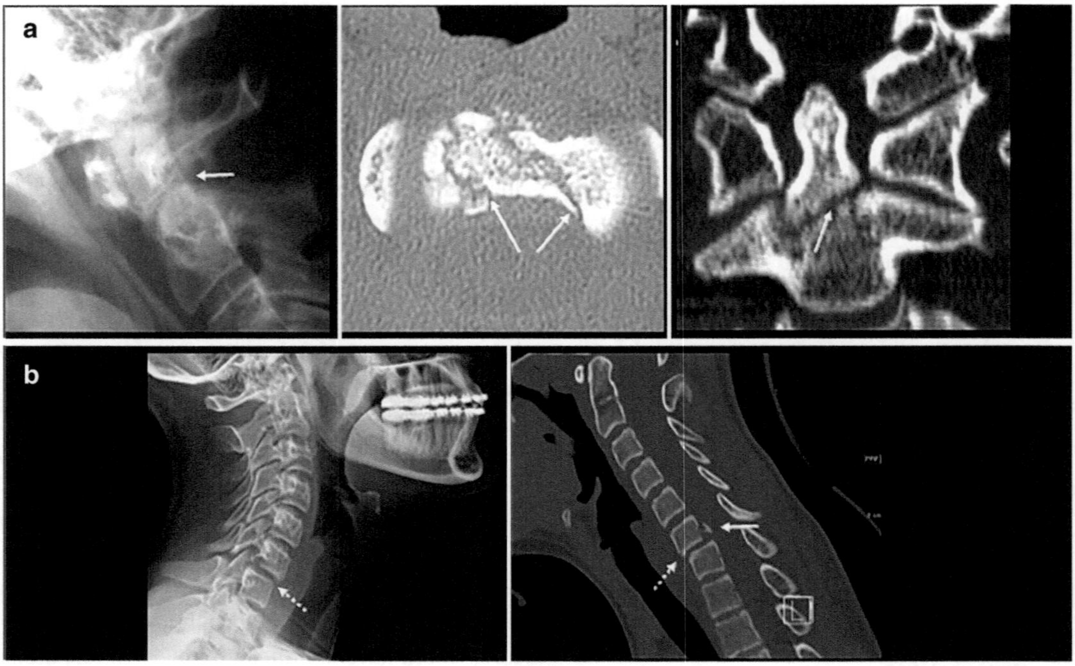

Fig. 9.3 Increased sensitivity of CT for spine trauma, relative to radiography. On top (Panel **a**), a type III odontoid fracture that can be reasonably well-appreciated on radiography, but is impossible to miss on CT. On bottom (Panel **b**), images from a 14-year-old who fell off a trampoline. A subtle, focal anterolisthesis can be seen at C6/C7 on radiography (dotted line) suggestive of trauma. The traumatic anterolisthesis is substantially more obvious on CT, and an associated fracture with retropulsion (solid arrow) is readily visible

to cervical spine trauma, the role of radiography in thoracolumbar trauma has fallen out of favor owed to the increased speed and accuracy of MDCT [20, 33].

Despite the high NPV of these clinical tools and their sound foundation in evidence-based medicine, in practice CT has become a near-ubiquitous part of the acute trauma workup. Obtaining accurate histories in the trauma bay can be a challenge, and some exclusion criteria (e.g., age > 65) will triage a large fraction of the population into "high risk" for many hospital catchment populations. As the MDCT "trauma pan-scan" has resulted in dramatically increased CT volumes at major trauma centers, efficient analysis of this information has become increasingly central to rapid turnaround times for these studies. At our institution, we employ a high-resolution helical technique with 0.625 mm thin sections with a field of view extending from the skull base at approximately the external auditory meatus superiorly to below the thoracic inlet near T1/T2 inferiorly (**Protocol Table**). The raw data is reconstructed in bone and soft tissue kernel for both 0.625 and 2.5 mm axial slices, with sagittal and coronal reconstructions also routinely provided.

The ABS of Spine: A Systematic Approach to Spine CT

A pragmatic approach to spine trauma cases requires a simple, reproducible heuristic. Although a more nuanced understanding of specific fracture patterns and mechanisms of injury (described below) will certainly improve diagnostic sensitivity, a simple albeit meticulous search pattern will usually identify the most important findings—and provides a solid foundation for any radiological read. The classic "ABCs" mnemonic for musculoskeletal trauma (**A**lignment, **B**ony integrity, **C**artilage, and **S**oft tissues) also can be readily applied to spine. We streamline this approach to **A-B-S**, since cartilage, ligaments, and disks can all be considered soft tissues and are all best assessed using soft tissue kernels and windows on CT.

Alignment A careful examination of alignment is absolutely critical to any spine evaluation, and its importance is often overlooked by less experienced radiologists. Traumatic malalignment may be the only indication of an unstable injury, placing the cord at risk. Always remember: YOU ARE THE GUARDIAN OF THE CORD. From the patient's perspective, nondisplaced hairline fractures matter far less than a traumatic malignment -- which could potentially result in life-altering tetraplegia. Thus, although identifying subtle fractures is important, finding them should never come at the expense of a careful assessment of spine alignment.

Spine alignment is usually best assessed on sagittal reformatted CT images. Vertebral bodies should appear stacked like "blocks"—one on top of one another. Several smooth lines should be mentally traced along the vertebral bodies and posterior elements on the midsagittal view, namely the anterior vertebral line, the posterior vertebral line, the spinolaminar line, and the posterior spinous line (Fig. 9.4); the integrity of these lines is suggestive of proper alignment. Inspection of the facet joints in sagittal view should reveal that they are layered over one another like "shingles on a roof." The distance between facet joints should be similar level-to-level and no more than 2 mm (Fig. 9.5) [34]. In the axial view, the facet joints should smoothly articulate with one another, giving the appearance of a "hamburger bun." Disk spaces should be relatively symmetric.

When interpreting a cervical spine CT, alignment near the craniocervical junction should be particularly scrutinized. In addition to assessing the general alignment of the upper spine using the principles above, the distances between the basion and dens (BDI, basion-dens interval), between the anterior C1 arch and the dens (ADI, atlantodental interval), and between the posterior extent of the axis and the basion (BAI, basion-

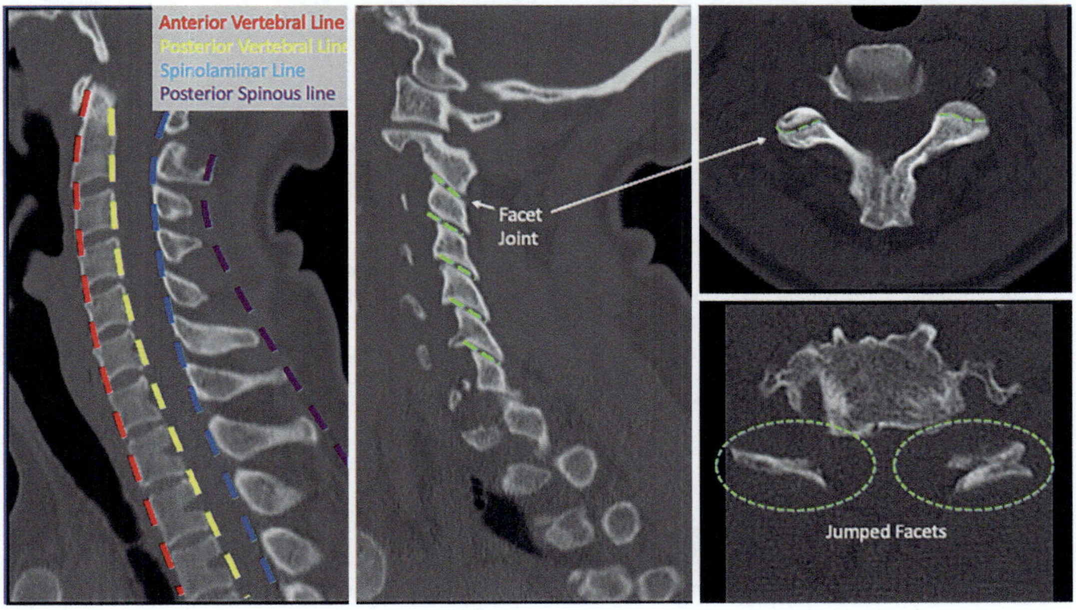

Fig. 9.4 Normal cervical spine alignment. Smooth curved lines can be traced along the vertebral bodies and posterior elements, and the facets should overlay like "shingles on a roof." Proper alignment is also shown on the axial view, with the appearance of "hamburger buns" to the hungry radiologist. An example of maligned facets is also shown on an axial CT slice (dotted circles)

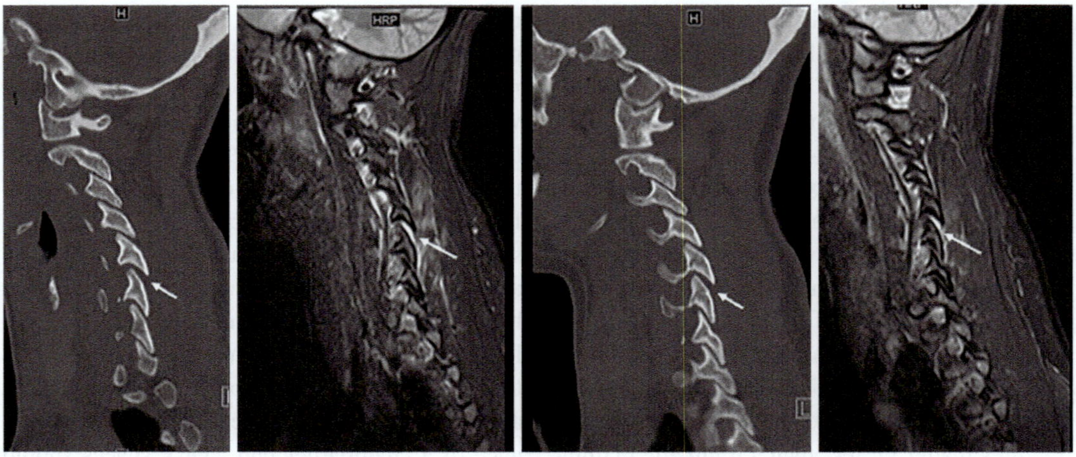

Fig. 9.5 Bilateral facet subluxation with MR correlates. Widening of several facet joints on either side of the neck can be seen on these sagittal reconstructions; the "shingles" appear to be falling off the roof. On the corresponding fluid sensitive MR, facet effusions and soft tissue edema surrounding the facet joints on both sides is readily apparent

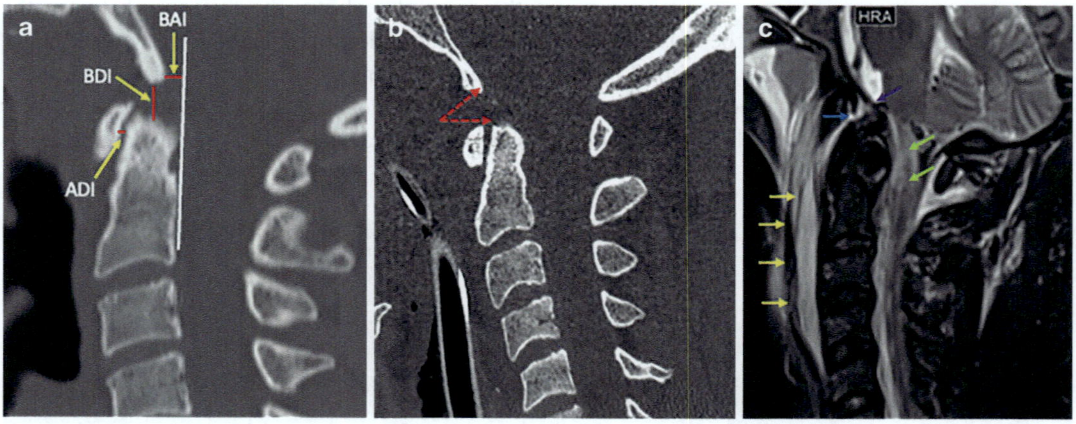

Fig. 9.6 Common measurements of the craniocervical junction. Panel **a** is a midsagittal CT reconstruction of the CCJ, in a normal adult patient. Measurements for the atlantodental interval (ADI), basion-dental interval (BDI), and basion-axial interval (BAI) shown in red. Panel **b** is a similar CT image from a 27-year-old involved in a high speed MVC. CT shows widening of the BDI (dotted arrows), as well as anterior displacement of the skull base relative to the spine. Both of these findings are indirect evidence of ligamentous injury. The corresponding fluid sensitive sagittal MRI sequence (STIR) is shown in Panel **c**. There is disruption of both the apical ligament (blue arrow) and the tectorial membrane (purple). Additional findings include cord edema (green) and prevertebral hematoma (yellow). Diagnosis? Craniocervical dissociation

axial interval) should be inspected (Fig. 9.6). The BDI is considered abnormal if >8.5 mm on CT, and the ADI is considered abnormal if >2 mm [35]; readers familiar with these measurements on radiography should note that these norms are smaller on CT. CT-derived BAI measurements are also not considered reliable. Additionally, it is important to remember that the ability to measure a simple distance is no replacement for a thoughtful analysis of all available data; for example, a borderline ADI in the setting of a questionable fracture or local soft tissue edema should raise concerns for the integrity of the transverse ligament—even if ADI is technically "normal."

If the radiologist observes an alignment abnormality, especially if disproportionate to other levels, then this region should be particularly scrutinized. This is especially true for younger patients where other causes of malalignment are rare. Assessment of traumatic malalignment in older patients can be more challenging given an increased prevalence of spondylosis, a common cause of nontraumatic listhesis. However, secondary findings should be present that suggest a nontraumatic cause (e.g., disproportionate facet arthrosis). Abnormally-widened interosseous distances near the CCJ may be indicative of ligamentous disruption near the skull base, and therefore MRI may be indicated for further evaluation.

Bony Integrity Assessment of bony integrity in the spine is similar to the assessment of the remainder of the musculoskeletal system. CT examination of the osseous structures is best assessed using bone kernels and windows. Acute fractures typically present as lucent lines with sharp margins, and cortical disruption and stepoffs are often visible. In contrast, chronic fractures, nutrient foramina, and other nontraumatic lesions will usually have smooth and often sclerotic margins (Fig. 9.7). Secondary findings of acuity (e.g., soft tissue edema) also will help lead to the appropriate diagnosis. When high-resolution MDCT data are available, the interpretating radiologist should take full advantage of the availabil-

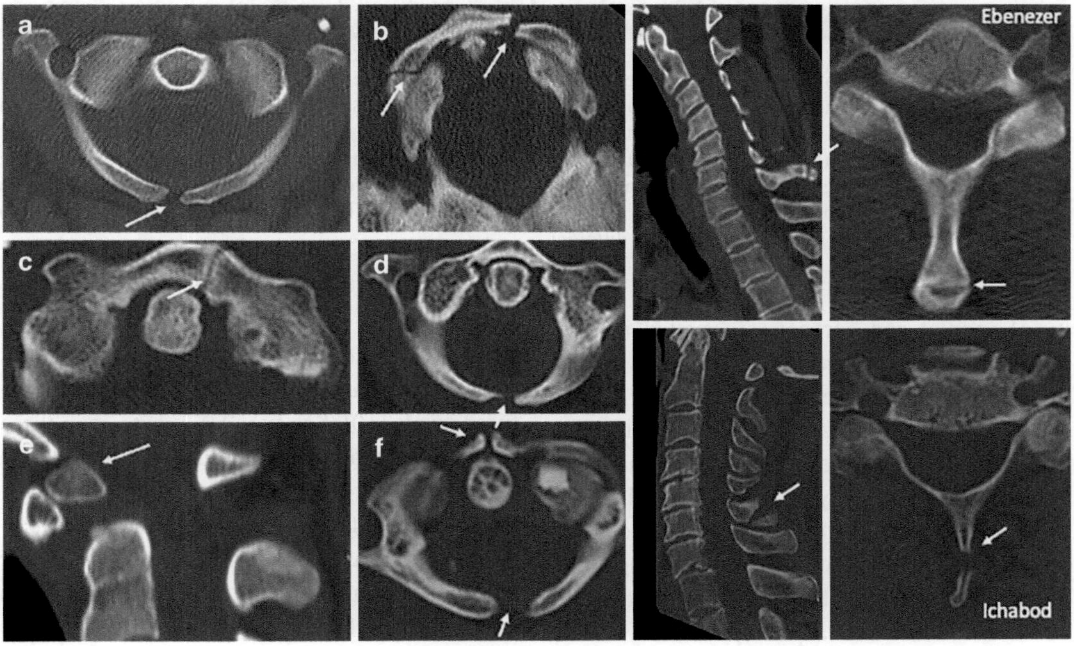

Fig. 9.7 Assessing bony integrity using basic MSK principles. On **left**, six CT images near the craniocervical junction from six trauma patients (Panels **a**–**f**). Which image shows an acute fracture? The correct answer is of course **b**, owed to the sharp margins of the lucencies and displaced fragments. Panel **a** represents congenital C1 rachischisis, a common developmental variant; note the smooth margins and midline location. Rachischisis can occur less commonly in the anterior arch (**c**), or both anterior and posterior arches (**f**), and need not be midline (although this is most common). Panel **e** represents an os odontoideum, which is occasionally misdiagnosed as a fracture fragment. However, note the smooth, sclerotic margins (and classic location). Panel **d** is a bit more challenging, but note lack of bone fragments and smooth margins. This represents an iatrogenic/surgical defect. On the **right** there are two patients (Ebenezer and Ichabod) of similar ages, both involved in motor vehicle collisions, and both with spinous process fractures (e.g., clay shoveler fracture). But which fracture is acute? Clearly, Ichabod's fracture is the acute one, given the lack of sclerosis of the fracture fragments. Clay shoveler's fractures often heal with nonunion, and incidental chronic spinous fractures will be seen in the trauma bay—if you look for them

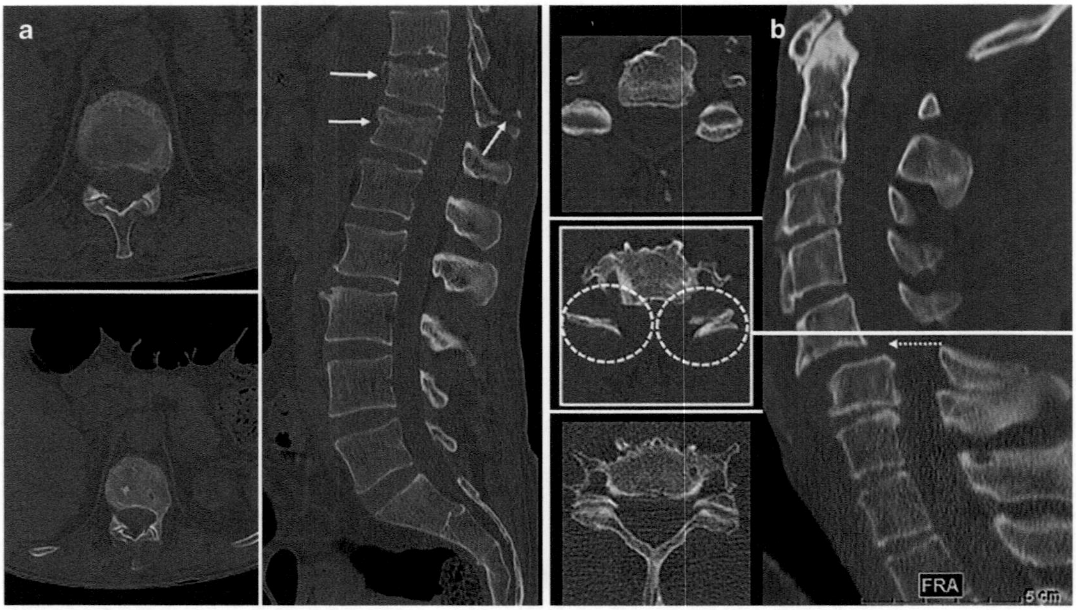

Fig. 9.8 The imperative of using multiplanar reformats, as demonstrated by two trauma patients. For the patient on the left (**a**), it is difficult to see fractures on the axial images, because they are in-plane to the slice. Yet they are readily apparent on the sagittal reformats, as is a distraction fracture of the T11 spinous process in this Chance-type injury. For Patient **b**, three axial images at different cervical levels are shown. Hopefully the abnormal level will be obvious, since we've already seen this image in Fig. 9.4 (middle axial slice, the "hamburger buns" are out of alignment). But how bad is the alignment? The true severity is much more apparent on sagittal, where there is borderline Grade III traumatic anterolisthesis (dotted line)

ity of sagittal and coronal reformatted images. Remember: subtle fractures may only be clearly visible in a single plane (Fig. 9.8). Vertebral body fractures should be assessed for posterior displacement into the spinal canal ("retropulsion"), and attempts to quantify the severity of spinal stenosis and associated soft tissue injury should be made. When the radiologist is assessing bony integrity in the cervical spine (using basic, tried-and-true musculoskeletal principles!), they should also pay particular attention to the integrity of the spinal canal walls and transverse foramina, as fractures in these areas may be indicative of cord or vertebral artery injury. In these cases, further workup using other imaging modalities (MRI, CTA, respectively) may be required.

Patients with inflammatory spondylarthritis or other causes of spine fusion (diffuse idiopathic skeletal hyperostosis or DISH, ossification of the posterior longitudinal ligament or OPLL, iatrogenic spine fusion) may have fractures in unusual locations due to altered biomechanics, particularly immediately superior and inferior to the fused levels [10]. See Fig. 9.9. Fractures in these patients also may be extraordinarily subtle due to osteoporosis or superimposed chronic findings. In these patients, the radiologist should be particularly cautious, taking extra effort to assess for small stepoffs and disruption of syndesmophytes or bridging osteophytes. Rarely, an acute spine fracture may present as a sclerotic line.

Soft Tissues Finally, every assessment of the spine should involve examination of its associated soft tissues (Fig. 9.10). While it is true that the spinal cord is often not well-visualized on CT, it would be an unfortunate mistake to assume that this means that it is not worth trying. On every cervical and thoracic spine case, an attempt should be made to identify the spinal cord and its position in the thecal sac. The epidural space should be examined for evidence of hematoma or

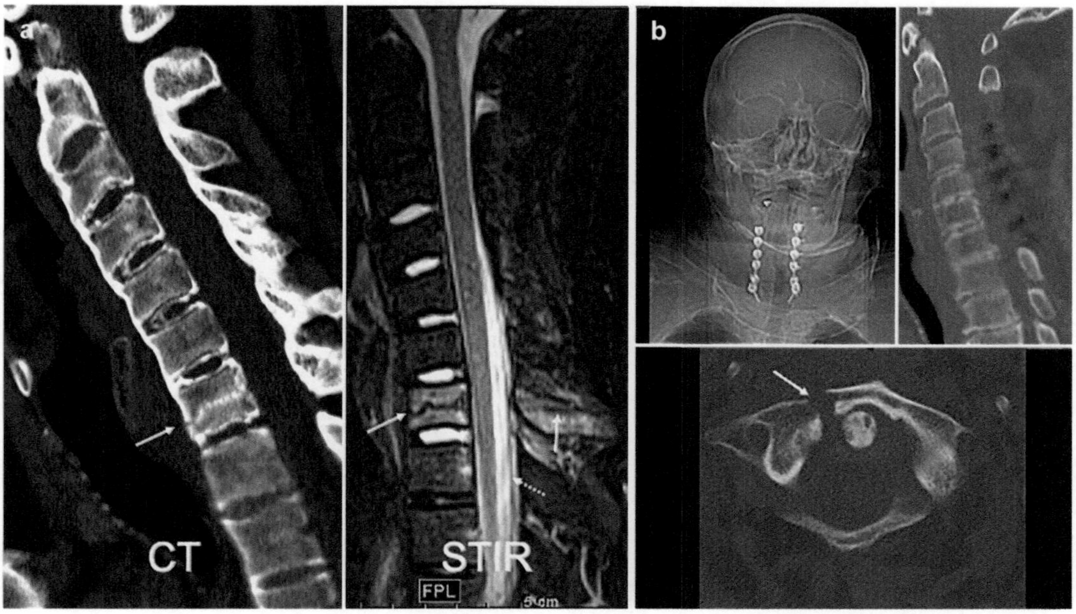

Fig. 9.9 Examples of unusual fracture patterns. Panel **a** shows CT and MR STIR sequences from a 43-year-old man with ankylosing spondylitis (AS) involved in a motor vehicle collision. Bridging syndesmophytes along the anterior spine, as well as fusion of the posterior elements confirm the diagnosis of AS. Note a C7 vertebral body fracture, presenting here as a sclerotic line rather than a lucency. The STIR shows the fracture, as well as surrounding marrow edema and a thin epidural hematoma (dotted arrow). MRI better also better demonstrates that the fracture extends into the posterior elements. Patients with AS will often present with unusual fracture patterns, including through vertebral bodies and disk spaces. Panel **b** shows CT from a 65-year-old man with a minor fall. Multi-level laminectomy and iatrogenic posterior fusion is evident. Altered biomechanics from the fusion likely contributed to the C1 anterior arch fracture (arrow)

other material in the extradural spinal canal. Although spodylotic disk disease is common and usually chronic, a traumatic disk extrusion should be considered if it appears disproportionate to the remainder of the spine, particularly if the patient has acute localizing symptoms to this level. If the patient has vertebral body fractures with retropulsed fragments, then the severity of spinal canal stenosis should be estimated.

The prevertebral soft tissues should also be carefully examined. The retropharyngeal space is often considered abnormal if wider than 7 mm in the sagittal plane, and the retrotracheal space abnormal if wider than ~2 mm (14 mm in children), although again a reassuring measurement is never a license to turn off your brain. Minor focal prevertebral swelling combined with focal malalignment or a questionable fracture should raise red flags—regardless of what the numbers are telling you.

Classic Mechanisms of Spine Injury

While adherence to a systemic heuristic like "**ABS** of Spine" will identify most acute trauma findings, a fundamental understanding of *classic mechanisms* of spine injury will also improve diagnostic sensitivity. Correctly identifying the mechanism of injury (either radiographically or based on the provided clinical history) will suggest a pattern of injury that will be particularly useful in complex cases where there are numerous potential findings to make [36]. However, the radiologist must always be aware that reality does not always follow these textbook patterns, and actual injuries will often be a mixture of multiple "classic" mechanisms.

Axial Loading Injuries Axial loading injuries result in the propagation of force along the long axis of the spine (e.g., diving injury), typically

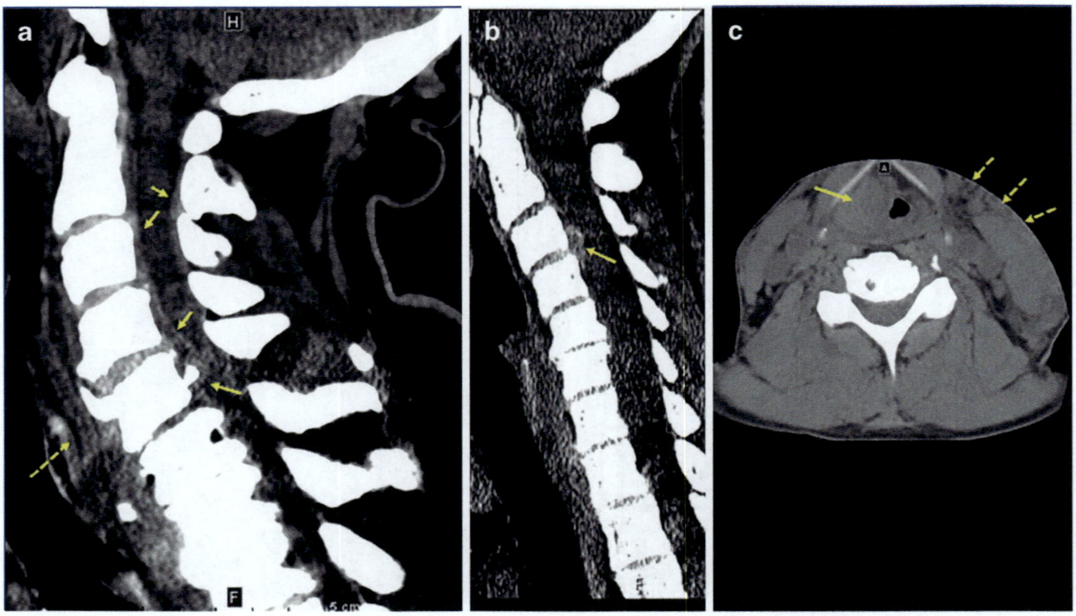

Fig. 9.10 Soft tissue injuries on CT. Panel **a** shows a moderate epidural hematoma (arrows) as well as prevertebral edema (dotted arrow), Panel **b** with a traumatic disk extrusion, and Panel **c** shows a laryngeal hematoma, airway displacement and narrowing, and associated soft tissue swelling (dotted arrow)

with the spine straight relative to the direction of force at the time of impact. Since the vertebral body and disk spaces are the principal structures bearing axial loads normally, they therefore often receive the brunt of the axial loading damage. This typically results in compression fractures. With severe axial loading, an intervertebral disk may herniate into the vertebral body, producing internal forces that cause the bone to explode from within. In the cervical spine, axial loading may also result in fractures to the occipital condyles, C1 ring, and lateral masses of C1. Significant axial loading usually results in unstable injuries.

Flexion Injuries Flexion injuries of the cervical spine are most associated with motor vehicle accidents, falls, and sports related injuries. Flexion of the spine beyond its intended range of motion can increase the compressive load on the anterior spinal column and "pull apart" the posterior elements from each other, resulting in increased tensile forces on the ligaments of the posterior column. Therefore, not surprisingly, extreme flexion results in compression fractures and traumatic narrowing of the disk space anteriorly and ligamentous injuries and dislocations posteriorly (Fig. 9.11). Teardrop fractures of the anterior vertebral bodies are usually flexion-related, and therefore in these cases the posterior elements should be inspected for alignment problems (e.g., widening of the intraspinous spaces). Flexion-distraction injuries can also result in fractures that extend throughout the posterior vertebral body endplates secondary to avulsions from the PLL, resulting in fracture fragments in the spinal canal.

Flexion also produces increased strain on the facet joints. In milder cases of flexion, the facet joints may be merely subluxed, with <50% overlap of the articular surfaces and mild widening of the joint space [11]. More extreme flexion can result dislocation of the facet joints. Facet dislocations are commonly classified into either *perched* (in which one facet is locked on top of the other) and *jumped* (in which the superior facet is dislocated anterior to the inferior facet), with the later indicative of a more serious injury (Fig. 9.12).

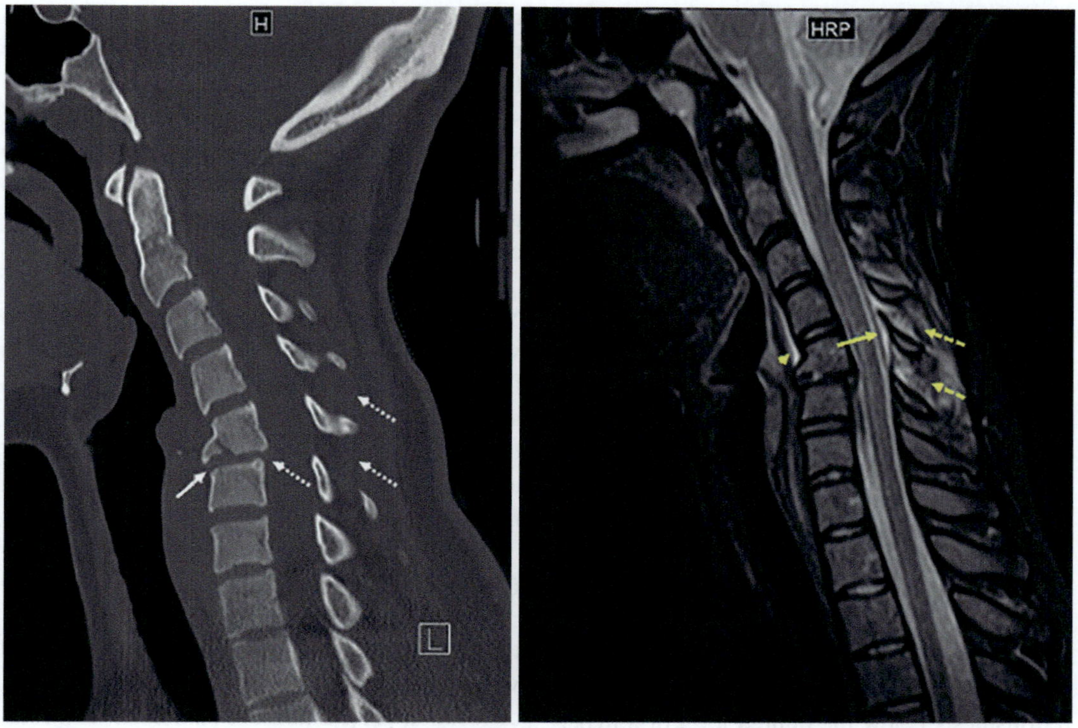

Fig. 9.11 Flexion pattern injury. 19-year-old woman who fell from approximately 10 feet. CT (left) shows a flexion teardrop fracture and subtle retrolisthesis at C5/C6 and widening of the intraspinous spaces (dotted arrows) disproportionate to the remainder of the spine. The corresponding MRI also shows findings of acute soft tissue injury, including a small prevertebral hematoma (arrowhead), small posterior epidural hematoma (arrow), and intraspinous edema suggestive of acute ligamentous injury (dotted arrows)

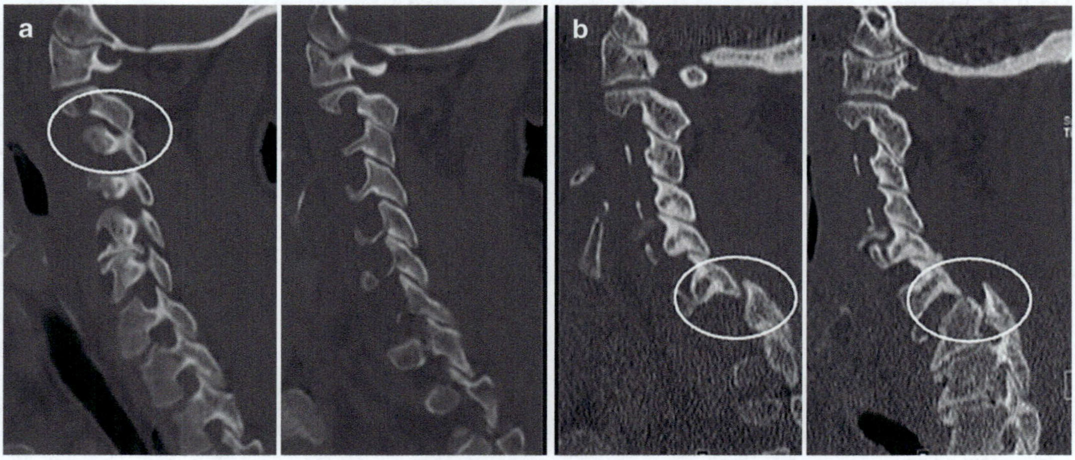

Fig. 9.12 Bilateral parasagittal CT from two patients with facet trauma. Patient **a** has unilateral perched facets, while Patient **b** has bilateral jumped facets

Jumped/perched facets are often associated with fractures of the facets themselves. The lack of ligamentous support in the posterior spine will often result in anterolisthesis of the vertebral body at the injured level.

Extension Injuries Extension pattern injuries are naturally somewhat of a mirror image to the flexion pattern (with a few notable exceptions). In hyperextension, compressive forces are focused on the posterior elements, while the anterior ligamentous complex undergoes tensile strain. This can result in compression fractures of the spinous processes or neural arches, as well as tearing of the anterior longitudinal ligament and associated malalignment (Fig. 9.13). Because the ALL may be more resistant to tensile forces than the vertebral bodies, avulsion fractures of the anterior vertebral body ("extension teardrop" fractures, see below) can be seen. Severe hyperextension can result in facet dislocation. Although retrolisthesis below the injured level of a hyperextension injury is common, traumatic anterolisthesis can also be observed on CT. This is because when the patient returns to a more neutral position following the hyperextension force, disruption of the anterior ligamentous complex can result in anterior slumping of the spine. While flexion injuries are common throughout the spine, serious extension injuries are usually only seen in the cervical spine. This is partly owed to differing morphology of the facet joints, which are more resistant to hyperextension in the thoracolumbar spine.

Shearing Injuries Shearing forces slide one vertebral body over another, and usually result in the horizontal distraction and dislocation, as well as avulsion fractures [36]. They most commonly occur in the thoracic and lumbar spine, and usually are associated with flexion injuries (i.e., a mixed pattern).

Rotational Injuries When traumatic forces are do not align with a single spine axis, then rotational injuries may occur. Rotation combined with hyperflexion may result in unilateral facet dislocation [11]. Extension combined with rotation may result in fractures of the articular pillar. Since the thoracic and lumbar spine are both designed to resist rotation [37], rotational injuries are most common in the cervical spine.

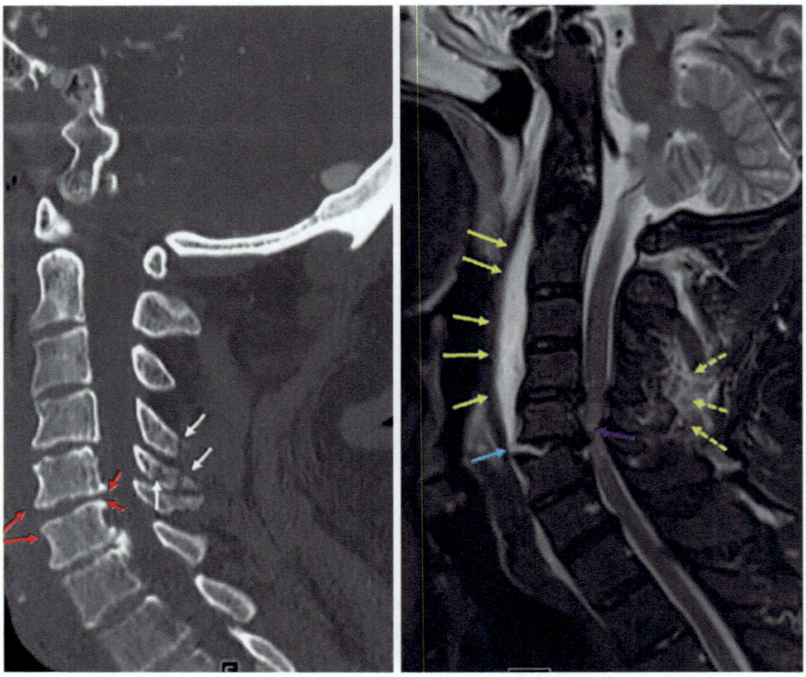

Fig. 9.13 Extension pattern injury. CT shows focally unequal widening of the anterior C5/C6 disk space relative to posterior (red arrows) associated with numerous acute fractures of the spinous processes (white arrows). MRI shows additional soft tissue findings including rupture of the ALL (blue), prevertebral edema (yellow), cord edema (purple), and intraspinous edema (dotted yellow)

Specific Fracture and Dislocation Patterns

The intersection between common mechanisms of injury and regional variations in spine anatomy results in several "classic" fracture and dislocation patterns, listed below. The perceptive reader will realize that many of these injuries can be inferred, based on the fundamental principles described in prior sections of this chapter. Nevertheless, a familiarity with these more specific patterns will further improve diagnostic accuracy, as well as potentially provide a greater understanding of more general concepts in spine trauma.

Craniocervical Dissociation (CCD) CCDs are commonly caused by high velocity motor vehicle collisions (Fig. 9.6c), are the cause of 6–8% of all motor vehicle deaths, and are usually fatal with a survivability of only about 1% [38]. They are often associated with high cord injuries and severe intracranial trauma. The diagnosis of CCD is rare on imaging, in part owed to an ascertainment bias (since these patients typically expire in the field). The short-term survivability of CCD is improving, however, and there likely will be a corresponding increase in patients with CCD who survive to imaging. Atlantooccipital dissociations can be divided into dislocations and subluxations. Subluxations are also severe injuries, but are more commonly survivable. CCDs can be particularly challenging to identify on CT, because there may be no fractures; subtle alignment abnormalities near the skull base may be the only diagnostic clue [39].

Occipital Condylar Fracture (C0) The occipital condyles articulate with the atlas and are functionally part of the upper spine. We often refer to the condyles as "C0," in order to remind trainees to evaluate them on every cervical spine case. Condylar fractures are rare, but are likely underdiagnosed [14]. They are usually associated with high impact axial loading injuries and are often found in combination with head and/or maxillofacial trauma, as well as fractures elsewhere in the spine (Fig. 9.14). Anderson and Montesanto described the most commonly-used classification system, with Type I representing comminuted fractures that do not involve foramen magnum, Type II represent occipital bone fractures that extend into the occipital condyle, and Type III representing avulsion injuries of the alar ligament [40].

Jefferson Fracture (C1) The Jefferson fracture is a burst fracture of the C1 vertebral body, typically caused by high energy traumas, and involves disruption and displacement of anterior and posterior arches resulting in an unstable fracture (Fig. 9.15). It can be caused by falls, car accidents, and sports related injuries (e.g., diving). On CT, disruption to the transverse ligament is suggested by widening of the ADI, and Jefferson fractures can be associated with fracture of the odontoid process [41]. An isolated nondisplaced fracture of the C1 arch is technically not a Jefferson fracture and may be stable, although MRI will nevertheless be required to assess ligamentous integrity.

Odontoid Fracture (C2) Fracture of the dens (i.e., odontoid process) is the most common unstable fracture near the CCJ, and accounts for approximately 60% of all C2 fractures [42]. Anderson described three types of odontoid fracture [40], and this a particularly useful classification system for the radiologist to know. Type I fractures are rare and represent a small avulsion fracture from the tip of the dens. Type II fractures are most common and extend through the body of the dens (Fig. 9.16a). Type III fractures occur near the base of the dens (Fig. 9.16c), with the fracture line extending through the C2 vertebral body. The distinction between Type II and III fractures is important, because while Type II fractures have a high rate of nonunion (~30–50%, Fig. 9.16b), Type III fractures often heal completely (Fig. 9.16d).

Hangman's Fracture (C2) The Hangman's fracture also occurs at C2 (Fig. 9.17) but is less common than an odontoid fracture. It involves bilateral pars interarticularis or posterior vertebral body fractures [43]. A Hangman's fracture

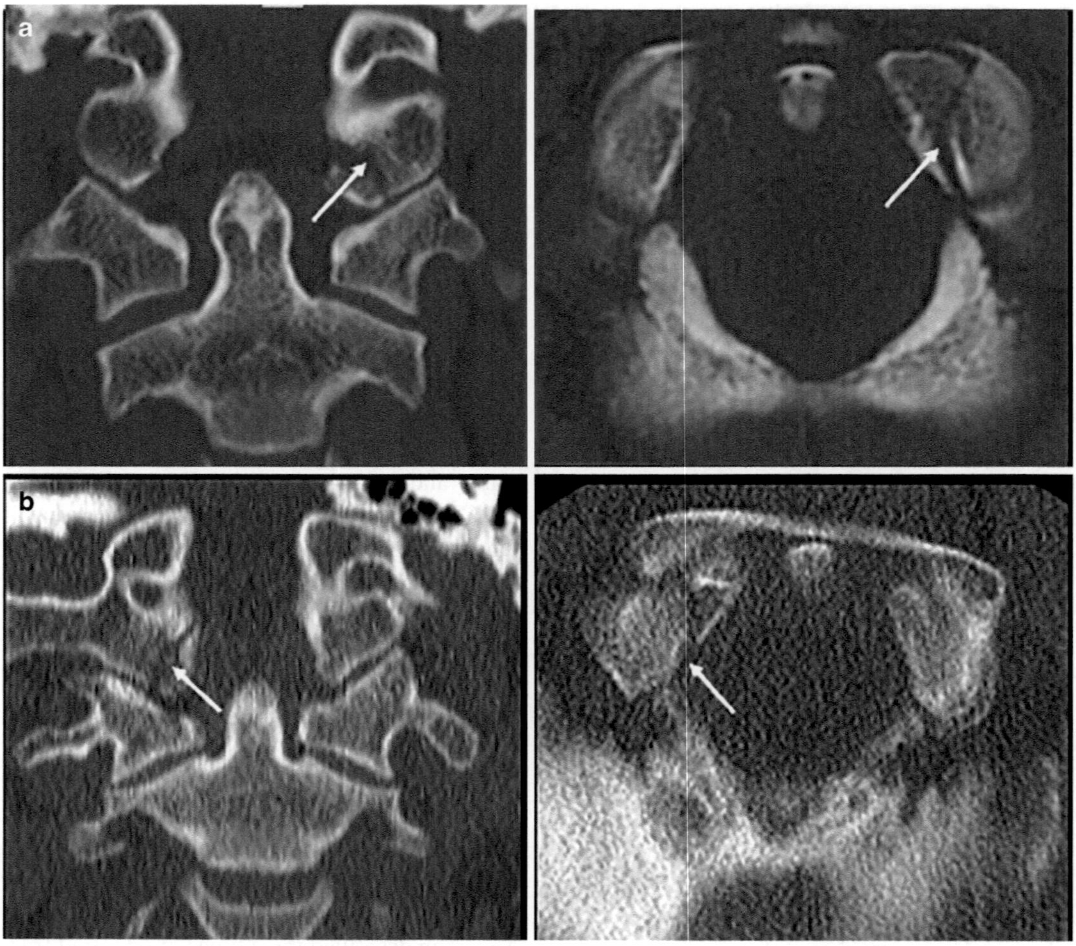

Fig. 9.14 Two patients with occipital condyle fractures, one with a left-sided fracture (**a**) and one on the right (**b**)

classically results in canal *autodecompression* and is therefore not usually associated with neurological symptoms. The Effendi classification divides Hangman's fractures into three types, based on an assessment of stability from 131 patients [44]. Type I fractures (<3 mm of translation of C2 on C3) are usually stable, while type II fractures (>3 mm translation) suggest disruption of the posterior longitudinal ligament—and therefore are unstable injuries. Type III are the most serious and are associated with bilateral facet dislocation.

Clay Shoveler's Fracture (C7-T1) Fracture of a spinous process near the cervicothoracic junction, most commonly C7. The eponym was originally used to describe an avulsion due to repetitive shear injury (e.g., from clay shoveling). However, in modern society, spinous process fractures more commonly involve direct trauma [45]. Examples of clay shoveler's fractures were shown in Fig. 9.7b. This is considered a stable fracture.

Burst Fractures Comminuted fractures of the vertebral body associated with extension through the superior and inferior endplates, typically associated with extreme axial loading (Fig. 9.18). Burst fractures result in displacement of fracture fragments including retropulsion into the spinal canal [3, 19, 34]. These fractures most commonly occur in the thoracic and lumbar spine (particularly near the thoracolumbar junction) but they also can be seen in the cervical spine. Burst frac-

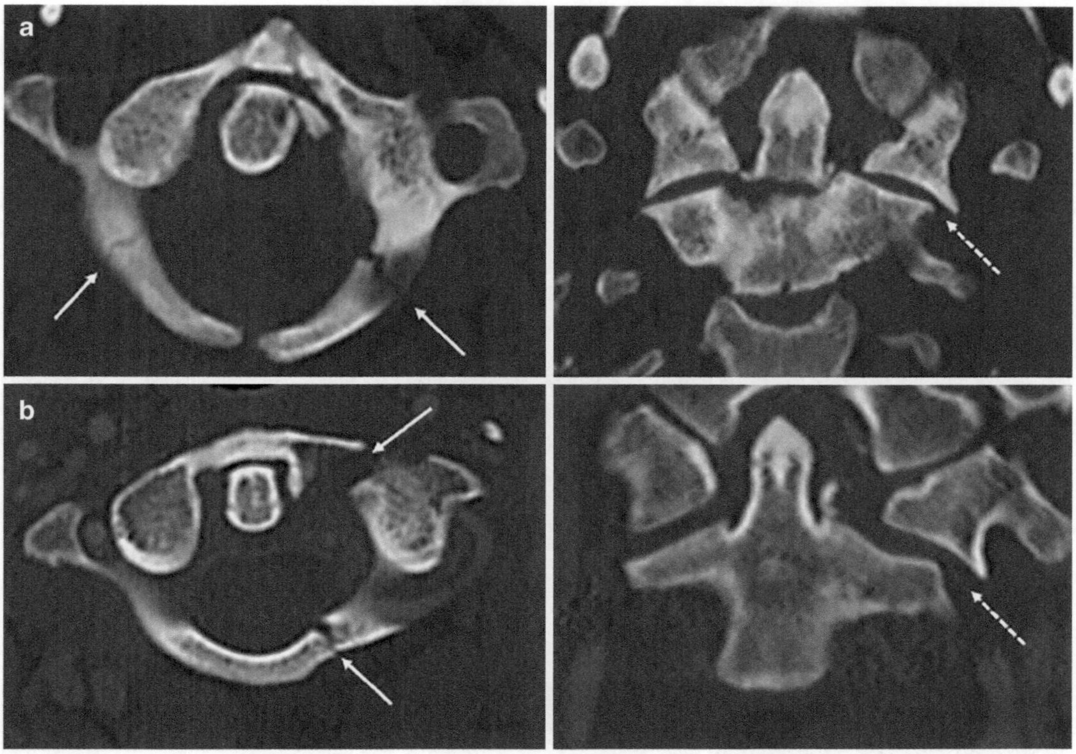

Fig. 9.15 Two patients with Jefferson fractures (solid lines). In both cases, there is displacement of the lateral masses relative to the dens (dotted line) which is indirect evidence of ligamentous disruption. Additional findings for Patient **a** include a type III odontoid fracture and congenital rachischisis of the posterior arch

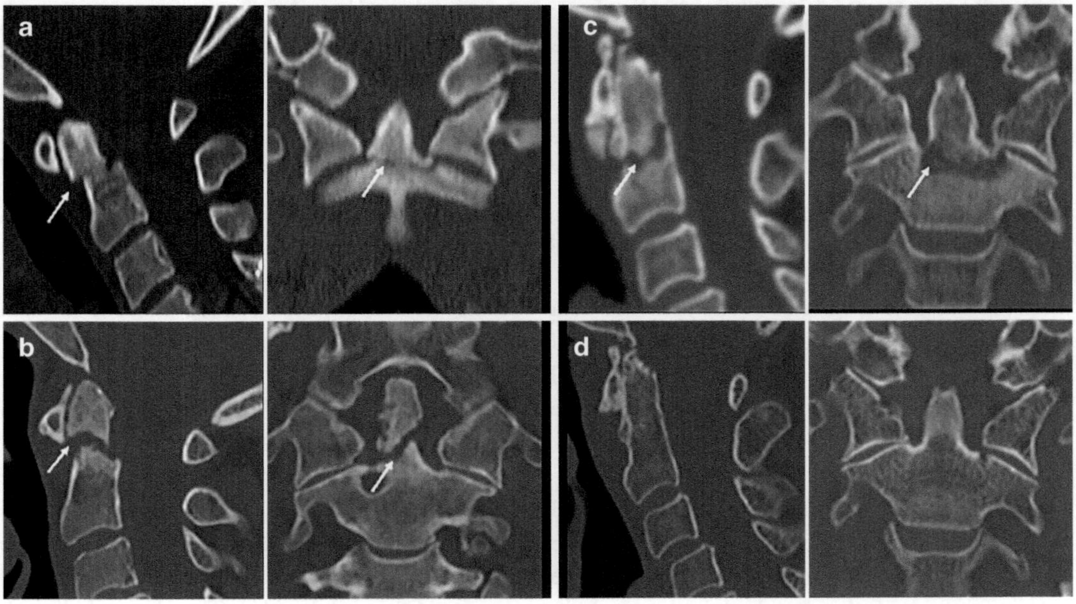

Fig. 9.16 Sagittal and coronal CT reformats of odontoid process fractures. Panel **a** has an acute type II fracture. Panel **b** is a different patient with a chronic type II fracture with nonunion. Panel **c** shows an acute type III odontoid fracture, with the fracture line through the body of the dens. Panel **d** is from the same patient approximately 2 months later; note significant interval healing

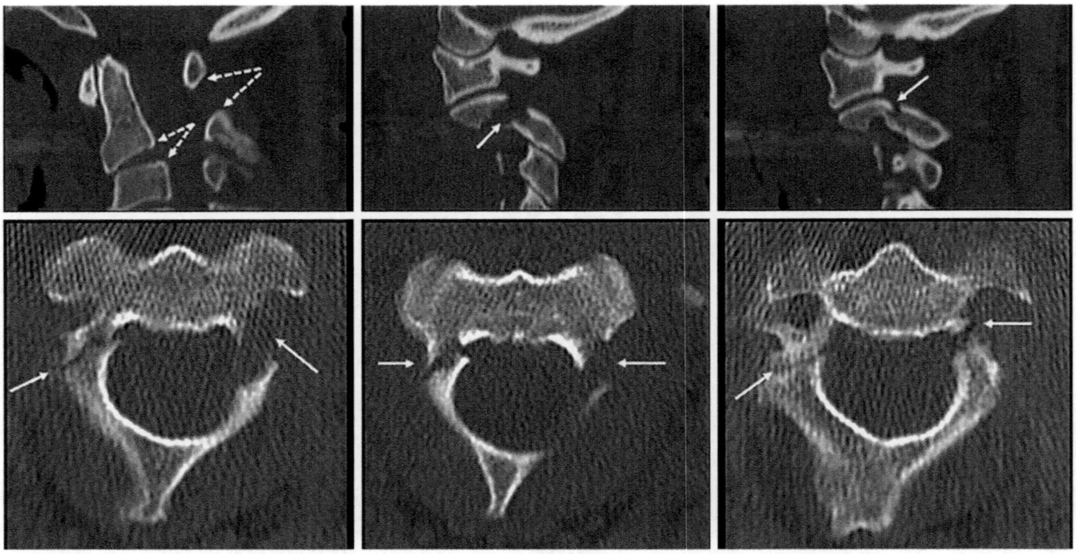

Fig. 9.17 Hangman's fracture (traumatic spondylolisthesis), with fractures labeled with solid arrows. Dotted arrows indicate areas of traumatic malignment

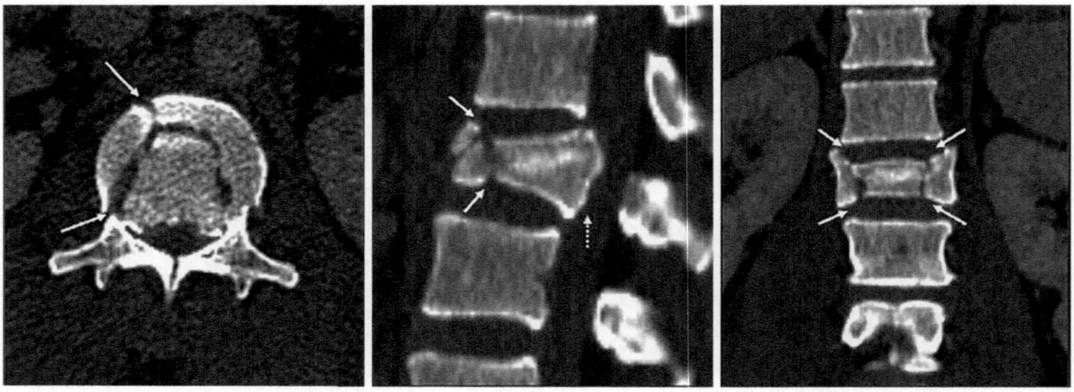

Fig. 9.18 Axial, sagittal, and coronal images from a trauma patient with a thoracolumbar burst fracture involving both endplates (arrows), with retropulsion into the spinal canal (dotted arrow)

tures are unstable (Fig. 9.19). The presence of a burst fracture is suggestive of high impact axial loading, and other fractures throughout the axial and appendicular skeleton (skull <->feet) are likely.

Flexion Teardrop Fracture Flexion-related fractures are relatively common throughout the spine (Fig. 9.11). Compressive forces on the anterior aspect of the vertebral body result in focal fractures, often resulting in a triangular fracture fragment (i.e., the "teardrop"). Less severe flexion injuries can be associated with nondisplaced fractures.

Extension Teardrop Fracture The extension teardrop fracture is far less common than its flexion counterpart. It represents an avulsion fracture of an anterior vertebral body corner owed to the higher tensile strength of the ALL relative to the adjacent bone (Fig. 9.20). They most commonly occur at C2 in adults [46]. The classic hallmark of an extension teardrop is that the length of the fracture fragment is longer than its width.

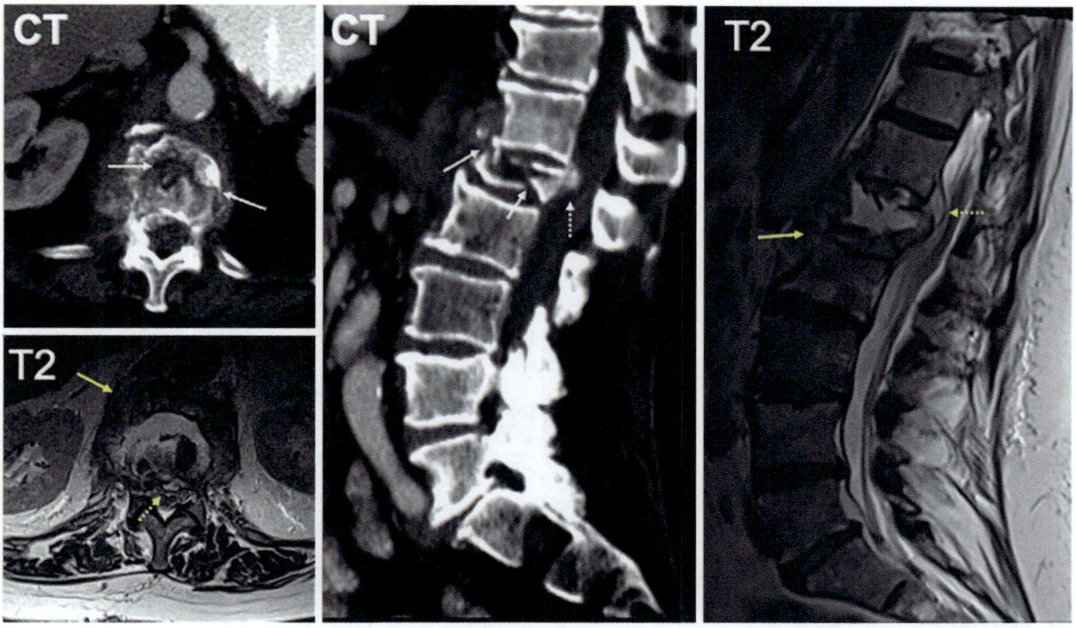

Fig. 9.19 L1 Burst fracture on abdominal CT, with MR correlates. Markedly comminuted vertebral body fracture (white arrows) and retropulsion (white dotted) are readily apparent on CT and there is suggestion of both prevertebral and epidural hematomas. T2-weighted MR sequences show the soft tissue findings to better effect, as well as marked marrow edema in the fractured vertebral body

Chance Fractures The Chance fracture is a hyperflexion injury of the thoracolumbar spine [47], first described following the widespread use of lap seat belts in the 1950s. It is characterized by fracture of the vertebral body extending into the posterior elements, usually associated with distraction of the posterior fracture fragments (Fig. 9.21). It has been estimated that approximately 80% of Chance-type fractures occur near the thoracolumbar junction, although they have been reported from T4-L5 [47]. They are unstable 2–3 column injuries and are often associated with serious intraabdominal trauma [48].

Special Considerations for Thoracic and Lumbar Trauma

There are over 160,000 thoracolumbar spine fractures in the USA annually [47]. Given that the thoracolumbar spine is intimately associated with the chest and abdomen, evidence of trauma in these regions usually will precipitate a wider field of view CT—in order to assess for associated visceral injuries. Therefore, dedicated trauma CT of the thoracic or lumbar spine is far less common than it is for the cervical spine. If necessary, high-resolution reconstructions of the thoracic and lumbar spine can be generated from MDCT chest, abdomen, and pelvis raw data [49, 50], and this practice is far more common at our institution than dedicated thoracolumbar imaging. However, in most trauma patients, the spine will be assessed as a component of thoracic and abdominal trauma CT, and even targeted spine reconstructions will not be necessary.

CT is clearly superior to radiography for detecting thoracolumbar fractures, with a sensitivity nearing 95–100% [20, 51]. Although spine injuries are in general more common in the cervical spine, fractures are most common in the lumbar followed by the thoracic spine [52], with an incidence of about 4–7% as compared to 3–4% in the cervical spine [53, 54]. Given transitional biomechanics, fractures are particularly common near the thoracolumbar junction [20]. Although

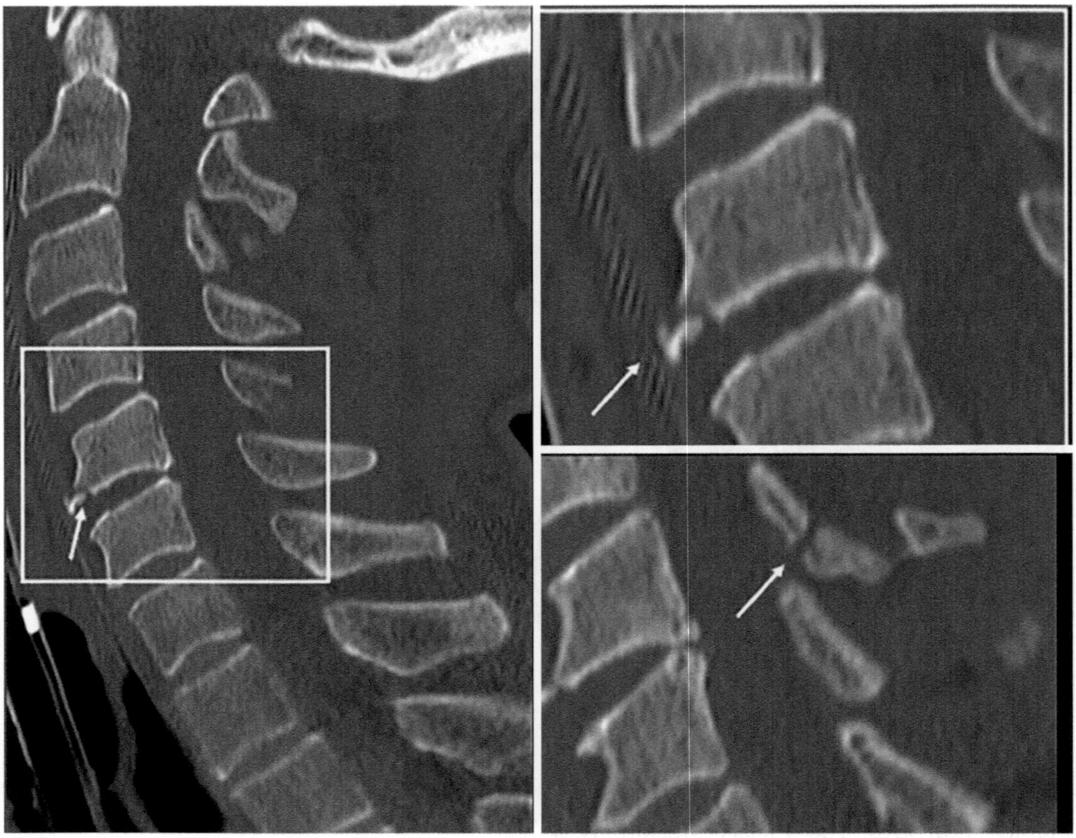

Fig. 9.20 Extension teardrop fracture in a bicyclist struck by a motor vehicle. A mildly displaced fracture of the C6 vertebral body is shown on left, with a magnified view in the white box (top right). Although flexion injuries are more common, the morphology of this fracture (fracture length longer than width) is suggestive of avulsion from hyperextension. An additional fracture in the posterior elements (bottom right) also suggests extension pattern

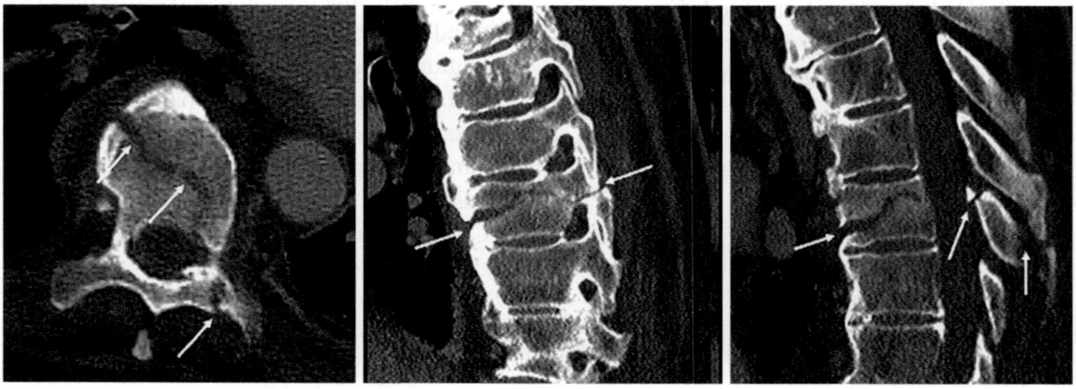

Fig. 9.21 Chance-type fracture in the thoracic spine. Patient has large bridging osteophytes with relative preservation of disk height, likely owed to DISH. Acute findings include transverse fracture through the vertebral body, osteophytes, and posterior elements (arrows)

thoracolumbar fractures are slightly more common, patterns of injury are essentially a subset of those seen in the cervical spine (in other words, there are slightly more thoracolumbar fractures, but fewer "kinds" of fractures as compared to the cervical spine). Approximately half of thoracolumbar fractures are anterior vertebral body wedge deformities [55]. As described above, severe hyperflexion may result in chance-pattern injuries. Lateral vertebral body fractures also occur and are common in patients with osteoporosis. Transverse process fractures are common in the lumbar spine, and nearly half (46.6%) have associated visceral injuries [56].

Role of Other Imaging Modalities in Management of Spine Trauma

MRI is an essential tool in the evaluation of trauma patients, although its precise role remains controversial [26]. MRI undoubtedly provides far superior contrast resolution (i.e., soft tissue) compared to CT, and is therefore the gold standard for evaluating the spinal cord, ligaments, disks, and epidural spaces [57]. MRI clearly plays a critical role in patients with established spine injuries, providing both important prognostic information and facilitating treatment planning (Fig. 9.22). However, in the setting of a non-focal neurological exam and a negative CT, the added benefit of MRI remains unclear. Although several societal guidelines recommend cervical MRI in CT-negative trauma patients that are either obtunded or intubated, others advise against this practice [58]. Acute ligamentous injuries in the absence of fractures are rare, and CT has a high sensitivity for fractures [59]. In a meta-analysis of 13,327 patients with blunt trauma, Panczykowski et al. found that CT alone is sufficient to clear the spine even in in obtunded or intubated patients [60]. Given that a properly interpreted MDCT has a ~ 98.9% NPV for ligamentous injury and a ~ 100% NPV for unstable cervical spine injuries [61], it should come as no surprise that the added value of MRI in the setting of a negative CT is marginal. Nevertheless, there will be a small percentage of patients that will benefit from the added sensitivity of CT + MRI, which has been estimated at about 0.7% of obtunded/comatose trauma patients by meta-analysis [58]. Whether the added cost and increased morbidity from prolonged cervical precautions in other patients justifies a benefit to a small minority remains an open question.

Similarly, the exact role of cross-sectional angiography in trauma is somewhat controversial. The American College of Radiology (ACR) recommends against the routine use of CT angiography (CTA) as part of trauma workup [26], but notes that either CTA or Magnetic Resonance Angiography (MRA) is "usually appropriate" in the setting of positive spine findings on CT (or a high clinical suspicion for acute vascular injury). Recommendations from other medical societies vary, but many propose more relaxed thresholds (for example, neck CTA for *any* patient with suspicion of a high velocity trauma anywhere from the neck to the pelvis ([62]. Given their intimate association with the cervical spine, the vertebral arteries are particularly prone to traumatic dissections and pseudoaneurysms (Fig. 9.22). Approximately 0.5% of all trauma patients will have a vertebral artery injury, and only 70% of these will have an associated cervical spine fracture [63]. Since CTA data can be rapidly acquired as part of a CT pan-scan [64], there certainly is temptation to include CTA as part of routine screening, particularly if the patient is receiving contrast for other reasons. However, CTAs are extremely complicated studies that often include more than 2000 images and result in a significant resource burden on interpreting radiologists and also have a relatively high rate of false positives that has been estimated as high as >45% [65]. Similar to spine MRI, in the absence of a positive CT, the added benefit of cross-sectional angiography appears marginal, although the precise role of CTA in trauma patients is likely to evolve in the near future.

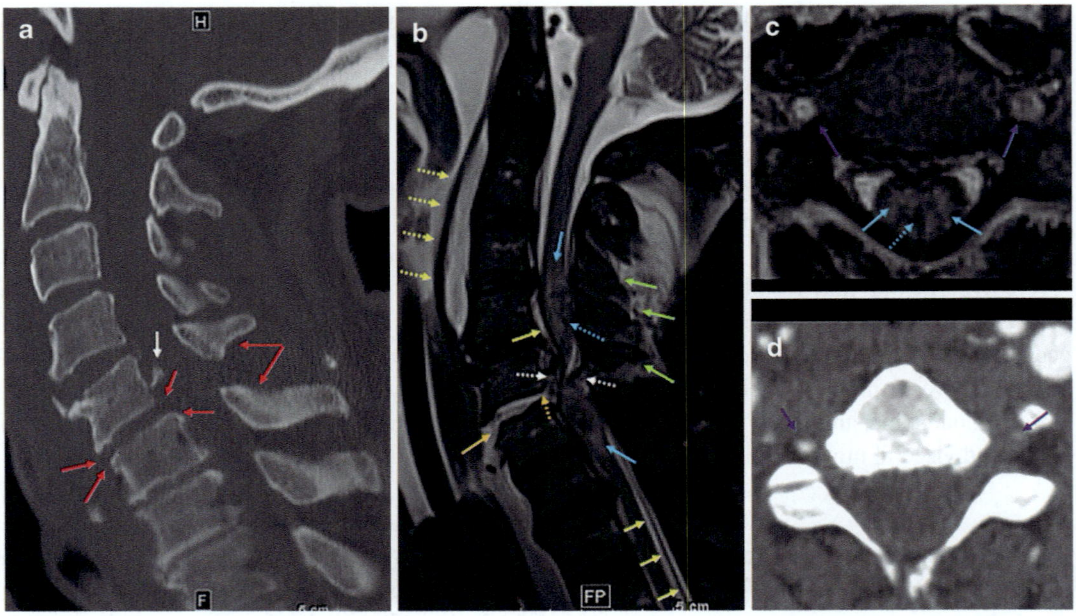

Fig. 9.22 The complementary role of imaging modalities in the assessment of trauma, and end-of-chapter "Final Exam." Panel **a** shows sagittal CT reformats from a patient who fell down a staircase. Focal **A**lignment abnormalities at C5/C6 are readily apparent (red), as is a small triangular **B**one fragment in the spinal canal (white) suggestive of PLL avulsion injury. Epidural and prevertebral hematoma are visible on **S**oft tissue windows (Fig. 9.10**a**). Overall *pattern of findings* suggests severe flexion-distraction injury, warranting further characterization with MRI. Sagittal STIR from MRI (Panels **b**, **c**) visualizes the epidural (yellow) and prevertebral (dotted yellow) hematomas to better effect. It also provides several additional soft tissue findings, including disruption of the ALL (orange), disk rupture (dotted orange), severe cord compression (dotted white), multi-segment cord edema (blue), intramedullary hemorrhage (dotted blue, a poor prognostic sign), and intraspinous and paraspinal edema (green). There also are absent flow voids in vertebral arteries (Panel **c**) concerning for bilateral dissection (purple). CTA performed in panel **d** confirms bilateral dissections, with irregularity and eventually complete absence of opacification of the vertebral arteries bilaterally

Conclusion

MDCT has become the indispensable diagnostic tool in the management of spine trauma. The decision to image should be based on evidence-based clinical tools which have high NPV. Spine CT studies should be read systematically, with careful attention to alignment, liberal use of multiplanar reformats, a fundamental understanding of mechanisms of injury, and particular attention to the CCJ.

Protocol

Protocol Name	Cervical Spine CT (revo_ct_22bc.50)
Indication	Spine Trauma
Protocol Designed for (scanner model)	GE Revolution CT
First Series	
Oral contrast	None
IV Contrast	None
Tube Settings	
kV	120
mA	251 mA
Dose modulation	Yes
Tube Rotation time (s)	0.7
Table Speed (mm/s)	56.25
Pitch Factor:	0.984375
Slice collimation	0.625
Reconstructed slice thickness	2.5 mm 0.625 mm (thins)
Reconstruction kernel	GE: Standard (at both 2.5 mm and 0.625 mm) GE: Boneplus (at both 2.5 mm and 0.625 mm)

Breath hold	No
Window settings	Window Center: 250 Window Width: 2000
Post processing	2.5 mm Sagittal Reformats (Standard kernel) 2 mm Sagittal Reformats (Boneplus kernel) 2 mm Coronal Reformats (Boneplus kernel)
Other	
Typical dose	
CTDIvol	19 mGy
DLP	480 mGy*cm

Acknowledgments This chapter is based on a lecture that I originally prepared for UPenn Radiology's ED Readiness Course. I would like to thank Drs. Alex Mamourian and Andrew McClelland for providing many of the conceptual seeds for this lecture, as well as to generations of UPenn residents for their valuable feedback over the years. I would also like to thank Daryn Youngblood for performing literature searches as part of preparation for this chapter.

References

1. Kumar R, Lim J, Mekary RA, Rattani A, Dewan MC, Sharif SY, Osorio-Fonseca E, Park KB. Traumatic spinal injury: global epidemiology and worldwide volume. World Neurosurg. 2018;113:e345–63.
2. Lee BB, Cripps RA, Fitzharris M, Wing PC. The global map for traumatic spinal cord injury epidemiology: update 2011, global incidence rate. Spinal Cord. 2014;52(2):110–6.
3. Guarnieri G, Izzo R, Muto M. The role of emergency radiology in spinal trauma. Br J Radiol. 2016;89(1061):20150833.
4. Sekhon LHS, Fehlings MG. Epidemiology, demographics, and pathophysiology of acute spinal cord injury. Spine (Phila Pa 1976). 2001;26:S2–S12.
5. Goldberg W, Mueller C, Panacek E, Tigges S, Hoffman JR, Mower WR. Distribution and patterns of blunt traumatic cervical spine injury. Ann Emerg Med. 2001;38(1):17–21.
6. Milby AH, Halpern CH, Guo W, Stein SC. Prevalence of cervical spinal injury in trauma. Neurosurg Focus. 2008;25(5):1–9.
7. Cairns C, Kang C. National Hospital Ambulatory Medical Care Survey: 2020 Emergency Department Summary Tables. 2022 Dec.
8. Riascos R, Bonfante E, Cotes C, Guirgui M, Hakimelahi R, West C. Imaging of atlanto-occipital and atlantoaxial traumatic injuries: what the radiologist needs to know. Radiographics. 2015;35(7): 2121–34.
9. Rosse C, Gaddum-Rosse P. Hollingshead's textbook of anatomy. 5th ed. Philadelphia, PA: Lippincott-Raven Publishers; 1997.
10. Shah NG, Keraliya A, Nunez DB, Schoenfeld A, Harris MB, Bono CM, et al. Injuries to the rigid spine: what the spine surgeon wants to know. Radiographics. 2019;39(2):449–66.
11. Izzo R, Popolizio T, Balzano RF, Pennelli AM, Simeone A, Muto M. Imaging of cervical spine traumas. Eur J Radiol. Elsevier Ireland Ltd. 2019;117:75–88.
12. Fassett DR, Dailey AT, Vaccaro AR. Vertebral artery injuries associated with cervical spine injuries: a review of the literature. J. Spinal Disord Tech. 2008;21(4):252–8.
13. Werndle MC, Myers J, Mortimer A. Missed cervical spine injuries: aim for the top. Emerg Radiol. 2022;29(3):491–7.
14. Leone A, Cerase A, Colosimo C, Lauro L, Puca A, Marano P. Occipital condylar fractures: a review. Radiology. 2000;216(3):635–44.
15. Bleys RLAW. Introduction anatomy of the cervical spine. In: Vialle LR, editor. AOSpine masters series, volume 5: cervical spine trauma. Georg Thieme Verlag; 2015. Aug 5.
16. de Almeida Prado RM, de Almeida Prado JL, Yamada AF, Correa Fernandes AR, Puertas EB, Ueta RH, Guimarães JB. Spine trauma: radiological approach and new concepts. Skelet Radiol. 2021;50:1065–79.
17. Liebsch C, Wilke HJ. Which traumatic spinal injury creates which degree of instability? A systematic quantitative review. Spine J. 2022;22(1):136–56.
18. Denis F. The three column spine and its significance in the classification of acute thoracolumbar spinal injuries. Spine. 1983;8(8):817–31.
19. Khurana B, Sheehan SE, Sodickson A, Bono CM, Harris MB. Traumatic thoracolumbar spine injuries: what the spine surgeon wants to know. Radiographics. 2013;33(7):2031–46.
20. Izzo R, Al Qassab S, Popolizio T, Balzano RF, Perri M, Cassar-Pullicino V, Guglielmi G. Imaging of thoracolumbar spine traumas. Eur J Radiol. 2022;1:110343.
21. Stiell IG, Wells GA, Vandemheen KL, Clement CM, Lesiuk H, De Maio VJ, Laupacis A, Schull M, McKnight RD, Verbeek R, Brison R. The Canadian C-spine rule for radiography in alert and stable trauma patients. JAMA. 2001;286(15):1841–8.
22. Hoffman JR, Mower WR, Wolfson AB, Todd KH, Zucker MI. Validity of a set of clinical criteria to rule out injury to the cervical spine in patients with blunt trauma. N Engl J Med. 2000;343(2):94–9.
23. Holmes JF, Akkinepalli R. Computed tomography versus plain radiography to screen for cervical spine injury: a meta-analysis. J Trauma Injury, Infection and Critical Care. 2005;58:902–5.
24. Adelgais KM, Grossman DC, Langer SG, Mann FA. Use of helical computed tomography for imaging the pediatric cervical spine. Acad Emerg Med. 2004;11(3):228–36.

25. McAllister AS, Nagaraj U, Radhakrishnan R. Emergent imaging of pediatric cervical spine trauma. Radiographics. 2019;39(4):1126–42.
26. Beckmann NM, West OC, Nunez D, Kirsch CFE, Aulino JM, Broder JS, et al. ACR appropriateness criteria ® suspected spine trauma. J Am Coll Radiol. 2019;16(5):S264–85.
27. Khurana B, Keraliya A, Velmahos G, Maung AA, Bono CM, Harris MB. Clinical significance of "positive" cervical spine MRI findings following a negative CT. Emerg Radiol. 2022;29(2):307–16.
28. Alessandrino F, Bono CM, Potter CA, Harris MB, Sodickson AD, Khurana B. Spectrum of diagnostic errors in cervical spine trauma imaging and their clinical significance. Emerg Radiol. 2019;26(4):409–16.
29. Fisher BM, Cowles S, Matulich JR, Evanson BG, Vega D, Dissanaike S. Is magnetic resonance imaging in addition to a computed tomographic scan necessary to identify clinically significant cervical spine injuries in obtunded blunt trauma patients? Am J Surg. 2013;206(6):987–94.
30. Hsu JM, Joseph T, Ellis AM. Thoracolumbar fracture in blunt trauma patients: guidelines for diagnosis and imaging. Injury. 2003;34(6):426–33.
31. Holmes JF, Panacek EA, Miller PQ, Lapidis AD, Mower WR. Prospective evaluation of criteria for obtaining thoracolumbar radiographs in trauma patients. J Emerg Med. 2003;24(1):1–7.
32. Inaba K, Nosanov L, Menaker J, Bosarge P, Williams L, Turay D, et al. Prospective derivation of a clinical decision rule for thoracolumbar spine evaluation after blunt trauma: an American Association for the Surgery of Trauma Multi-Institutional Trials Group Study. J Trauma Acute Care Surg. Lippincott Williams and Wilkins. 2015:459–67.
33. Wintermark M, Mouhsine E, Theumann N, Mordasini P, van Melle G, Leyvraz PF, et al. Thoracolumbar spine fractures in patients who have sustained severe trauma: depiction with multi-detector row CT. Radiology. 2003;227(3):681–9.
34. Vaccaro AR, Hulbert RJ, Patel AA, Fisher C, Dvorak M, Lehman RA Jr, Anderson P, Harrop J, Oner FC, Arnold P, Fehlings M. The subaxial cervical spine injury classification system: a novel approach to recognize the importance of morphology, neurology, and integrity of the disco-ligamentous complex. Spine. 2007;32(21):2365–74.
35. Rojas CA, Bertozzi JC, Martinez CR, Whitlow J. Reassessment of the craniocervical junction: normal values on CT. Am J Neuroradiol. 2007;28(9):1819–23.
36. Daffner RH, Deeb ZL, Rothfus WE. "Fingerprints" of vertebral trauma—a unifying concept based on mechanisms. Skelet Radiol. 1986;15:518–25.
37. Zhang S, Wadhwa R, Haydel J, Toms J, Johnson K, Guthikonda B. Spine and spinal cord trauma. Diagnosis and management. Neurol Clin. 2013;31:183–206.
38. Bellabarba C, Mirza SK, West GA, Mann FA, Dailey AT, Newell DW, et al. Diagnosis and treatment of craniocervical dislocation in a series of 17 consecutive survivors during an 8-year period. J Neurosurg Spine. 2006;4(6):429–40.
39. Chang W, Alexander MT, Mirvis SE. Diagnostic determinants of craniocervical distraction injury in adults. Am J Roentgenol. 2009;192(1):52–8.
40. Anderson LD, D'Alonzo RT. Fractures of the odontoid process of the axis. JBJS. 1974;56(8):1663–74.
41. Esses S, Langer F, Gross A. Fracture of the atlas associated with fracture of the odontoid process. Injury. 1981;12(4):310–2.
42. Greene KA, Dickman CA, Marciano FF, Drabier JB, Hadley MN, Sonntag VK. Acute axis fractures: analysis of management and outcome in 340 consecutive cases. Spine. 1997;22(16):1843–52.
43. Li XF, Dai LY, Lu H, Chen XD. A systematic review of the management of hangman's fractures. Eur Spine J. 2006;15:257–69.
44. Effendi B, Roy D, Cornish B, Dussault RG, Laurin CA. Fractures of the ring of the axis. A classification based on the analysis of 131 cases. J Bone Joint Surg Br. 1981;63(3):319–27.
45. Posthuma de Boer J, van Wulfften Palthe AFY, Stadhouder A, Bloemers FW. The clay Shoveler's fracture: a case report and review of the literature. J Emerg Med. 2016;51(3):292–7.
46. Dreizin D, Letzing M, Sliker CW, Chokshi FH, Bodanapally U, Mirvis SE, et al. Multidetector CT of blunt cervical spine trauma in adults. Radiographics. 2014;34(7):1842–65.
47. Bernstein MP, Mirvis SE, Shanmuganathan K. Chance-type fractures of the thoracolumbar spine: imaging analysis in 53 patients. Am J Roentgenol. 2006;187(4):859–68.
48. Tyroch AH, Mcguire EL, McLean SF, Kozar RA, Gates KA, Kaups KL, et al. The association between chance fractures and intra-abdominal injuries revisited: a multicenter review. Am Surg. 2005;71(5):434–8.
49. Kim S, Yoon CS, Ryu JA, Lee S, Park YS, Kim SS, Lee YH, Suh JS. A comparison of the diagnostic performances of visceral organ-targeted versus spine-targeted protocols for the evaluation of spinal fractures using sixteen-channel multidetector row computed tomography: is additional spine-targeted computed tomography necessary to evaluate thoracolumbar spinal fractures in blunt trauma victims? J Trauma Acute Care Surg. 2010;69(2):437–46.
50. Lee JY, Vaccaro AR, Lim MR, Öner FC, Hulbert RJ, Hedlund R, Fehlings MG, Arnold P, Harrop J, Bono CM, Anderson PA. Thoracolumbar injury classification and severity score: a new paradigm for the treatment of thoracolumbar spine trauma. J Orthop Sci. 2005;10:671–5.
51. Karul M, Bannas P, Schoennagel BP, Hoffmann A, Wedegaertner U, Adam G, et al. Fractures of the thoracic spine in patients with minor trauma: comparison of diagnostic accuracy and dose of biplane radiography and MDCT. Eur J Radiol. 2013;82(8):1273–7.

52. Luna LM, de Jesús Altamirano Mendoza R, Oropeza YM. Epidemiology of spine trauma in patients with polytrauma. Coluna/Columna. 2017;16(2):121–6.
53. Cooper C, Dunham CM, Rodriguez A. Falls and major injuries are risk factors for thoracolumbar fractures: cognitive impairment and multiple injuries impede the detection of back pain and tenderness. J Trauma Acute Care Surg. 1995;38(5):692–6.
54. Katsuura Y, Osborn JM, Cason GW. The epidemiology of thoracolumbar trauma: a meta-analysis. J Orthop. 2016;13(4):383–8.
55. Looby S, Flanders A. Spine trauma. Radiol Clin. 2011;49(1):129–63.
56. Shahriari M, Sadaghiani MS, Spina M, Yousem DM, Franck B. Traumatic lumbar spine fractures: transverse process fractures dominate. Clin Imaging. 2021;71:44–8.
57. Freund P, Seif M, Weiskopf N, Friston K, Fehlings MG, Thompson AJ, Curt A. MRI in traumatic spinal cord injury: from clinical assessment to neuroimaging biomarkers. Lancet Neurol. 2019;18(12):1123–35.
58. James IA, Moukalled A, Yu E, Tulman DB, Bergese SD, Jones CD, Stawicki SP, Evans DC. A systematic review of the need for MRI for the clearance of cervical spine injury in obtunded blunt trauma patients after normal cervical spine CT. J Emerg Trauma Shock. 2014;7(4):251.
59. Chiu WC, Haan JM, Cushing BM, Kramer ME, Scalea TM. Ligamentous injuries of the cervical spine in unreliable blunt trauma patients: incidence, evaluation, and outcome. J Trauma Acute Care Surg. 2001;50(3):457–64.
60. Panczykowski DM, Tomycz ND, Okonkwo DO. Comparative effectiveness of using computed tomography alone to exclude cervical spine injuries in obtunded or intubated patients: meta-analysis of 14,327 patients with blunt trauma: a review. J Neurosurg. 2011;115(3):541–9.
61. Hogan GJ, Mirvis SE, Shanmuganathan K, Scalea TM. Exclusion of unstable cervical spine injury in obtunded patients with blunt trauma: is MR imaging needed when multi-detector row CT findings are normal? Radiology. 2005;237(1):106–13.
62. Abu Mughli R, Wu T, Li J, Moghimi S, Alem Z, Nasir MU, et al. An update in imaging of blunt vascular neck injury. Can Assoc Radiol J. 2020;71(3):281–92.
63. Fassett DR, Dailey AT, Vaccaro AR. Vertebral artery injuries associated with cervical spine injuries: a review of the literature. Clin Spine Surg. 2008;21(4):252–8.
64. Langner S, Fleck S, Kirsch M, Petrik M, Hosten N. Whole-body CT trauma imaging with adapted and optimized CT angiography of the craniocervical vessels: do we need an extra screening examination? Am J Neuroradiol. 2008;29(10):1902–7.
65. Wirth S, Heberand J, Basilico R, Berger F, Blanco A, Calli C, et al. European Society of Emergency Radiology—Guideline on Radiological Polytrauma Imaging. Availablle at: https://www.eser-society.org/app/uploads/ESER-Guideline-Long-Version-15.11.2020.pdf. Accessed: 3/31/2023.
66. Yushkevich PA, Piven J, Hazlett HC, Smith RG, Ho S, Gee JC, et al. User-guided 3D active contour segmentation of anatomical structures: significantly improved efficiency and reliability. NeuroImage. 2006;31(3):1116–28.

The Bony Pelvis

10

Riti Kanesa-thasan and Antje Greenfield

Introduction

Evaluation of the osseous structures for fractures or malalignment is an essential component of the search algorithm for computed tomography (CT) performed for patients after trauma given the possible association with significant complications, morbidity, and mortality [1]. This chapter will first introduce our hospital's CT imaging technique for the pelvis followed by a review of pertinent anatomy. Injury patterns seen in the trauma setting will then be discussed, including pelvic ring injury, acetabular fractures, hip dislocation, femoral fractures, and sacral fractures. Although the femur is considered a part of the appendicular skeletal and lower extremity, traumatic injuries of the hip joint and proximal femur are commonly within the field of view of the pelvis CT and will thus be reviewed.

CT Imaging Technique

At our hospital, the CT protocol utilized is by default obtained as part of a chest, abdomen, and pelvis protocol as summarized in Table 10.1. Additional dedicated CT of the pelvis can also be performed on a case-by-case basis, such as a CT cystography or dedicated bony pelvis CT with thin section. The protocol our hospital uses for dedicated bony pelvis CT is summarized in Table 10.2. When obtained, surface-rendered 3D multidetector images (3D reconstructions typi-

Table 10.1 Chest, abdomen and pelvis protocol

Protocol	CT chest-abdomen-pelvis for polytrauma
Protocol designed for (scanner model)	GE revolution apex
Patient preparation	Arms elevated
Oral contrast	n/a
IV contrast (ml, ml/s)	70/3, 55/2, 20 NaCl 2 cc/s
	Delay: 65 s
Tube settings	
kV	120
mA	smartmA 120–550
Dose modulation	smartmA, Noise index 12
Tube rotation time (s)	0.5 s
Table speed (mm/s)	158.75 mm/s
Pitch	0.992
Slice collimation	0.625 mm
Recontructed slice thickness	5 mm
	0.625 True Fidelity
Anatomical coverage	Chest-abdomen-pelvis
Reconstruction kernel	STND, ASIR 50
Breath hold	Inspiration
Window settings	400/40
Post-processing	1 mm STND, Lung, 3 mm STND, Lung, 2 mm Sag and Cor

R. Kanesa-thasan (✉) · A. Greenfield
Department of Radiology, University of Pennsylvania, Philadelphia, PA, USA
e-mail: riti.kanesa-thasan@pennmedicine.upenn.edu; antje.greenfield@pennmedicine.upenn.edu

F. Knollmann (ed.), *Trauma Computed Tomography*, https://doi.org/10.1007/978-3-031-45746-3_10

Table 10.2 Dedicated bony pelvis CT

Protocol	Noncontrast CT bony pelvis
Protocol designed for (scanner model)	GE scanner
Patient preparation	Feet first with feet slightly internally rotated
Oral contrast	n/a
IV contrast (ml, ml/s)	None
kV	120
mA	smartmA 80–450
Dose modulation	smartmA
Tube rotation time (s)	0.5 s
Pitch	0.992
Reconstructed slice thickness	1.25 x 1.25 mm
Anatomical coverage	Pelvis (iliac crest to lesser trochanters)
Reconstruction kernel	ASIR-v
Field of view	Large (skin to skin)
Post processing	1.25 mm BONE, 1.25 mm STND, 1.5 mm BONE Sag and Cor, 1.5 mm ST sag and Cor

cally obtained from thin-section CT images) as well as maximal intensity projection images (MIP images) can offer a supplementary overall view of the pelvis to help in injury evaluation and surgical planning, noting that limitations exist (such as non-visualization of subtle fracture lines or artifact). Imaging of the pelvis should include the entirety of the pelvis (including the margins of the iliac wings) through to the lesser trochanters of the femur.

Anatomy: Bones of the Pelvis

The pelvic ring consists of the sacrum and two innominate bones of the pelvis. The innominate bones are the adult fusion of three components: the ilium, ischium, and pubis. In utero, these three components originated as primary ossification centers separated by the triradiate cartilage. During development, endochondral ossification of the three components with narrowing of the triradiate cartilage progresses until osseous fusion is complete. Thus, the triradiate cartilage disappears during the teenage years.

Joints of the pelvic ring include two sacroiliac joints posteriorly and the pubic symphysis anteriorly. The sacroiliac joints are formed by the junction of the innominate bones to the sacrum. The pubic symphysis is where the innominate bones articulate anteriorly. The sacroiliac joints, sacrum, and posterior ilium together are considered the "posterior arch." The pubic symphysis, superior, and inferior pubic rami are considered the "anterior arch." The posterior arch plays a larger role in overall pelvic stability compared to the anterior arch. The anterior arch contributes to approximately one-third or less of overall pelvic stability [2].

The connection of the bony pelvis to the lower extremities is provided by the bilateral hip joints. The acetabulum consists of the junction of the pelvis ilium, ischium, and pubis components which articulate at the hip joint with the femoral head. The acetabula are located at the junction of the posterior arch and anterior arch bilaterally. Secondary ossification centers such as the os acetabuli, posterior epiphysis, and acetabular epiphysis typically fuse with the acetabulum around the age of 18 years old [3].

The sacrum is a component of the vertebral column and posterior bony pelvis. It consists of five vertebrae/costal elements which fuse to form the central sacral body, sacral neuroforamina, and bilateral sacral ala. The sacrum cranially articulates with the lumbar spine at the lumbosacral junction at L5-S1 disc space and bilateral facet joints. The sacrum caudally articulates with the coccyx at the sacrococcygeal junction. The sacrum laterally articulates with the ilium at the bilateral sacroiliac joints.

The hip joint is formed by the junction of the acetabulum and the femur. Three ligaments (the iliofemoral, pubofemoral, and ischiofemoral ligaments) form and reinforce the joint capsule. A fibrocartilaginous labrum lines the acetabulum anteriorly, superiorly, and posteriorly with a transverse acetabular ligament inferiorly [3]. Hyaline cartilage lines the acetabulum and femoral head [3]. The ligamentum teres extends from the acetabulum to the fovea of the femur.

The proximal femur (from proximal to distal) consists of the femoral head, femoral neck, intertrochanteric region (between the trochanters), and subtrochanteric region. The greater trochanter laterally and the lesser trochanter inferomedially to the femoral neck provide for bony attachments of various tendons. The fovea capitis is a focal concavity of the femoral head at the attachment of the ligamentum teres. The subtrochanteric region of the femur spans approximately 5 cm caudal to the lesser trochanter or to the level of the narrowest region of the proximal diaphysis [4].

Multiple apophyses, bony crests, tubercles, trochanters, and spines about the pelvis, sacrum, and proximal femur function as origins, insertions, or attachments for various muscles, tendons, and ligaments. Note that avulsion fractures of these sites can occur with specific traumatic injuries, however, are beyond the scope of this chapter.

Anatomy: Ligaments

Pelvic stability is supported by multiple ligaments at the sacroiliac joint, posterior pelvis, and pubic symphysis. In the pelvic ring model, the posterior sacroiliac ligament is considered one of the most important stabilizers due to the higher degree of pelvic instability that arises when it is disrupted [2]. Muscles/tendons of the pelvic floor, trunk, hip, and thigh also contribute to pelvic stability.

Ligaments that support the sacroiliac joint include the posterior, interosseous, and anterior sacroiliac ligaments. The posterior sacroiliac ligaments play a larger role in overall stability compared to the anterior sacroiliac ligaments. The posterior sacroiliac ligaments impede internal rotation as well as vertical movement, while the anterior sacroiliac ligaments impede external rotation [2].

Ligaments that provide additional support to the sacroiliac joint and posterior pelvic ring include the sacrospinous ligament, the sacrotuberous ligament, and the iliolumbar ligament. The sacrotuberous ligament courses from the sacrum to the ischial tuberosity. The sacrospinous ligament courses from sacrum to the ischial spine. The iliolumbar ligament courses from the iliac crest to the lumbar spine (L5 or L4) transverse processes. Avulsion fractures at the attachment sites of these ligaments can signal unstable pelvic injury [5, 6].

Ligaments that support the pubic symphysis and its fibrocartilaginous central disc include the inferior (arcuate), superior, anterior, and posterior pubic ligaments. The arcuate ligament is the major ligamentous stabilizer and extends along the anterior-inferior aspect of the joint to the anterior-inferior pubic tubercles bilaterally [7]. The arcuate ligament joins with the rectus abdominus muscles and common adductor origins to form a fibrocartilaginous plate (aponeurosis) [8]. Injury of this ligamentous apparatus is known as athletic pubalgia (also referred to as "sports hernia" in the literature), and its discussion is beyond the scope of this chapter [9].

Pelvic Ring Injury

Pelvic ring injuries are commonly seen as a result of motor vehicle collision (or also collisions involving motorcycles, bicycles, or pedestrians), fall, or crush injury [2]. Similar to the concept that a ring typically breaks in two places, the pelvic ring biomechanical model emphasizes that the presence of one abnormality along the ring should raise suspicion for a second site of abnormality. These fractures can be subtle and thus an increased index of suspicion is needed to detect the second break of the ring. Exceptions to this rule include young patients with avulsions fractures or older patients with insufficiency fractures; discussion of these fractures is not included in this chapter [10]. The abnormalities can be fractures and/or joint malalignment. Unstable injuries are typically associated with vascular and visceral injuries. The degree of instability of the injured pelvis guides management decisions. For example, stable and nondeformed injuries can be managed conservatively (such as prompt weight-bearing and mobilization) [11]. Unstable or deformed injuries are often operative indications [11].

Multiple classification systems exist to help categorize findings of pelvic ring injury, some of which categorizing degree of stability versus instability. A few notable classification systems include the Letournel and Judet, Pennal, Tile, and Young and Burgess classification systems [2, 12–16]. Some injuries may still demonstrate inherent variability in stability despite categorization [11]. Significant displacement greater than 1 cm and/or posterior sacroiliac ligament disruption are typically considered unstable [2].

An overall understanding of the injury patterns associated with certain force mechanisms can help guide imaging detection. This chapter will focus on the Young-Burgess Classification given its predominant usage. The Young-Burgess Classification describes four injury patterns based on force vectors: Lateral Compression Injury, Anterior–Posterior (AP) Compression Injury, Vertical Shear Injury, and Complex Injury. Lateral compression injuries occur most frequently, followed by AP compression and vertical shear injuries, respectively [2]. Note that complex injury represents a combination of bony/joint abnormalities seen in lateral compression, AP compression, and vertical shear injuries and can have variable stability and management implications. Younger patients with stronger cancellous bone tend to demonstrate more ligamentous disruption/joint abnormalities, while patients with weaker bones tend to fracture [2].

Lateral compression injury occurs when a side-impact force results in lateral compression of the pelvic ring. Examples include T-bone motor vehicle collision (vehicle hit from side) or side-impact fall. Resultant hemipelvis internal rotation toward the contralateral side and decreased pelvic volume can be associated with bladder rupture or nerve injury to the sacral, sciatic or superior gluteal nerves [2]. Significant hemorrhage is not mechanistically expected compared to the other injury patterns, but can occur (such as direct laceration of the iliac vessels adjacent fracture margin) [2]. Lateral compression injuries are subdivided into type 1, 2 or 3 based on suspected increasing degrees of instability. All types of lateral compression injury demonstrate fracture(s) of the inferior and/or superior pubic rami in conjunction with other findings. Type 1 lateral compression injury demonstrates ipsilateral sacral buckle (impaction) fracture. Nondisplaced type 1 injury can be treated nonoperatively. Type 2 lateral compression injury typically demonstrates ipsilateral iliac wing fracture or posterior sacroiliac joint diastasis. Rotational instability resulting from type 2 injury can be an indication for surgical intervention. Type 3 lateral compression injury (often referenced as "windswept" pelvis) demonstrates contralateral injury superimposed on type 1 or 2 injury patterns secondary to contralateral AP compression injury/external rotation of the contralateral pelvis (such as a patient run over by a car). Rotational and vertical instability resulting from type 3 injury (due to disruption of the sacrotuberous and/or sacrospinous ligaments) is typically treated operatively. See Figs. 10.1, 10.2, and 10.3, for example, of lateral compression injuries.

AP compression injury (also referred to as "open book fracture") occurs when front-impact force results in anterior–posterior compression of the pelvic ring. Examples include crush injury or head-on traffic motor vehicle accidents. Resultant unilateral or bilateral hemipelvis external rotation and increased pelvic volume can be associated with significant vascular hemorrhage as well as genitourinary or lumbosacral plexus injury. AP compression injuries are subdivided into type 1, 2, or 3 based on suspected increasing degree of instability. All types of AP compression injury demonstrate varying degrees of widening of the pubic symphysis, the primary location of pelvic ring failure in this type of injury. Type 1 injury demonstrates less than 25 cm widening of the pubic symphysis with possible pubic rami fracture(s). Pure type 1 injury may be treated nonoperatively as the posterior ligaments are likely intact. Type 2 injury demonstrates widening of the pubic symphysis greater than 2.5 cm with additional widening of the anterior sacroiliac joint. Rotational instability resulting from type 2 injury (typically due to anterior sacroiliac, sacrospinous, and sacrotuberous ligamentous disruption) can be an indication for surgical treat-

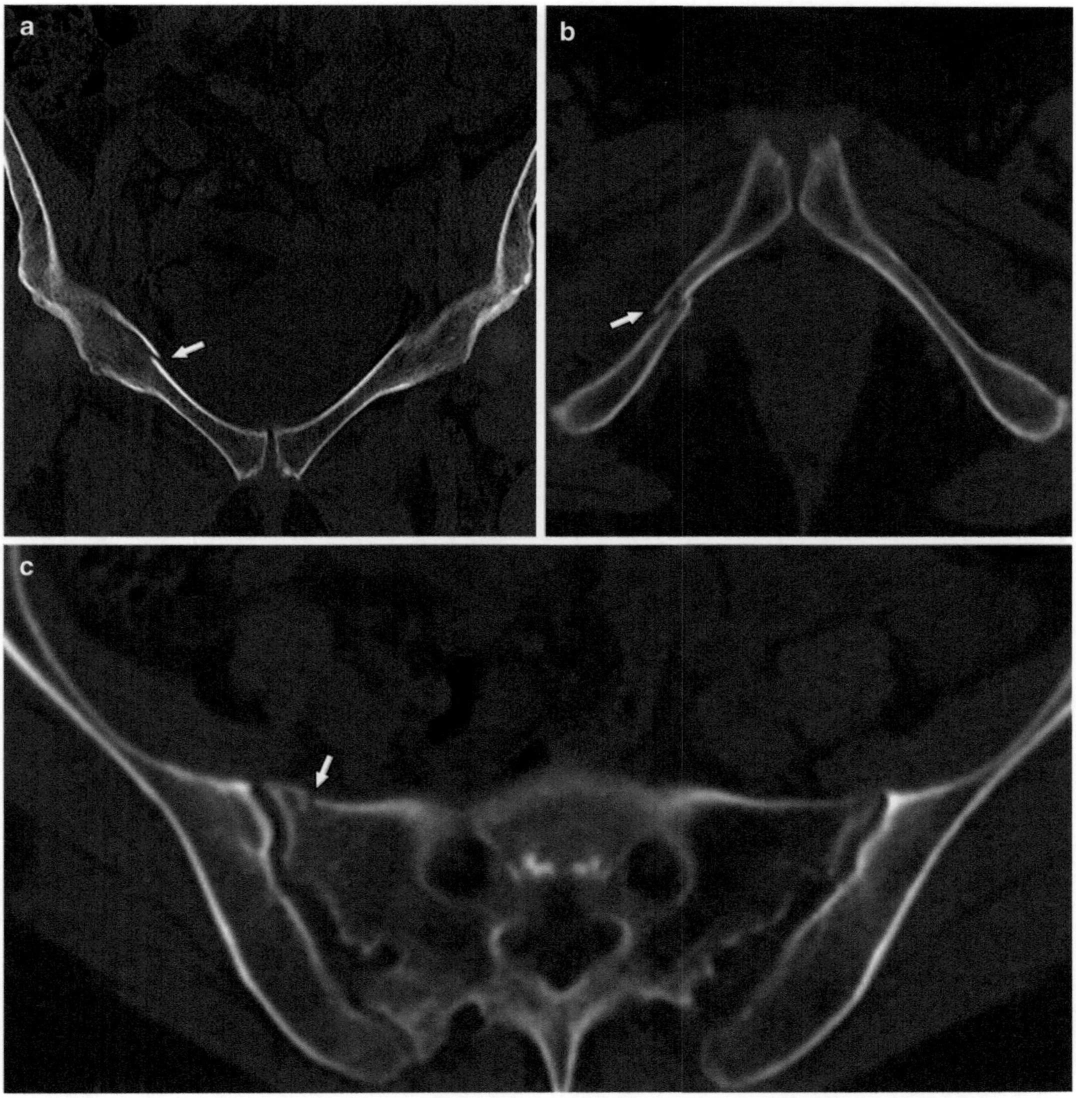

Fig. 10.1 Lateral compression type 1 pelvic ring injury in a 63 year old after a fall with side-impact. (**a**) Coronal CT image shows a nondisplaced transverse fracture of the right superior pubic ramus (arrow). (**b**) Axial CT image shows an additional fracture of the ipsilateral right inferior pubic ramus (arrow). (**c**) Axial CT image shows a buckle fracture of the ipsilateral right sacral ala (arrow)

ment. (Type 2 injuries are considered vertically stable due to intact posterior sacroiliac joint ligament). Type 3 injury demonstrates widening of the pubic symphysis (typically greater than 2.5 cm), widening of the anterior and posterior sacroiliac joint, and possible pubic rami fracture(s). Rotational and vertical instability resulting from type 3 injury (secondary to multiligamentous disruption that includes the posterior sacroiliac ligament) is typically treated operatively. See Figs. 10.4, 10.5, and 10.6, for example, of AP compression injuries.

Vertical shear injury occurs secondary to a craniocaudally directed force. An example

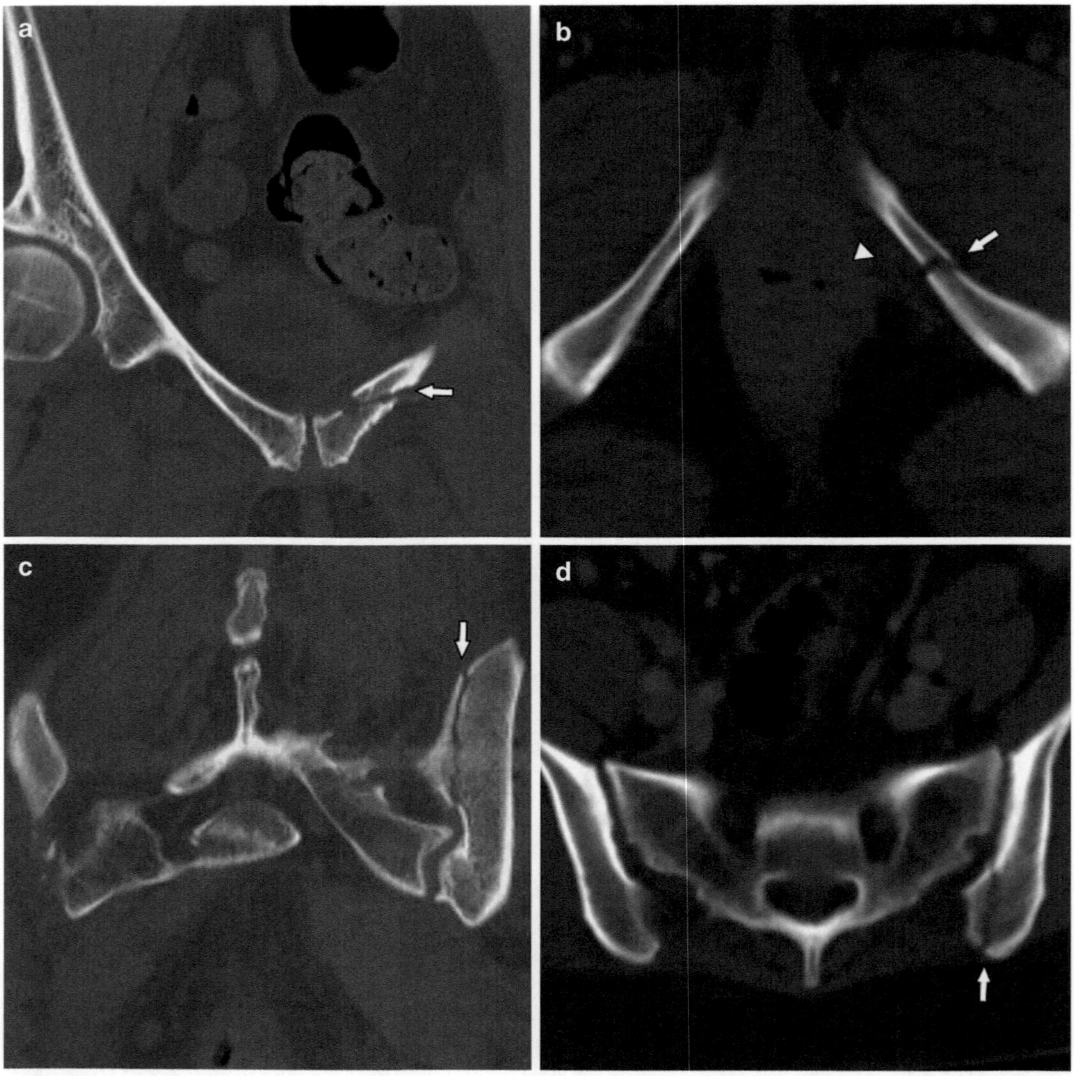

Fig. 10.2 Lateral compression type 2 pelvic ring injury in a 57 year old. (**a**) Coronal CT image shows a transverse fracture of the left superior pubic ramus (arrow). (**b**) Axial CT image shows an additional fracture of the ipsilateral left inferior pubic ramus (arrow). Note adjacent muscle hemorrhage (arrowhead). (**c**) Coronal CT image and (**d**) axial CT image show a fracture of the ipsilateral left posterior ilium with extension to the sacroiliac joint (arrows)

includes fall from height with extended legs where one leg hits the ground before the other. Associated visceral injuries commonly include vascular injury, genitourinary complications, or nerve abnormality. At the anterior arch, vertical shear injury demonstrates underlying disruption of the pubic symphysis (similar to AP compression fractures) or vertically oriented pubic symphysis fracture. At the posterior arch, vertical shear injury demonstrates disruption of the sacroiliac joint or sacral fracture. Vertical shear injury demonstrates superimposed superior displacement of the hemipelvis, typically of the posterior arch at the sacroiliac joint, sacrum or iliac wing. Vertical shear injury is considered rotationally and vertically unstable. See Fig. 10.7, for example, of a vertical shear injury.

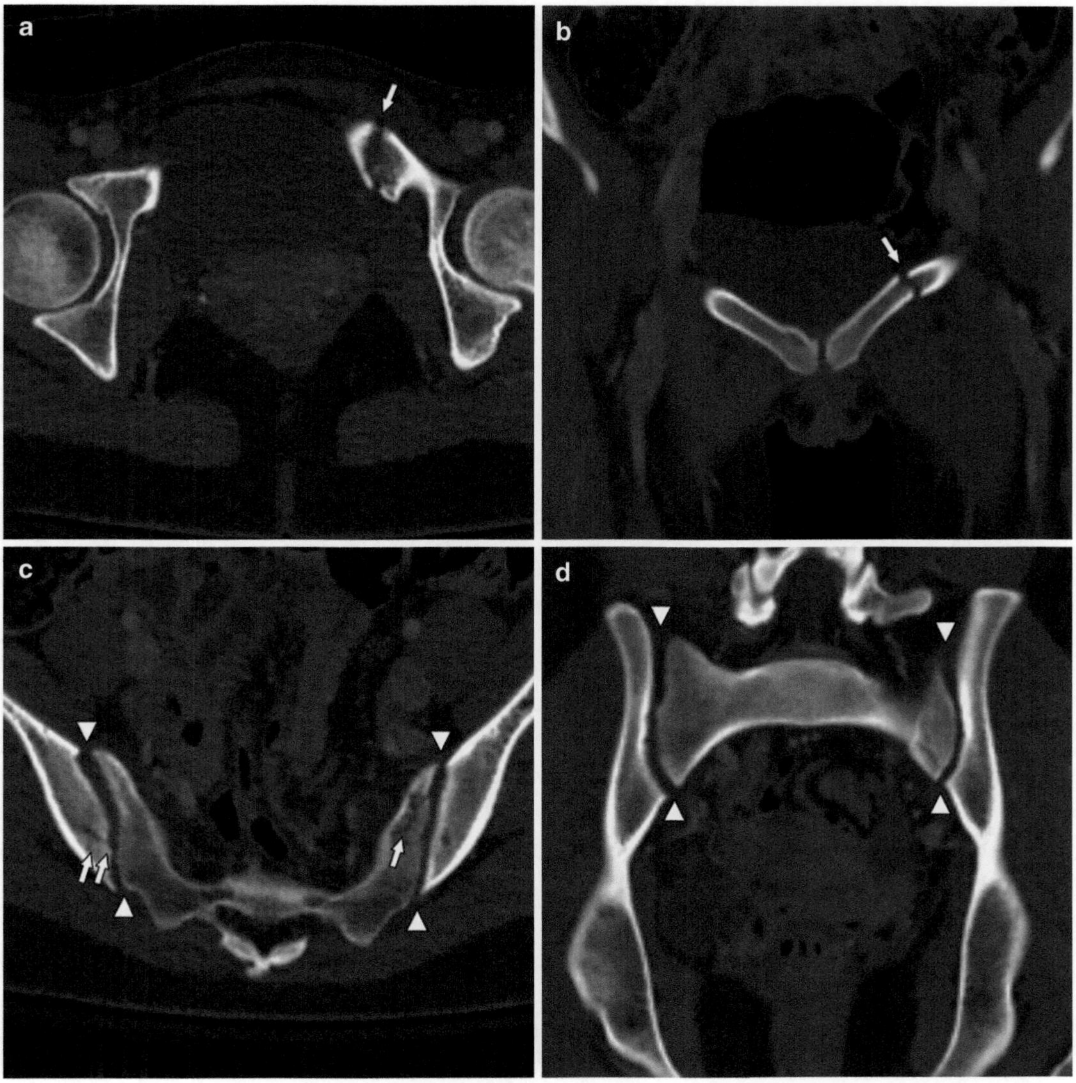

Fig. 10.3 Lateral compression type 3 pelvic ring injury in a 20 year old. (**a**) Axial and (**b**) coronal CT images show a fracture of the left superior pubic ramus (arrow). (**c**) Axial and (**d**) coronal CT images show a fracture of the ipsilateral left sacral ala (arrow) with extension to the adjacent sacroiliac joint (arrowheads). There is widening of the anterior greater than posterior sacroiliac joints bilaterally (arrowheads), worse on the contralateral right side, consistent with underlying injury to the posterior sacroiliac ligaments. Partially visualized is a fracture of the contralateral right posterior ilium (two arrows)

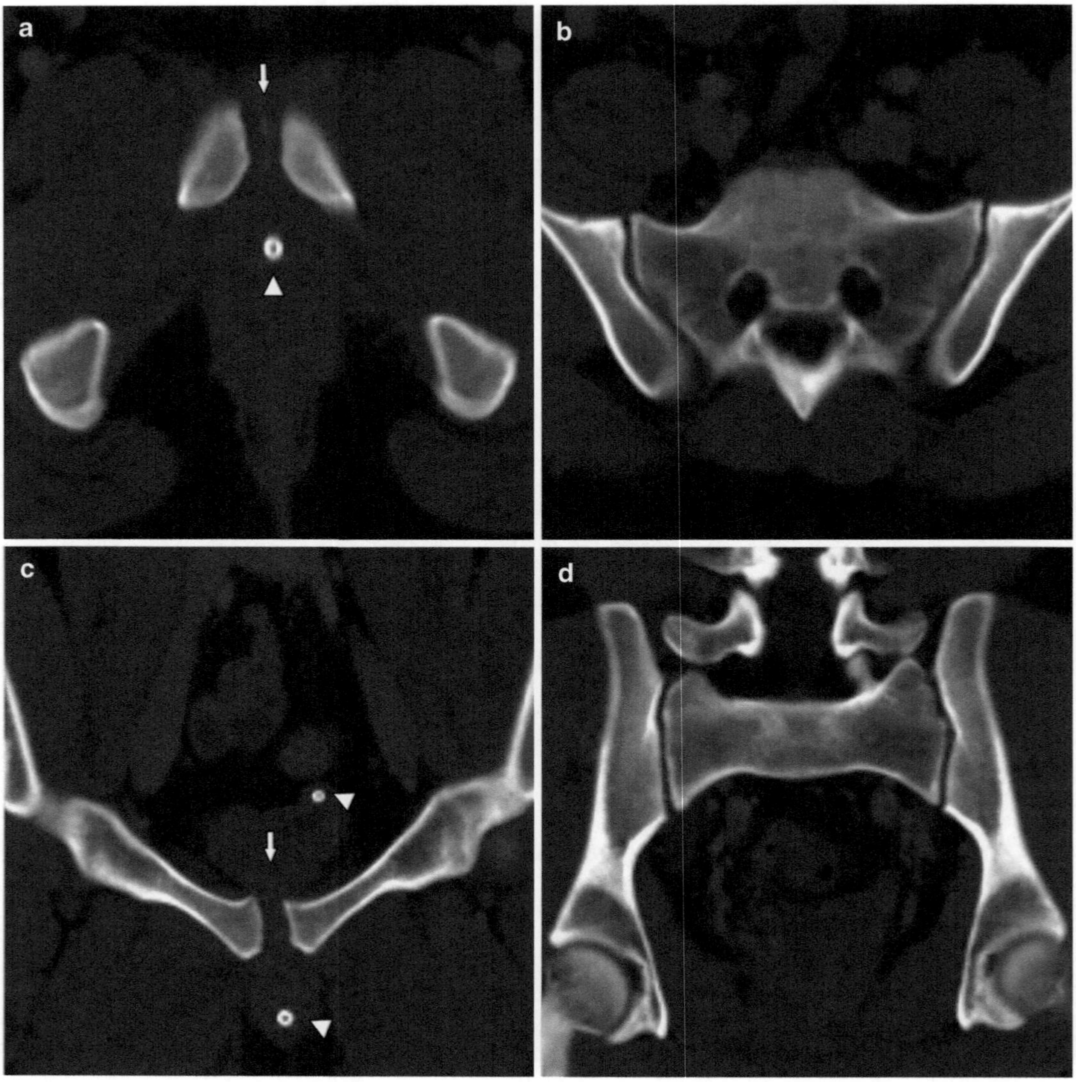

Fig. 10.4 AP compression type 1 pelvic ring injury in a 23 year old male. (**a**) Axial and (**c**) coronal CT images show 1.1 cm widening of the pubic symphysis with faint thin avulsion fracture fragment at midline (arrow). A foley catheter is incidentally noted (arrowheads). (**b**) Axial and (**d**) coronal CT images show an intact posterior arch without any abnormalities of the ilium, sacrum, or sacroiliac joints

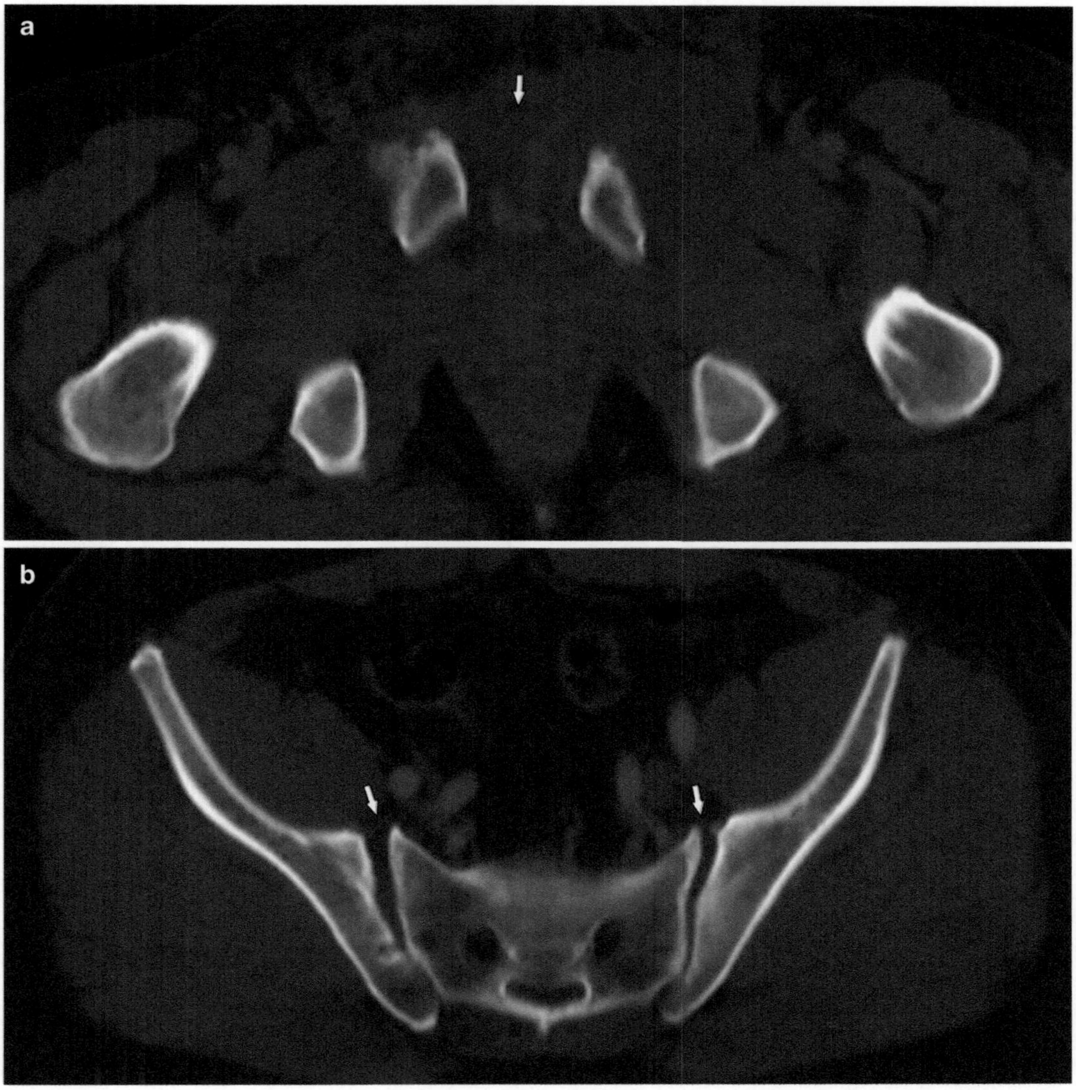

Fig. 10.5 AP compression type 2 pelvic ring injury in a 69 year old after motorcycle accident. (**a**) Axial CT image demonstrates widening of the pubic symphysis to 2.6 cm (arrow). The high density within the central portion of the pubic symphysis is consistent with active vascular extravasation and hematoma formation. The source branch from the anterior division of the left internal iliac artery was subsequently embolized to control hemorrhage. (**b**) Axial CT image demonstrates widening of the right greater than left anterior sacroiliac joints (arrows), with associated avulsion fracture of the anterior margin of the left ilium at the sacroiliac joint

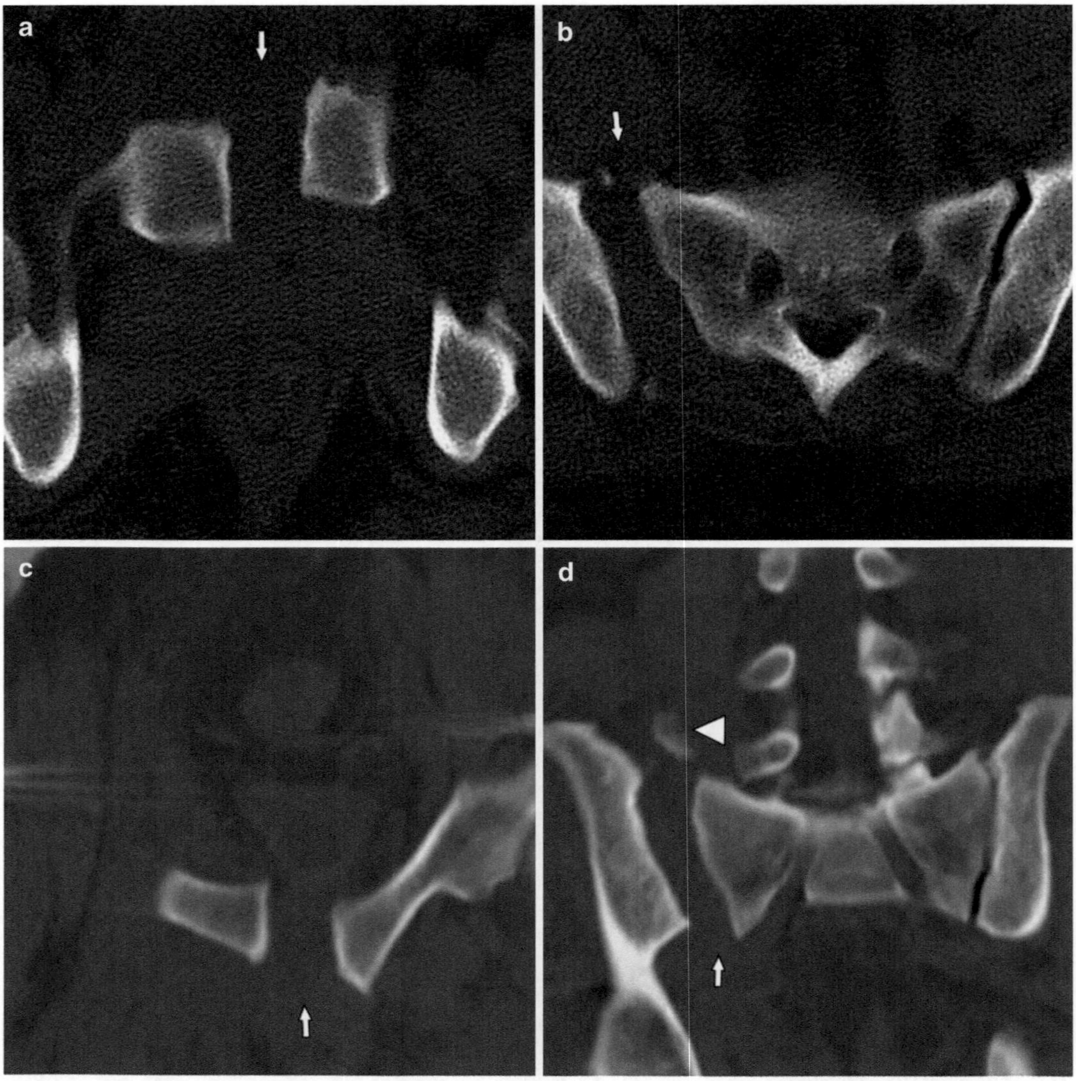

Fig. 10.6 AP compression type 3 pelvic ring injury in a 51 year old after motor vehicle accident. (**a**) Axial and (**c**) coronal CT images demonstrate widening and malalignment of the pubic symphysis. (**b**) Axial and (**d**) coronal CT images demonstrate widening of the right sacroiliac joint anteriorly and posteriorly with adjacent avulsion fracture fragments, indicating disruption of the anterior and posterior sacroiliac ligaments (arrows). Note avulsion fracture of the right L5 transverse process (arrowhead) consistent with injury to the iliolumbar ligament

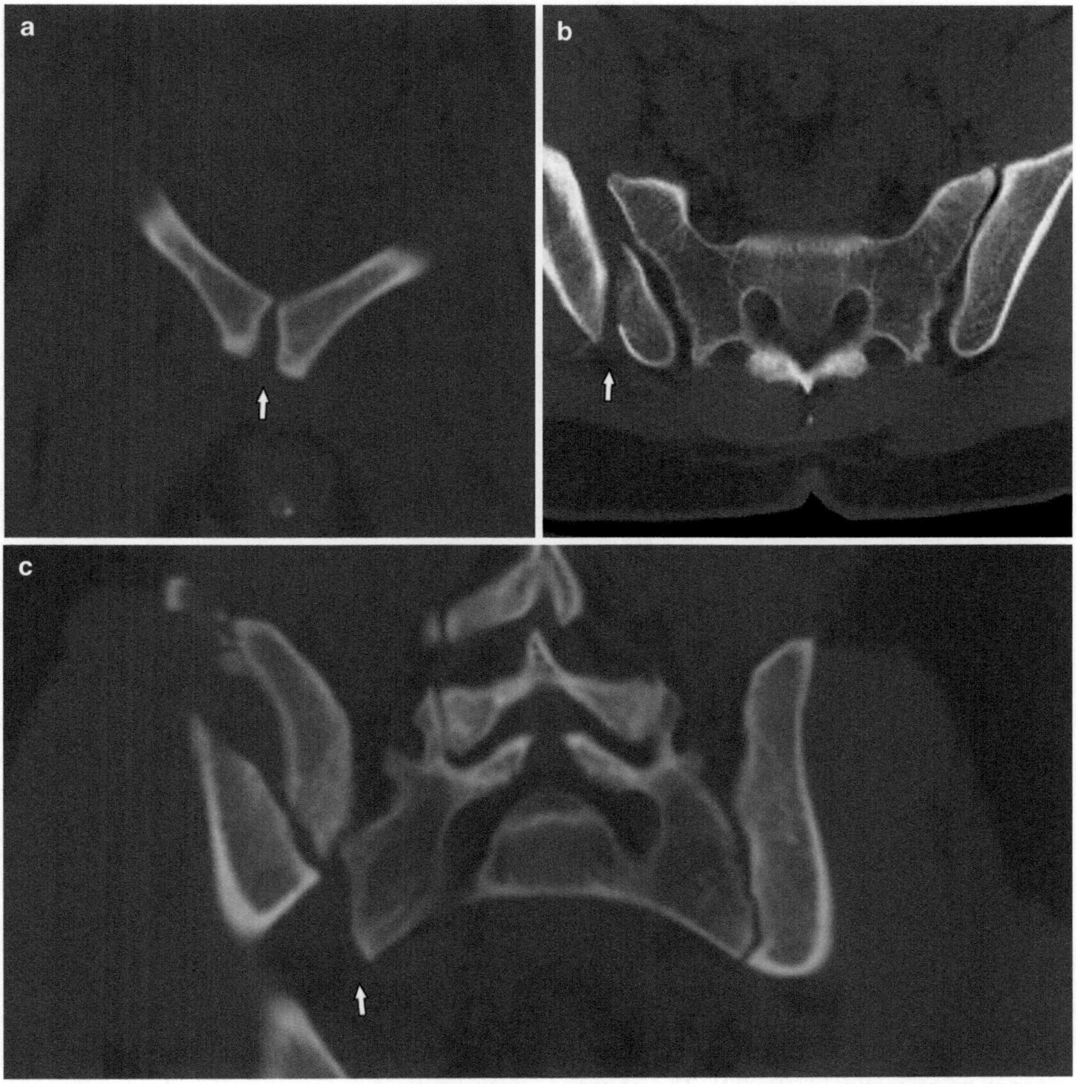

Fig. 10.7 Vertical shear fracture in a 25-year-old electrician who fell 25 feet from a lift while at work. (**a**) Coronal CT image demonstrates malalignment and asymmetric widening of the pubic symphysis with superior displacement of the right pubic body. (**b**) Axial CT image demonstrates widening of the right sacroiliac joint with fracture of the right posterior ilium (arrow). (**c**) Coronal CT image demonstrates widening of the right sacroiliac joint with fracture of the right posterior ilium (arrow) and superior displacement of the right hemipelvis. Clinically suspected ureteral and bladder injury was excluded by subsequently performed retrograde urethrogram and CT cystogram performed

Acetabular Fractures

Multiple classification systems exist for acetabular fractures, including the Judet and Letournel classification and the Arbeitsgemeinschaft für Osteosynthesefragen/Orthopedic Trauma Association (AO/OTA) classification, as well as the more recently proposed CT-based Harris classification system [3, 17–20]. The Judet and Letournel classification system is a commonly used shared framework for evaluating acetabular fractures and will be reviewed in this chapter. However, it should be noted that the original intent of Judet and Letournel classification system was to guide surgical exposure and not necessarily to guide fracture management [11]. Fracture variants can exist beyond this framework and treatment planning is highly patient-centered with consideration of additional multiple factors, including but not limited to fracture classification, presence of additional injury, and functional status before the injury [11]. These categories are conventionally based on the projection of the fracture lines when viewing the acetabulum en face.

The Letournel classification system identifies multiple key portions of the acetabulum and pelvis based on anatomy and radiographs. The anterior column is composed of the anterior wall of the acetabulum, anterior two-thirds of the iliac wing (including the anterior-superior iliac spine, anterior-inferior iliac spine, and pelvic brim), and superior pubic ramus [3, 21, 22]. The posterior column is composed of the posterior wall of the acetabulum, ischial tuberosity, and ischium along the sciatic notch [3, 21, 22]. The columns are characteristically described as forming the shape of a greek letter "lambda" (λ), with the posterior column representing the smaller component of the letter [3, 21, 22]. The sciatic buttress is the portion of the posterior, superomedial innominate bone located adjacent to the sacroiliac joint and above the sciatic notch that serves as the junction of both columns and the axial skeleton [3, 21, 22]. The quadrilateral surface (or plate) is the medial surface of the acetabulum adjacent the pelvic viscera and obturator internus muscle [21]. The anterior wall consists of the anterior acetabular articular surface and rim, with the Judet and Leteournel classification definition also including a portion of the anterior column such as extension to the quadrilateral surface [3]. The posterior wall consists of the posterior acetabular articular surface and rim [3]. The ischiopubic ramus (the inferior pubic ramus and inferior ischial ramus) bridges the anterior and posterior columns along the inferior aspect of the obturator foramen [3, 21, 22].

The Judet and Letournel classification system divides acetabular fractures into 10 categories: 5 elementary (anterior wall, posterior wall, anterior column, posterior column, and transverse) and 5 associated acetabular fractures (T-shaped, transverse with posterior wall, posterior column with posterior wall, both column, and anterior column/wall with posterior hemitransverse). The elementary fractures divide the pelvis into two parts while the associated fractures divide the pelvis into three parts [3]. Wall fractures are separated from the acetabulum. Column fractures are separated from the sciatic buttress and include fracture line extension across the obturator foramen/ring. Transverse fractures travel across the acetabulum and typically separate the acetabulum into superior and inferior parts. T-shaped fractures are transverse fractures with additional fracture line extension through the obturator foramen/ring.

The most common Judet and Letournel categories are the posterior wall fracture, both column fracture, and transverse with posterior wall fracture [3, 23, 24]. Posterior wall fractures include the posterior articular surface/rim of the acetabulum (Fig. 10.8), without extension of the fracture line to the quadrilateral plate/medial surface of the acetabulum or across the obturator foramen/ring. Both column fractures disconnect the entire acetabulum from the sciatic buttress with dominant fracture line(s) separating the anterior and posterior columns (Fig. 10.9). Transverse with posterior wall fractures are a combination of the elementary transverse fracture with superimposed comminuted posterior wall fracture component (Fig. 10.10); note the lack of fracture line extension across the obturator foramen/ring.

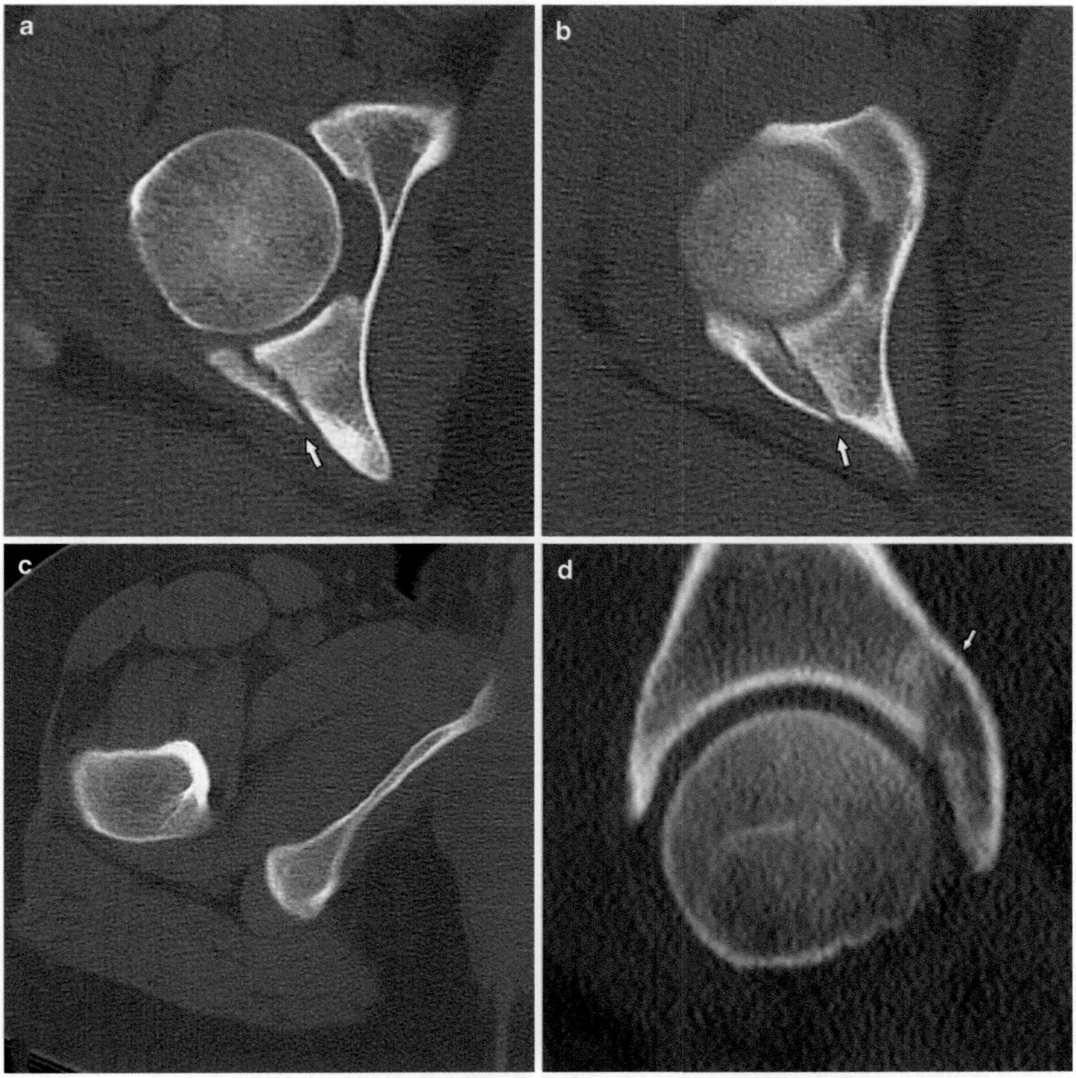

Fig. 10.8 Posterior wall right acetabular fracture in a 40 year old. Consecutive axial CT images of the right acetabulum from caudal (**a**) to cranial (**b**) demonstrate acute fracture of the posterior wall of the right acetabulum (arrow). (**c**) Axial CT image demonstrates intact right ischiopubic ramus. (**d**) Sagittal CT image demonstrates fracture of the posterior wall (arrow)

For the purposes of comparison to the posterior wall fracture described above, note the less frequently seen posterior column with posterior wall fracture in Fig. 10.11. The fracture line extends to the medial margin of the acetabulum with fracture line extension across the obturator foramen, and posterior column separation from the sciatic buttress.

For the purposes of comparison to the both column fractures described above, the less frequently seen anterior column fracture is depicted in Fig. 10.12. The fracture lines in an anterior column fracture separate it from the sciatic buttress, extend to the quadrilateral surface, and cross the obturator foramen/ring. The cranial-most extent of the fracture line in an anterior column fracture does not necessarily have to extend through the iliac crest/pelvic brim; in fact, the cranial-most fracture line can be as low as the iliopectineal eminence [3].

Additional details to include when evaluating an acetabular fracture is presence of impaction,

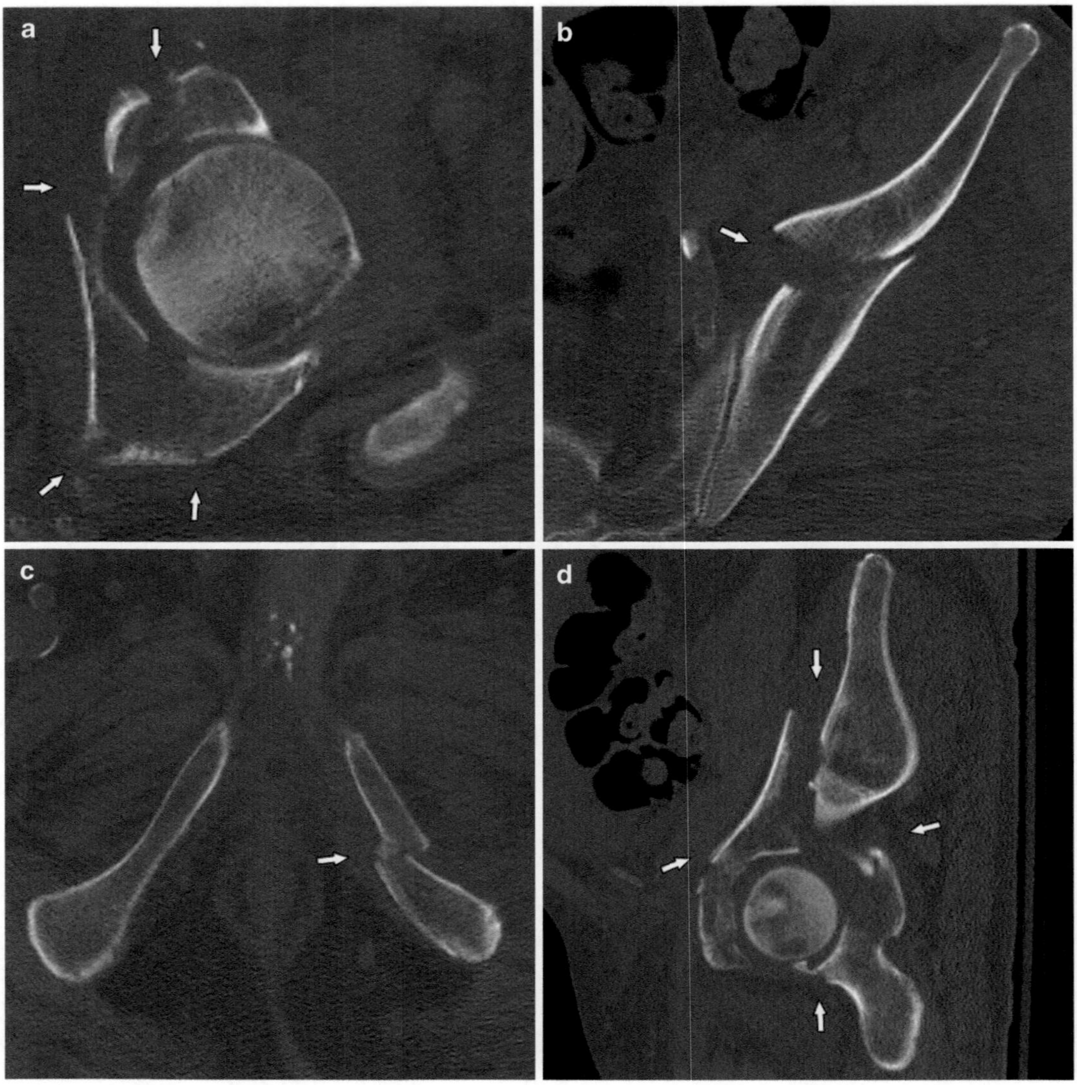

Fig. 10.9 Both column left acetabular fracture in a 66 year old. (**a**) Axial CT image at the level of the left acetabulum demonstrates comminuted fracture with fracture lines (arrows) extending to the anterior column, anterior wall, posterior column, posterior wall, and quadrilateral surface. (**b**) Axial CT image demonstrates extension of the fracture line to the left iliac wing superiorly (arrow). (**c**) Axial CT image demonstrates extension of the fracture line to the left ischiopubic ramus (arrow). (**d**) Sagittal CT image demonstrates comminuted acetabular fracture lines (arrows) separating both columns from the sciatic buttress region

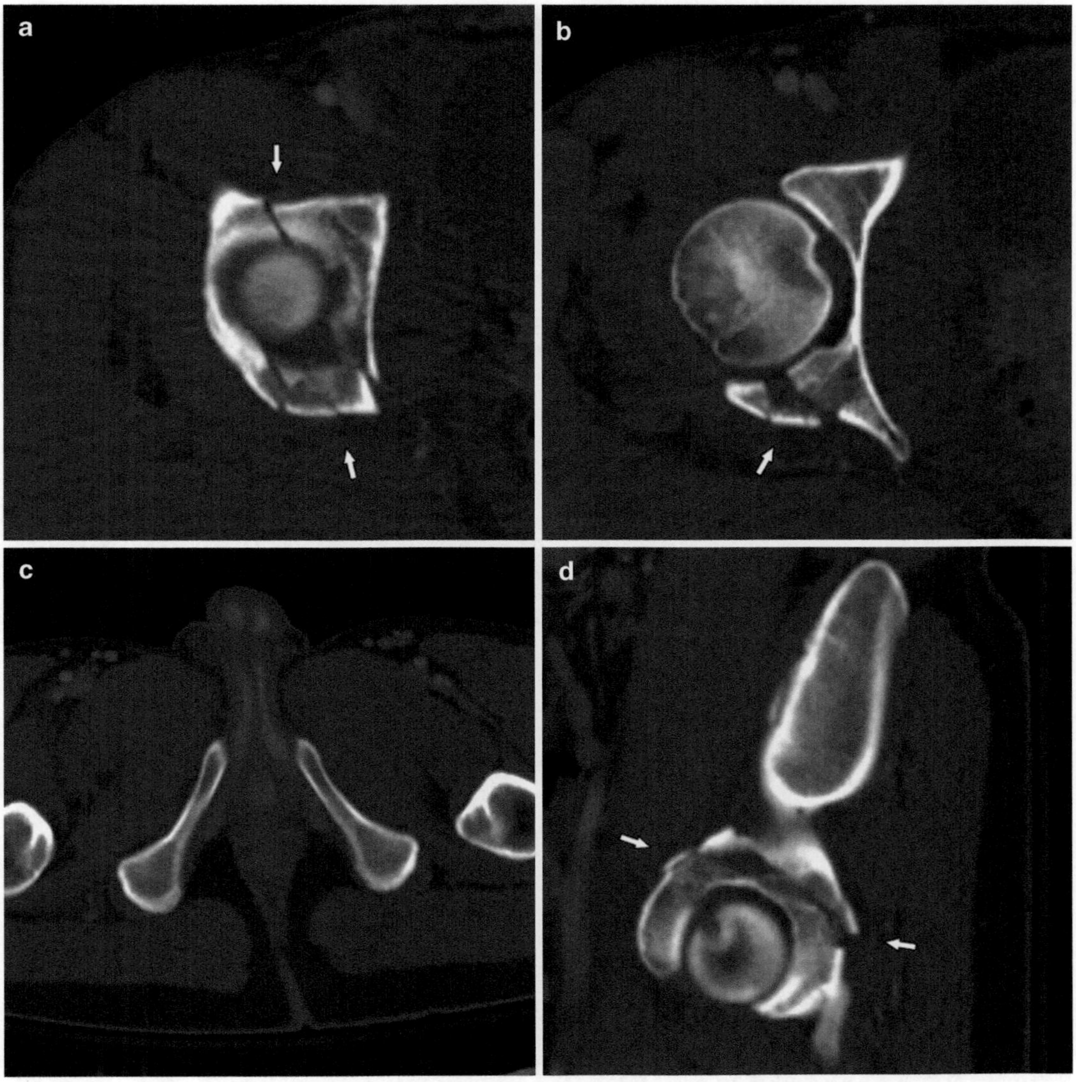

Fig. 10.10 Transverse with posterior wall right acetabular fracture in a 30 year old. Consecutive axial CT images of the right acetabulum from cranial (**a**) to caudal (**b**) demonstrate transverse fracture with superimposed comminuted fracture of the posterior wall of the right acetabulum (arrow). (**c**) Axial CT image demonstrates intact ischiopubic ramus. (**d**) Sagittal CT image demonstrates transverse fracture line component (arrows)

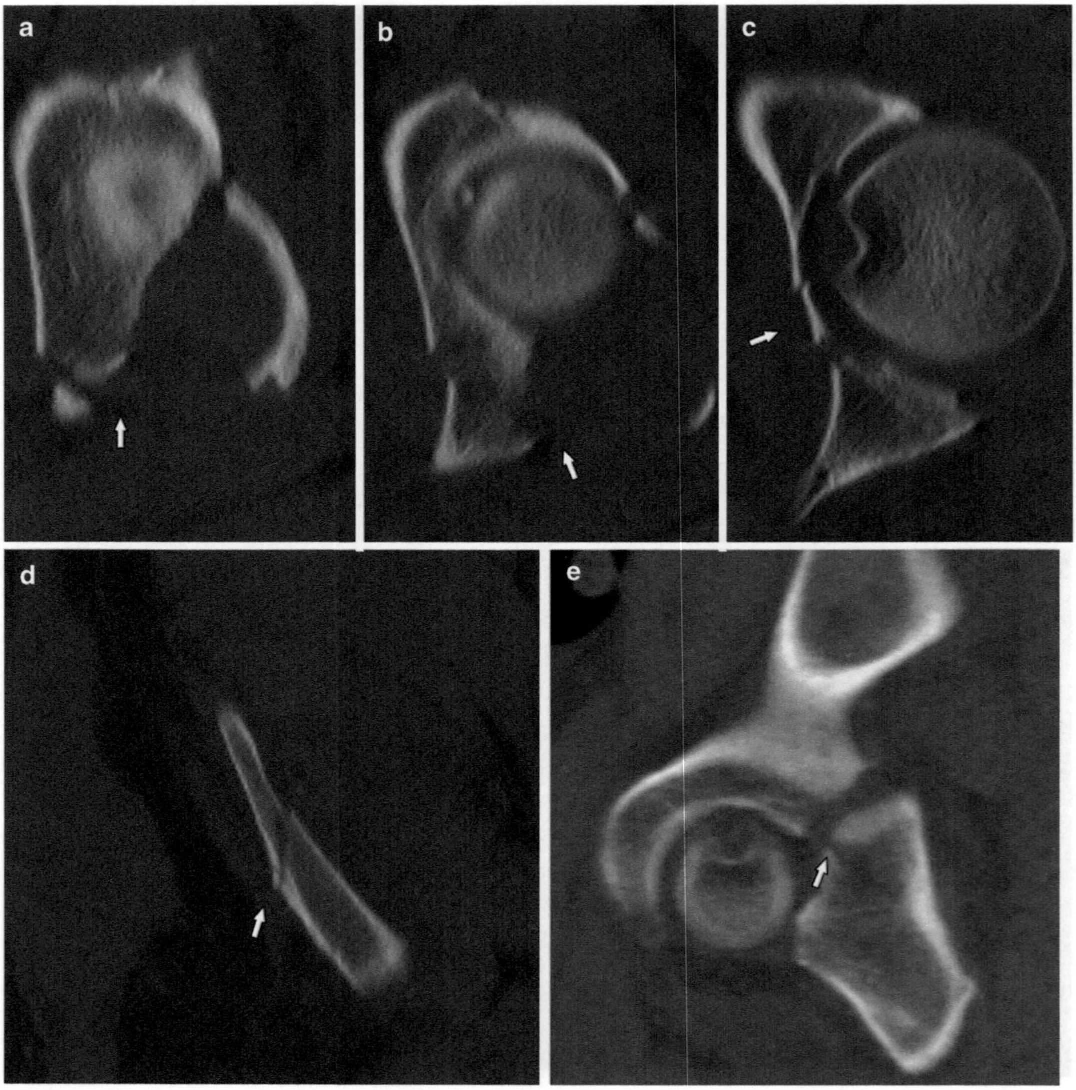

Fig. 10.11 Posterior column with posterior wall acetabular fracture in a 50 year old. Consecutive axial CT images of the left acetabulum from cranial to caudal (**a**–**c**) demonstrate comminuted, displaced fracture of the left posterior column and posterior acetabular wall. (**d**) Axial CT image demonstrates fracture of the left ischiopubic ramus. (**e**) Sagittal CT image demonstrates comminuted fracture line involving the posterior column and acetabular wall (arrow). Note the intact anterior column

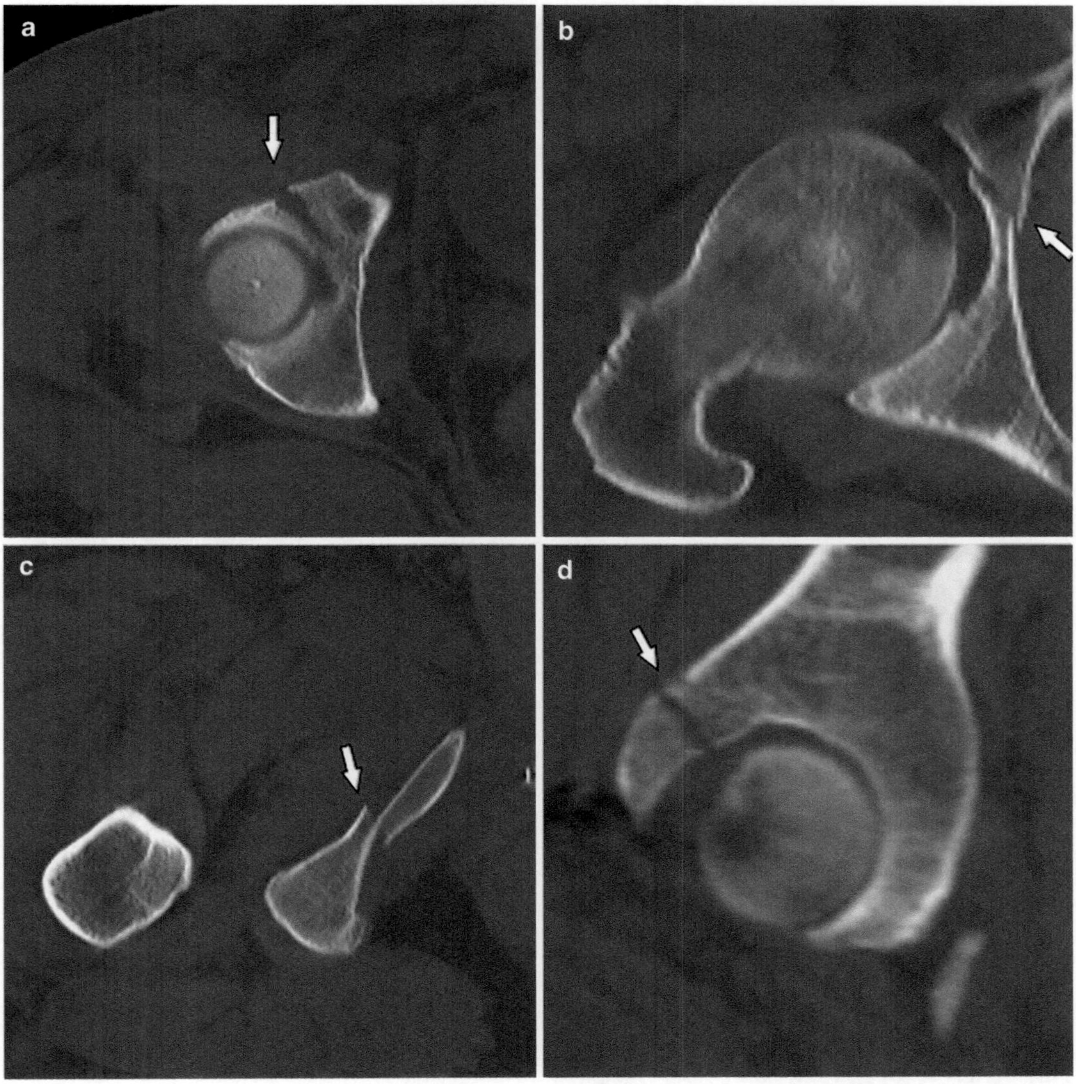

Fig. 10.12 Anterior column right acetabular fracture in a 44 year old. Consecutive axial CT images of the right acetabulum from cranial (**a**) to caudal (**b**) demonstrate fracture of the right anterior column (arrow in a) with extension to the quadrilateral plate (arrow in **b**). (**c**) Axial CT image demonstrates fracture of the right ischiopubic ramus. (**d**) Sagittal CT image demonstrates fracture line involving the anterior column of the acetabulum (arrow). Note the intact posterior column

comminution, displacement/angulation/rotation, intra-articular loose fracture fragments, superior acetabular dome involvement, posterior wall involvement percentage, secondary congruence with the femoral head in the setting of both column fractures (which can impact management), femoral head fracture, sacral fracture, and/or soft tissue injury [3, 25]. Comment on their multiplanar or 3D reconstructions are often needed to recognize the full extent of injury.

Fractures of the Sacrum

Fractures of the sacrum can occur secondary to multiple mechanisms, including high-energy trauma, low-energy trauma in the setting of older patients, insufficiency fractures, or stress fractures [26–28]. Although nondisplaced and stable sacral fractures can be treated conservatively (such as in the case of a lateral compression type 1 pelvic ring injury), unstable and/or displaced sacral fractures are treated with surgical fixation (such as in the case of vertical shear pelvic ring injury) [26]. Multiple classification systems exist for sacral fractures.

Intrinsic sacral fractures are frequently categorized using the Denis classification system of three zones (Fig. 10.13), with zone 1 located lateral to the neuroforamina (Fig. 10.14), zone 2 fractures involving the neuroforamina (Fig. 10.15), and zone 3 fractures extending into the spinal canal (Fig. 10.16) [26]. Denis Zone 3 fractures are frequently subclassified using the Roy-Camille and Strange-Vognsen and Lecech classification systems based on degree of instability, displacement, or impaction.

The Isler classification system classifies sacral fractures involving the lumbosacral junction into three types [26]. Type 1 injury is located lateral to the L5-S1 facet joint, often impacting pelvic stability [26]. Type 2 injury involves the L5-S1 facet joint, often associated with displacement and neurologic injury [26]. Type 3 injury extends medial the facet joint with involvement of the spinal canal, often associated with instability

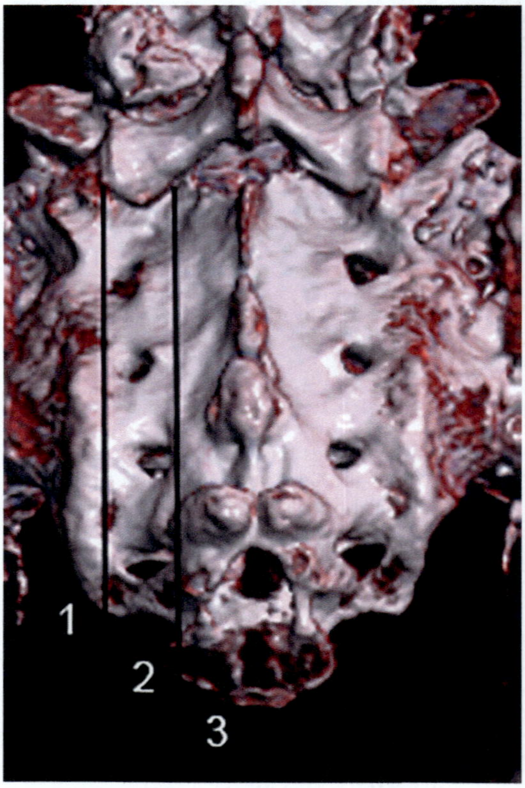

Fig. 10.13 Surface-rendered 3D image of the posterior sacrum demonstrates the Denis classification system for sacral fractures. Zone 1 fractures are lateral to the neuroforamina. Zone 2 fractures involve the neuroforamina. Zone 3 fractures involve the spinal canal

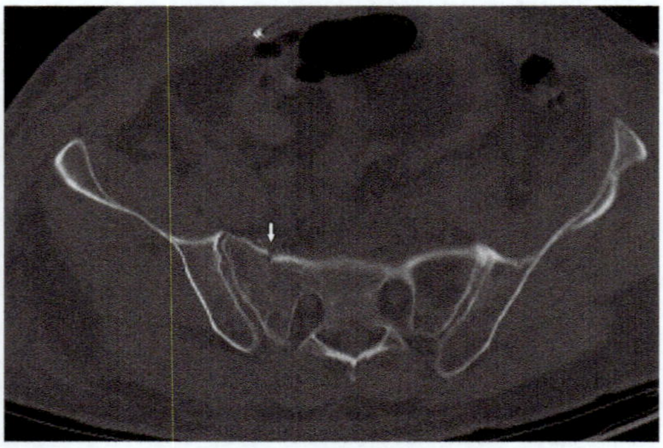

Fig. 10.14 Denis zone 1 right sacral fracture in a 50 year old. Axial CT image demonstrates mildly comminuted, impaction fracture of the right sacral ala (arrow)

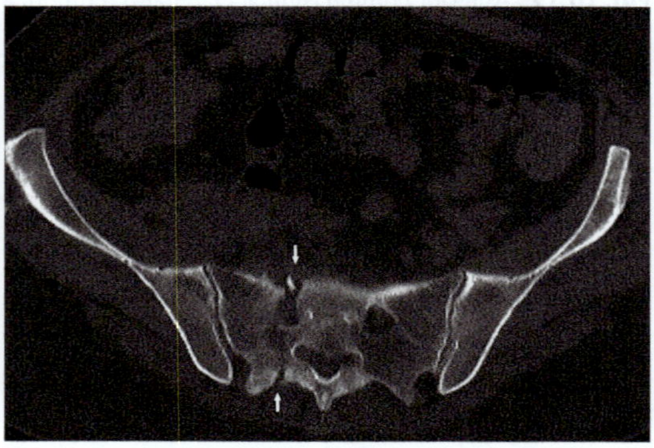

Fig. 10.15 Denis zone 2 right sacral fracture in a 47 year old. Axial CT image demonstrates mildly comminuted fracture of the right sacrum involving the S1 neuroforamen (arrows)

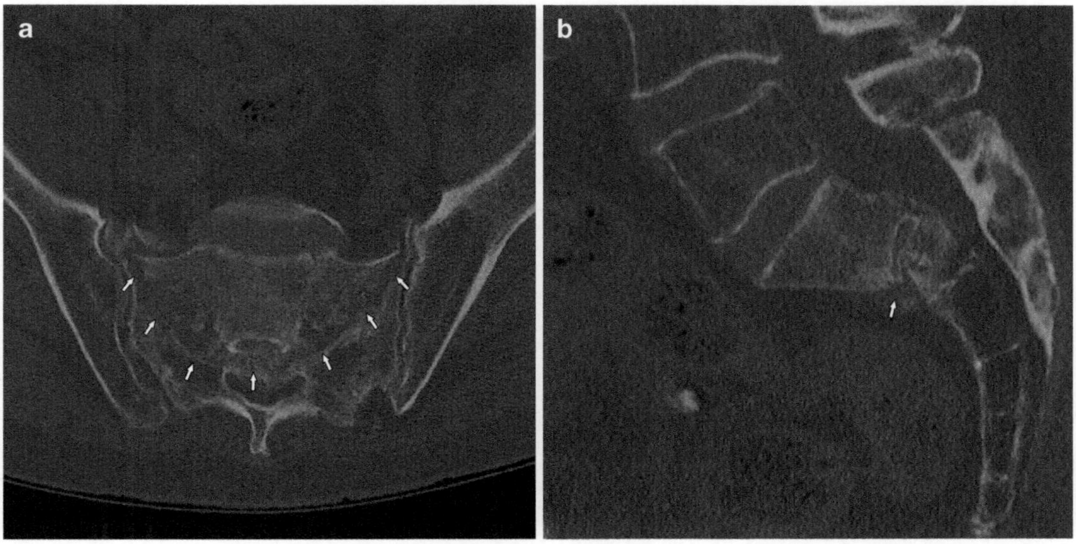

Fig. 10.16 Denis Zone 3 sacral fracture with U-shape in a 93 year old. (**a**) Axial CT image demonstrates U-shaped fracture of the sacrum (arrows). (**b**) Sagittal CT image demonstrates kyphotic angulation and mild anterior displacement at the level of the fracture (arrow)

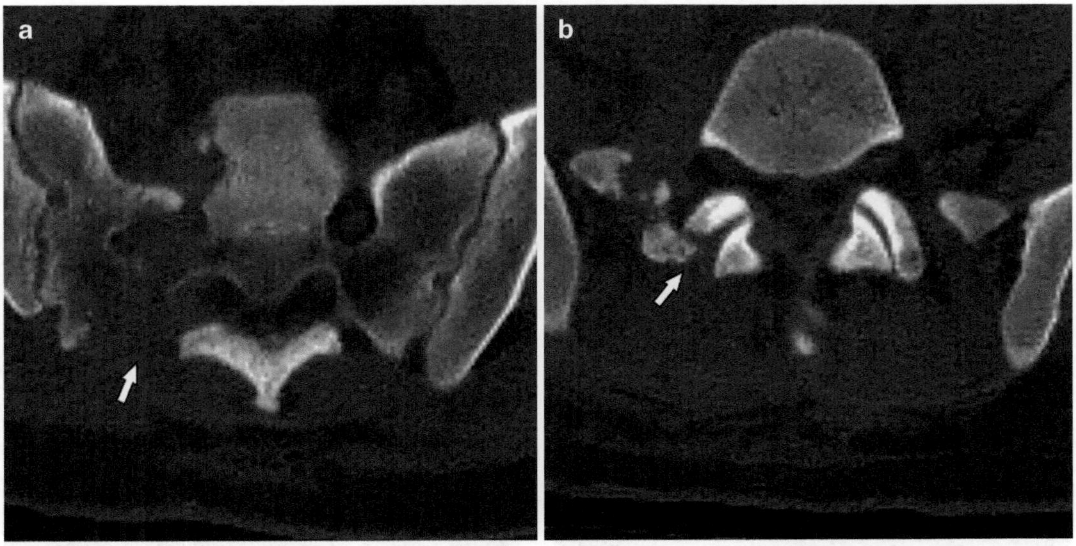

Fig. 10.17 Isler type 2 right sacral fracture in a 32 year old with extension into the neuroforamen and L5-S1 facet joint. (**a**) Axial CT image demonstrates right sacral fracture involving multiple neuroforamina (arrow). (**b**) Axial CT image at the level of the L5-S1 facet demonstrates extension of the comminuted sacral fracture into the L5-S1 facet joint (arrow)

[26]. See Fig. 10.17, for example, of an Isler type 2 sacral fracture.

Sacral fractures associated with pelvic ring injury are frequently categorized using the Letournel, Tile and AO-ASIF classification systems [26]. The letter of the alphabet (H, U, Lambda, or T) can also be used to describe sacral fractures (see Fig. 10.16, for example, of an U-shaped sacral fracture).

Hip Dislocation

Hip dislocations occur when the femoral head is abnormally forced outside of its normal concentric position within the acetabular socket. Posterior hip dislocation (Fig. 10.18) occurs when the femoral head is forced posteriorly and typically superolaterally upon comparison to the acetabulum [29]. Anterior hip dislocation (Fig. 10.19) occurs when the femoral head is forced anteriorly and typically inferomedially in relationship to the acetabulum (however, there are rare reports of anterior-superior hip dislocations) [29]. Posterior hip dislocation accounts for the majority of hip dislocations and it occurs typically due to abnormal force exerted on a flexed knee (such as in a dashboard injury) [29]. Multiple classification systems exist, including the Thompson-Epstein, Stewart-Milford, and Levin classification systems.

Hip dislocation can be noted on the initial CT scan of a patient after trauma. However, CT imaging is also frequently obtained after closed reduction. Post-reduction evaluation of the hip joint should include assessment for congruent alignment of the joint, femoral fractures (including osteochondral fractures, femoral head fractures, or femoral neck fractures), acetabular fracture (including presence of marginal impaction, medial wall involvement, and percentage of posterior wall involvement), intra-articular fracture fragments, or other soft tissue abnormalities [29]. Figure 10.20 demonstrates an intra-articular loose fracture fragment interposed between the femur and acetabulum after an unsuccessful attempt at closed reduction. Figure 10.21 demonstrates piriformis hematoma along the course of the expected sciatic nerve, which was contused upon surgical evaluation. For acetabular fractures, commenting on whether the percentage of posterior wall involvement is greater than or less than 20% may help guide management [29]. For femoral fractures, the Pipkin classification system discussed in the subsequent section can be used to categorize findings in the setting of hip dislocation [4, 29, 30]. Note that in the setting of an unsuccessful reduction, CT is limited in evaluation for displaced labral tear, displaced chondral fragments or capsular injury which may prevent adequate congruence of the joint during closed

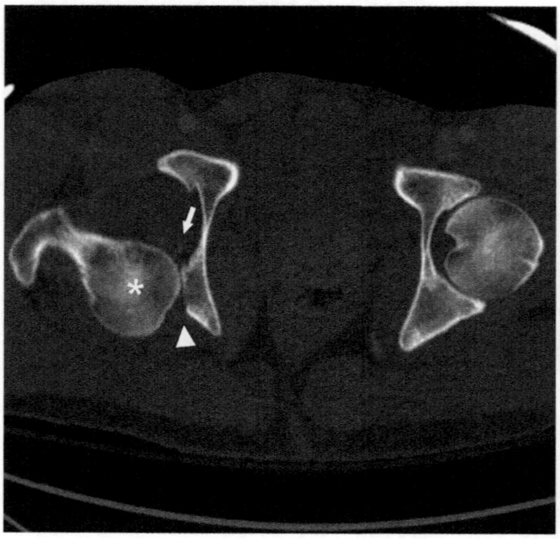

Fig. 10.18 Posterior hip dislocation in a 38 year old. Axial CT image demonstrates posterior dislocation of the femoral head (asterisk) of the right hip joint. Note associated osteochondral fracture of the femoral head and marginal impaction fracture of the posterior acetabulum (arrowhead). Note the subcentimeter intra-articular fracture fragments (arrow)

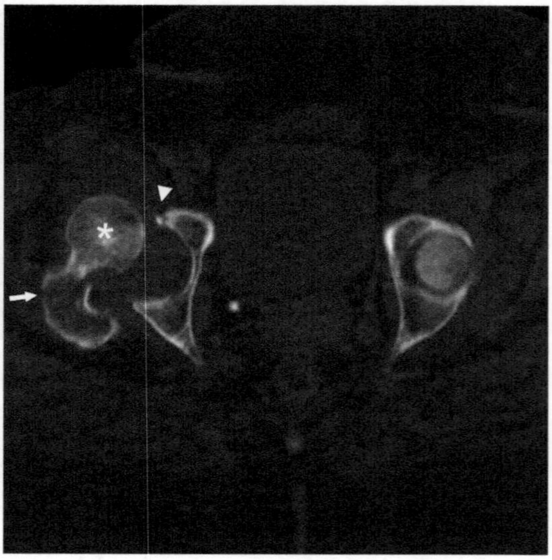

Fig. 10.19 Anterior hip dislocation in a 65 year old. Axial CT image demonstrates anterior dislocation of the right femoral head (asterisk) at the right hip joint. Note associated fractures of the acetabulum (arrowhead) and the greater trochanter (arrow)

reduction. Magnetic resonance imaging can be useful in these scenarios. Surgery and open reduction may be needed for management.

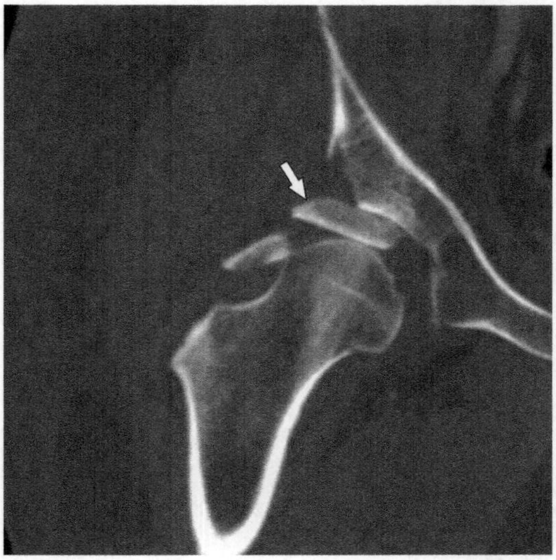

Fig. 10.20 Loose intra-articular fracture fragment in a 48 year old after attempted closed reduction for posterior hip dislocation. Coronal CT image demonstrates a displaced, intra-articular acetabular fracture fragment interposed between the femoral head and the acetabulum (arrow) which is interfering with adequate closed reduction

Proximal Femoral Fractures

CT scan of the pelvis should include the proximal femur from the femoral head to the subtrochanteric region such that the lesser trochanter is fully visualized. Femoral fractures can be divided into of the femoral head, femoral neck, intertrochanteric, and subtrochanteric fractures.

Fractures of the femoral head are intracapsular. Multiple classification systems exist. The Pipkin classification system is a commonly used categorization based on fracture location relative to the fovea/ligamentum teres insertion (type 1 is located caudal to the fovea and type 2 extends cranial to the fovea centralis), additional femoral neck fracture (type 3; Fig. 10.22), or additional acetabular fracture (type 4; Fig. 10.23) [30]. Pipkin type 3 is typically associated with worse prognosis. Presence of Pipkin type 3 fracture is a contraindication for closed reduction and requires open reduction due to risk of additional displacement of the femoral neck fracture and avascular necrosis. Osteochondral impaction fractures also occur in the femoral head and are frequently associated with hip dislocation.

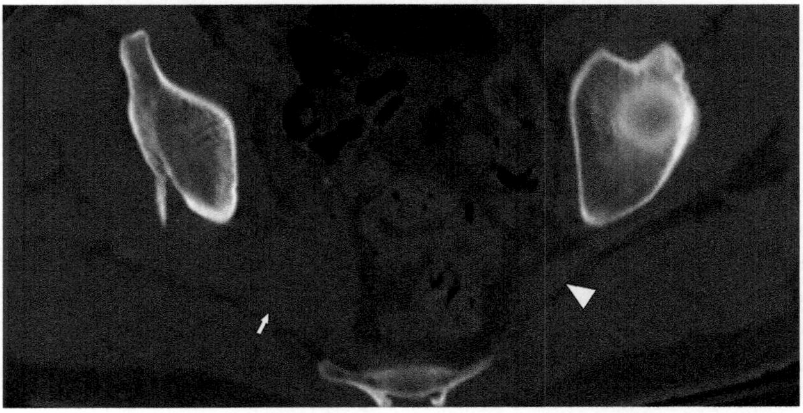

Fig. 10.21 Intramuscular hematoma of the right piriformis muscle in a 24-year-old patient with right posterior hip dislocation and acetabular fracture. Axial CT image demonstrates asymmetric enlargement and loss of definition of the right piriformis muscle (arrow) compared to the left piriformis muscle (arrowhead). An associated contusion of the right sciatic nerve was noted intraoperatively

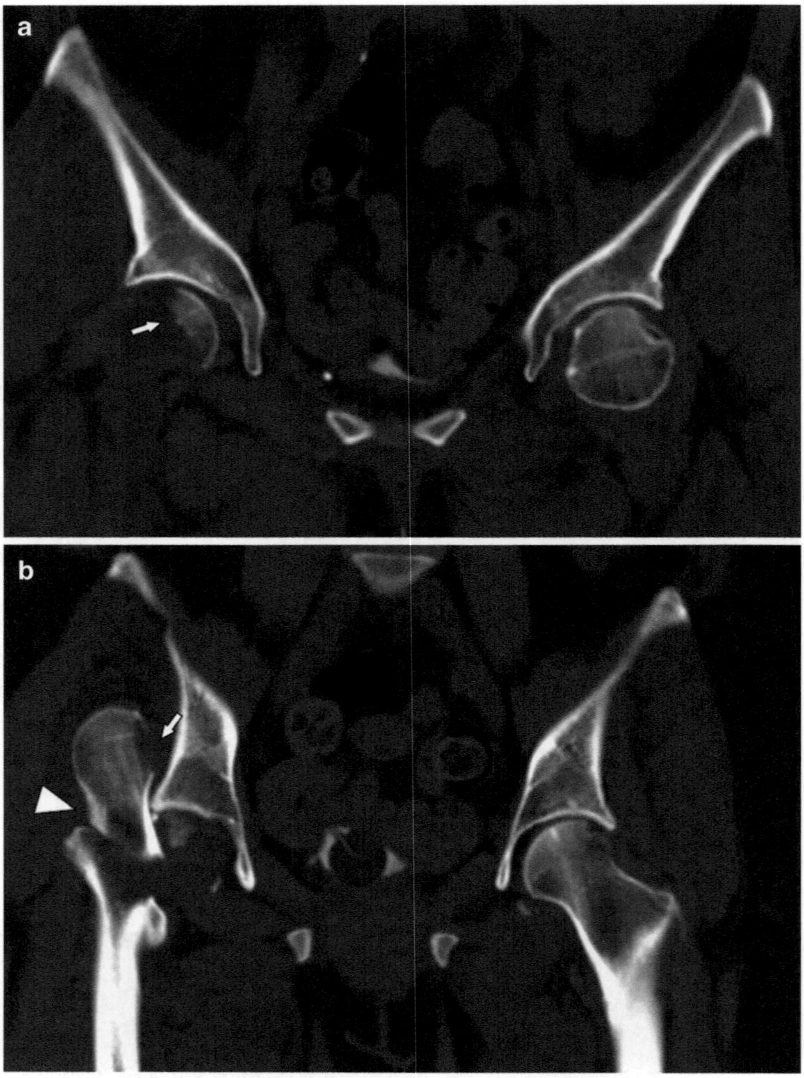

Fig. 10.22 Pipkin type 3 femoral head and neck fracture in a 58-year old patient with posterior hip dislocation. Coronal CT images of the pelvis from anterior (**a**) to posterior (**b**) demonstrate posterosuperior dislocation of the femur with displaced fracture of the femoral head (arrow) and displaced fracture of the femoral neck (arrowhead)

Femoral neck fractures can be described based on location as subcapital (Fig. 10.24), transcervical, and basicervical along the proximal to distal femoral neck. Subcapital and transcervical fractures are intracapsular and more likely to be associated with avascular necrosis. Basicervical fractures may be intracapsular or extracapsular and are less frequently associated with avascular necrosis. The Garden classification system and Pauwels classification system for subcapital femoral neck fractures can help guide management [4, 31, 32]. It is important to report the presence of incomplete fractures or displacement as this can guide management.

Intertrochanteric fractures are extracapsular and centered between the greater and lesser trochanters (Fig. 10.25). Multiple classification systems exist, including the Evans-Jensen classification system [33, 34]. It is important to report comminution, displacement, and/or extension to the greater trochanter, lesser trochanter, and subtrochanteric region.

Subtrochanteric fractures can be seen in the setting of trauma. However, fractures in this location can also result secondary to insufficiency, stress, or bisphosphonate medication. It is important to recognize incomplete fractures in this region to avoid risk of completion with continued

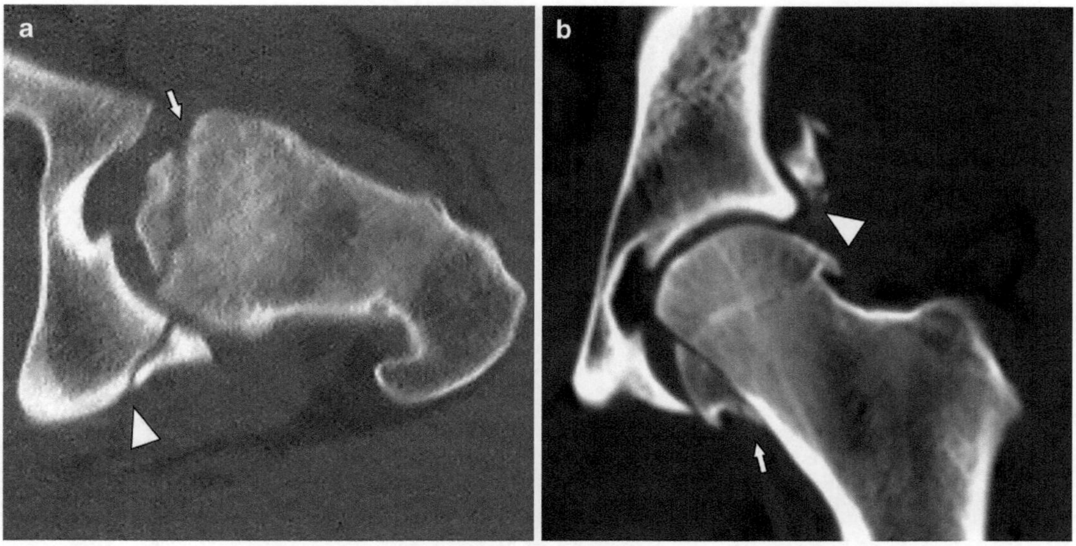

Fig. 10.23 Pipkin type 4 femoral head fracture with associated acetabular fracture in a 34 year old with posterior hip dislocation status post-reduction. (**a**) Axial and (**b**) coronal CT images demonstrate mildly displaced fracture of the femoral head located below the level of the fovea capitis/ligamentum teres insertion (arrow). Note the mildly displaced fracture of the posterior acetabulum (arrowhead)

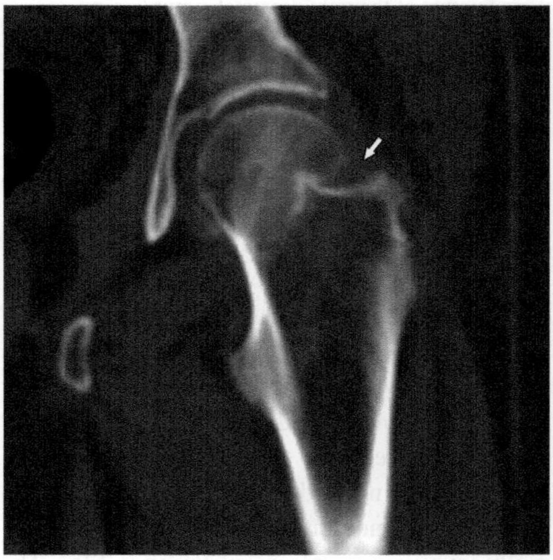

Fig. 10.24 Subcapital fracture in an 80 year old. Coronal CT image demonstrates an impacted, incomplete subcapital fracture of the left femur (arrow)

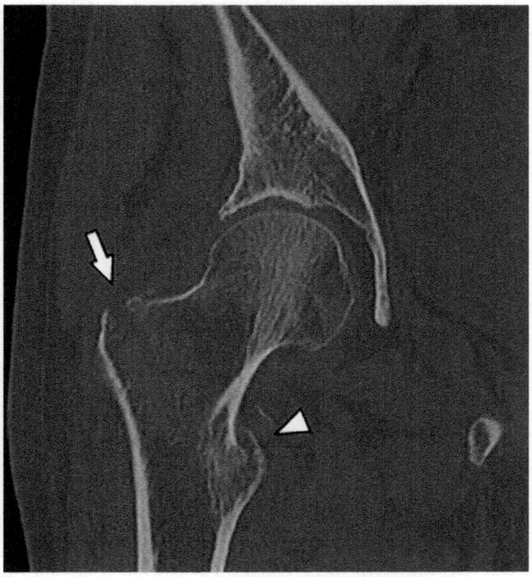

Fig. 10.25 Intertrochanteric fracture in a 74 year old. Coronal CT image of the right hip demonstrates mildly comminuted intertrochanteric fracture of the right femur with extension of the fracture line to the greater trochanter (arrow) and lesser trochanter (arrowhead)

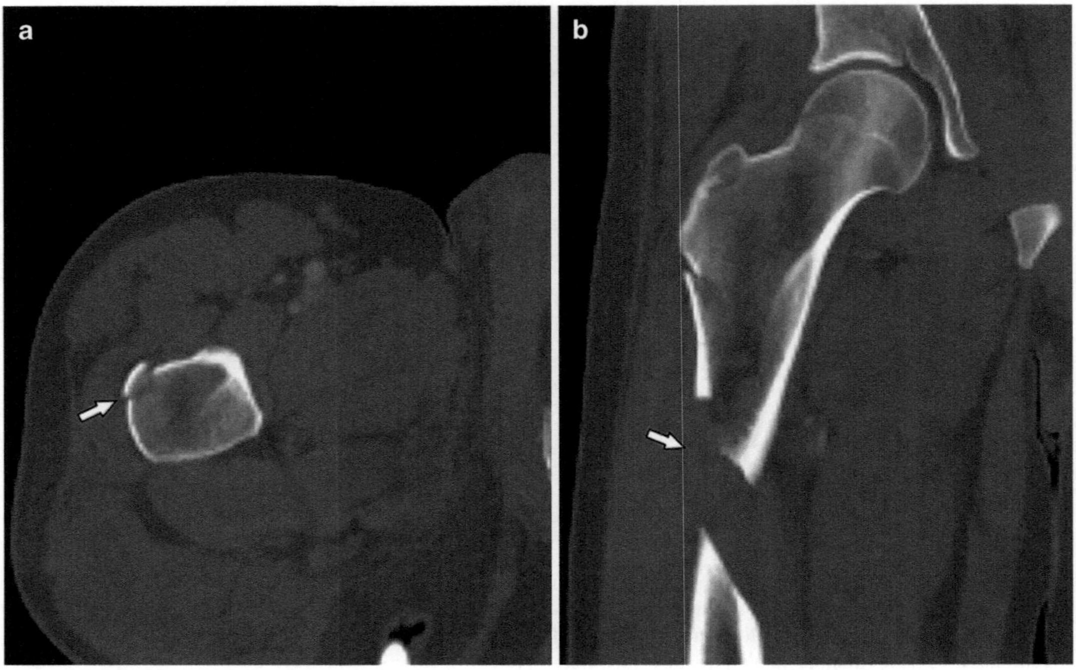

Fig. 10.26 Subtrochanteric fracture in a 43 year old after a motor vehicle collision. (**a**) Axial CT image and (**b**) coronal CT image demonstrate mildly comminuted, spiral subtrochanteric fracture of the right proximal femur (arrow)

weight-bearing. It is also important to evaluate the osseous structures on the most caudal images of the CT scan, as a subtrochanteric/proximal diaphyseal fracture may be partially visualized (Fig. 10.26).

Soft Tissues

The identification of soft tissue findings associated with pelvic trauma is important. Multiple soft tissue injuries can occur, including muscle/tendon strain, ligamentous sprain, hematomas, genitourinary injuries, and neurovascular injury. One noteworthy post-traumatic injury is a fascial closed degloving injury, also known as a Morel-Lavallee lesion (Fig. 10.27). These lesions result from a shearing force (such as from motor vehicle accident) causing abrupt separation of the skin/subcutaneous soft tissues from the underlying fascia [35]. Associated vascular and lymphatic injury results in a collection of blood, lymphatic fluid, and/or lobules of interspersed fat [35]. These lesions can occur in the greater trochanter, thigh, pelvis, gluteal, or lumbosacral regions [35]. On CT, these lesions appear as lentiform fluid collections/hematomas along the fascia with or without lobules of fat density [35]. Morel-Lavallee lesions occur due to shear injury along fascial planes and can present with slowly enlarging collections. These may encapsulate, become superinfected, and may not respond to conservative measures, often requiring minimally invasive or surgical intervention [35]. The presence of these lesions is also important to communication because it can affect surgical planning for the more acute underlying pelvic injury; some surgeons may prefer to avoid traversing this lesion due to possible risk of infection and poor wound healing [26].

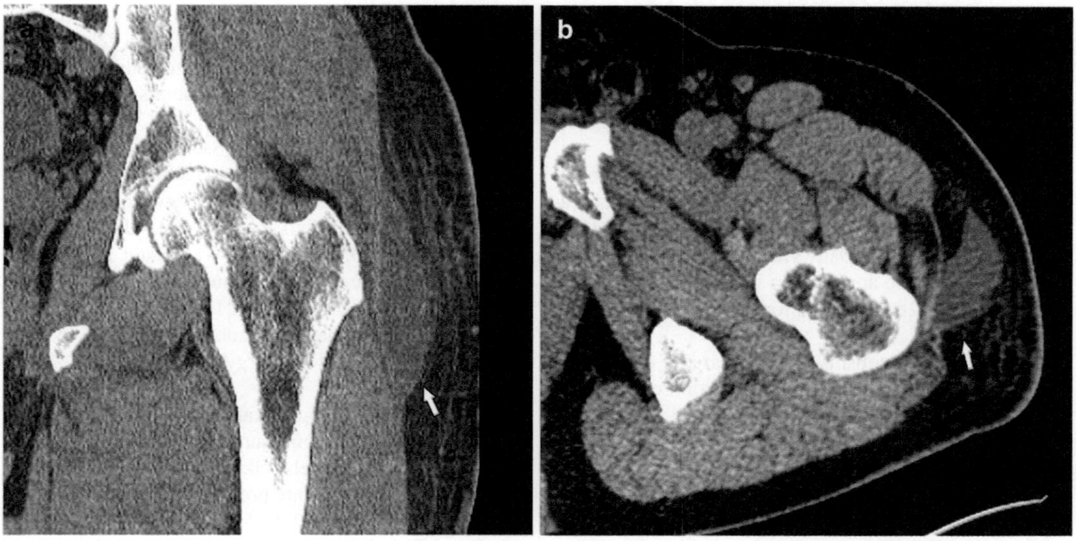

Fig. 10.27 Morel-Lavallee lesion in a 58-year-old patient with left lateral hip pain and ecchymosis status post-bike accident. (**a**) Coronal CT image and (**b**) axial CT image demonstrate 3.7 × 2.8 × 8.6 cm lentiform subcutaneous fluid collection (arrow) along the interface of the superficial fascia overlying the greater trochanter of the femur and subcutaneous fascia. There is surrounding soft tissue infiltration

References

1. Falchi M, Rollandi GA. CT of pelvic fractures. Eur J Radiol. 2004;50(1):96–105.
2. Khurana B, Sheehan SE, Sodickson AD, Weaver MJ. Pelvic ring fractures: what the orthopedic surgeon wants to know. Radiographics. 2014;34(5):1317–33.
3. Scheinfeld MH, Dym AA, Spektor M, Avery LL, Dym RJ, Amanatullah DF. Acetabular fractures: what radiologists should know and how 3D CT scan aid classification. Radiographics. 2015;35(2):555–77.
4. Sheehan SE, Shyu JY, Weaver MJ, Sodickson AD, Khurana B. Proximal femoral fractures: what the Orthopedic surgeon wants to know. Radiographics. 2015;35(5):1563–84.
5. Lee MJ, Wright A, Cline M, Mazza MB, Alves T, Chong S. Pelvic fractures and associated genitourinary and vascular injuries: a multisystem review of pelvic trauma. AJR Am J Roentgenol. 2019;213(6):1297–306.
6. Starks I, Frost A, Wall P, Lim J. Is a fracture of the transverse process of L5 a predictor of pelvic fracture instability? J Bone Joint Surg Br. 2011;93(7):967–9.
7. Kanesa-Thasan RM, Zoga AC, Meyers WC, Roedl JB. Postoperative MR imaging of the pubic symphysis and athletic Pubalgia. Magn Reson Imaging Clin N Am. 2022;30(4):689–702.
8. Omar IM, Zoga AC, Kavanagh EC, Koulouris G, Bergin D, Gopez AG, et al. Athletic pubalgia and "sports hernia": optimal MR imaging technique and findings. Radiographics. 2008;28(5):1415–38.
9. Mizrahi DJ, Poor AE, Meyers WC, Roedl JB, Zoga AC. Imaging of the pelvis and lower extremity: demystifying uncommon sources of pelvic pain. Radiol Clin N Am. 2018;56(6):983–95.
10. Leone E, Garipoli A, Ripani U, Lanzetti RM, Spoliti M, Creta D, et al. Imaging review of pelvic ring fractures and its complications in high-energy trauma. Diagnostics (Basel). 2022;12(2):384.
11. Ricci WM, Mehta S. Orthopaedic knowledge update: trauma. Wolters Kluwer; 2022. book
12. Raniga SB, Mittal AK, Bernstein M, Skalski MR, Al-Hadidi AM. Multidetector CT in vascular injuries resulting from pelvic fractures: a primer for diagnostic radiologists. Radiographics. 2019;39(7):2111–29.
13. Pennal GF, Tile M, Waddell JP, Garside H. Pelvic disruption: assessment and classification. Clin Orthop Relat Res. 1980;151:12–21.
14. Tile M. Acute pelvic fractures: I. Causation and classification. J Am Acad Orthop Surg. 1996;4(3):143–51.
15. Young JW, Burgess AR, Brumback RJ, Poka A. Pelvic fractures: value of plain radiography in early assessment and management. Radiology. 1986;160(2):445–51.
16. Burgess AR, Eastridge BJ, Young JW, Ellison TS, Ellison PS, Poka A, et al. Pelvic ring disruptions: effective classification system and treatment protocols. J Trauma. 1990;30(7):848–56.
17. Letournel E. Acetabulum fractures: classification and management. Clin Orthop Relat Res. 1980;151:81–106.
18. Meinberg EG, Agel J, Roberts CS, Karam MD, Kellam JF. Fracture and dislocation classification

Compendium-2018. J Orthop Trauma. 2018;32(Suppl 1):S1–170.
19. Harris JH, Lee JS, Coupe KJ, Trotscher T. Acetabular fractures revisited: part 1, redefinition of the Letournel anterior column. AJR Am J Roentgenol. 2004;182(6):1363–6.
20. Harris JH, Coupe KJ, Lee JS, Trotscher T. Acetabular fractures revisited: part 2, a new CT-based classification. AJR Am J Roentgenol. 2004;182(6):1367–75.
21. Bodanapally UK, Dattwyler M. Acetabular fractures: a stepwise approach to identification and classification on 2D computed tomography. Appl Radiol. 2019;48(4):17–24.
22. Durkee NJ, Jacobson J, Jamadar D, Karunakar MA, Morag Y, Hayes C. Classification of common acetabular fractures: radiographic and CT appearances. AJR Am J Roentgenol. 2006;187(4):915–25.
23. Giannoudis PV, Grotz MRW, Papakostidis C, Dinopoulos H. Operative treatment of displaced fractures of the acetabulum. A meta-analysis. J Bone Joint Surg Br. 2005;87(1):2–9.
24. Geijer M, El-Khoury GY. Imaging of the acetabulum in the era of multidetector computed tomography. Emerg Radiol. 2007;14(5):271–87.
25. Alton TB, Gee AO. Classifications in brief: letournel classification for acetabular fractures. Clin Orthop Relat Res. 2014;472(1):35–8.
26. Mehta S, Auerbach JD, Born CT, Chin KR. Sacral fractures. J Am Acad Orthop Surg. 2006;14(12):656–65.
27. Santolini E, Kanakaris NK, Giannoudis PV. Sacral fractures: issues, challenges, solutions. EFORT Open Rev. 2020;5(5):299–311.
28. Hak DJ, Baran S, Stahel P. Sacral fractures: current strategies in diagnosis and management. Orthopedics. 2009;32:10. orthosupersite.com/view.asp?rID=44034
29. Mandell JC, Marshall RA, Weaver MJ, Harris MB, Sodickson AD, Khurana B. Traumatic hip dislocation: what the orthopedic surgeon wants to know. Radiographics. 2017;37(7):2181–201.
30. Pipkin G. Treatment of grade IV fracture-dislocation of the hip. J Bone Joint Surg Am. 1957;39-A(5):1027–42. passim
31. Garden RS. Low-angle fixation in fractures of the femoral neck. J Bone Joint Surg. 1961;43-B(4):647–63.
32. Bartonícek J. Pauwels' classification of femoral neck fractures: correct interpretation of the original. J Orthop Trauma. 2001;15(5):358–60.
33. Evans EM. The treatment of trochanteric fractures of the femur. J Bone Joint Surg Br. 1949;31B(2):190–203.
34. Jensen JS. Classification of trochanteric fractures. Acta Orthop Scand. 1980;51(5):803–10.
35. Spain JA, Rheinboldt M, Parrish D, Rinker E. Morel-Lavallée injuries: a multimodality approach to imaging characteristics. Acad Radiol. 2017;24(2):220–5.

The Extremities

11

Elana B. Smith, Kyle Costenbader,
and David Dreizin

Abbreviations

3D	Three-dimensional
ABI	Ankle-brachial index
API	Arterial pressure index
AVF	Arteriovenous fistula
AVN	Avascular necrosis
CPR	Curved planar reformats
CT	Computed tomography
CTA	Computed tomography angiography
DSA	Digital subtraction angiogram
MIP	Maximum intensity projection
MPR	Multiplanar reformat
MRI	Magnetic resonance imaging
ORIF	Open reduction and internal fixation
PTFE	Polytetrafluoroethylene
TVS	Temporary vascular shunt
VR	Volume rendering

E. B. Smith (✉) · D. Dreizin
Trauma and Emergency Radiology, Department of Diagnostic Radiology and Nuclear Medicine, R Adams Cowley Shock Trauma Center, University of Maryland School of Medicine, Baltimore, MD, USA
e-mail: elana.smith@umm.edu

K. Costenbader
Department of Diagnostic Radiology and Nuclear Medicine, University of Maryland School of Medicine, Baltimore, MD, USA
e-mail: Kyle.Costenbader@umm.edu

Introduction

The clinical relevance of findings related to vascular and soft tissue injury stems from management principles with respect to the threatened and mangled extremity. An extremity with a vascular injury posing a risk for ischemia is considered *threatened* [1]. The term *mangled extremity* is used to describe a multisystem extremity injury with significant involvement of at least three of the following: soft tissue, nerves, vessels, and bones [2]. Management of multisystem extremity trauma is complex, potentially requiring a team of general, vascular, orthopedic, and plastic surgeons, in addition to interventional and diagnostic radiologists.

This chapter explores the clinical principles and imaging findings guiding osseous, neurovascular, and soft tissue injury management, the CT principles used to optimize scanning in the setting of extremity trauma, and the spectrum of traumatic and post-operative imaging findings associated with severe extremity injuries.

Extremity Trauma: An Overview

Long bone fractures can be described by their location (epiphysis, metaphysis, or diaphysis [proximal, middle, or distal third]), articular involvement, degree of comminution (simple, wedge, or comminuted/multifragmentary), and

F. Knollmann (ed.), *Trauma Computed Tomography*, https://doi.org/10.1007/978-3-031-45746-3_11

degree of displacement [3]. Open fractures are associated with soft tissue defects, allowing for communication with the environment, while closed fractures do not [4]. The degree of soft tissue injury and wound contamination associated with open fractures (which can be particularly severe in farm and industrial accidents) impacts clinical course and management, placing patients at an increased risk for compartment syndrome, soft tissue infection, and amputation [5, 6].

Vascular injuries may accompany extremity trauma and affect surgical management. This is a frequent imaging indication and a focus of this chapter. Although arterial injuries account for less than 1% of traumatic injuries, half of all arterial injuries are associated with extremity trauma, leading to increased morbidity, mortality, and amputation [7, 8]. The risk of associated arterial injuries varies by fracture site and injury type. For example, there is a less than 0.1% risk of arterial injury in closed long bone diaphysis fractures (Fig. 11.1), a 9% risk in open tibial fractures (Fig. 11.2), and an up to 60% risk of popliteal artery injury in the setting of knee dislocations (Fig. 11.3) [9–11]. Fractures on either side of a joint (i.e. floating joints) (Fig. 11.4) and trauma in the region of major neurovascular bundles (Fig. 11.5) also increase the risk of arterial injury [12].

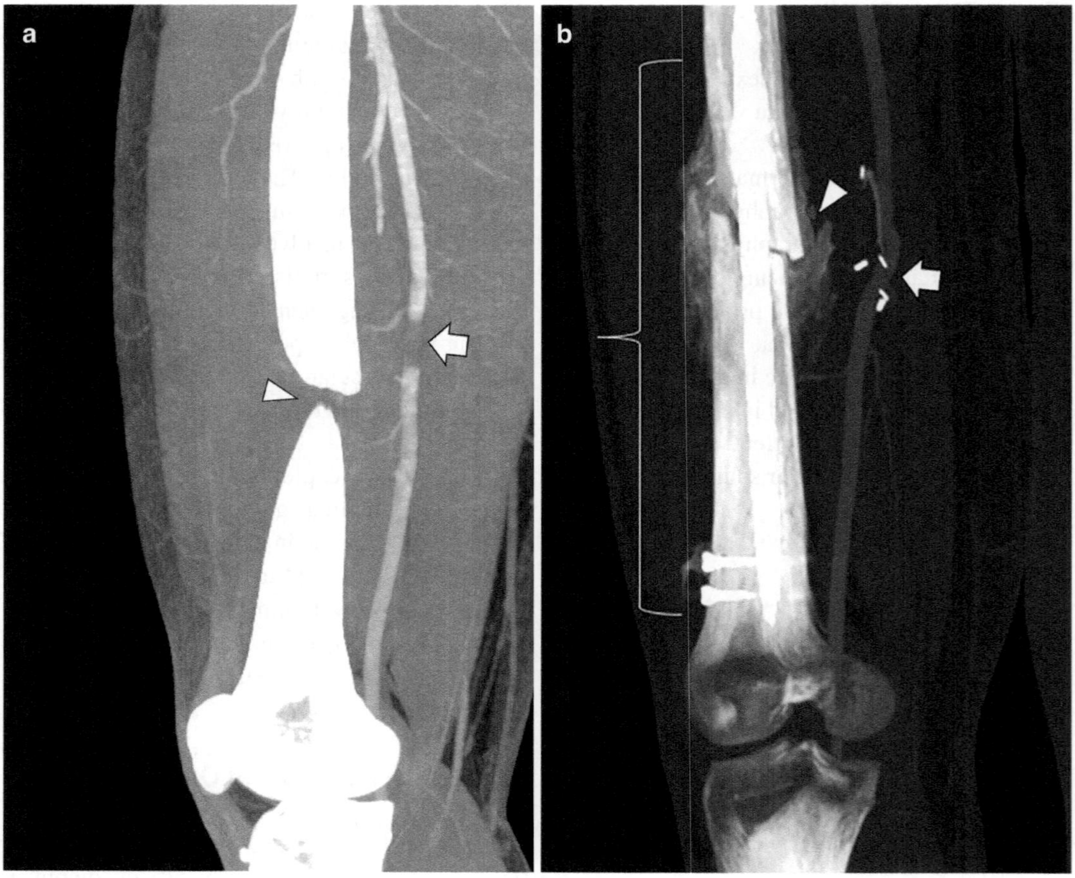

Fig. 11.1 Vascular injury in a closed femoral diaphysis fracture. Sagittal oblique CTA MIP image (**a**) demonstrates a short segment occlusion of the right superficial femoral artery (arrow, **a**) in a patient with a closed femoral diaphysis fracture (arrowhead, **a**) after being struck by a vehicle. The vascular injury was repaired with a reverse saphenous vein graft from the contralateral leg and the fracture was treated with open reduction and internal fixation. A coronal MIP image from a follow-up CTA (**b**) demonstrates the patent graft (arrow, **b**), intramedullary nail and screws (brace, **b**), and heterotopic bone formation (arrowhead, **b**)

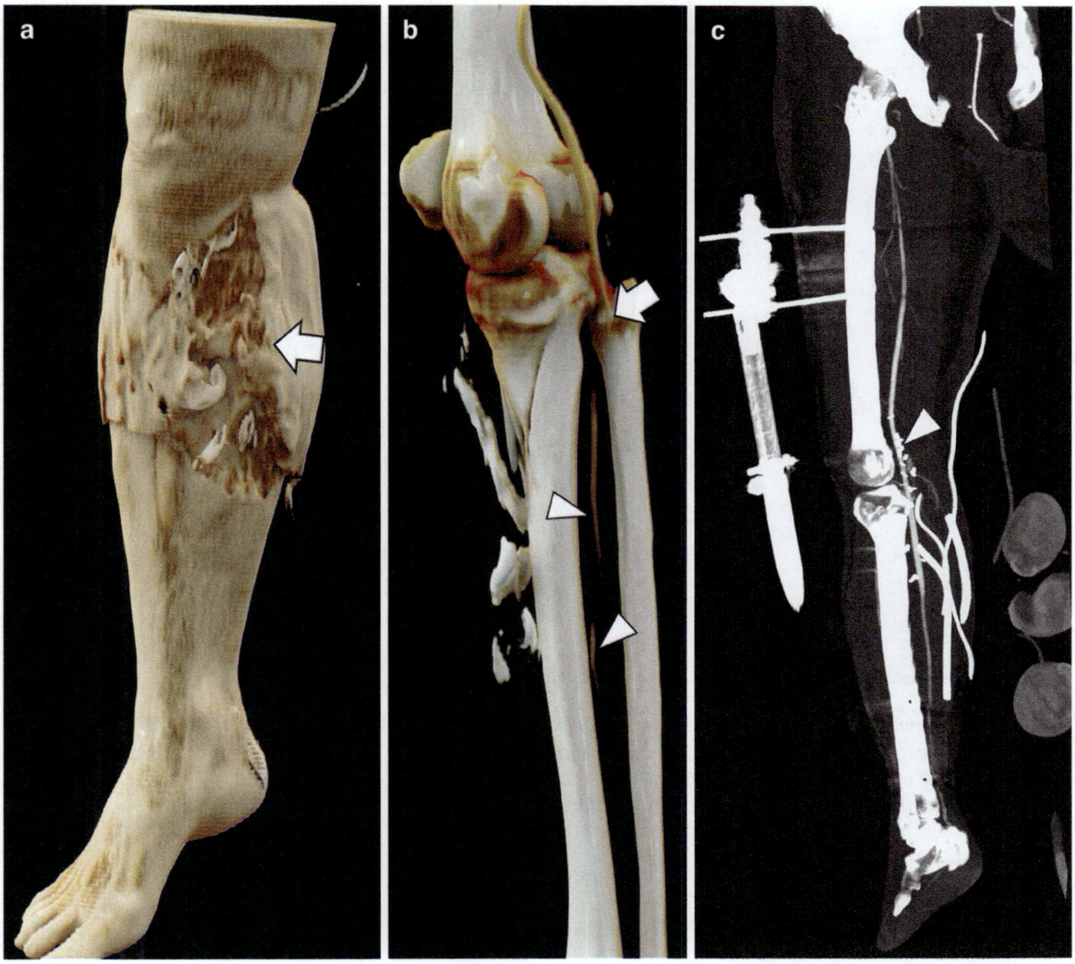

Fig. 11.2 Open tibial plateau fracture. Cinematic 3D volume rendered images of the lower extremity (**a**, **b**) demonstrate an anteromedial leg degloving injury (arrow, **a**), a trifurcation injury with cutoff at the distal popliteal artery (white arrow, **b**), and intermittent visualization of short segments of the posterior tibial artery (arrowhead, **b**). A patent reverse saphenous vein graft from the popliteal to the posterior tibial artery (arrowhead, **c**) is shown on a sagittal oblique MIP CTA image (**c**). Several months later, the graft became occluded

The Gustilo-Anderson Fracture Classification

The combination of osseous, soft tissue, and vascular injuries significantly impacts patient management [5, 6, 13]. The Gustilo-Anderson fracture classification system was developed to classify the mangled extremity, predict complications, and optimize treatment strategies. This system categorizes extremity injuries into three broad types, accounting for soft tissue and vascular injuries [6]. Type I fractures have subcentimeter wounds and limited contamination. Type II fractures are associated with a 1–10 cm soft tissue wound [6]. Type III fractures are the most severe and are further subdivided to account for the wide array of associated injuries and complications. Type IIIA includes fractures with soft tis-

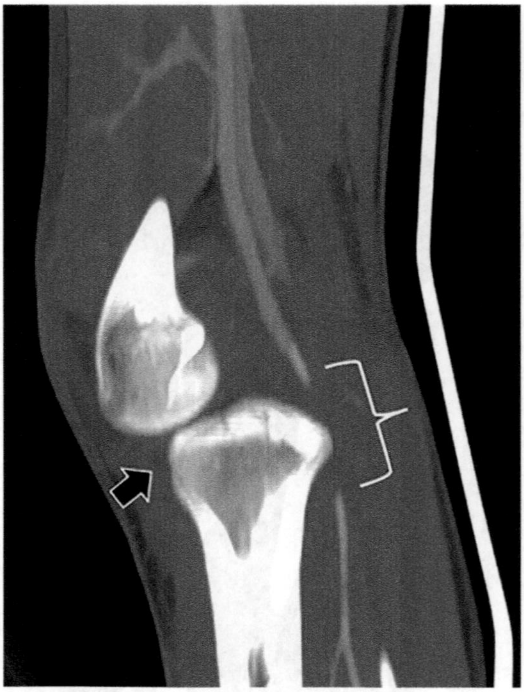

Fig. 11.3 Popliteal artery occlusion. Sagittal CTA through the knee shows a segmental popliteal artery occlusion (brace) associated with a posterior knee dislocation (arrow) after a motor vehicle collision. The popliteal artery injury was treated with a reverse saphenous vein graft and four-compartment fasciotomy

sue defects larger than 10 cm that still retain adequate soft tissue coverage, as well as farm-related injuries and gunshot wounds with smaller soft tissue defects [5, 14]. Type IIIB fractures are characterized by extensive soft tissue injury with massive contamination, periosteal stripping, and bony exposure [5, 14]. Type IIIC fractures are open fractures with concomitant arterial injuries requiring repair [5].

Owing to extensive soft tissue contamination, types IIIB and IIIC fractures are at particularly high risk for infection, nonunion, and delayed or impaired return of function that may require skin grafts or flaps, or secondary amputation [5, 6, 14]. In one study, all patients with type IIIC fractures developed complications, with 78% of patients ultimately requiring amputation (Fig. 11.6) [14].

Definitive classification used to guide treatment is best determined intraoperatively and should be based on injury mechanism and the overall appearance of the soft tissue envelope. However, CT plays a role in the initial evaluation, assessing for the extent of soft tissue injuries, localization of debris, and identification of associated arterial injuries [14].

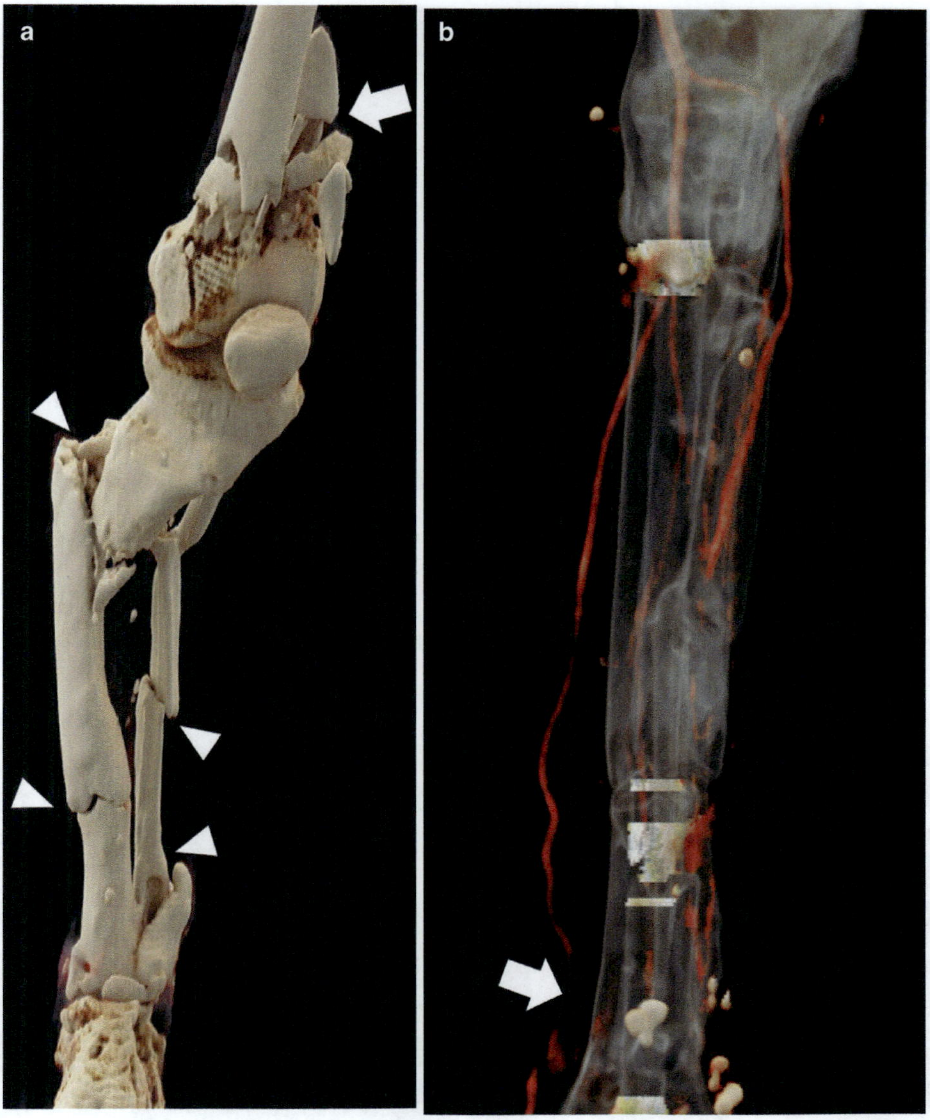

Fig. 11.4 Floating joint. Cinematic 3D volume rendered images of the left lower extremity from a patient involved in a motor vehicle collision show a comminuted fracture of the distal femur (arrow, **a**) and segmental fractures of the tibia and fibula (arrowheads, **a**) consistent with floating knee. There is single-vessel runoff from the posterior tibial artery (arrow, **b**). Nonunion resulted and amputation was considered; however, the patient suffered cardiac arrest prior to further management

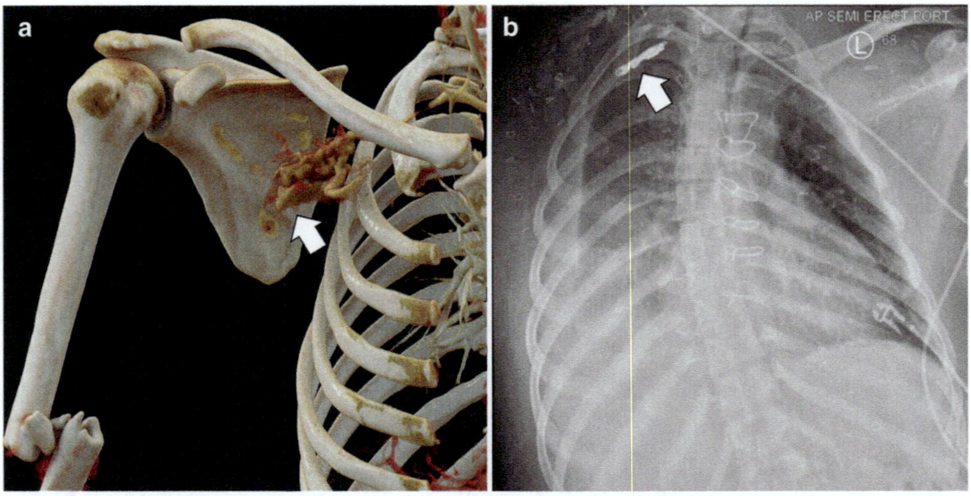

Fig. 11.5 Axillary artery pseudoaneurysm. Cinematic 3D volume rendered image of the right upper extremity (**a**) and AP chest radiograph (**b**) in a patient with right upper extremity injury and absent pulses following a motorcycle collision. There is an axillary artery pseudoaneurysm with active hemorrhage (arrow, **a**) and distal occlusion. At surgery, the brachial plexus was found to be avulsed. Amputation of the right upper extremity was required due to significant muscular ischemia from the injury and the right subclavian artery was coiled (arrow, **b**)

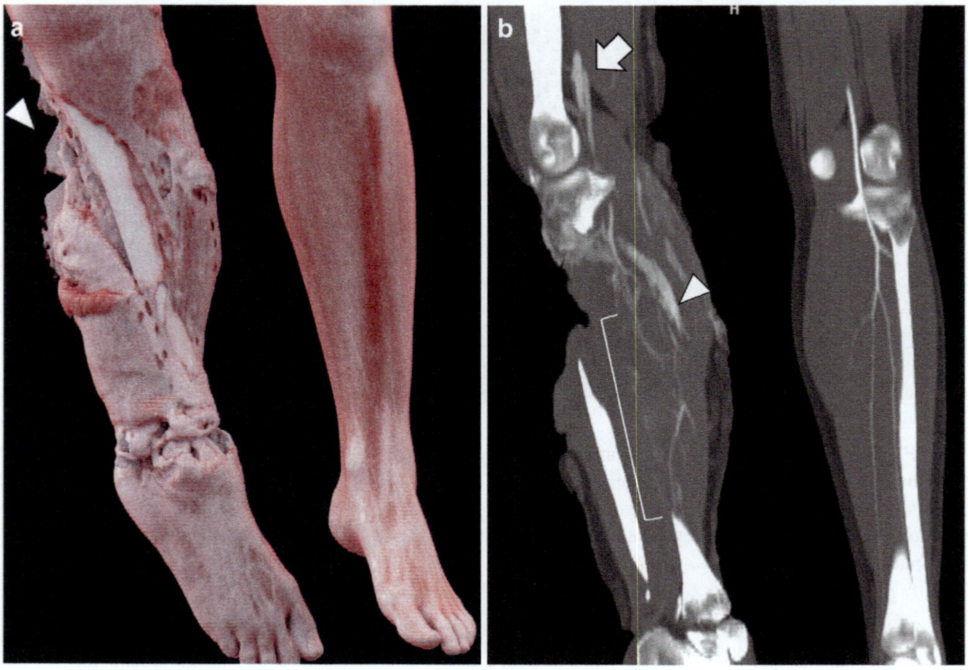

Fig. 11.6 Dysvascular injury requiring amputation. Type IIIC fracture in a pedestrian struck by a vehicle. A cinematic 3D volume rendered image (**a**) shows significant right lower extremity soft tissue defect with exposure of the underlying bone (arrowhead, **a**). Early venous filling in the thigh (arrow, **b**), active contrast extravasation (arrowhead, **b**), and lack of arterial enhancement below the knee (bracket, **b**) are demonstrated on a coronal MIP CTA image (**b**). The patient ultimately required a through-knee amputation due to the dysvascular nature of the injury

Imaging Extremity Injuries

Osseous Injuries

Fracture evaluation typically begins with radiographs, which are highly sensitive, cost-effective, and have superior spatial resolution when compared to CT [15]. While CT is often not necessary for fracture detection, it is frequently requested by orthopedic surgeons for operative planning. CT better visualizes fracture lines and the degree of comminution and displacement, which can predict complications [16]. In the proximal humerus, for instance, non-comminuted fractures can be managed conservatively, while four-part fractures require surgery to minimize the risk of avascular necrosis (AVN), pain, and disability [17]. CT can improve the detection of fracture lucencies through the medial aspect of the proximal metaphysis, which also increases the risk for AVN [17]. In the setting of hip dislocations, CT can determine if an associated femoral head fracture extends superior to fovea centralis, a risk factor for AVN requiring open reduction and internal fixation (ORIF) [18]. In the femoral neck, CT improves detection of posteromedial comminution and better depicts fractures that extend through the head–neck junction, another risk factor for AVN [18]. Preoperative CT is also used to identify large bone defects, for which bone grafting may be required [19].

To detect clinically suspected, radiographically occult fractures, magnetic resonance imaging (MRI) is considered the gold standard. If MRI is not readily available, dual-energy CT (DECT) techniques can be used to improve fracture detection using calcium and virtual noncalcium images to generate bone marrow edema color maps (Fig. 11.7) [20]. A meta-analysis by Wilson et al. demonstrated a very high sensitivity and specificity for the detection of bone marrow edema using this technique [21]. Although there are some limitations based on injury location, particularly in the foot and ankle, DECT can potentially eliminate the additional time and cost of an MRI if a CT has already been obtained through the area of interest [21–23].

Vascular Injuries

CTA plays a key role in the diagnosis of vascular injuries and management of complex extremity fractures. Most patients with hard signs of arterial occlusion—pulselessness, pallor, paresthesias, pain, paralysis, and a cool blue extremity—will go to surgery without preoperative imaging [12, 13, 24]. Patients with hard signs such as a palpable thrill, audible bruit, or presumed arteriovenous fistula (AVF) may benefit from preoperative imaging to aid in surgical planning [24].

Soft signs of vascular trauma include hemorrhage, asymmetrically decreased pulse amplitude, wound trajectories less than 5 mm from a vessel, and neurological symptoms and are associated with a 3–25% risk of vascular injuries on CTA [25, 26]. Patients with soft signs are screened for vascular injury with ankle-brachial index (ABI) or arterial pressure index (API) [12, 27, 28]. The ABI is the ratio between the peak ankle and brachial artery systolic pressure [28], while the API compares the systolic blood pressure in the injured ankle or wrist to the contralateral limb [12]. Patients without hard signs of arterial injury and an ABI or API $\geq$0.9 can be observed, while those with an ABI or API <0.9 will benefit from CTA [29, 30]. Recent studies support decreasing the ABI threshold to 0.6 [28] and 0.7 [31] in blunt and penetrating lower extremity trauma, respectively. While this potentially would allow for a decrease in the amount of imaging performed, there has not been widespread adoption of these lower thresholds.

The use of hard and soft signs of vascular injury to stratify the need for CTA had been an integral part of the clinical evaluation prior to the ubiquitous availability of CT. Today, however, patients with hard signs may undergo extremity CTA for surgical planning in order to reduce operative time and unnecessary exploration [32]. In patients with a radial or ulnar artery injury, for instance, CTA can serve as an imaging analog to the Allen test to assess arterial flow to the hand [33]. A complete palmar arch suggests that ligation of the distal radial or ulnar artery will be well-tolerated, while arterial repair may be nec-

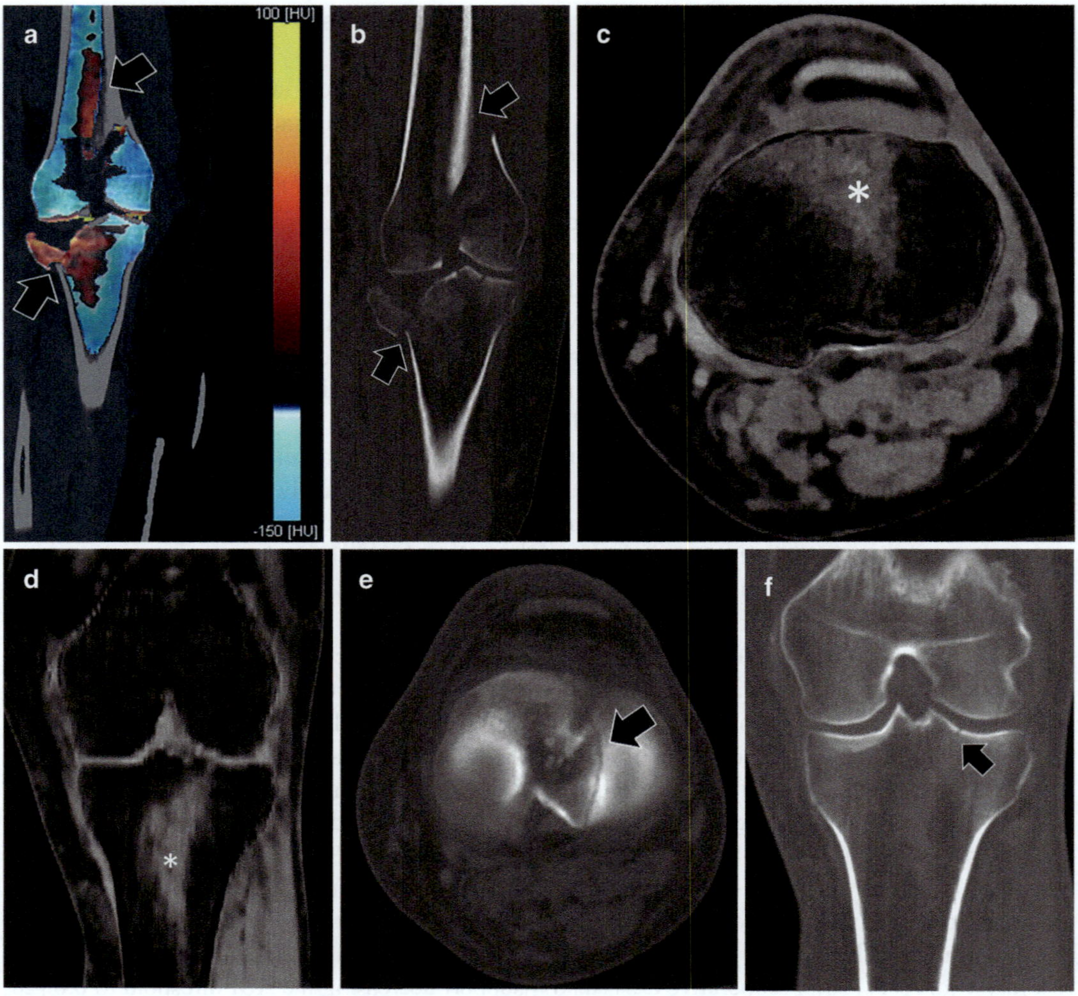

Fig. 11.7 Bone marrow edema detection using dual-energy CT technique. Post-processed bone marrow edema map illustrating edema in the distal femur and lateral tibial plateau (arrows, **a**) related to associated fractures shown on a coronal CT image (arrows, **b**) following a motor vehicle accident. Axial and coronal calcium-suppressed images show areas of marrow edema (asterisks, **c** and **d**) surrounding a nondisplaced lateral tibial plateau fracture (arrows, **e** and **f**) in a different patient who sustained a fall

essary to maintain distal blood flow in the setting of an incomplete arch [34].

Patients who have no hard or soft signs may be scanned to decrease the risk of missing a clinically occult injury. For instance, 60% of patients with significant axillosubclavian artery injuries requiring repair may have normal pulses due to collaterals [35, 36]. At level 1 trauma centers, where most polytrauma patients with shock undergo CT, an extremity CTA can easily be added to a whole-body CT, saving time, avoiding the need for an additional contrast bolus, and providing improved definition and scope of injury (Fig. 11.8) [37, 38].

In a meta-analysis, Patterson et al. found that CTA is 95–100% sensitive and 87–99% specific in detecting blunt and penetrating traumatic peripheral arterial injury [39]. CTA has high accuracy rates, low rates of nondiagnosis, and excellent inter-observer agreement [40]. Advantages over conventional angiogram include noninvasive three-dimensional (3D) assessment

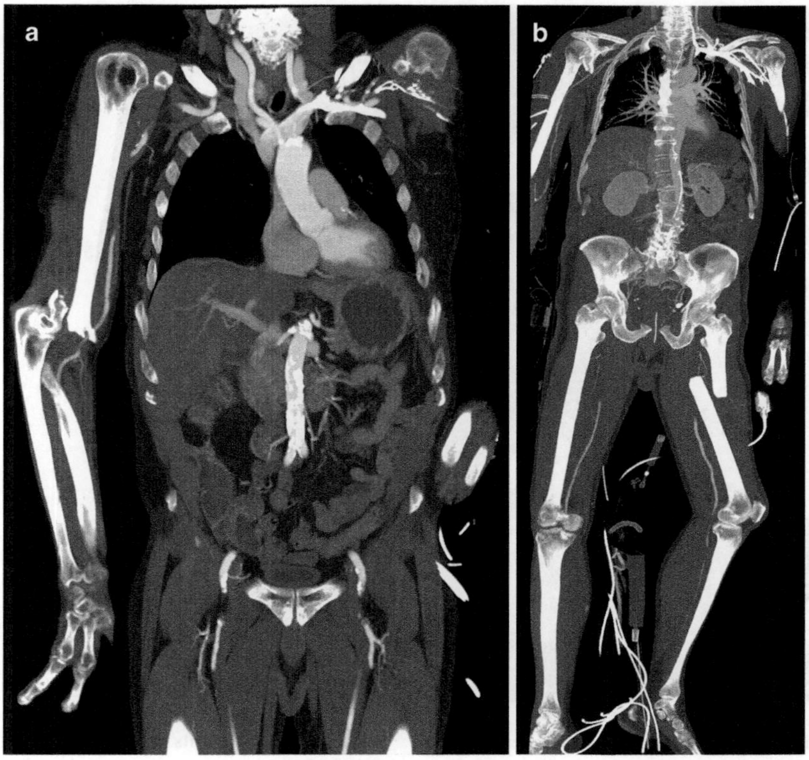

Fig. 11.8 Whole-body CT with runoff. Whole-body coronal MIP CTA image with concurrently obtained upper (**a**) and lower (**b**) extremity runoffs, performed using a single contrast bolus

of vasculature, characterization of concomitant soft tissue and osseous injuries and their relationship to vascular injuries, and rapid acquisition time [41]. A normal CTA essentially excludes the need for surgical or endovascular intervention due to its high negative predictive value [42]. Additionally, CTA can aid in triaging clinically occult findings, such as sub-5 mm vascular lesions or injuries with small intimal flaps, which can be observed for signs of ischemia or hemorrhage (Fig. 11.9) [8, 13, 42].

Following the acute management of life and limb-threatening injuries, patients may require soft tissue reconstruction with a free or pedicled flaps or grafts [43]. Prior to a flap reconstruction, many surgeons will request a preoperative CTA to assess the vascular pedicle or recipient vessels, confirming they lie outside the zone of injury to reduce the risk of complications [19, 44, 45].

Technical Considerations

Contrast Bolus Timing

The utility of a CTA is predicated on the performance of a high-quality exam. Optimal contrast bolus timing for extremity CTAs is critically important; a suboptimally timed contrast bolus may lead to nondiagnosis of vascular injuries and distal arterial injuries may be missed if the scanner outruns the bolus.

Arterial phase enhancement may be achieved with fixed time delays, bolus tracking, or a test bolus [46]. With a fixed time delay, a scan is performed at a designated time following the contrast injection [46]. While studies have shown low rates of nondiagnosis using this technique, it cannot account for hemodynamic variability between patients and is generally not well suited to today's faster CT scanners, unless the table speed is decreased [47, 48].

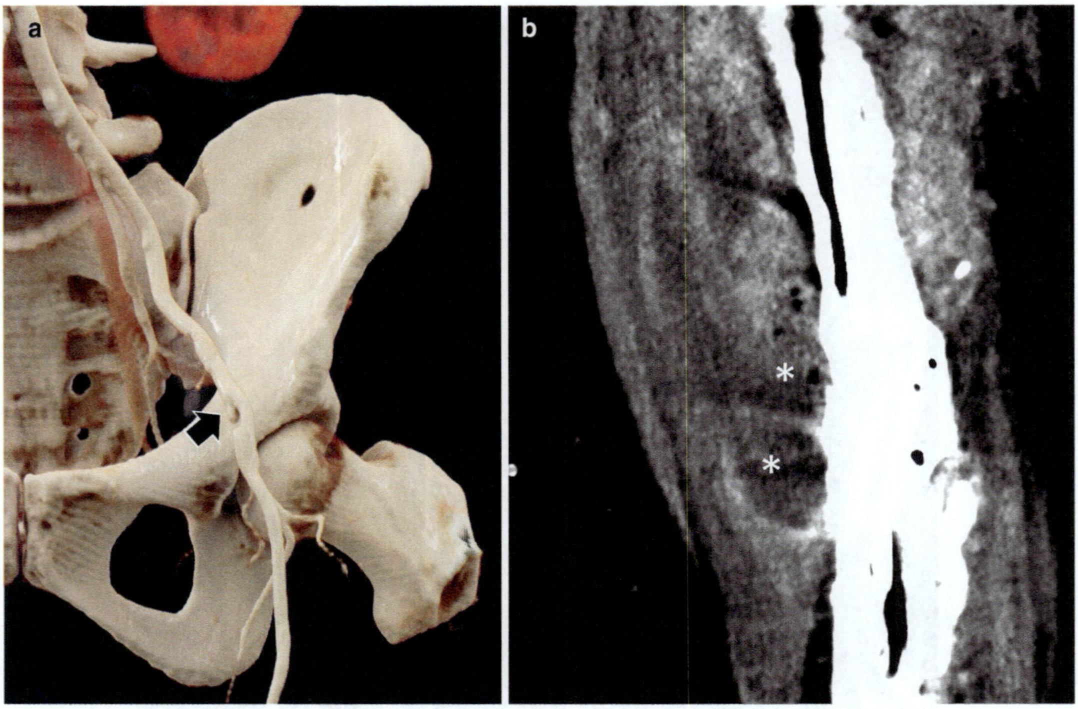

Fig. 11.9 Conservatively managed pseudoaneurysm. An asymptomatic left common femoral artery pseudoaneurysm is seen on cinematic 3D volume rendered CT (arrow, **a**) in a patient sustaining a ground level fall with a subtrochanteric fracture. The vascular injury was managed conservatively, owing to its small size. The patient underwent ORIF, after which the patient developed a complex multiloculated fluid and gas collection in the left thigh (asterisks, **b**), suspicious for superinfected hematoma, as shown on sagittal CTA (**b**)

In bolus tracking, a region of interest (ROI) is placed over a target vessel on a noncontrast image. Low-dose scans follow the contrast bolus injection, triggering a full scan after a predetermined Hounsfield unit is reached [46, 49]. With a test bolus, a small volume of contrast is injected and a major artery just proximal to the level of suspected injury is selected. A time-enhancement curve is plotted to determine the time to peak enhancement, to which a 5–8 s delay is added prior to the start of the scan [49, 50]. Compared to bolus tracking, more contrast medium is used with a test bolus technique and has the disadvantage of early enhancement of other organs [48].

At the authors' institution, extremity CTAs are often performed concurrently with the whole-body CT, using bolus tracking following a single contrast bolus injected at a rate of 5 mL/s. As modern scanners frequently outrun the bolus, delayed images through the distal extremities are acquired at the discretion of the technologist (Fig. 11.10) [32, 51].

Venous injuries frequently accompany arterial injuries and may go undetected if venous phase imaging is not performed [32, 52]. If there is specific concern requiring the visualization of a venous injury, venous phase imaging can be considered [25, 32]. Although not routinely performed at the authors' institution, delayed phase scanning (5–7 min post-injection) may be useful in differentiating between active hemorrhage and pseudoaneurysm, particularly in hypotensive or unstable patients in whom the transit of contrast may be delayed [53].

In the trauma setting, the inclusion of noncontrast images is not typically necessary for an extremity CTA, as it serves to increase the radiation dose without improving the diagnostic yield [25]. When dual-energy techniques are employed, virtual noncontrast CT images could alternatively be used to problem solve (Fig. 11.11).

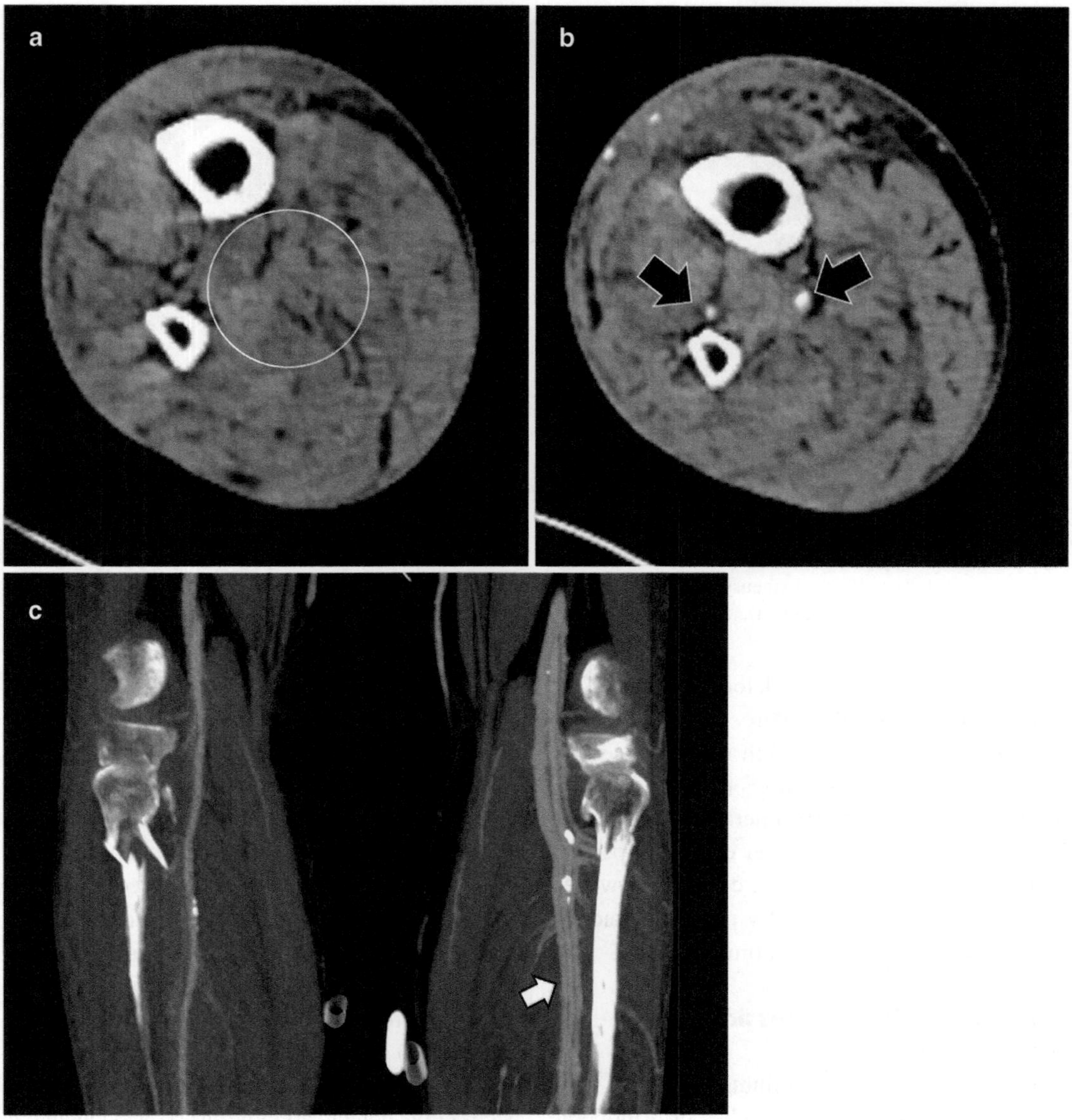

Fig. 11.10 Contrast bolus timing and hyperemia. Axial CTA images (**a**, **b**) of the right lower extremity in a patient with bilateral tibia and fibula fractures. There is nonenhancement of the right lower leg arteries on the arterial phase (circle, **a**) which opacify when this region was rescanned 60 s later (arrows, **b**). Early venous filling of the left leg is seen on a follow-up coronal CTA MIP image (arrow, **c**). The patient had a normal pulse exam and these findings were attributed to hyperemia

Intravenous Access

The location of a patient's intravenous (IV) access should be assessed prior to performing an extremity CTA. Intravenous contrast should not be administered through an IV in an injured extremity as the presence of a vascular injury may lead to contrast extravasation, increasing the risk for compartment syndrome [25]. There is also a risk of nondiagnosis resulting from beam hardening artifact from the dense contrast bolus that can obscure arterial injuries [25].

Obtaining vascular access in hypotensive trauma patients can be challenging. If adequate peripheral IV access cannot be obtained, a patient's only vascular access may be through an introducer sheath, for which safety for power

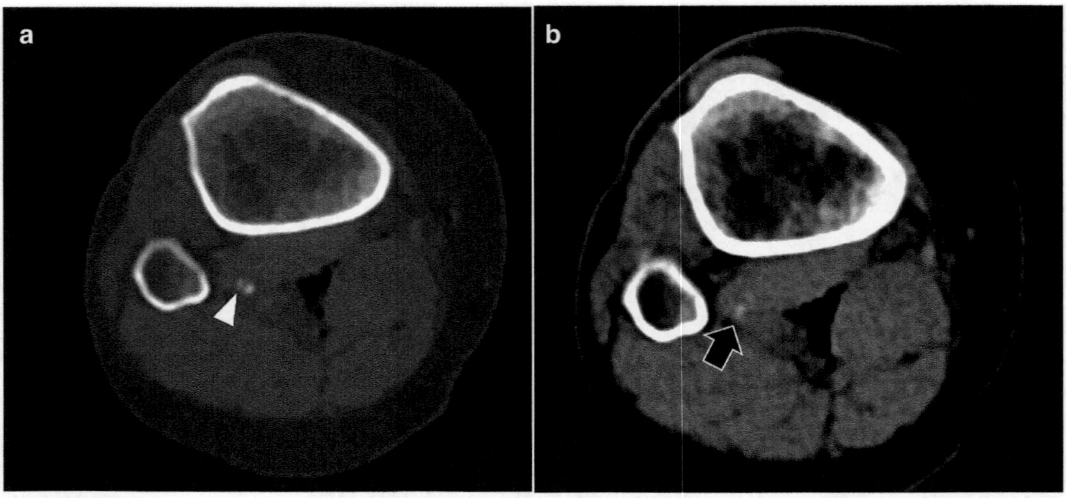

Fig. 11.11 Virtual noncontrast imaging. Following a right lower extremity gunshot wound, an axial CTA image shows a suspected small pseudoaneurysm arising from the tibioperoneal trunk (arrowhead, **a**). This study was performed using dual energy and on the virtual noncontrast axial CT image, a small hyperdensity is present in this region (arrow, **b**) compatible with a calcification, rather than a pseudoaneurysm

injections has not yet been determined [54]. Due to concerns for sheath rupture, leak, and migration, power injections through these devices are prohibited at many institutions [54]. If an appropriate upper extremity peripheral IV or a central line cannot be placed, a lower extremity peripheral IV may be used to inject contrast, however, as CT protocols are generally not optimized for this, the study may not be optimally timed.

Artifacts and Post-processing Techniques

Streak artifact from comminuted fracture fragments and metallic foreign bodies or orthopedic hardware can limit evaluation, although this may be somewhat mitigated with DECT techniques [8, 55]. To decrease perivenous streak artifact from the contrast bolus, a small bolus of saline should immediately follow the contrast injection [55]. To reduce motion artifact, extremities should be immobilized if the patient is unable to remain still during the exam [50, 51, 55].

Although not always feasible in the upper extremities, CTAs performed for unilateral lower extremity injury should always include the contralateral lower extremity. This allows for the assessment of anatomic variants and can differentiate outpacing the contrast bolus from true pathology [56]. In the upper extremities, the arms should be placed overhead, palms up with fingers extended. If the arms cannot be raised, the patient can be scanned with the arms and palms down [38]. If performed as part of a single bolus whole-body CT, the arm can be placed on a pillow resting on the torso to reduce the effect of streak artifact on thoracoabdominal structures [57].

The creation of multiplanar reformats (MPR), curved planar reformats (CPR), maximum intensity projections (MIPs), and volume rendered (VR) images should be routinely used in conjunction with source images to efficiently and accurately detect abnormalities and visualize anatomic relationships [55]. At the authors' institution, MIPs are routinely provided by the technologists for all extremity CTAs. Three-dimensional reconstructions for fracture visualization are created and sent to PACS by the technologists at the request of the ordering physicians for operative planning. Radiologists also routinely create and manipulate MIP, CPR, and VR images from the source data using the PACS system and post-processing software contemporaneously during initial image interpretation.

Bone removal, atherosclerotic plaque removal, and the creation of iodine maps and virtual noncontrast images using dual-energy techniques can aid in detection of vascular abnormalities (see Fig. 11.11) [55, 58]. Dual-energy post-processing can also be useful in differentiating a focus of contrast extravasation or pseudoaneurysm from an adjacent bony fragment or foreign body [38]. As mentioned previously, post-processing software can also be used to aid in the detection of radiographically occult fractures on DECT scans. At the authors' institution, these dual-energy post-processing techniques are not routinely included in extremity CTAs, but can be created as needed.

Imaging Findings: Vascular Injury

Direct signs of vascular injury on CTA include occlusive and non-occlusive thrombus, active contrast extravasation, pseudoaneurysm, and early proximal venous opacification from an AVF (Figs. 11.12, 11.13, and 11.14) [50, 59].

Post-traumatic vascular occlusion may result from in situ thrombus secondary to intimal injury or embolization from a proximal source (see Figs. 11.12 and 11.15) [25]. On imaging, an AVF appears as a direct venous connection to a single vein with early venous enhancement (see Fig. 11.14) [38]. Venous density approaching that of the adjacent artery favors an AVF, while a more diffuse pattern of venous enhancement may be seen in traumatic hyperemia (see Fig. 11.10c). Differentiating between these entities can be challenging and may require ultrasound or diagnostic angiogram for definitive diagnosis [25, 38, 60].

Blunt trauma frequently results in intimal injuries, arterial dissection, or partial occlusion, while penetrating trauma often leads to active hemorrhage [37, 41, 61, 62]. Active contrast extravasation results from focal or circumferential disruption of all the vessel walls (see Fig. 11.6b). Focal disruptions (i.e. lacerations) may also appear as a segmental occlusion (see Fig. 11.12), while transections (circumferential disruptions) may show a vascular cutoff with surrounding hematoma [25]. Segmental injuries less than 2 cm in length can be treated with primary or endovascular repair (Fig. 11.15), while longer

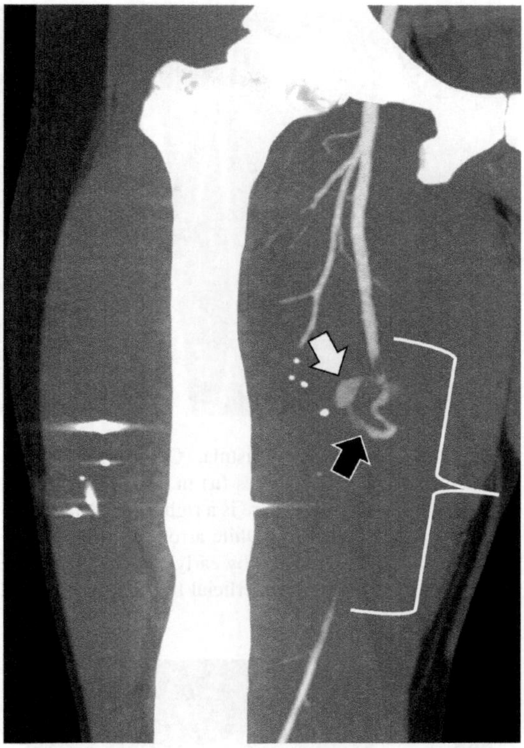

Fig. 11.12 Active bleeding and segmental occlusion. A coronal MIP CTA image of the right lower extremity following a gunshot wound to the right lower extremity shows a pseudoaneurysm (white arrow) with active contrast extravasation from the right superficial femoral artery (black arrow) and segmental occlusion (brace). These injuries were treated with an interposition graft and fasciotomies

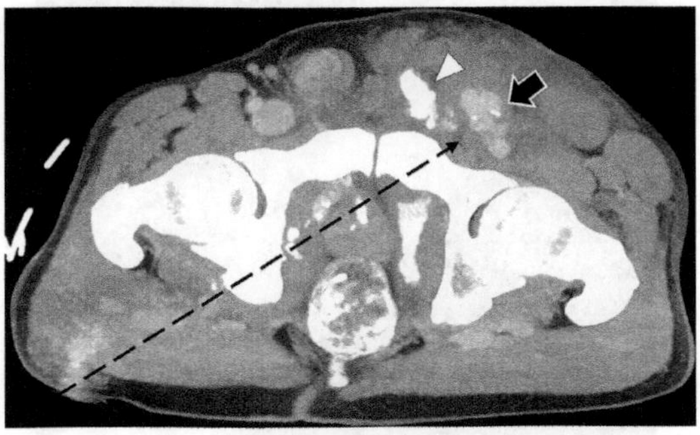

Fig. 11.13 Pseudoaneurysm. An axial MIP CTA image demonstrates a ballistic course extending from the right gluteal region, ultimately terminating in the left lower extremity (black dashed arrow). The injury resulted in a large, multilobulated left common femoral artery pseudoaneurysm (arrow). Adjacent dense contrast extravasation (arrowhead) is related to an associated extraperitoneal bladder rupture (not shown)

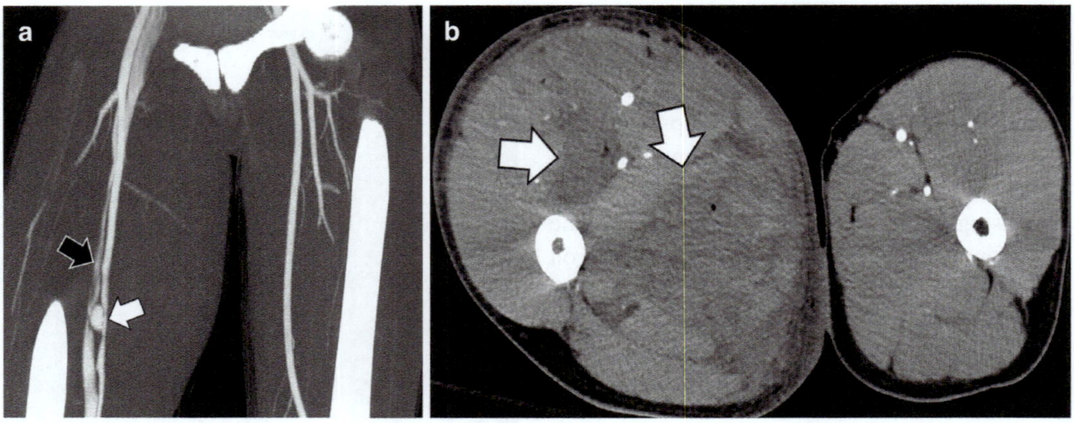

Fig. 11.14 Arteriovenous fistula. Coronal MIP CTA image of the lower extremities (**a**) in a patient who sustained a gunshot wound. There is a right superficial femoral artery pseudoaneurysm (white arrow, **a**) with an AVF (black arrow, **a**) as evidenced by early venous filling. The injury was treated with a superficial femoral artery stent, after which the patient developed clinical signs and symptoms of compartment syndrome. On follow-up, an axial CTA image of the lower extremities (**b**) shows edema and geographic hypoenhancement in the anterior and medial compartments of the right thigh (arrows, **b**). The patient underwent fasciotomy and hematoma evacuation

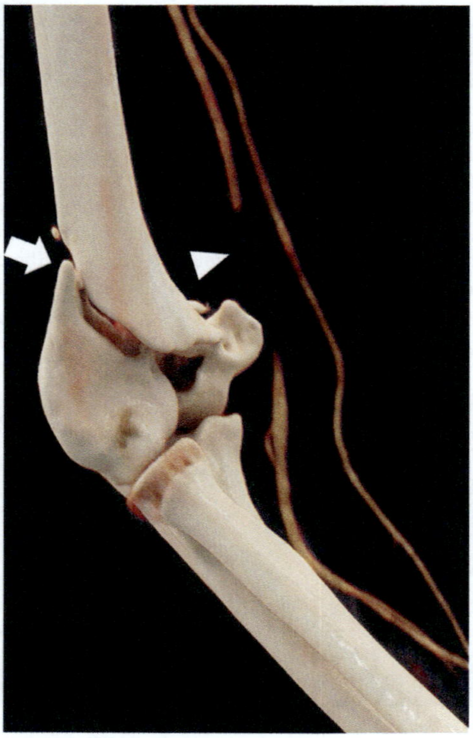

Fig. 11.15 Short segment arterial occlusion. Oblique 3D cinematic rendered CT image of the right upper extremity demonstrates a bicondylar fracture (arrow) with segmental nonenhancement of the distal brachial artery (arrowhead) following a stab wound. A 1 cm brachial artery defect found at surgery, which was repaired primarily with an end-to-end anastomosis

injuries may require a bypass graft (see Figs. 11.1 and 11.16) [8, 25, 63]. Although the length of a vascular injury should be reported, imaging may over- or underestimate the true length of vascular injury when it is definitively characterized at surgery (see Fig. 11.15) [56].

A pseudoaneurysm is a round, often smooth-walled focus of contrast contained by the adventitia (see Figs. 11.13 and 11.17). Enhancement follows the blood pool on multiphase imaging [25]. A collection of extraluminal contrast in the arterial phase that changes size and shape on multiphase imaging is consistent with arterial hemorrhage; contrast extravasation seen only in the venous phase may be due to a slow arterial or venous hemorrhage [25]. Active extravasation from small branch vessels may be managed conservatively, while proximal arterial injuries may require surgical or endovascular intervention. Occult vascular injury can be suggested in the presence of a perivascular hematoma or penetrating tract or shrapnel less than 5 mm from a vessel [50, 59].

On CTA, vasospasm appears as a concentric, smooth tapering (Fig. 11.18), whereas stenoses are eccentric and irregular (Fig. 11.19) [41]. Although this distinction may be possible in proximal vessels, it can be impossible to differen-

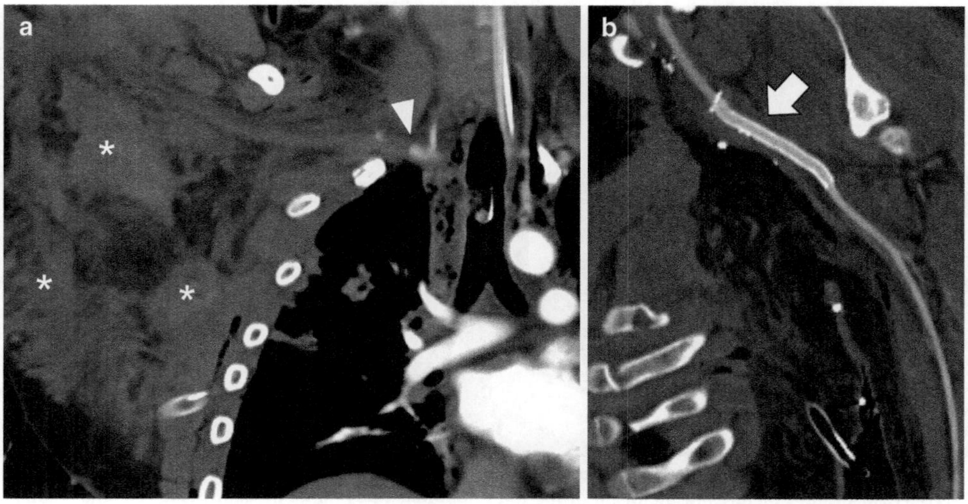

Fig. 11.16 Axillary hematoma and brachial plexus injury. A coronal MIP CTA image (**a**) demonstrates complete occlusion of the right subclavian artery (arrowhead, **a**) and a large axillary hematoma (asterisks, **a**), in a patient with a cool right upper extremity and an absent radial pulse following a motor vehicle collision. At surgery, a 6–7 cm disruption of the brachial plexus was also identified. The subclavian artery was successfully treated with a self-expanding stent graft (arrow, **b**), as shown on the post-operative curved planar reformat CTA image (**b**)

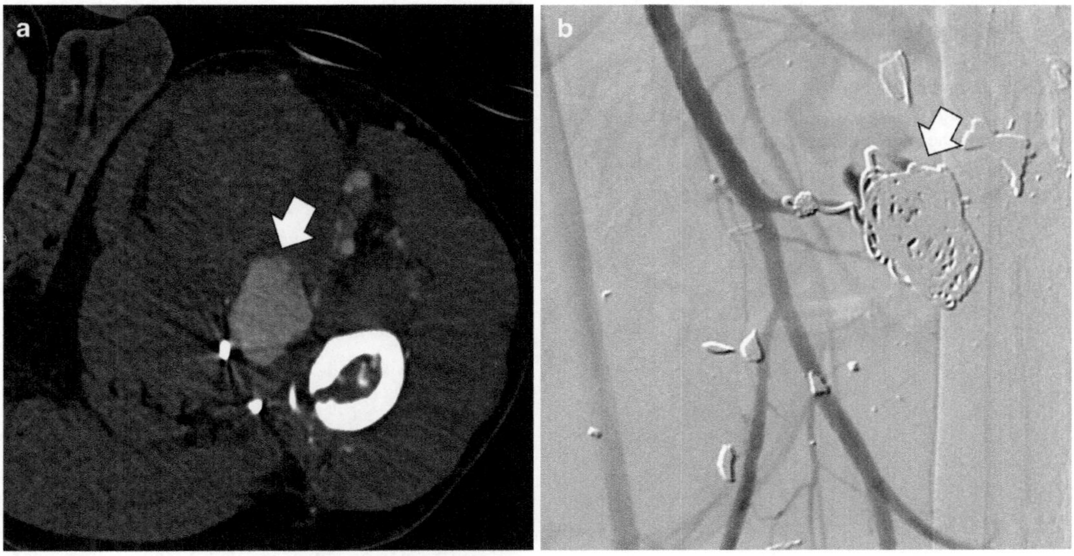

Fig. 11.17 Pseudoaneurysm treated with coil embolization. There is a large left profunda femoris artery pseudoaneurysm (arrow, **a**) on an axial CTA of the pelvis (**a**), successfully treated with coil embolization (arrow, **b**), as shown on DSA

tiate between intimal injury, vasospasm, external compression, and occlusion distally [25, 41, 59]. A stable patient may be observed or undergo a repeat CTA if initial imaging shows decreased or absent distal arterial enhancement. If immediate, definitive characterization is needed, a conventional angiogram performed with vasodilator injection may be required [41, 50, 59].

Limb ischemia in the setting of an odd number of bullet wounds (indicating retained ballistic

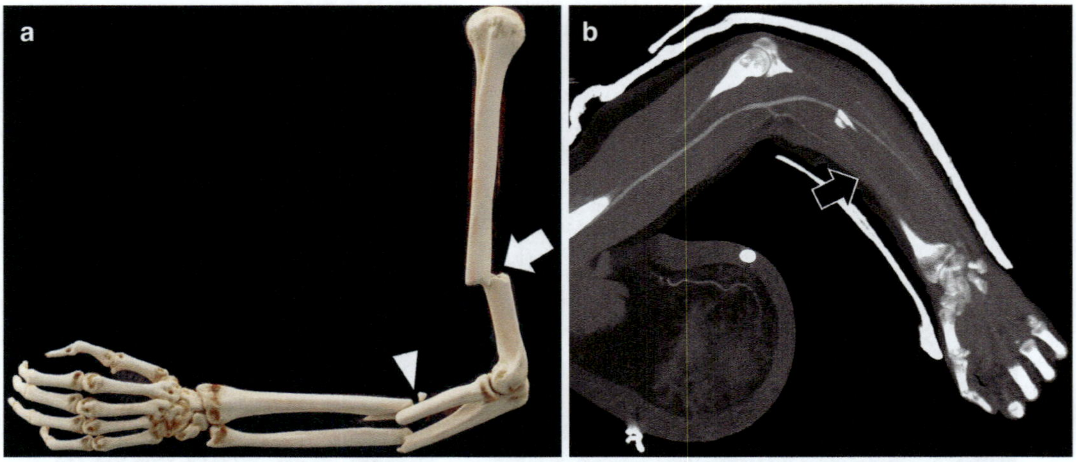

Fig. 11.18 Vasospasm. Fractures of the distal of the left humerus (white arrow, **a**) and proximal radius and ulna (arrowhead) constitute a floating elbow, as seen on 3D cinematic rendered CT (**a**) in a patient who had been in a motor vehicle collision. An oblique MIP CTA image (**b**) demonstrates smooth narrowing of the radial artery (arrow, **b**). Pulses on exam were only slightly diminished and this was attributed to vasospasm rather than occlusion. No vascular intervention was required

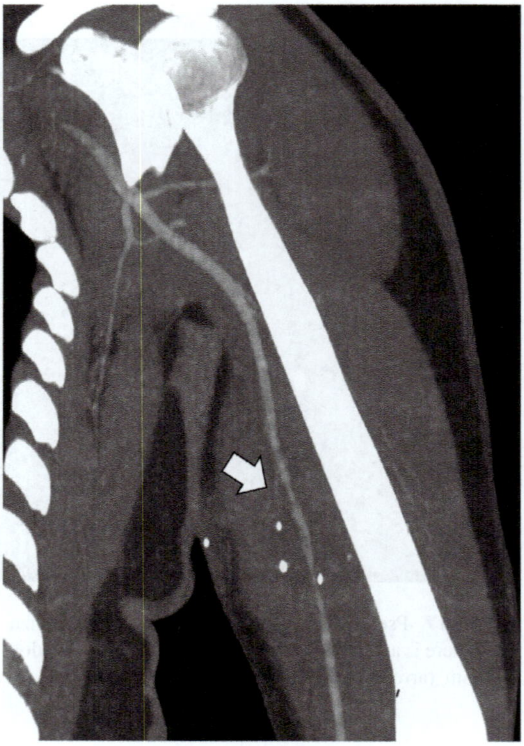

Fig. 11.19 Traumatic arterial narrowing. Irregular luminal narrowing (arrow) with adjacent shrapnel from a gunshot wound to the arm is demonstrated on this coronal MIP CTA image. The patient had decreased motor function in the left upper extremity and numbness in all fingers. At surgery, there was a brachial sheath hematoma compressing the adjacent nerves, as well as brachial vein transection and brachial artery contusion. The patient's symptoms improved following brachial vein ligation and hematoma evacuation

fragments) raises the possibility of a bullet embolus. Bullet embolization to a peripheral artery typically originates from the heart or aorta, but occasionally may embolize from peripheral arteries or veins [64–66]. Bullet emboli are rare; however, the risk is increased if a bullet smaller than the affected vessel caliber enters a vessel with low kinetic energy [65, 67]. On CTA, this will appear as intraluminal shrapnel and can show absent or diminished distal flow (Fig. 11.20).

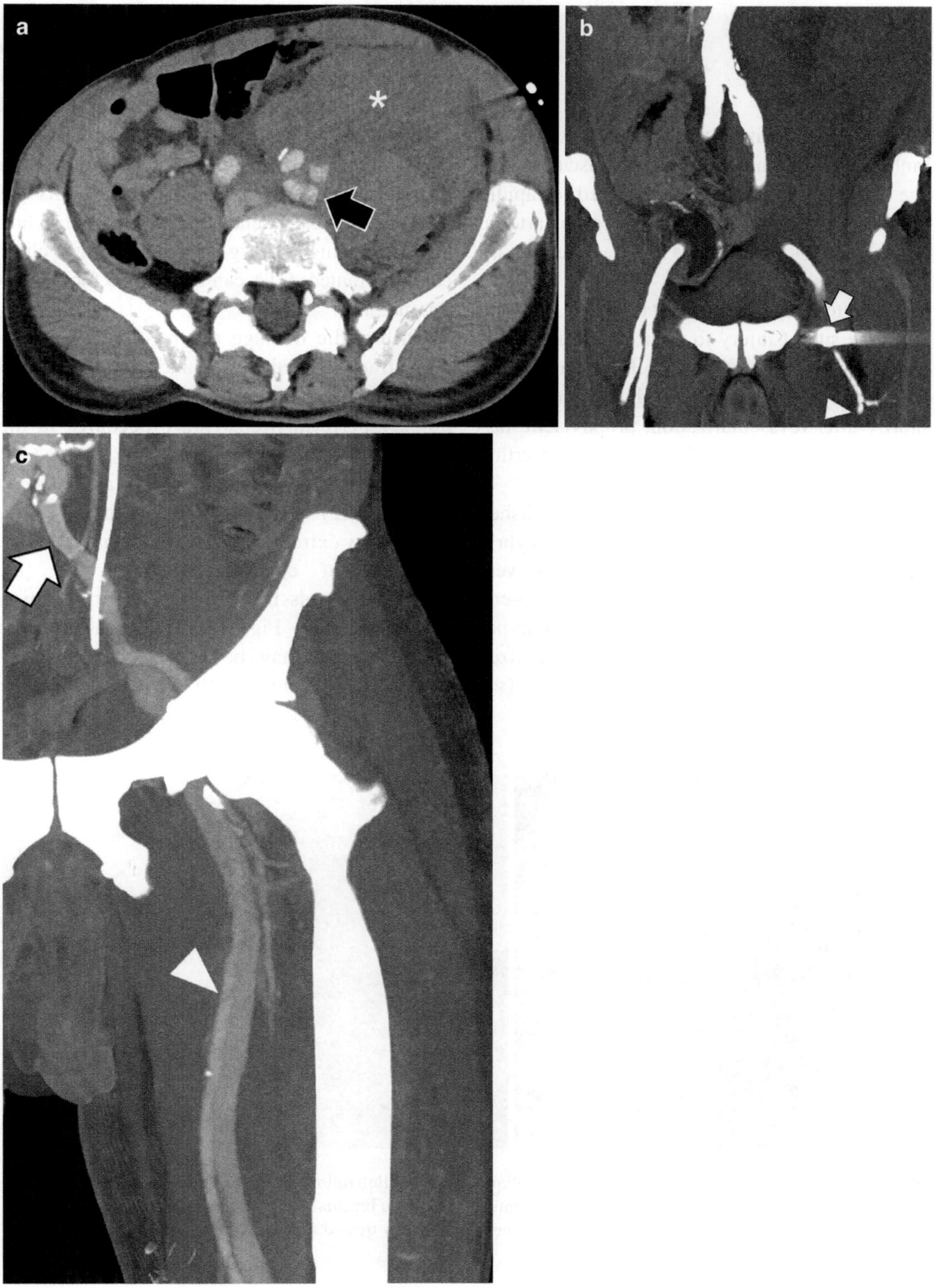

Fig. 11.20 Bullet embolus. Pelvis CTA axial (**a**) and coronal (**b**) MIP images demonstrate a left common iliac artery pseudoaneurysm (arrow, **a**) and large pelvic hematoma (asterisk, **a**). There is a bullet embolus (arrow, **b**) in the left superficial femoral artery with flow only seen in the profunda femoris (arrowhead, **b**). A post-operative coronal MIP CTA image of the left lower extremity (**c**) demonstrates a patency of the left common iliac artery stent (arrow, **c**) and superficial femoral artery (arrowhead, **c**) after removal of bullet embolus

Management

Damage Control

In a polytraumatized patient with concurrent limb and life-threatening injuries, vascular damage control procedures are performed to rapidly treat ongoing peripheral hemorrhage or arterial occlusion. This may include the use of temporary vascular shunts (TVS)—plastic conduits designed to temporarily maintain blood flow distal to the site of injury to reduce ischemic times [68, 69]. To reduce the risks for compartment syndrome and secondary shunt thrombosis shortly after revascularization, prophylactic fasciotomies are performed after TVS insertion [69].

Definitive vascular repair can be accomplished through an open, endovascular, or hybrid approach. Open repair techniques include vein patch grafting for partial transection, end-to-end anastomosis (see Fig. 11.15), and venous interposition or bypass graft (often a valvulotomized contralateral saphenous or cephalic vein) (see Fig. 11.1) [34, 52].

Compared to open repair, endovascular embolization and stent grafting are associated with fewer complications and shorter hospital stays [70]. Permanent embolization can be achieved with coils (see Figs. 11.5 and 11.17), while temporary embolization can be performed with absorbable gelatin powder [70]. Stent grafts can be used to treat pseudoaneurysms, AVFs, and vascular occlusions (Fig. 11.21) [70, 71]. If clinically warranted, CTA can be utilized for follow-up imaging.

Orthopedic damage control—early, temporary fracture reduction and stabilization—reduces primary operative time and is used to quickly perform life-saving procedures in the acute phase of trauma through the use of debridement, external fixation, and splints (Fig. 11.22) [72–75]. Fasciotomies often accompany extremity injury treatment to reduce the risk of compartment syndrome [8]. Antibiotic beads may be placed for infection prevention (see Fig. 11.22). Extra-anatomic reconstruction may be warranted in grossly contaminated wounds with extensive soft tissue injury [8, 76].

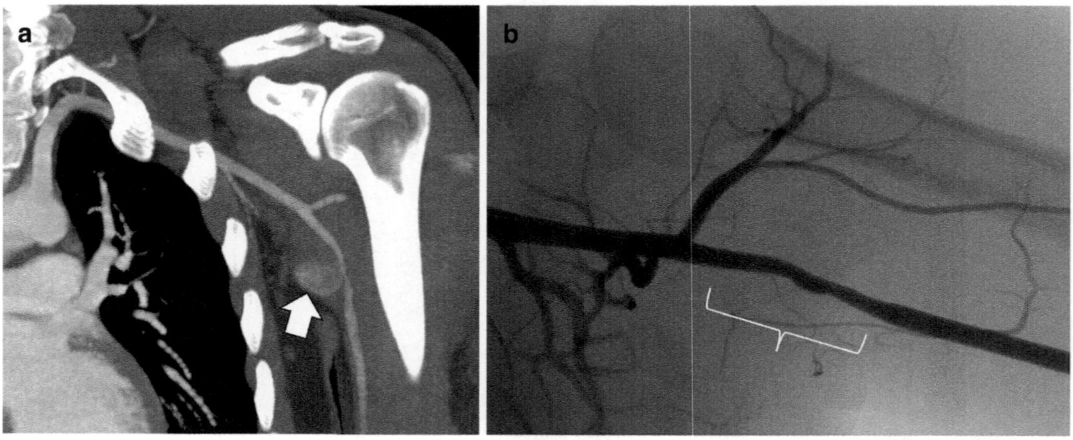

Fig. 11.21 Stented pseudoaneurysm. Coronal oblique CTA (**a**) and DSA (**b**) images of the left upper extremity in a patient presenting with left upper extremity numbness and tingling following a gunshot wound to the back. There is a large brachial artery pseudoaneurysm (arrow, **a**), successfully treated with a stent (brace, **b**)

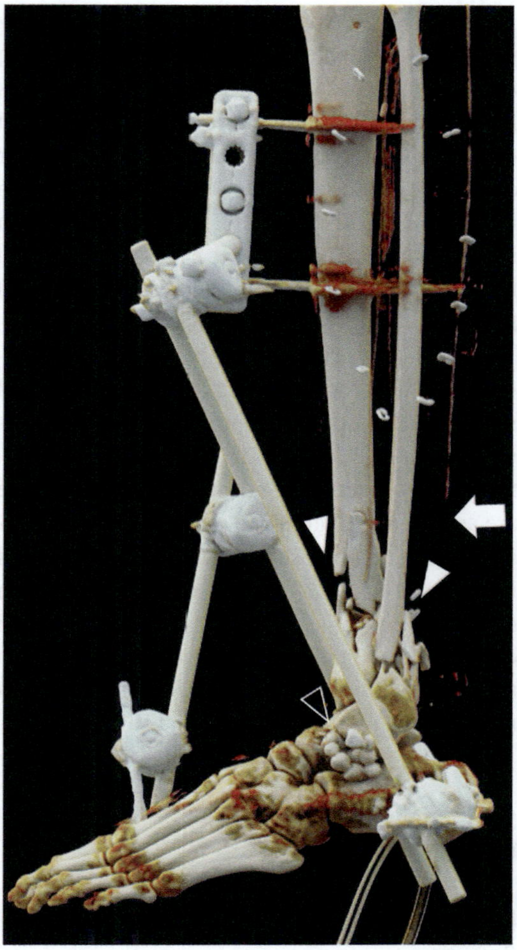

Fig. 11.22 External fixator and antibiotic beads. Sagittal 3D cinematic rendered image of the left lower extremity from a patient with open distal tibial and fibula fractures (white arrowheads) after a motorcycle collision. Proximal to the ankle, there is complete occlusion of the posterior tibial (white arrow) and anterior tibial arteries (black arrow). The fractures were initially stabilized with an external fixator device and antibiotic beads were placed for infection prevention (black arrowhead). Complications following the posterior tibial artery repair necessitated a below-the-knee amputation

Complications

Early Post-traumatic Period

Compartment Syndrome

Patients with complex extremity fractures are at risk for developing compartment syndrome, a condition that results from soft tissue hemostasis disruption, increasing tissue pressure and reducing capillary blood flow causing local hypoxia and tissue necrosis [77]. Blood products and fluid accumulate in the myofascial compartments, leading to venous hypertension and venous ischemia. When cells lyse, they release their contents into the interstitium, increasing interstitial fluid and compartment pressure. Arteriolar pressures eventually rise, causing irreversible myonecrosis and nerve damage. After 6–8 h, amputation will likely be required if compartment syndrome is untreated [78, 79].

Compartment syndrome is a clinical diagnosis based on (1) symptoms such as pain, paresthesia, and paresis, (2) increased intracompartmental pressure, and (3) elevated biomarkers such as myoglobin, serum creatinine, or creatine phosphokinase [80]. The nonspecific imaging findings of geographic soft tissue edema and compartmental hypoenhancement are a late manifestation and should not determine the need for fasciotomy (see Fig. 11.14b) [81]. Similarly, a normal CT does not exclude compartment syndrome [82].

Post-traumatic compartment syndrome is commonly associated with tibial diaphysis and distal radius fractures [77]. Patients under 35 years of age are at the greatest risk of developing compartment syndrome due to increased muscle mass [77, 83].

Neurovascular Complications

Combined neurovascular and musculoskeletal injuries increase the risk of limb loss. Although several predictive models have been developed to identify candidates for amputation and successful limb salvage, none has been successfully validated in large scale prospective studies and all have failed to predict functional recovery of patients who undergo successful limb reconstruction [84–86]. Relative indications for primary amputation include ischemia for more than 6 h, extensive nerve disruption, extensive soft tissue loss, multiple comminuted fractures with bone loss, or other life-threatening injuries that preclude limb salvage [8, 84, 87, 88]. Currently, however, the only absolute indication for primary amputation is irreparable vascular injury in an ischemic limb [4, 89].

In the proximal upper extremity, the axillo-subclavian arteries and veins and brachial plexus course closely together, frequently resulting in concurrent neurovascular injuries [90]. The presence of an axillary hematoma or axillary artery pseudoaneurysm on CT is highly suggestive of brachial plexus transection or external nerve compression (see Figs. 11.5 and 11.16) [34, 90, 91]. Compared to open repair, endovascular treatment of axillosubclavian injuries reduces the risk of brachial plexus injury and is associated with improved recovery [71, 92–94].

In the setting of supracondylar humerus fractures with associated brachial artery injury, Volkmann ischemic contracture may result from occlusion proximal to the deep brachial artery origin and doubles the risk of amputation [34, 95, 96]. The median nerve courses with the brachial artery, which passes deep to the bicipital aponeurosis, forming a tight compartment [34]. On CT, a hematoma in the antecubital fossa or more proximally along the brachial sheath may explain distal ischemia or neuropathy resulting from brachial artery or median nerve compression, respectively (Fig. 11.19) [34, 97]. If not successfully treated with fasciotomy, irreversible muscle ischemia and necrosis occur between 6 and 12 h and irreversible nerve damage occurs after 12 h [95, 98].

Popliteal artery injury is frequently associated with knee dislocations (see Fig. 11.3), particularly when there is a concurrent open tibial plateau, distal femoral metadiaphyseal, or femoral bicondylar fracture [10]. Prompt reduction of the dislocated knee and CTA are necessary to identify popliteal artery dissection and thrombosis [62].

In the distal leg, an isolated anterior tibial artery injury significantly increases the risk of amputation (odds ratio, 22.39) [52]. This particularly poor prognosis may be attributed to an association with more extensive soft tissue or osseous injuries and the increased susceptibility of the anterior tibialis muscle to ischemia and myonecrosis [52]. A higher incidence of osteomyelitis and nonunion has also been associated with posterior tibial artery injury, a branch of which supplies the tibial periosteum (Fig. 11.23) [99].

Outcomes in below-knee arterial injury are poor with secondary amputation rates ranging from 5.5% to 28% following revascularization. Increased complications are often secondary to myonecrosis, infection, distal thrombus, and poor collaterals, and these patients are frequently followed with CT [99]. The risk of amputation increases proportionally to the number of below-knee arterial injuries in the leg (see Fig. 11.23) [52].

Vascular injuries resulting from ankle fractures are uncommon [100]. Although universal screening for vascular injuries in this setting is unnecessary, a CTA may be warranted in the setting of asymmetric pedal pulses [100]. If there are sufficient collaterals to maintain distal perfusion, patients are observed, or the injured vessel is ligated (Fig. 11.24) [88]. Revascularization in the lower leg, ankle, and foot is rarely performed due to high complication rates; however, when necessary, a reverse saphenous vein bypass graft may be used to restore perfusion [101].

Subacute and Late-Stage Complications

Infection

Soft tissue infections and osteomyelitis may complicate fractures and amputations (see Figs. 11.9b and 11.25) either through local infection from overlying soft tissue ulcerations or hematologic seeding [102]. The rate of infection is significantly higher with Gustilo IIIC fractures, compared to IIIA and IIIB fractures [99]. Soft tissue infections may require revision surgery and are associated with increased morbidity and mortality [103]. The use of negative pressure wound therapy has been shown to improve wound healing and decreased rates of soft tissue infection and osteomyelitis by increasing regional blood flow and an increased formation of granulation tissue [104, 105].

On imaging, the radiologist should assess for implant loosening, nonunion (see Fig. 11.23) periostitis, osteolysis, and the presence of a sequestrum [106]. Soft tissue abscesses or sinus tracts may also be present (see Fig. 11.25) [106].

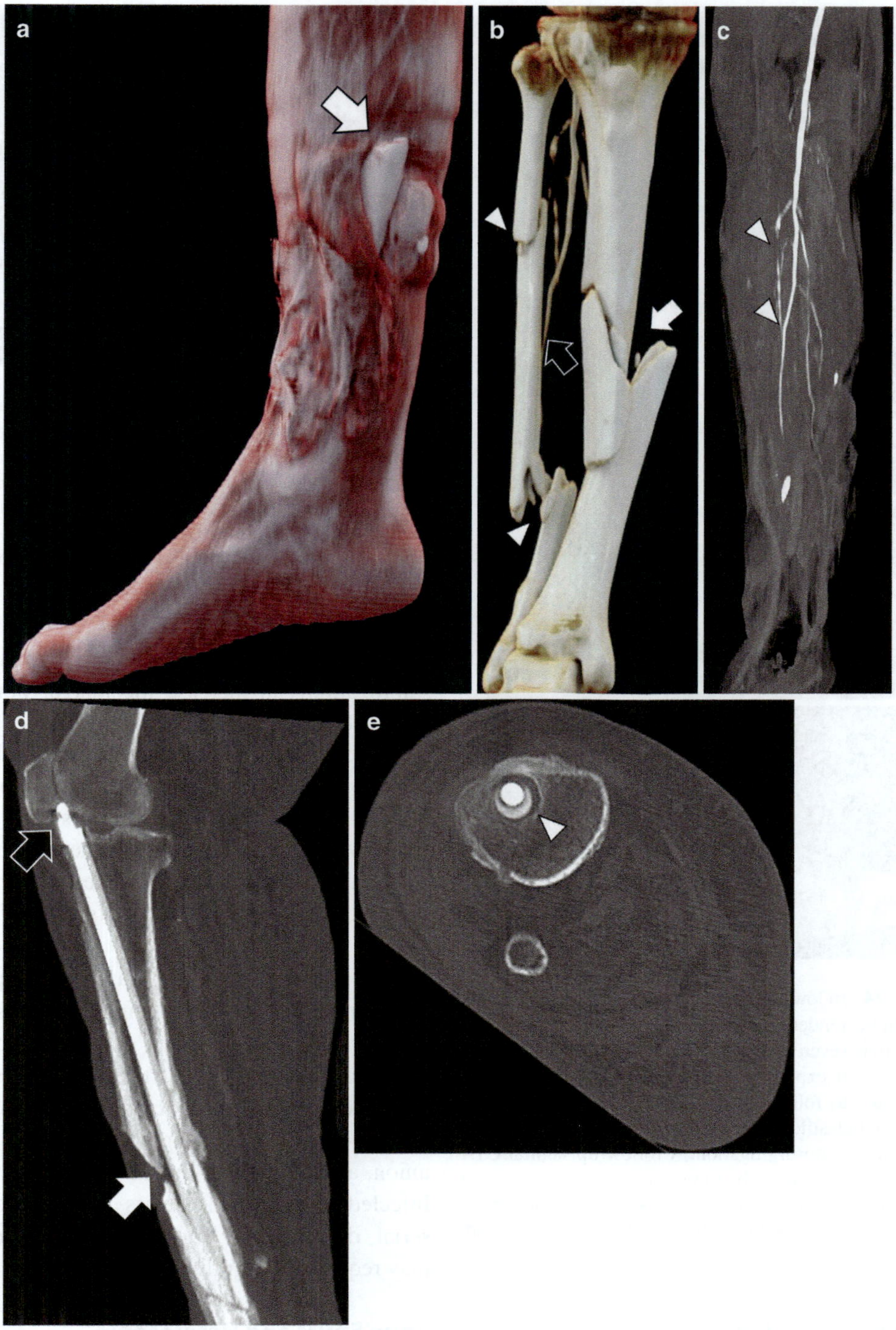

Fig. 11.23 Single-vessel runoff. Pedestrian struck by a motor vehicle. Cinematic 3D volume renderings (**a**, **b**) show an open, comminuted fracture of the tibia (white arrows, **a** and **b**) and fibula (arrowheads, **b**) with occlusion of the anterior tibial artery (black arrow, **b**). Coronal MIP CTA image (**c**) demonstrates anterior tibial artery occlusions (arrowheads, **c**). The tibial fracture was definitively treated with an intramedullary nail, while a rotational flap and skin graft were used to close the large soft tissue defect; the arterial injuries were not treated. The patient required multiple debridements and hardware revision due to recurrent osteomyelitis and soft tissue infections. Sagittal MIP (**d**) and axial (**e**) CT images of the right lower extremity obtained 2 years later show nonunion (white arrow, **d**) and hardware loosening, evidenced by proximal hardware migration into the knee joint (black arrow, **d**) and periprosthetic lucency (arrow, **e**)

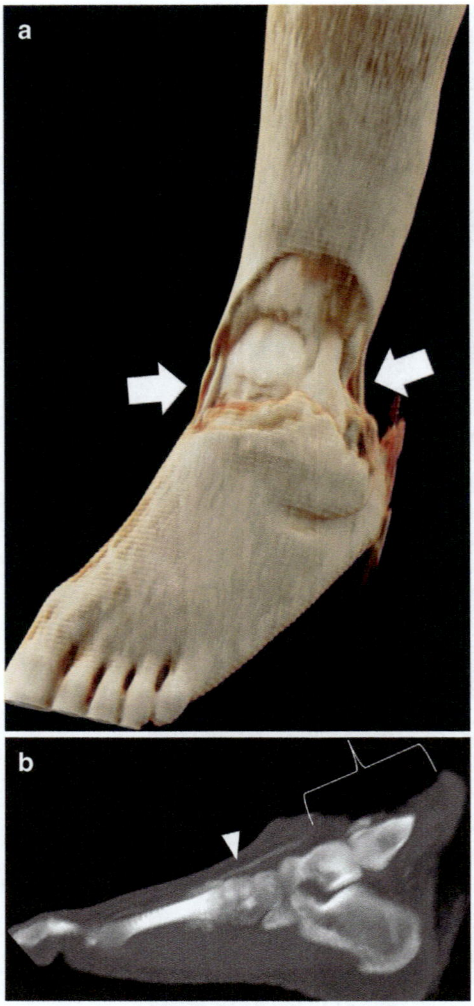

Fig. 11.24 Below the knee arterial ligation. Cinematic 3D volume rendered (**a**) and sagittal CTA (**b**) images demonstrate severe degloving injury of the medial and lateral ankle with exposure of the mortise and lateral malleolus (arrows, **a**) following a cycling accident. At bedside, there was pulsatile bleeding from the proximal dorsalis pedis artery requiring ligation. A follow-up sagittal CTA MIP image of the foot (**b**) shows nonenhancement of the proximal dorsalis pedis artery at the site of ligation (brace, **b**) with distal reconstitution from collaterals (arrowhead, **b**)

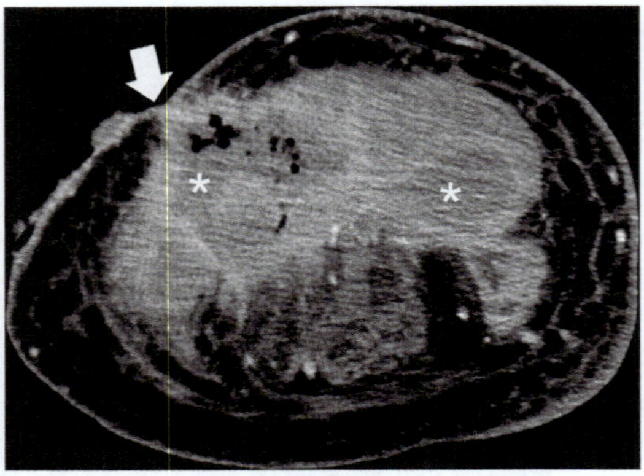

Fig. 11.25 Stump abscess. Draining wounds in a patient involved in a motor vehicle collision following amputation for a Gustilo IIIC injury of the lower leg. A contrast-enhanced axial CT of the right lower extremity proximal to the stump demonstrates peripherally enhancing fluid- and gas-containing collections in the anterior soft tissues, compatible with abscesses (asterisks) and a sinus tract that extends to the skin surface (arrow)

Osseous Nonunion

Nonunion is defined as a fracture that persists for at least 9 months without signs of healing for 3 or more months [107]. Wound size, degree of soft tissue damage and contamination, high degree of fracture displacement at presentation, the presence or development of infection, and inadequate stabilization can increase the risk of nonunion [43, 108–111]. Type III fractures have a high incidence of nonunion, infection, and prolonged healing times [108]. Nonunion rates are particularly high in open tibial fractures due to the extensive soft tissue defects (further exacerbated by multiple debridements) and severe periosteal and associated vascular injuries (see Fig. 11.23d) [43, 99, 108].

CT is more sensitive than radiographs in detecting early healing changes, such as early bone bridging, or persistent cortical defects and bony sclerosis [111]. A fracture gap and the presence of single-cortex continuity on immediate post-operative imaging are predictive of nonunion, as is early post-operative infection [108]. Infected nonunited fractures are treated with serial debridement, fracture stabilization, and may require bone grafting.

Bone Spurs and Heterotopic Ossification

Bone spurs along a stump margin result from post-traumatic or post-operative periosteal stripping [103]. They can cause damage to the overlying soft tissues and lead to infection [103].

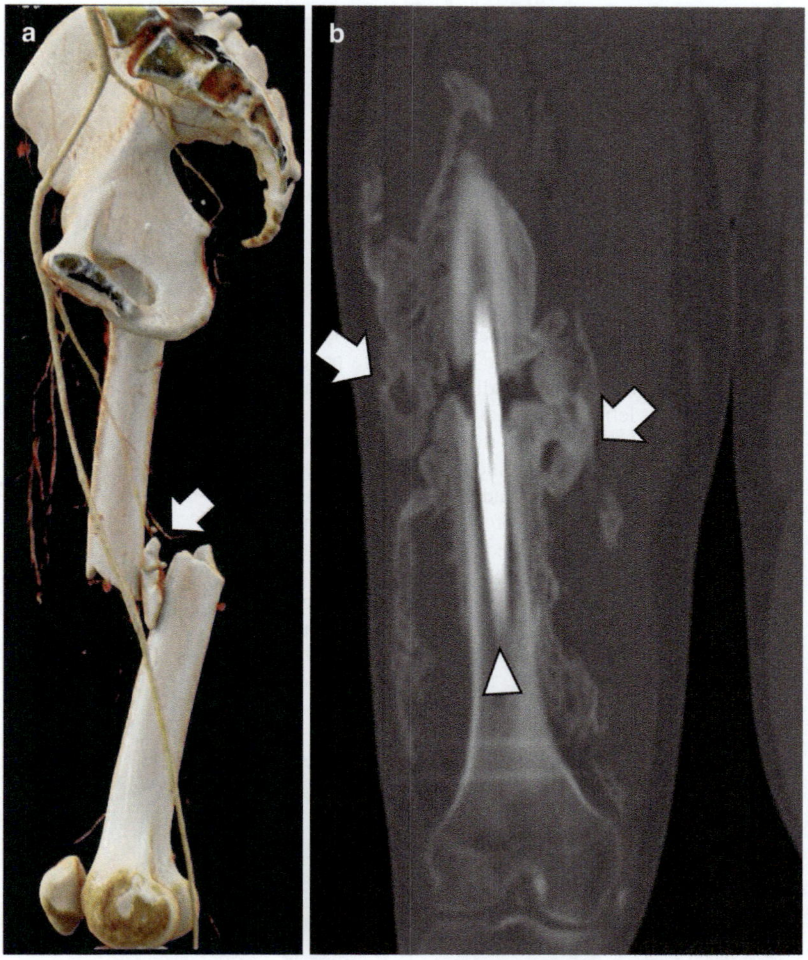

Fig. 11.26 Heterotopic ossification. A displaced femur fracture (arrow, **a**) following a motor vehicle collision is demonstrated on a cinematic 3D volume rendered image of the right lower extremity (**a**). A coronal CT image obtained 6 months later (**b**) demonstrates the presence of an intramedullary nail (arrowhead, **b**) and extensive heterotopic ossification (arrows, **b**)

Heterotopic ossification may result from muscular ischemia and excessive periosteal stripping, frequently developing at amputation sites or around hardware (see Figs. 11.1 and 11.26). It results in limited joint movement and may require surgical excision [103].

Both bone spurs and heterotopic ossification can lead to pain and result in an ill-fitting prosthesis [103]. CT and radiographs readily identify established heterotopic ossification, while bone scintigraphy is sensitive to early development of heterotopic ossification [103].

Endovascular Complications

Early complications following endovascular repair include pseudoaneurysms, stent thrombosis, endoleaks, and thromboembolic events (Fig. 11.27). Infection, endoleaks, device migration, intimal hyperplasia, occlusion, and stent failure are late complications (Fig. 11.28) [70, 71, 92, 93]. Endovascular thrombolysis, angioplasty, or repeat stenting may be required to recanalize an occluded stent [71]. If complications are suspected, CTA will often be performed for the purposes of diagnosis and operative planning.

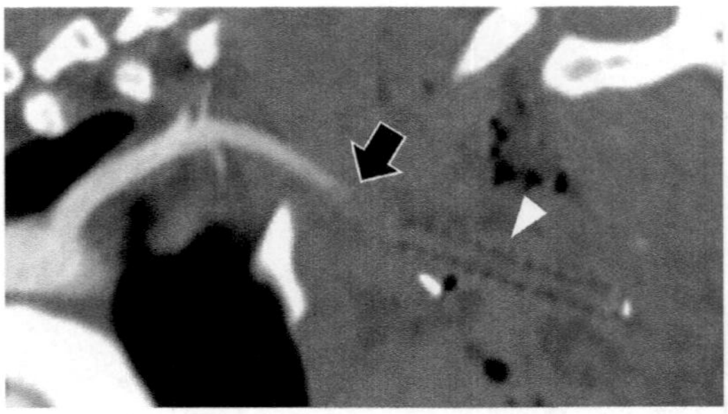

Fig. 11.27 Acute polytetrafluoroethylene (PTFE) graft thrombosis. Gunshot wound to the left chest in a patient with a pulsatile hemorrhage, axillary hematoma, and diminished pulses left upper extremity pulses. The patient emergently went to the operating room, where a left axillary artery transection was identified. A PTFE interposition bypass graft was placed and left upper extremity pulses were detected at the end of the case. Several hours later, the left upper extremity became pulseless and the patient developed symptoms of compartment syndrome. A coronal oblique CTA image through this region demonstrates occlusion of the left axillary artery (arrow) and graft (arrowhead). The axillary artery was revascularized with a new PTFE graft and the patient underwent fasciotomies

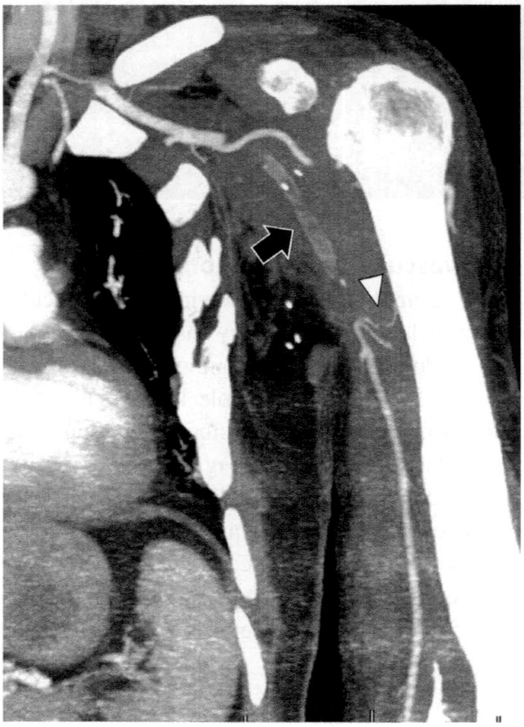

Fig. 11.28 Chronically occluded stent graft. Coronal MIP CTA image shows a chronically occluded left axillary artery stent graft (arrow) with distal flow supplied by collaterals (arrowhead) in a patient with a remote history of vascular injury from a motorcycle accident

Conclusion

The management of open extremity fractures is a complex multidisciplinary process. An understanding of this multifaceted topic will aid the radiologist in optimizing imaging techniques, making accurate diagnoses, and improving communications through the creation of clinically relevant reports for our surgical colleagues.

Disclosure Statement The authors have nothing to disclose.

Trauma CT Protocols

Protocol name	CTA upper extremity
Indication	Vascular injury
Protocol designed for (scanner model)	Siemens Somatom Force
Patient preparation	None
First series	
Oral contrast	None
IV contrast	100 mL iohexol 350
Tube settings	
kV	100 kVp
mA	200 mAs
Dose modulation	Yes
Tube rotation time (s)	0.5 s
Table speed (mm/s)	118.5 mm/s
Slice collimation	128 × 0.6
Reconstructed slice thickness	2 mm/1 mm
Anatomical coverage	Thoracic inlet to finger tips
Reconstruction kernel	BV40
Breath hold	None
Window settings	W360/L60
Post-processing	Coronal and sagittal MIPS 5 mm/2 mm

Protocol name	CTA lower extremity
Indication	Vascular injury
Protocol designed for (scanner model)	Siemens Somatom Force
Patient preparation	None
First series	
Oral contrast	None
IV contrast	100 mL iohexol 350
Tube settings	
kV	100 kVp
mA	230 mAs
Dose modulation	Yes

Protocol name	CTA lower extremity
Tube rotation time (s)	0.5 s
Table speed (mm/s)	216 mm/s
Slice collimation	128 × 0.6
Reconstructed slice thickness	2 mm/1 mm
Anatomical coverage	Diaphragm to toes
Reconstruction kernel	BV36
Breath hold	Stop breathing
Window settings	W360/L60
Post-processing	Coronal and sagittal MIPS 2 mm/2 mm

References

1. Rutherford RB, Baker JD, Ernst C, Johnston KW, Porter JM, Ahn S, et al. Recommended standards for reports dealing with lower extremity ischemia: revised version. J Vasc Surg. 1997;26(3):517–38.
2. Gregory RT, Gould RJ, Peclet M, Wagner JS, Gilbert DA, Wheeler JR, et al. The mangled extremity syndrome (M.E.S.): a severity grading system for multisystem injury of the extremity. J Trauma. 1985;25(12):1147–50.
3. Meinberg EG, Agel J, Roberts CS, Karam MD, Kellam JF. Fracture and dislocation classification compendium-2018. J Orthop Trauma. 2018;32(Suppl 1):S1–70.
4. Iyer KM. Amputations. In: Iyer KM, Khan WS, editors. General principles of orthopedics and trauma. Cham: Springer; 2019. p. 385–406.
5. Gustilo RB, Mendoza RM, Williams DN. Problems in the management of type III (severe) open fractures: a new classification of type III open fractures. J Trauma. 1984;24(8):742–6.
6. Gustilo RB, Anderson JT. Prevention of infection in the treatment of one thousand and twenty-five open fractures of long bones: retrospective and prospective analyses. J Bone Joint Surg Am. 1976;58(4):453–8.
7. Diamond S, Gaspard D, Katz S. Vascular injuries to the extremities in a suburban trauma center. Am Surg. 2003;69(10):848–51.
8. Franz RW, Shah KJ, Halaharvi D, Franz ET, Hartman JF, Wright ML. A 5-year review of management of lower extremity arterial injuries at an urban level I trauma center. J Vasc Surg. 2011;53(6):1604–10.
9. Medina O, Arom GA, Yeranosian MG, Petrigliano FA, McAllister DR. Vascular and nerve injury after knee dislocation: a systematic review. Clin Orthop Relat Res. 2014;472(9):2621–9.
10. Bernhoff K, Michaelsson K, Bjorck M. Incidence and outcome of popliteal artery injury associated with knee dislocations, ligamentous injuries, and close to knee fractures: a Nationwide population based cohort study. Eur J Vasc Endovasc Surg. 2021;61(2):297–304.
11. Halvorson JJ, Anz A, Langfitt M, Deonanan JK, Scott A, Teasdall RD, et al. Vascular injury associated with extremity trauma: initial diagnosis and management. J Am Acad Orthop Surg. 2011;19(8):495–504.
12. Levy BA, Zlowodzki MP, Graves M, Cole PA. Screening for extremity arterial injury with the arterial pressure index. Am J Emerg Med. 2005;23(5):689–95.
13. Monazzam S, Goodell PB, Salcedo ES, Nelson SH, Wolinsky PR. When are CT angiograms indicated for patients with lower extremity fractures? A review of 275 extremities. J Trauma Acute Care Surg. 2017;82(1):133–7.
14. Kim PH, Leopold SS. In brief: Gustilo-Anderson classification. [corrected]. Clin Orthop Relat Res. 2012;470(11):3270–4.
15. Huda W, Abrahams RB. X-ray-based medical imaging and resolution. AJR Am J Roentgenol. 2015;204(4):W393–7.
16. Martin J, Marsh JL, Nepola JV, Dirschl DR, Hurwitz S, DeCoster TA. Radiographic fracture assessments: which ones can we reliably make? J Orthop Trauma. 2000;14(6):379–85.
17. Bao MH, DeAngelis JP, Wu JS. Imaging of traumatic shoulder injuries—understanding the surgeon's perspective. Eur J Radiol Open. 2022;9:100411.
18. Sheehan SE, Shyu JY, Weaver MJ, Sodickson AD, Khurana B. Proximal femoral fractures: what the orthopedic surgeon wants to know-erratum. Radiographics. 2015;35(5):1624.
19. Zeiderman MR, Pu LLQ. Contemporary approach to soft-tissue reconstruction of the lower extremity after trauma. Burns. Trauma. 2021;9:tkab024.
20. Gosangi B, Mandell JC, Weaver MJ, Uyeda JW, Smith SE, Sodickson AD, et al. Bone marrow edema at dual-energy CT: a game changer in the emergency department. Radiographics. 2020;40(3):859–74.
21. Wilson MP, Lui K, Nobbee D, Murad MH, McInnes MDF, McGrath TA, et al. Diagnostic accuracy of dual-energy CT for the detection of bone marrow edema in the appendicular skeleton: a systematic review and meta-analysis. Eur Radiol. 2021;31(3):1558–68.
22. Narayanan A, Dettori N, Chalian M, Xi Y, Komarraju A, Chhabra A. Dual-energy CT-generated bone marrow oedema maps improve timely visualisation and recognition of acute lower extremity fractures. Clin Radiol. 2021;76(9):710.e9–14.
23. Li M, Qu Y, Song B. Meta-analysis of dual-energy computed tomography virtual non-calcium imaging to detect bone marrow edema. Eur J Radiol. 2017;95:124–9.
24. Feliciano DV. Pitfalls in the management of peripheral vascular injuries. Trauma Surg Acute Care Open. 2017;2(1):e000110.
25. Fritz J, Efron DT, Fishman EK. Multidetector CT and three-dimensional CT angiography of upper extremity arterial injury. Emerg Radiol. 2015;22(3):269–82.
26. Feliciano DV. Management of peripheral arterial injury. Curr Opin Crit Care. 2010;16(6):602–8.

27. Johansen K, Lynch K, Paun M, Copass M. Non-invasive vascular tests reliably exclude occult arterial trauma in injured extremities. J Trauma. 1991;31(4):515–9; discussion 9–22.
28. Hemingway J, Adjei E, Desikan S, Gross J, Tran N, Singh N, et al. Lowering the ankle-brachial index threshold in blunt lower extremity trauma may prevent unnecessary imaging. Ann Vasc Surg. 2020;62:106–13.
29. Peng PD, Spain DA, Tataria M, Hellinger JC, Rubin GD, Brundage SI. CT angiography effectively evaluates extremity vascular trauma. Am Surg. 2008;74(2):103–7.
30. Lynch K, Johansen K. Can Doppler pressure measurement replace "exclusion" arteriography in the diagnosis of occult extremity arterial trauma? Ann Surg. 1991;214(6):737–41.
31. Hemingway J, Adjei E, Desikan S, Gross J, Tran N, Singh N, et al. Re-evaluating the safety and effectiveness of the 0.9 ankle-brachial index threshold in penetrating lower extremity trauma. J Vasc Surg. 2020;72(4):1305–11.e1.
32. Gakhal MS, Sartip KA. CT angiography signs of lower extremity vascular trauma. AJR Am J Roentgenol. 2009;193(1):W49–57.
33. O'Toole RV, Hardcastle J, Garapati R, Andrew Eglseder W. Fracture of the distal radius with radial artery injury: injury description and outcome of vascular repair. Injury. 2013;44(4):437–41.
34. McCready RA. Upper-extremity vascular injuries. Surg Clin North Am. 1988;68(4):725–40.
35. Spitler CA, Patch DA, McFarland GE, Smith WR. Assessment and interventions for vascular injuries associated with fractures. J Am Acad Orthop Surg. 2022;30(9):387–94.
36. Merchant N, Scalea T, Stein D. Can CT angiography replace conventional bi-planar angiography in the management of severe scapulothoracic dissociation injuries? Am Surg. 2012;78(8):875–82.
37. Huber-Wagner S, Kanz KG, Hanschen M, van Griensven M, Biberthaler P, Lefering R. Whole-body computed tomography in severely injured patients. Curr Opin Crit Care. 2018;24(1):55–61.
38. Paes FM, Munera F. Computer tomography angiography of peripheral vascular injuries. Radiol Clin N Am. 2023;61(1):141–50.
39. Patterson BO, Holt PJ, Cleanthis M, Tai N, Carrell T, Loosemore TM, et al. Imaging vascular trauma. Br J Surg. 2012;99(4):494–505.
40. Jens S, Kerstens MK, Legemate DA, Reekers JA, Bipat S, Koelemay MJ. Diagnostic performance of computed tomography angiography in peripheral arterial injury due to trauma: a systematic review and meta-analysis. Eur J Vasc Endovasc Surg. 2013;46(3):329–37.
41. Rieger M, Mallouhi A, Tauscher T, Lutz M, Jaschke WR. Traumatic arterial injuries of the extremities: initial evaluation with MDCT angiography. AJR Am J Roentgenol. 2006;186(3):656–64.
42. Frykberg ER. Advances in the diagnosis and treatment of extremity vascular trauma. Surg Clin North Am. 1995;75(2):207–23.
43. Parrett BM, Matros E, Pribaz JJ, Orgill DP. Lower extremity trauma: trends in the management of soft-tissue reconstruction of open tibia-fibula fractures. Plast Reconstr Surg. 2006;117(4):1315–22; discussion 23–4.
44. Yu JL, Tolley PD, Kneib C, Miller EA, Crowe CS. Current concepts in microsurgical soft tissue reconstruction of lower extremity trauma in a single-vessel extremity. Plast Aesthet Res. 2022;9(5):37.
45. Stranix JT, Lee ZH, Jacoby A, Anzai L, Avraham T, Thanik VD, et al. Not all Gustilo type IIIB fractures are created equal: arterial injury impacts limb salvage outcomes. Plast Reconstr Surg. 2017;140(5):1033–41.
46. Adler C, Hangge PT, Albadawi H, Knuttinen MG, Alzubaidi SJ, Naidu SG, et al. Multi-detector computed tomography imaging techniques in arterial injuries. J Clin Med. 2018;7(5):88.
47. Keeling AN, Farrelly C, Carr JC, Yaghmai V. Technical considerations for lower limb multidetector computed tomographic angiography. Vasc Med. 2011;16(2):131–43.
48. Fleischmann D. CT angiography: injection and acquisition technique. Radiol Clin N Am. 2010;48(2):237–47, vii.
49. Murphy DJ, Aghayev A, Steigner ML. Vascular CT and MRI: a practical guide to imaging protocols. Insights Imaging. 2018;9(2):215–36.
50. Uyeda JW, Anderson SW, Sakai O, Soto JA. CT angiography in trauma. Radiol Clin N Am. 2010;48(2):423–38, ix–x.
51. Miller-Thomas MM, West OC, Cohen AM. Diagnosing traumatic arterial injury in the extremities with CT angiography: pearls and pitfalls. Radiographics. 2005;25(Suppl 1):S133–42.
52. Scalea JR, Crawford R, Scurci S, Danquah J, Sarkar R, Kufera J, et al. Below-the-knee arterial injury: the type of vessel may be more important than the number of vessels injured. J Trauma Acute Care Surg. 2014;77(6):920–5.
53. Raniga SB, Mittal AK, Bernstein M, Skalski MR, Al-Hadidi AM. Multidetector CT in vascular injuries resulting from pelvic fractures: a primer for diagnostic radiologists. Radiographics. 2019;39(7):2111–29.
54. Khatri GD, Robinson JD. Is it safe to inject contrast through the side arm of an introducer sheath? An in vitro study. Emerg Radiol. 2020;27(3):303–6.
55. Bozlar U, Ogur T, Norton PT, Khaja MS, All J, Hagspiel KD. CT angiography of the upper extremity arterial system: part 1—anatomy, technique, and use in trauma patients. AJR Am J Roentgenol. 2013;201(4):745–52.
56. Dreizin D, Smith EB, Champ K, Morrison JJ. Roles of trauma CT and CTA in salvaging the threatened or mangled extremity. Radiographics. 2022;42(2):E50–67.

57. Karlo C, Gnannt R, Frauenfelder T, Leschka S, Bruesch M, Wanner GA, et al. Whole-body CT in polytrauma patients: effect of arm positioning on thoracic and abdominal image quality. Emerg Radiol. 2011;18(4):285–93.
58. Madhuripan N, Mehta P, Smolinski SE, Njuguna N. Computed tomography angiography of the extremities in emergencies. Semin Ultrasound CT MR. 2017;38(4):357–69.
59. Pieroni S, Foster BR, Anderson SW, Kertesz JL, Rhea JT, Soto JA. Use of 64-row multidetector CT angiography in blunt and penetrating trauma of the upper and lower extremities. Radiographics. 2009;29(3):863–76.
60. Nagpal K, Ahmed K, Cuschieri R. Diagnosis and management of acute traumatic arteriovenous fistula. Int J Angiol. 2008;17(4):214–6.
61. Colip CG, Gorantla V, LeBedis CA, Soto JA, Anderson SW. Extremity CTA for penetrating trauma: 10-year experience using a 64-detector row CT scanner. Emerg Radiol. 2017;24(3):223–32.
62. Hundersmarck D, Hietbrink F, Leenen LPH, De Borst GJ, Heng M. Blunt popliteal artery injury following tibiofemoral trauma: vessel-first and bone-first strategy. Eur J Trauma Emerg Surg. 2022;48(2):1045–53.
63. Modrall JG, Weaver FA, Yellin AE. Diagnosis and management of penetrating vascular trauma and the injured extremity. Emerg Med Clin North Am. 1998;16(1):129–44.
64. Devlin BA, Lee JJ, Hutchinson CM, Ring AC, Kainth AS, Horn CB. Multiple gunshot wounds with bullet embolus to the right iliac artery. J Trauma Acute Care Surg. 2021;90(5):e113–5.
65. Biswas S, Cadot H, Abrol S. Gunshot wound of the thoracic aorta with right popliteal artery embolization: a case report of bullet embolism with review of relevant literature. Case Rep Emerg Med. 2013;2013:198617.
66. Rich NM, Collins GJ Jr, Andersen CA, McDonald PT, Kozloff L, Ricotta JJ. Missile emboli. J Trauma. 1978;18(4):236–9.
67. Castater C, Noorbakhsh S, Harousseau W, Klingensmith N, Koganti D, Nguyen J, et al. Missing bullets: bullet embolization case series and review of the literature. Vasc Endovasc Surg. 2022:15385744221141295.
68. Feliciano DV, Subramanian A. Temporary vascular shunts. Eur J Trauma Emerg Surg. 2013;39(6):553–60.
69. Hornez E, Boddaert G, Ngabou UD, Aguir S, Baudoin Y, Mocellin N, et al. Temporary vascular shunt for damage control of extremity vascular injury: a toolbox for trauma surgeons. J Visc Surg. 2015;152(6):363–8.
70. Khurana A, Quencer K, Saini A, Sill A, Albadawi H, Jamal L, et al. Endovascular interventions in the management of acute extremity trauma: a narrative review. Ann Transl Med. 2021;9(14):1197.
71. DuBose JJ, Rajani R, Gilani R, Arthurs ZA, Morrison JJ, Clouse WD, et al. Endovascular management of axillo-subclavian arterial injury: a review of published experience. Injury. 2012;43(11):1785–92.
72. Hildebrand F, Giannoudis P, Kretteck C, Pape HC. Damage control: extremities. Injury. 2004;35(7):678–89.
73. Jansen JO, Thomas R, Loudon MA, Brooks A. Damage control resuscitation for patients with major trauma. BMJ. 2009;338:b1778.
74. Taeger G, Ruchholtz S, Waydhas C, Lewan U, Schmidt B, Nast-Kolb D. Damage control orthopedics in patients with multiple injuries is effective, time saving, and safe. J Trauma. 2005;59(2):409–16; discussion 17.
75. Guerado E, Bertrand ML, Cano JR, Cervan AM, Galan A. Damage control orthopaedics: state of the art. World J Orthop. 2019;10(1):1–13.
76. Asensio JA, Kuncir EJ, Garcia-Nunez LM, Petrone P. Femoral vessel injuries: analysis of factors predictive of outcomes. J Am Coll Surg. 2006;203(4):512–20.
77. Shadgan B, Menon M, Sanders D, Berry G, Martin C Jr, Duffy P, et al. Current thinking about acute compartment syndrome of the lower extremity. Can J Surg. 2010;53(5):329–34.
78. Schmidt AH. Acute compartment syndrome. Injury. 2017;48(Suppl 1):S22–S5.
79. Oprel PP, Eversdijk MG, Vlot J, Tuinebreijer WE, den Hartog D. The acute compartment syndrome of the lower leg: a difficult diagnosis? Open Orthop J. 2010;4:115–9.
80. Osborn PM, Schmidt AH. Diagnosis and management of acute compartment syndrome. J Am Acad Orthop Surg. 2021;29(5):183–8.
81. Neal E. Imaging findings in the setting of rhabdomyolysis. Appl Radiol. 2021;50(2):20–5.
82. Shadgan B, Menon M, O'Brien PJ, Reid WD. Diagnostic techniques in acute compartment syndrome of the leg. J Orthop Trauma. 2008;22(8):581–7.
83. McQueen MM, Gaston P, Court-Brown CM. Acute compartment syndrome. Who is at risk? J Bone Joint Surg Br. 2000;82(2):200–3.
84. Scalea TM, DuBose J, Moore EE, West M, Moore FA, McIntyre R, et al. Western Trauma Association critical decisions in trauma: management of the mangled extremity. J Trauma Acute Care Surg. 2012;72(1):86–93.
85. Ly TV, Travison TG, Castillo RC, Bosse MJ, MacKenzie EJ, Group LS. Ability of lower-extremity injury severity scores to predict functional outcome after limb salvage. J Bone Joint Surg Am. 2008;90(8):1738–43.
86. Bosse MJ, MacKenzie EJ, Kellam JF, Burgess AR, Webb LX, Swiontkowski MF, et al. A prospective evaluation of the clinical utility of the lower-extremity injury-severity scores. J Bone Joint Surg Am. 2001;83(1):3–14.

87. Black CK, Ormiston LD, Fan KL, Kotha VS, Attinger C, Evans KK. Amputations versus salvage: reconciling the differences. J Reconstr Microsurg. 2021;37(1):32–41.
88. Burkhardt GE, Cox M, Clouse WD, Porras C, Gifford SM, Williams K, et al. Outcomes of selective tibial artery repair following combat-related extremity injury. J Vasc Surg. 2010;52(1):91–6.
89. American Academy of Orthopedic Surgeons. Limb salvage or early amputation evidence-based clinical practice guideline. AAOS.org/lsacpg. Published 6 Dec 2019.
90. Johnson SF, Johnson SB, Strodel WE, Barker DE, Kearney PA. Brachial plexus injury: association with subclavian and axillary vascular trauma. J Trauma. 1991;31(11):1546–50.
91. Bradley MJ, Franklin BR, Renninger CH, Graybill JC, Bowyer MW, Andreatta PB. Upper-extremity vascular exposures for trauma: comparative performance outcomes for general surgeons and orthopedic surgeons. Mil Med. 2022;188:e1395.
92. Branco BC, Boutrous ML, DuBose JJ, Leake SS, Charlton-Ouw K, Rhee P, et al. Outcome comparison between open and endovascular management of axillosubclavian arterial injuries. J Vasc Surg. 2016;63(3):702–9.
93. Carrafiello G, Lagana D, Mangini M, Fontana F, Recaldini C, Piacentino F, et al. Percutaneous treatment of traumatic upper-extremity arterial injuries: a single-center experience. J Vasc Interv Radiol. 2011;22(1):34–9.
94. Gilani R, Tsai PI, Wall MJ Jr, Mattox KL. Overcoming challenges of endovascular treatment of complex subclavian and axillary artery injuries in hypotensive patients. J Trauma Acute Care Surg. 2012;73(3):771–3.
95. Asensio JA, Kessler JJ 2nd, Miljkovic SS, Kotaru TR, Dabestani PJ, Kalamchi LD, et al. Brachial artery injuries operative management and predictors of outcome. Ann Vasc Surg. 2020;69:146–57.
96. Debakey ME, Simeone FA. Battle injuries of the arteries in World War II: an analysis of 2,471 cases. Ann Surg. 1946;123(4):534–79.
97. Teixeira PGR, DuBose J. Surgical management of vascular trauma. Surg Clin North Am. 2017;97(5):1133–55.
98. Pettitt DA, McArthur P. Clinical review: Volkmann's ischaemic contracture. Eur J Trauma Emerg Surg. 2012;38(2):129–37.
99. Soni A, Tzafetta K, Knight S, Giannoudis PV. Gustilo IIIC fractures in the lower limb: our 15-year experience. J Bone Joint Surg Br. 2012;94(5):698–703.
100. Wynes J, Kirksey L. Assessing vascular status and risk of latent ischemia with ankle fracture: a case report and algorithm for treatment. J Foot Ankle Surg. 2014;53(3):353–5.
101. Georgakarakos E, Papatheodorou N, Keskinis A, Karaolanis GI, Georgoulas P. Anterior tibial to dorsalis pedis bypass to manage acute ischemia attributed to pilon fracture. Vasc Endovasc Surg. 2023;57(1):64–8.
102. Ukai T, Hamahashi K, Uchiyama Y, Kobayashi Y, Watanabe M. Retrospective analysis of risk factors for deep infection in lower limb Gustilo-Anderson type III fractures. J Orthop Traumatol. 2020;21(1):10.
103. Subedi N, Heire P, Parmer V, Beardmore S, Oh C, Jepson F, et al. Multimodality imaging review of the post-amputation stump pain. Br J Radiol. 2016;89(1068):20160572.
104. Virani SR, Dahapute AA, Bava SS, Muni SR. Impact of negative pressure wound therapy on open diaphyseal tibial fractures: a prospective randomized trial. J Clin Orthop Trauma. 2016;7(4):256–9.
105. Argenta LC, Morykwas MJ. Vacuum-assisted closure: a new method for wound control and treatment: clinical experience. Ann Plast Surg. 1997;38(6):563–76; discussion 77.
106. Govaert GAM, Kuehl R, Atkins BL, Trampuz A, Morgenstern M, Obremskey WT, et al. Diagnosing fracture-related infection: current concepts and recommendations. J Orthop Trauma. 2020;34(1):8–17.
107. Lynch JR, Taitsman LA, Barei DP, Nork SE. Femoral nonunion: risk factors and treatment options. J Am Acad Orthop Surg. 2008;16(2):88–97.
108. Ford AN, Harkin EA, Lyons MM, Summers HD, Hecht GG, Lack WD, et al. Clinical and radiographic predictors of nonunion in open tibial shaft fractures. Orthopedics. 2021;44(3):142–7.
109. Bell A, Templeman D, Weinlein JC. Nonunion of the femur and tibia: an update. Orthop Clin North Am. 2016;47(2):365–75.
110. Santolini E, West R, Giannoudis PV. Risk factors for long bone fracture non-union: a stratification approach based on the level of the existing scientific evidence. Injury. 2015;46(Suppl 8):S8–S19.
111. Fayad LM, Patra A, Fishman EK. Value of 3D CT in defining skeletal complications of orthopedic hardware in the postoperative patient. AJR Am J Roentgenol. 2009;193(4):1155–63.

12 Pediatric Trauma Computed Tomography: A Comprehensive Guide

Neal Joshi, Kathleen E. Schenker, Rahul Nikam, and Vinay Kandula

Introduction

Trauma is the leading cause of morbidity and mortality in children over 1 year of age, with motor vehicle collisions being a major contributor [1]. Other mechanisms include falls, bicycle injuries, sports injuries, or child abuse. Approximately 90% of injuries are from blunt trauma. Head, spine, and limb injuries are most common, followed by chest and abdominal injuries. It can be especially difficult to differentiate accidental trauma from nonaccidental trauma, a differentiation with drastic social and legal implications for the patient, families, and clinicians. CT has become an important guidance tool in evaluation and management of trauma in pediatric patients. However, because children are at increased risk of harmful radiation effects, CT must be used more judiciously. The increased risk of radiation effects in children can be attributed to two major factors. First, children have a longer life expectancy allowing more time for radiation-induced cancers to manifest. Second, radiation damage preferentially affects dividing and proliferating cells in growing children [2]. Furthermore, children are less likely to require operative intervention for solid organ injuries than adults. Thus, the need for CT imaging in a pediatric trauma patient must be carefully considered to maximize clinically relevant diagnostic information but minimize radiation exposure.

Recent strategies have been employed to decrease CT utilization and radiation dose. The Image Gently campaign has raised awareness in healthcare for the need to reduce CT dose in children and has promoted dose reduction protocols [2–4]. Corresponding to the rollout of these awareness campaigns, CT use in pediatric patients has finally started to decline over the last decade [5]. Various clinical guidelines and algorithms have been also developed and have proven successful in decreasing rate of CT utilization in pediatric trauma patients without missing addi-

Neal Joshi and Kathleen E. Schenker contributed equally.

N. Joshi
Department of Radiology, Thomas Jefferson University Hospital, Philadelphia, PA, USA
e-mail: nxj058@jefferson.edu

K. E. Schenker · R. Nikam · V. Kandula (✉)
Department of Medical Imaging, Nemours Children's Hospital, Wilmington, DE, USA
e-mail: Kathleen.Schenker@nemours.org; Rahul.Nikam@nemours.org; vinay.kandula@nemours.org

F. Knollmann (ed.), *Trauma Computed Tomography*, https://doi.org/10.1007/978-3-031-45746-3_12

tional clinically important injuries [6–8]. However, studies have shown that there is still significantly higher usage of CT in adult or mixed population trauma centers as opposed to pediatric trauma centers [9].

This chapter will guide trainees of all levels and practicing physicians in imaging workup and diagnosis of pediatric accidental and nonaccidental trauma, with a focus on CT imaging. Special considerations for pediatric specific protocols will be discussed. Trauma mimics, including developmental and anatomic variants are important diagnostic pitfalls and will be reviewed. This chapter will include the common pediatric trauma diagnoses as well as some uncommon diagnoses which are important to consider.

Pediatric CT Protocols

Pre-scan preparation for children is important and should focus on making the environment comfortable for the child to minimize motion and need to repeat scanning. Sedation can be used if necessary. Multiphase scanning is used conservatively, primarily in the setting of suspected urinary tract injury where delayed scans are needed to assess for extravasation from the collecting system or bladder. A strategy for minimizing multiphase scanning is using a split bolus of contrast to simultaneously opacify the collecting system and the renal parenchyma [10, 11]. Pre-contrast CT is rarely needed. Oral contrast is not routinely used in the emergency setting. Specific protocol parameters are outlined below.

Protocol name	CTA chest	Chest/ abdomen/ pelvis with contrast	Abdomen/ pelvis with contrast	CT C-Spine	CT T-Spine	CT L-Spine	CTA head/neck	CTA neck	CT head without contrast	CT facial bones and orbits	CT temporal bones
Indication	Trauma	Trauma	Trauma	Trauma	Trauma	Trauma	Trauma	Cervical trauma	Trauma	Trauma	Trauma
Protocol designed for (scanner model)	Siemens Somatom Definition Flash	Siemens Somatom Definition Flash	Siemens Somatom Definition Flash	Siemens Somatom Definition Flash	Siemens Somatom Definition Flash	Siemens Somatom Definition Flash	Siemens Somatom Definition Flash	Siemens Somatom Definition Flash	Siemens Somatom Definition Flash	Siemens Somatom Definition Flash	Siemens Somatom Definition Flash
Patient preparation	No, contrast screening form	No, contrast screening form, pregnancy test (if applicable)	No, contrast screening form, pregnancy test (if applicable)	No	No	No	No	No	No	No	No
First series											
Oral contrast	No	No	No	No	No	No	No	No	No	No	No
IV contrast	OMNIPAQUE 350 contrast 2 mL/kg at 75%	OPTIRAY 320 contrast 2 mL/kg	OPTIRAY 320 CONTRAST 2 mL/kg	No	No	No	OMNIPAQUE 2 mL/kg of body weight	OMNIPAQUE 2 mL/kg of body weight	No	No	No
Tube settings											
kV	80–120 kV (depending on age)	80–120 kV (depending on age)	80–120 kV (depending on age)	80–120 kV (depending on age)	80–120 kV (depending on age)	80–120 kV (depending on age)	70 or 80 kV	70 or 80 kV	120 kV	120 kV	120kV
mA	100–400 mAs	100–400 mAs	100–400 mAs	100–230 mAs	100–230 mAs	100–230 mAs	200–400 mAs	200–400 mAs	100–300 mAs	125 mAs	180 mAs
Dose modulation	Whenever possible	Off	Off	Whenever possible	Whenever possible	Whenever possible	Whenever possible	Whenever possible	Off	Off	Off
Tube rotation time (s)	0.5	0.5	0.5	1	1	1	0.5	0.5	1	1	1
Table speed (mm/s)	46	53	46	30	30	30	46	46	8.4	30	3.6
Slice collimation	0.6 mm	0.6 mm	0.6 mm	0.6 mm	0.6 mm		0.6 mm	0.6 mm	0.6 mm	0.6 mm	0.6 mm
Reconstructed slice thickness	Soft tissue 2 mm axial	Soft tissues 5 mm axial	Soft tissues 5 mm axial	Soft tissue and bone 2 mm axial	Soft tissue and bone 2 mm axial	Soft tissue and bone 2 mm axial	Soft tissue 2 mm axial	Soft tissue 2 mm axial	Soft tissue 5 mm and bone sharp kernel 2 mm	Soft tissue 2 mm and bone sharp kernel 1–2 mm	Soft tissue 0.6 mm and bone sharp kernel 0.6 mm

Protocol name	CTA chest	Chest/ abdomen/ pelvis with contrast	Abdomen/ pelvis with contrast	CT C-Spine	CT T-Spine	CT L-Spine	CTA head/neck	CTA neck	CT head without contrast	CT facial bones and orbits	CT temporal bones
Anatomical coverage	Top of the apices to mid-adrenals	Top of the shoulders through lesser trochanter, Delay 55–60 s	Top of the liver through lesser trochanter, Delay 55–60 s	Base of the skull to T1, craniocaudal	Mid C7 through L1, craniocaudal	Mid T12 through tip of coccyx, craniocaudal	Aortic arch through vertex, caudocranial	Aortic arch through mid-orbits, include nose, caudocranial	Base of skull through vertex	Facial bones: Below mandible through frontal sinus, behind EAC	Below tip of mastoid to above temporal bone
										Orbits: Below maxillary sinus through frontal sinus, behind IAC	
Reconstruction kernel	Body Regular—Sharpness Level 40	Body Regular—Sharpness Level 40	Body Regular—Sharpness Level 40	Body Regular—Sharpness Level 62	Body Regular—Sharpness Level 62	Body Regular—Sharpness Level 62	Head Crisp—Sharpness Level 40	Head Crisp—Sharpness Level 40	Head Regular—Sharpness Level 38	Head Regular—Sharpness Level 68	Ultra-High Res—Regular—Sharpness Level 70
Breath hold	Yes	Yes	Yes	No	No	No	No	No	No	No	No
Window settings	C: 40 W: 400	C: 40 W: 400	C: 40 W: 400	C:250 W:2000	C:250 W:2000	C:250 W:2000	C:80 W:700	C:40 W:400	Brain: C: 35 W:80 Bone: C: 250 W: 2000	Soft tissues: C: 40 W; 400, Bone: C: 250 W: 2000	Soft tissues: C: 40 W; 400, Bone: C: 700 W: 4000
Post-processing	2 mm coronal and sagittal soft tissue reformats	2 mm coronal and sagittal soft tissue reformats, 2 mm axial bone	2 mm coronal and sagittal soft tissue reformats, 2 mm axial bone	1 mm coronal and sagittal reformats in soft tissue and bone	1 mm coronal and sagittal reformats in bone and axial soft tissue	1 mm coronal and sagittal reformats in bone and axial soft tissue	2 mm axial, coronal and sagittal reformats in soft tissue	2 mm axial, coronal, and sagittal reformats in soft tissue	3D volume rendered reconstructions skull	3D volume rendered reconstructions facial bones	Axial and coronal bone sharp kernel 0.6 mm
Other											

Protocol name	CTA chest	Chest/abdomen/pelvis with contrast	Abdomen/pelvis with contrast	CT C-Spine	CT T-Spine	CT L-Spine	CTA head/neck	CTA neck	CT head without contrast	CT facial bones and orbits	CT temporal bones
Typical dose											
CTDIvol	4.4	7.3	7.7	4.4	6	12	12	4	24	15.6	39.04
DLP	77	470	180	80	110	231	185	80	431	284	181
Eff. dose	3.47	4.08	4.38	1.4	4.9	4.9	1.22	1.52	0.76	0.275	0.391
Second series											
Oral contrast											
IV contrast											
Tube settings											
kV											
mA											
Dose modulation											
Tube rotation time (s)											
Table speed (mm/s)											
Slice collimation											
Reconstructed slice thickness											
Anatomical coverage											
Reconstruction kernel											
Breath hold											
Window settings											
Post-processing											
Other											
Typical dose											
CTDIvol											
DLP											
Eff. dose											
Third series											
Oral contrast											
IV contrast											
Tube settings											
kV											

Protocol name	CTA chest	Chest/abdomen/pelvis with contrast	Abdomen/pelvis with contrast	CT C-Spine	CT T-Spine	CT L-Spine	CTA head/neck	CTA neck	CT head without contrast	CT facial bones and orbits	CT temporal bones
mA											
Dose modulation											
Tube rotation time (s)											
Table speed (mm/s)											
Slice collimation											
Reconstructed slice thickness											
Anatomical coverage											
Reconstruction kernel											
Breath hold											
Window settings											
Post-processing											
Other											
Typical dose											
CTDIvol											
DLP											
Eff. dose											

Dual Energy CT (DECT) in Children

Dual-energy CT has many important uses, mostly in the adult population where much of the literature comes from. However, dual-energy CT is also useful in pediatric patients and its use is emerging. Two main reconstruction algorithms in DECT are material-decomposition images and virtual monoenergetic images. Material decomposition can either use two-material or three-material decomposition (e.g., iodine and water, or in the abdomen soft tissue, fat, and iodine). With material decomposition, virtual unenhanced images can be obtained, which are helpful in confidently identifying blood or calcium on an enhanced CT. Virtual monoenergetic images can help improve iodine contrast in small children with paucity of visceral fat at low kiloelectron volt (keV) data sets. Conversely, higher keV data help reduce beam hardening and artifacts from metal [12, 13].

The basis of DECT is obtaining a high- and low-peak voltage acquisition to differentiate changes in attenuation of various material compositions such as iodine, hemorrhage, bone, and calcium, even if they are of similar density on a single energy CT. DECT can differentiate these materials from each other and soft tissue due to intrinsic properties such as atomic number, unique k-edge characteristics, and different linear attenuation coefficients at different energies [12]. Dual-energy bone removal CT (BRCT) is superior for intracranial hemorrhage detection [14]. It may also help detect trace subdural hemorrhage adjacent to bone, which otherwise can easily be mistaken for cupping artifact. One study, though performed on adults, found that the detection of epidural/subdural hemorrhages and contusions using DECT with the bone removal protocol was superior to standard CT [14].

Metal artifact can severely degrade CT image quality and obscure important pathology. A common metal artifact in children is spinal fusion hardware which can obscure abnormalities in solid organs, especially the kidneys. Virtual monoenergetic images between 110 and 150 keV can remove low-energy photons that contribute to beam hardening [15]. One example of the utility of DECT is its use in imaging the neck arteries in a child with a gunshot wound and retained bullet fragments in the neck. Similarly, with DECT angiogram the axial and appendicular skeleton can be removed, allowing better visualization of the contrast enhanced vessels. Virtual monoenergetic images can be utilized for iodine maps for solid organ perfusion.

Pediatric Head, Neck, and Spine Trauma

Imaging Appropriateness Criteria for Pediatric Head Trauma

The American College of Radiology (ACR) Appropriateness Criteria rates imaging procedures for specific clinical situations on a scale of 1–9, with 1 being not at all appropriate and 9 being highly appropriate. These criteria can be used to guide imaging decisions. Non-enhanced computed tomography (NECT) remains the gold standard for imaging acute head trauma in pediatric and adult patients. The ACR appropriateness criteria for imaging children with acute head trauma is based on risk stratification into low, intermediate, and high-risk groups established by the Pediatric Emergency Care Applied Research Network criteria (PECARN) (Table 12.1) [16, 17]. NECT is indicated for all high-risk children due to high risk of clinically important traumatic brain injury if any of the following are present: GCS <15, altered mental status, or signs of basilar skull fracture. CT may be considered for intermediate risk children <2 years old who have GCS 15, but may have loss of consciousness, severe mechanism of injury, or non-frontal scalp hematoma. CT may be considered for intermediate risk children >2 years old who do not meet the high-risk criteria but may have vomiting, loss of consciousness, severe headache, or severe mechanism of injury. CT is not indicated in low-risk children who do not meet any of the above criteria. Other appropriateness criteria are outlined for subacute and chronic head trauma, in which MRI is more frequently indicated [16]. Imaging appropriateness criteria differ for sus-

Table 12.1 ACR Appropriateness Criteria for noncontrast head CT in pediatric head trauma, based on PECARN risk classification

PECARN risk classification	NECT	Child <2 years old	Child >2 years old
High	Appropriate	GCS <15 **or** altered mental status, signs of basilar skull fracture	GCS <15 **or** altered mental status, signs of basilar skull fracture
Intermediate	May be appropriate	GCS 15 **With any of:** nonfrontal scalp hematoma, loss of consciousness >5 seconds, severe mechanism of injury, not acting normally No signs of altered mental status or palpable skull fracture	GCS 15 **with any of:** any loss of consciousness, vomiting, severe mechanism of injury, severe headache No signs of altered mental status or basilar skull fracture
Low	Not appropriate	GCS 15 **With none of following:** palpable skull fracture, nonfrontal scalp hematoma, loss of consciousness >5 s, severe mechanism of injury, not acting normal, other signs of altered mental status	GCS 15 **With none of following:** signs of basilar skull fracture, loss of consciousness, vomiting, severe mechanism of injury, severe headache, signs of altered mental status

pected child abuse and are discussed later with non-accidental trauma.

Pitfalls in the Interpretation of Pediatric Head CT

Pitfalls in the interpretation of pediatric CT are encountered due to anatomic and developmental differences in pediatric patients. Increased water content in the neonatal brain can be misinterpreted as cerebral edema [18]. Increased water density reduces the contrast between normal and abnormal tissue, making detection of subtle hypoxic-ischemic injuries and cerebral edema difficult. Using narrower window levels can improve the contrast between white and gray matter, helping to avoid this pitfall. If equivocal, MRI can be performed for further clarification. Pseudosubarachnoid hemorrhage can be seen in the setting of diffuse cerebral edema due to a relative increase in attenuation within the basal cisterns in the absence of hemorrhage. Increased ICP causes hyperdense extra-axial vascular engorgement coupled with reduced hypodense CSF spaces due to effacement. The juxtaposition of the basal cisterns with adjacent hypodense, edematous cerebral parenchyma creates the pseudosubarachnoid hemorrhage appearance. Calvarial sutures, accessory sutures, or Wormian bones can often be mistaken for fractures. Sutures and Wormian bones have interdigitating, zig-zag contours with sclerotic margins, while fractures tend to be linear with sharp, non-sclerotic margins and adjacent scalp swelling. Multiplanar and volume rendered reconstructions are helpful in assessing the calvarium for fractures and differentiating from sutures.

Birth-Related Trauma

Birth is an inherently traumatic process with mechanical forces occurring that can lead to intracranial or extracranial hemorrhage, spinal cord injuries, peripheral or cranial nerve injuries, or skeletal injuries. One study found that intracranial hemorrhage was present in 26% of asymptomatic neonates [19]. Ultrasound, CT, and MRI all play a role in initial work-up and follow-up. Rapid skull molding during birth may result in rapid or severe skull deformation, which can tear the dural folds or bridging veins resulting in extra-axial hemorrhage that may be epidural, subdural, or subarachnoid. Birth-related SDH is relatively common, occurring in 38% of births, and can be seen with or without the use of instrumentation during delivery [20]. Most birth related subdural hemorrhages occur in both the supratentorial and infratentorial compartments [20]. Birth related SDH must be considered as an alternative explanation for hemorrhage in the workup for abusive head trauma in neonates. If AHT is suspected, MRI should be obtained. Fat-suppressed sequences can improve the detection of subtle subdural collections and spinal trauma [21]. Additionally, adding T2* or SWI and FLAIR in addition to routine sequences may help with subtle findings as well, including small hemorrhages [22, 23].

Birth-related intraparenchymal hemorrhage, small cortical contusions, and shearing axonal injuries may also occur [24]. Arterial stroke is a rare but serious birth complication that can occur due to vascular compression from a large intraparenchymal hematoma or from arterial stretching injury during birth [24]. Although CT can evaluate for intra- or extracranial hemorrhages and is more feasible in most clinical scenarios, MRI (specifically susceptibility-weighted imaging) is superior for the evaluation of extracranial and posterior fossa hemorrhages [19, 24].

CT with multiplanar and 3D reconstructions is also particularly useful in assessing the calvarium for birth-related skull fractures. The most common patterns include linear fractures, depressed skull fractures, or occipital osteodiastasis. Occipital osteodiastasis occurs in breech babies where there is excessive pressure on subocciput during birth, resulting in separation of the squamous and lateral aspect of the occipital bone, often associated with posterior fossa subdural hemorrhage. Skull fractures can occasionally result in leptomeningeal cysts, in which the leptomeninges are trapped within the fracture defect and CSF pulsations result in the subsequent enlargement of the fractures (commonly referred to as growing fractures). These can be imaged using high-resolution ultrasound and followed up by CT or MRI [24].

Extracranial/scalp hemorrhages are relatively common after birth and include cephalohematoma, caput succedaneum, and subgaleal hemorrhage, depending on which layer of the scalp the hemorrhage occurs. In most cases, these resolve spontaneously. Subgaleal hematomas, however, can have more serious complications. A minority may cause extensive blood loss requiring transfusion and evacuation of the hematoma. Imaging and follow-up usually consist of high-resolution head ultrasound. The relation of the hematoma to adjacent sutures on imaging is important to proper classification. Cephalohematomas are subperiosteal, often over the parietal convexity between the outer table of the calvarium and overlying periosteum. Thus, cephalohematomas do not cross sutures. On the other hand, a subgaleal hematoma occurs from rupture of emissary veins between the dural sinus and scalp veins and can cross sutures [25]. Caput succedaneum occurs in the superficial subcutaneous scalp, external to the galea aponeurosis and crosses sutures, usually at the vertex.

Spinal cord injuries can also result from birth-related trauma, caused by excessive traction, rotation, and hyperextension and may be accompanied by vertebral fractures or subluxations. Neonates are prone to craniocervical ligamentous injuries due to ligamentous laxity and relatively large head size. Initially, a lateral radiograph of the spine is helpful to detect fractures or subluxation, though MRI is needed to assess for ligamentous or spinal cord injury. Brachial plexus birth injuries and fractures, particularly clavicle, rib or humerus fractures are other potential birth complications [24]. CT does not routinely play a role in the workup for these injuries.

Traumatic Injuries of the Head, Neck, and Spine

Cerebral Contusions

One of the most common manifestations of traumatic brain injury in the pediatric population is cerebral contusions. In adults, contusions are usually located in rigid areas of the cranial fossa such as frontal and temporal lobes at skull bases. However, in the pediatric population, they can be present anywhere due to a lack of formation of skull base ridges [18, 26]. On NECT, cerebral contusions may appear as single or multiple hyperdense foci, though they may be occult initially. Subtle cortical hypodense areas can reflect edema in the setting of contusions. MRI can further characterize these injuries. It is important to identify scalp contusions or skull fractures since cerebral contusion patterns may occur in a coup-contrecoup mechanism [18, 26].

Diffuse Axonal Injury

Diffuse axonal injury (DAI) is caused by rapid acceleration-deceleration forces that lead to the shearing of axonal fibers and is associated with traumatic brain injury (TBI), both accidental and non-accidental. DAI is most commonly seen in severe TBI cases but can also be seen in some cases of mild and moderate TBI. These injuries usually occur at the gray-white matter interface, appearing as microhemorrhages. CT has low sensitivity for detection of DAI and MRI is the gold standard for diagnosis. Nonspecific findings on CT such as interhemispheric fissure or perimesencephalic cistern subarachnoid hemorrhage may suggest DAI [26]. Larger or hemorrhagic DAI lesions may be seen on NECT. Otherwise, NECT has a low sensitivity for non-hemorrhagic lesions. MR findings for DAI include blood products on SWI or GRE for hemorrhagic lesions and T2/FLAIR hyperintense foci for non-hemorrhagic lesions, indicating edema. Small lesions on NECT suggesting DAI should alert the radiologist to recommend further MRI, since the extent of the injury is likely much greater than seen on NECT. In general, deeper DAI lesions, particularly involving the brainstem, are associated with worse functional outcomes [27].

Craniovertebral Junction Injuries

Although cervical spine injuries only account for 1–2% of pediatric trauma, there is a high risk of significant neurologic injury because the mechanism of injury typically involves high force. It is crucial to accurately diagnose and grade severity of spinal injuries to decrease the risk of permanent neurological damage and death. Spinal injuries differ from adults due to marked differences in anatomy and physiology in young children. Overall, the cervical spine in children is hypermobile and tends to dislocate rather than fracture. Predisposing biomechanics include horizontal uncovertebral and facet joints, ligamentous laxity, weak musculature, increased head-to-body ratio, and underdeveloped/incompletely ossified bones with higher fulcrum [28]. Vertebral bodies are more wedge-shaped compared to the rectangular shape seen in adults. By the age of 8–10, the biomechanics of the pediatric cervical spine become more adult-like and by 10–12 years, injuries are similar to adults [29].

Although the incidence of cervical spine injury is lower in children, the sequelae are more severe. The younger the child, the greater likelihood of an upper cervical spine injury between the occiput and C3. Atlanto-occipital dislocation injuries are three times more common in children [30]. Often injuries are ligamentous and not bony. Careful attention for cervical spine malalignment on radiographs or CT is needed, as this suggests underlying ligamentous injury. Confusing developmental or anatomic variants for cervical spine injury is an important pitfall to avoid. McAllister et al. discuss ossification variants in the cervical spine in more detail, which is beyond the scope of this chapter [29]. Pseudosubluxation of the cervical spine, especially at C2–C3 is an important pitfall to recognize. Pseudosubluxation is a normal finding in children that occurs from increased ligamentous laxity resulting in appearance of subluxation. However, in contrast to true subluxation, the posterior spinolaminar line is maintained [30]. Spine radiographs remain the initial imaging modality of choice, though CT may be the initial modality when patients are obtunded, experience polytrauma, or have a high-risk mechanism of injury.

Craniovertebral junction (CVJ) and upper cervical distraction injuries are more common in young children with potentially grave consequences, given the relative instability of the upper cervical spine. The mechanism of injury is most often rapid deacceleration and hyperflexion during motor vehicle crash. Knowledge of the normal development and ossification patterns of the atlas and axis is necessary to avoid false positives or misclassifying the extent of the injury. Vertebral body alignment is usually abnormal in CVJ injuries because most injuries are ligamentous and not bony. The occipital condyle-C1 interval is the most sensitive and specific for detecting atlanto-occipital (AO) dislocation [31–33]. Although there are many other methods of detecting AO dislocation such as the Powers ratio, C1-2 interspinous space, and Wackenheim line, the most sensitive measurement is the basion-dens interval and interspinous ratio. Regarding atlantoaxial (AA) injuries, asymmetry of the C1–C2 joint space is crucial for diagnosis. On the coronal CT plane, greater than 4 mm space between the C1 and C2 lateral masses, or greater than a 5 mm odontoid-lateral mass interval is indicative of ligamentous injury. At times, these measurements can be difficult to obtain if some of the landmarks are not yet ossified or partially ossified; therefore, multiple methods need to be in the radiologist's arsenal.

There should be low threshold for MRI when signs of CVJ injury are visualized on CT or radiographs. Soft tissue planes on MR are best visualized on the sagittal plane, and associated findings include but are not limited to fat stranding between the basion and dens, the elevation of the posterior AO membrane or atlantoaxial (AA) membrane, retroclival hematoma, and extrathecal collections/hemorrhage [29]. Coronal STIR MR sequence can show edema/hyperintensity, confirming ligamentous injury. Other areas of signal abnormality can be seen between the clivus and dens, between the anterior arch of C1 and the dens, and along the interspinous ligaments. If a retroclival hemorrhage is noted on CT, then further evaluation with an MR should be obtained as this may a ligamentous injury at the craniocervical junction (Fig. 12.1).

Spinal Cord Injury Without Radiographic Abnormality (SCIWORA)

Children are more prone to spinal cord injuries without radiographic abnormality (SCIWORA). Ligamentous laxity of the cervical spine and hypermobility of the osseous spine predisposes to direct spinal cord injuries without bony abnormalities during flexion-extension injury [30]. Not surprisingly, SCIWORA is inversely proportional to age [32, 34]. Radiographs and cervical spine CT are characteristically normal. However, MRI shows T2 signal hyperintensity with or without hemorrhage in the cervical cord with edema in the soft tissues and/or ligaments [28, 30]. MRI may also show other clinically significant findings such as traumatic herniated disc or epidural hematoma that may compress the cord [28]. MRI has become the gold standard in patients with suspected spinal cord injury to detect soft tissue and spinal cord abnormalities which may be present in the absence of bony abnormalities. Treatment is typically immobilization [30] (Fig. 12.2)

C1 Synchondrosis Fracture

The C1 cervical vertebra is unique in that it is mainly a cartilaginous structure and incompletely ossified at birth. C1 consists of an anterior and two posterolateral ossification centers with cartilaginous bridges known as synchondroses. The ossification centers appear at varying ages and can completely ossify at different ages. It appears that the closure of the anterior neurocentral synchondrosis usually occurs later than the posterior. Depending on the study, the anterior synchondrosis typically closes around 5 to 6 years of age, but may be incomplete even after age 9 [35]. Unsurprisingly, in the setting of trauma, C1 synchondrosis fractures may be seen (Fig. 12.3). For isolated anterior C1 arch fractures, 6 weeks of rigid immobilization has been used with success [36].

C2/Odontoid Synchondrosis Fracture

In the setting for cervical spine trauma, it is important to consider possible congenital anomalies, variants, and normal synchondroses/ossification centers that may mimic a traumatic injury. For example, congenital agenesis/hypoplasia of the posterior arch of the atlas, although usually asymptomatic and incidentally discovered on radiographs in the trauma setting, may be associated with neck pain or present with more severe neurologic symptoms from atlanto-occipital instability. In cases where radiograph is unequivocal, CT is the gold standard to detect differences in ossified and nonossified portions of C1 and other more minor defects [37]. Congenital absence of the posterior elements of C1–C4,

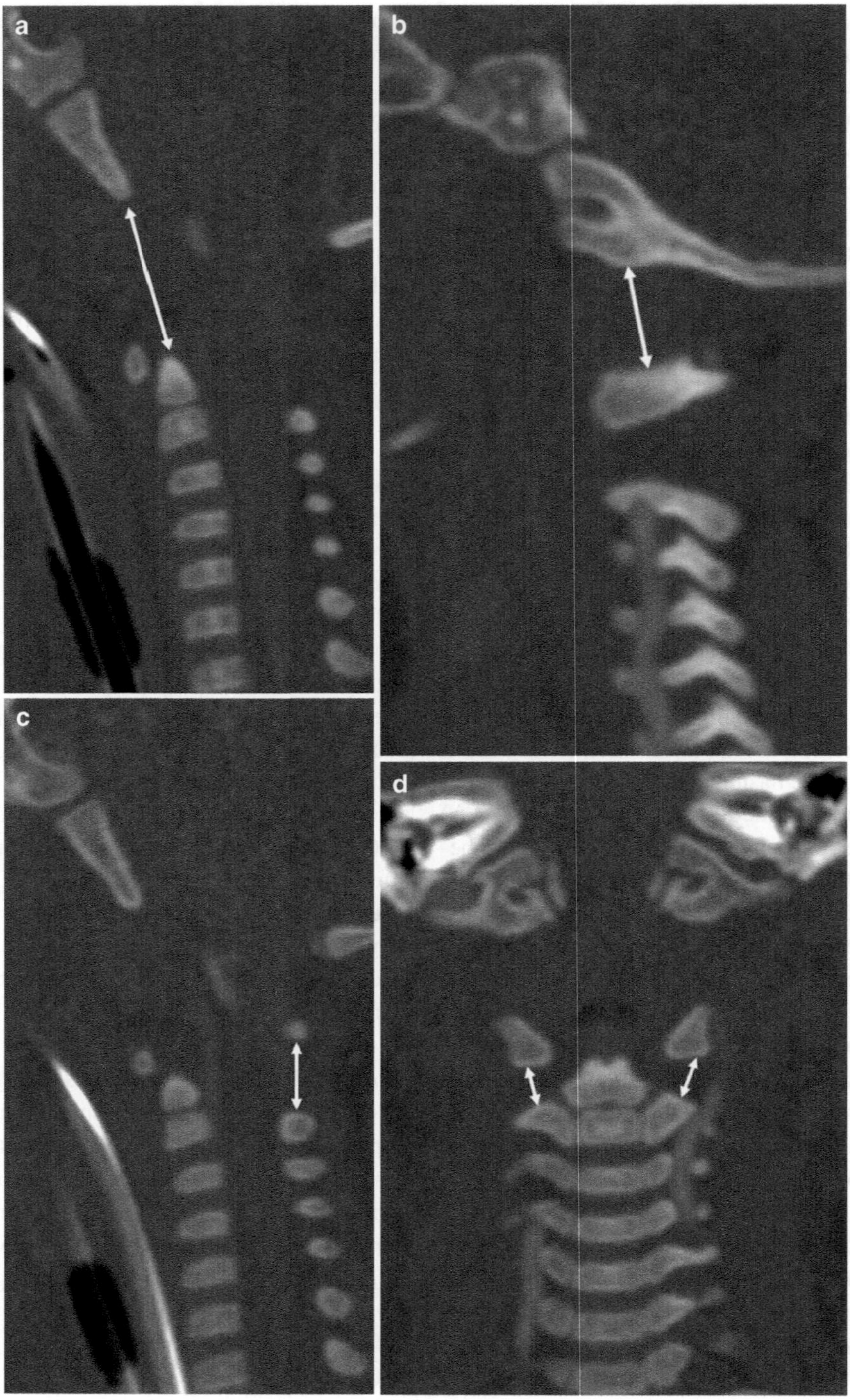

Fig. 12.1 Sagittal midline (**a**), parasagittal (**b**, **c**), and coronal (**d**) CT scans bone windows: 8-month-old girl involved in MVC, inappropriately restrained, found suspended by her neck from her seatbelt. Figure (**a**) midline image demonstrates an increase in basion-dens interval of 25 mm (normal is less than 12 mm). Figure (**b**) parasagittal image demonstrates increase in atlanto-occipital interval of 11 mm (normal is 4 mm in younger children and 2.5 mm in older children). Figure (**c**) demonstrates increase in interspinous ratio of 4.4 [11/2.5 mm] (C1–C2 interspinous space divided by C2–C3 interspinous space with a normal interspinous ratio is less than 2.5) and C1–C2 space measuring 11 mm (and normal interspinous measurement is less than 12 mm). Figure (**d**) Coronal CT image shows widening of the atlantoaxial space. Features are in keeping with Occipito-Atlanto-Axial distraction injury

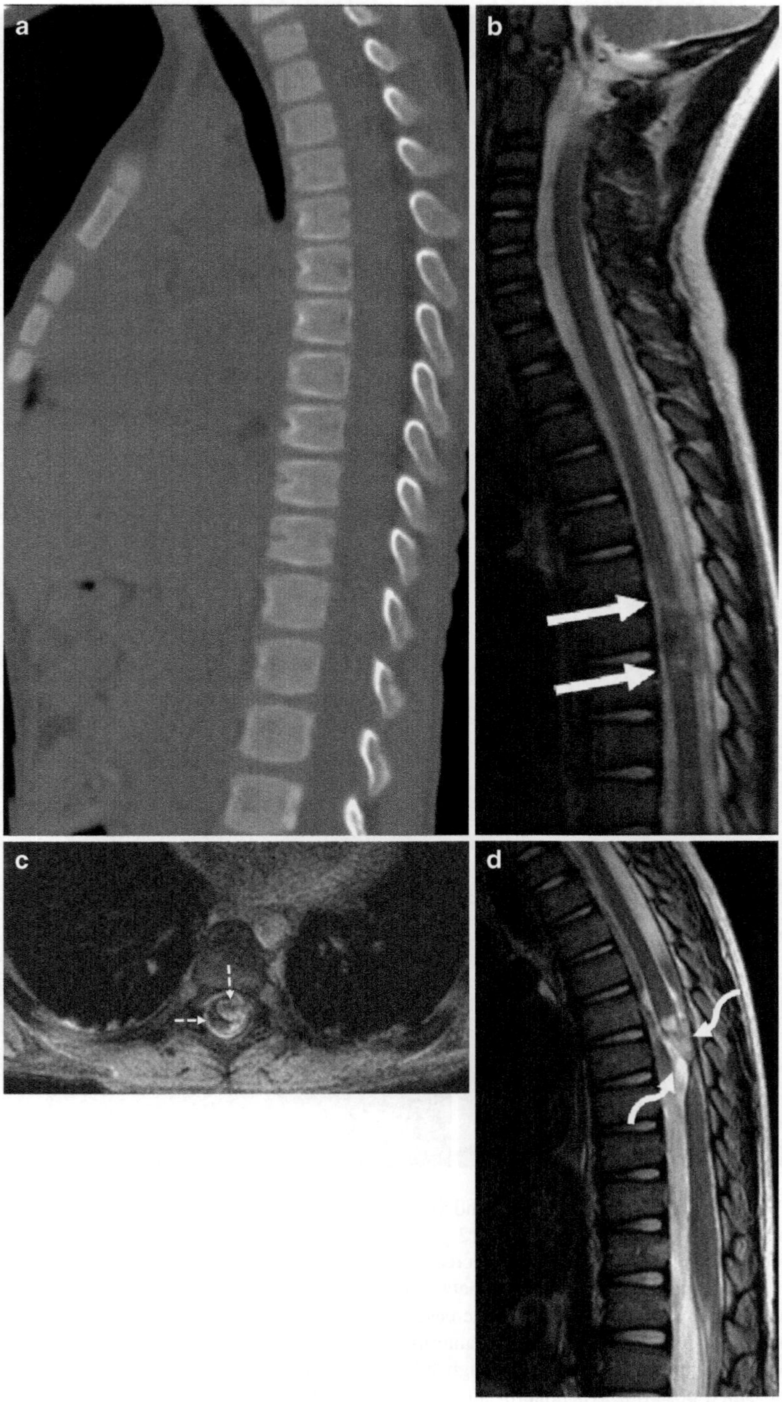

Fig. 12.2 Sagittal CT (**a**), Sagittal T2 (**b**), axial gradient (**c**), and Sagittal T2 (**d**) 6 weeks after the initial scan: 4-year-old male unrestrained passenger in MVA not moving his legs and had no apparent sensation in the lower limbs 12 hours after injury. No fractures on CT. At T6-T8, there is increased T2 signal intensity within the cord with increase in diameter (arrows). Gradient echo images at this level show evidence of blood products (dashed arrows) both within and surrounding the cord. No bone marrow or ligamentous/soft tissue signal abnormality was appreciated in keeping with SCIWORA (Spinal Cord Injury Without Radiological Abnormality). Follow-up imaging (**c**) demonstrates severe myelomalacia and atrophy of the cord (curved arrows) from inferior aspect of the T6 vertebral body to the superior aspect of the T8 vertebral body

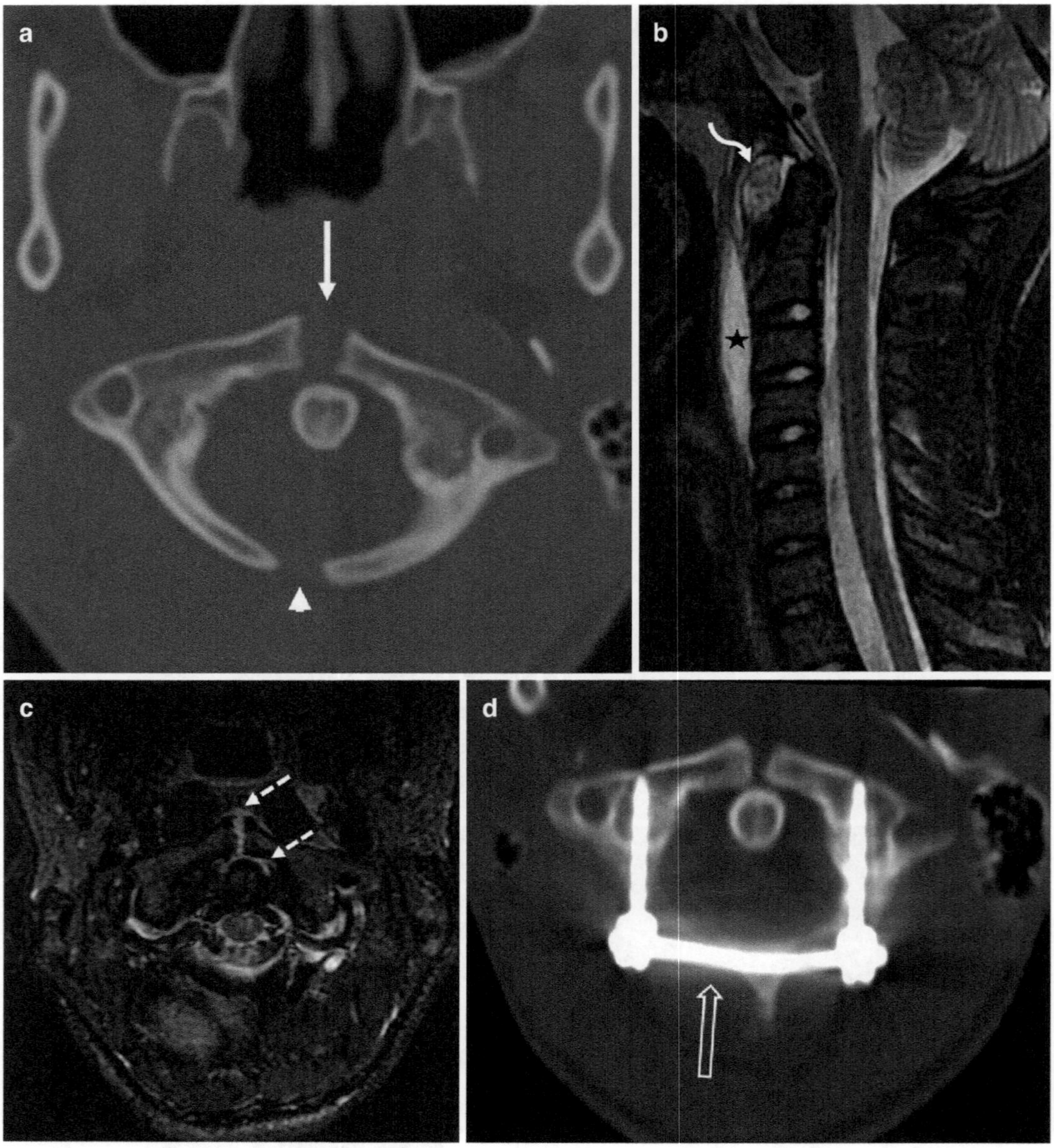

Fig. 12.3 Axial CT bone windows (**a**), Sagittal and axial STIR images (**b**, **c**), axial CT post fixation (**d**): 12-year-old male with neck injury (football game) and decreased range of motion. Asymmetric distance is noted between the dens and the lateral mass of the C1 with increased separation through the unossified cartilage of the anterior ring of C1 (arrow) suspicious for fracture through this region. Note, unossified posterior synchondrosis (arrowhead). T2 hyperintensity in the midline unossified cartilage of the anterior arch of C1 most likely representing an acute fracture (curved arrow). Small amount of fluid is identified anterior and posterior to the fracture (dashed arrow) and significant prevertebral soft tissue swelling and fluid extending from C2–C5 vertebral body levels (star). Due to potential unstable nature of the fracture, fixation was performed along the posterior arch of C1 with plate and screws (open arrow)

including the absence of C4 pedicles and double spinous apophysis of the axis, may also be seen [38]. Although outside the scope of this paper, Karawacki and Scheider published an extensive review of normal ossification patterns of the atlas and axis using CT [39]. One clue to help differentiate these normal synchondroses/ossification centers from fractures is that they are well-corticated, symmetric, and in expected locations without adjacent soft tissue swelling. Odontoid-equivalent fractures in ages seven or younger usually occur through the subdental synchondrosis before fusion (Fig. 12.4). The fractured dens typically are displaced anteriorly to some degree with the attachment of the alar ligament. Due to differences in the biomechanics of a pediatric spine, the odontoid cartilaginous synchondrosis is most commonly involved, and the axis contains multiple ossification centers and synchondroses, which may not be fully ossified until ages 7–10 [40]. Rusin et al. have developed a classification system based on odontoid synchondrosis fracture location and degree of angulation [41].

Os Odontoideum

Os odontoideum is well-defined bony ossicle at the superior aspect of the dens, which may be congenital or sequelae of prior odontoid synchondrosis fracture (a subtype of a discoligamentous injury) and should not be confused for an unfused odontoid tip ossification center. The unfused odontoid tip typically begins to ossify around 3 years of age and fuses by 12 years. If it persists after age 12, it is called ossiculum terminale. An os terminale typically much smaller than os odontoideum. Os odontoideum is commonly seen incidentally but can present with neck pain, myelopathy or quadriparesis (Fig. 12.5). Flexion and extension radiographs of the cervical spine can show the instability of the os odontoideum, depending on location. In patients with neurological deficits, pain or gross instability, surgical intervention is indicated [42].

Ring Apophysis Fracture

Lumbar disc herniations (LDHs) occur in children with a prevalence of 0.2–3.2%, albeit at a much lower prevalence compared to adults [43]. In children, LDHs are more common with trauma and are more commonly associated with ring apophysis fractures (Fig. 12.6). The apophyseal ring typically ossifies between 6 and 13 years of age and is fully fused with the vertebral body by approximately 17–18 years. Fusion of the ring apophyses in the lumbar spine occurs last. The ring apophysis is a weak point where the intervertebral ligaments and outermost layer of the intervertebral disc attach to the vertebral body. Any trauma can result in injury to the ring apophysis and intervertebral disc. Given the incomplete fusion of the ring apophysis, adolescent children have a much higher incidence of ring apophyseal fractures than adults. One retrospective study found that 38% of pediatric patients with LDHs had ring apophyseal fractures, which were more common amongst males and were associated with central disc herniations [43].

Chance Fracture

Chance fractures are flexion-distraction injuries that involve all three columns of the spine, are highly unstable, and typically associated with motor vehicle crashes [44]. They are also known as seat belt fractures since the rapid deceleration results in spine hyperflexion and subsequent distraction of the middle and posterior elements when two point restraint lap belts are used (Fig. 12.7). Although initially described as purely osseous, variants can include soft tissue injury involving discoligamentous structures. Chance fractures are often associated with intraabdominal injuries adjacent to the thoracolumbar spine as well as spinal cord injury due to their high velocity nature (Fig. 12.8). One retrospective review showed that in the pediatric population, chance fractures are more likely to have concomitant intraabdominal injury compared to adults [45]. The pancreas, bladder, spleen, liver, and mesentery can also be involved and must be scrutinized [46]. According to the ACR criteria for suspected spine trauma in a child, the initial study of choice is a radiograph of the thoracic and lumbar spine. Although there are no consensus guidelines, CECT of the abdomen and pelvis might be

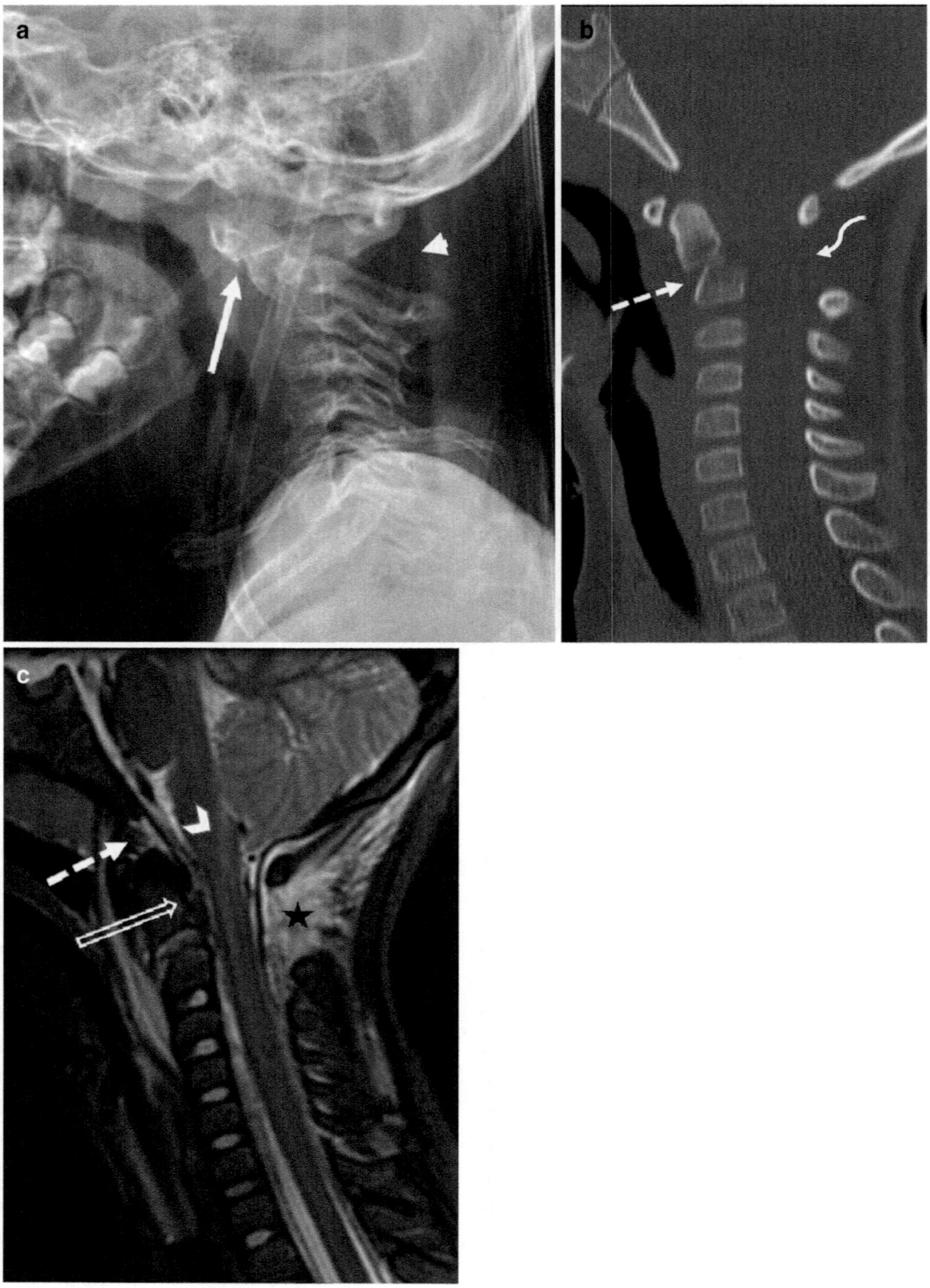

Fig. 12.4 Cervical X-ray (**a**), sagittal CT (**b**), and sagittal STIR (**c**): 4-year-old in MVC: There is a displaced fracture extending through the odontoid process (arrow) with widening of space between the spinous processes of C1 and C2 (arrowhead). CT demonstrates displaced C2 fracture through the odontoid synchondrosis with anterior dislocation of the odontoid process. In addition, there is disruption of the spinolaminar line at C1–C2 (curved arrow) with anterior subluxation of C1 with respect to the body and posterior elements of C2. There is also disruption of the anterior vertebral line (dashed arrow) at this level and significant widening of the posterior elements between C1 and C2. MRI demonstrates edema within the expected location of the apical ligament (dashed arrow) and cruciform ligament (open arrow) suggesting injury. In addition, there is discontinuity involving the anterior and posterior longitudinal ligaments at the level of the C2 fracture. Disruption of the posterior atlantoaxial ligament with significant edema (black star) surrounding the posterior atlantooccipital membrane. Patchy edema within the cervical cord (chevron arrow) at the craniocervical junction to the level of the odontoid process fracture

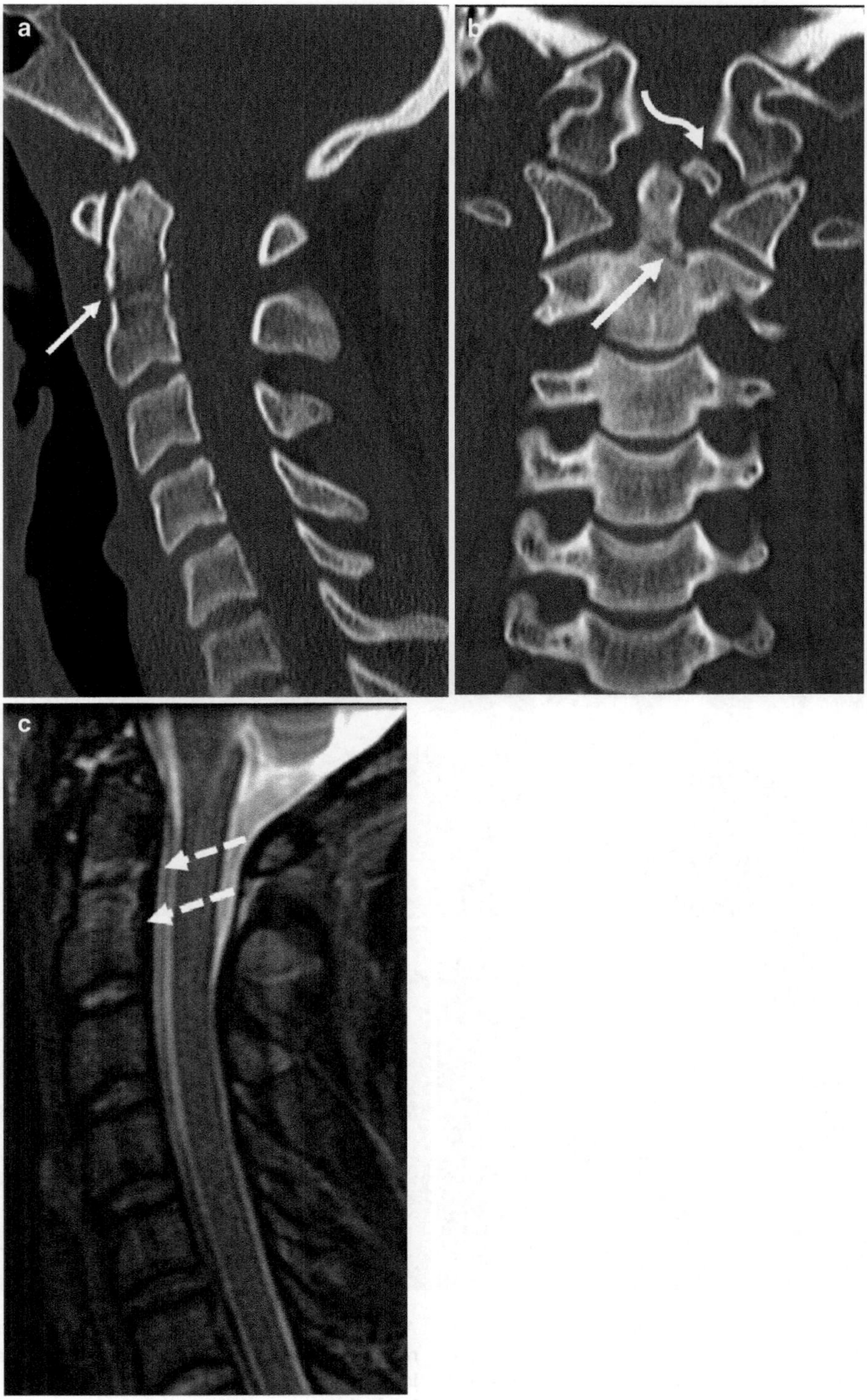

Fig. 12.5 Sagittal CT (**a**), coronal CT (**b**), and sagittal STIR (**c**): 15-year-old status post-MVA, unrestrained, with neck pain. There is a horizontal comminuted non-displaced fracture (arrows) through the base of the dens in keeping with type 2 fracture. On the coronal image, a well corticated bone is seen to the left of the dens (curved arrow) in keeping with os odontoideum, which should not be confused with tip of the dens type 1 fracture. MRI demonstrates acute type II fracture of the odontoid with bone marrow edema (dashed arrows). No edema is demonstrated at the site of the os odontoideum (not shown)

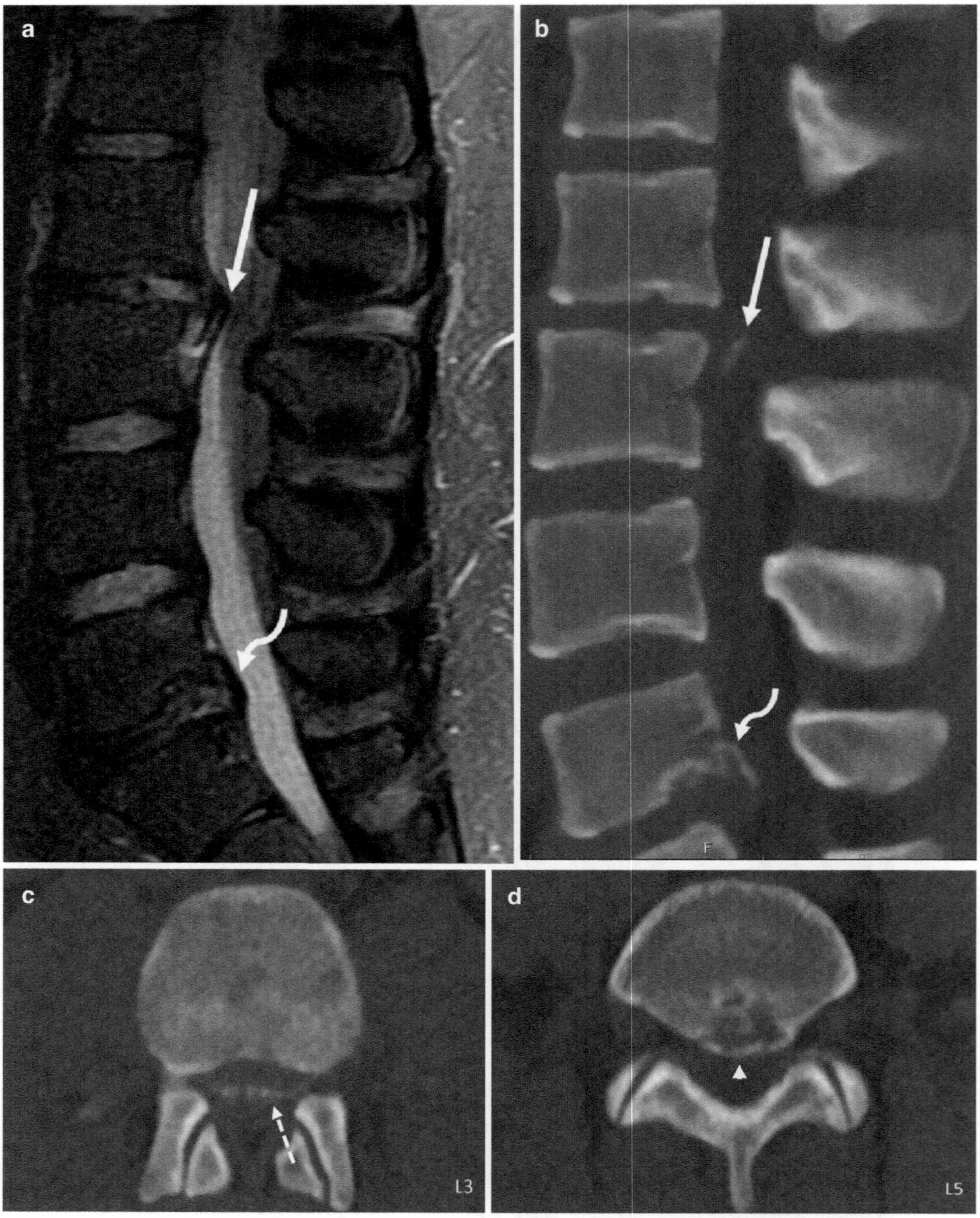

Fig. 12.6 Sagittal STIR (**a**), sagittal CT (**b**), axial CT scans at L3 and L5 (**c**, **d**): 16-year-old injured back doing dead lifts. There is a crescentic sliver of bone separated from the posterior superior margin of the L3 vertebral body associated with the large disc herniation seen on MRI consistent with apophyseal fracture (arrows). This bone sliver is relatively broad-based, extending from near the superior medial margin of both pedicles measuring approximately 2.7 cm transverse (dashed arrow). Additional ring apophyseal fracture is seen at the posterior inferior margin of L5 with extensive endplate irregularity and depression (curved arrows). Similar to the L3 level, the separated bone fragment is relatively broad-based measuring approximately 2.4 cm transverse (arrowhead). Along with the disc material seen on MRI, these bone fragments extend into the spinal canal causing central canal and lateral recess stenosis

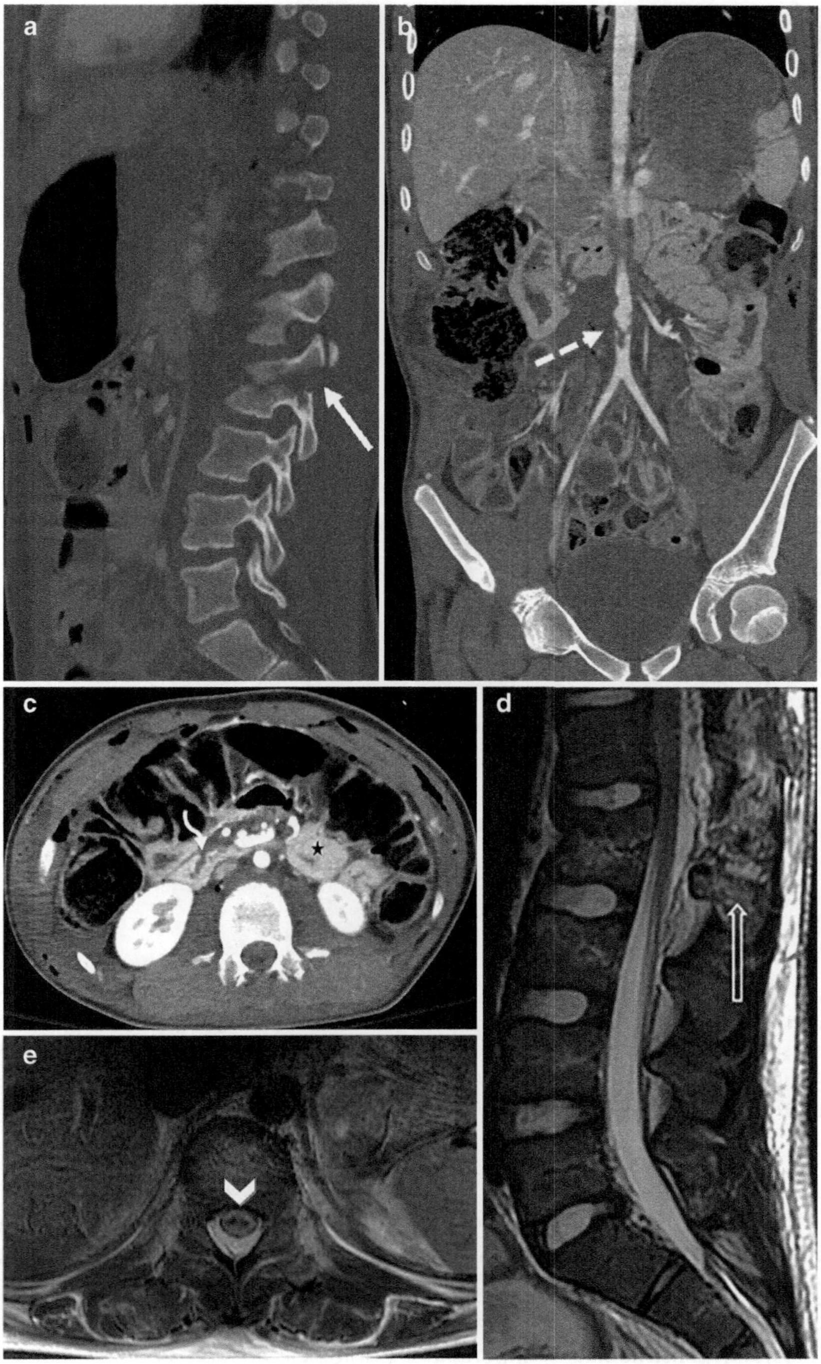

Fig. 12.7 Sagittal CT bone window (**a**), coronal and axial contrast enhanced CT (**b**, **c**), sagittal and axial T2 MRI (**d**, **e**): 13-year-old male in MVC. There is a chance fracture at L2 with approximately 1.3 cm craniocaudad distraction of the posterior elements (arrow). Complex acute transection of the lower abdominal aorta around the level of the IMA origin extends with intraluminal thrombus (dashed arrow) but no active contrast extravasation. There is narrowing of the distal aorta and iliac arteries. Focal disruption of the anteroinferior wall of the proximal third portion of duodenum (curved arrow) and left upper quadrant small bowel wall thickening and hyperenhancement (star) with small volume free intraperitoneal gas. Chance fracture of L2 with associated posterior soft tissue/ligamentous injury (open arrow). There is intramedullary spinal cord hemorrhage at the level of T10-11 with surrounding cord edema (chevron arrow). In addition, there is mild compression fracture/marrow contusion involving superior aspect of the L3 vertebral body

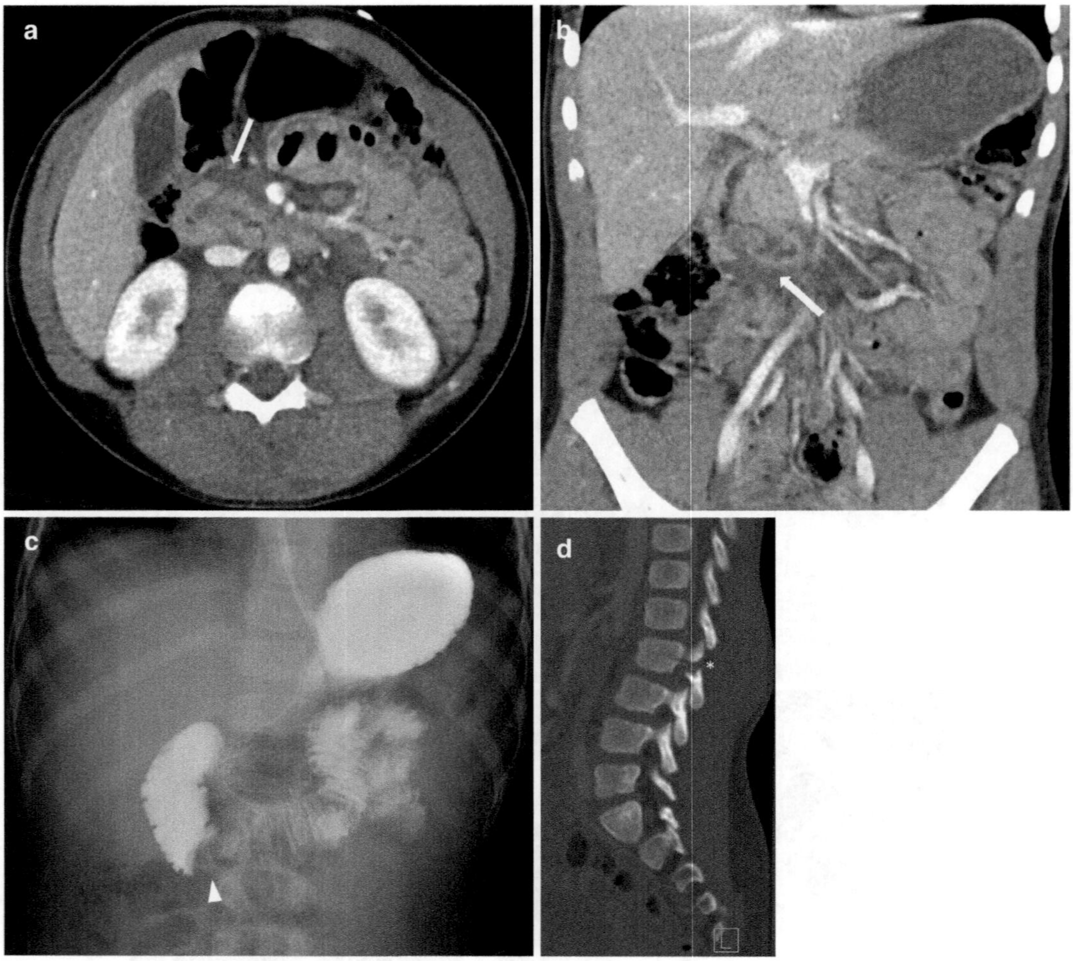

Fig. 12.8 Axial (**a**) and coronal (**b**) contrast-enhanced CT of the abdomen in a child presenting after a motor vehicle accident shows a linear laceration of the wall of the duodenum with adjacent mural hematoma (arrows). There is focal mass effect on the duodenum and luminal narrowing at the site of the hematoma (arrowhead) seen on fluoroscopic upper gastrointestinal series (**c**). Sagittal bone reformatting CT images of the spine from the same CT (**d**) shows associated hyperflexion injuring with a Chance fracture through the posterior elements (asterisk)

obtained if there is concern for intra-abdominal injury, and the spine should be scrutinized for associated fractures. Due to the horizontal nature of chance fractures, they can be easily missed on standard axial planes. Thus, careful review of coronal and sagittal reconstructions is important. MRI is undoubtedly the best modality for soft tissue and discoligamentous injury.

Craniocervical Arterial Dissection

Craniocervical arterial dissection (CCAD) in children can affect the carotid or vertebral artery and is commonly related to trauma. In fact, half of all cases are the result of trauma [47]. Etiologies include contact sports, skull/spine fractures, direct trauma though the oropharynx (such as falling with an object in the mouth), hyperextension of the neck, or motor vehicle accident [47, 48]. Carotid artery or vertebral artery dissections have also occurred after chiropractic treatments [49]. They can be categorized multiple ways including the location (intracranial versus extracranial) or circulation affected (anterior or posterior). Symptoms of acute ischemic stroke or transient ischemic attack (TIA) can be seen. Most carotid artery dissections in the presence of blunt trauma occur due to fractures at the skull base. The gold standard for CCAD diagnosis is CTA or time of flight MRA. CTA may be difficult in children due to optimal bolus timing and higher administration rates [48]. Dual energy CTA could be used if necessary to remove bone and metal artifacts if children have dental implants, though there is not much literature to support this in the pediatric population yet. In some cases, internal carotid artery dissection may cause thrombosis, and a clot may propagate to cause a large vessel occlusion.

Carotid-Cavernous Fistula

Carotid-cavernous fistula (CCF) is an abnormal connection between cavernous segment of the internal carotid artery and the cavernous venous plexus, resulting in high flow through the cavernous sinus. There are four types, types A–D. The most common to be associated with trauma is type A, where there is a skull fracture with a bony fragment causing a tear in the cavernous segment of the internal carotid artery. Types B–D are out of the scope of this chapter as they are mainly spontaneous or associated with dural anomalies. MRA or CTA is typically required to diagnose a CCF though digital subtraction angiography is the definitive gold standard. Findings include an enlarged cavernous plexus, dilated superior ophthalmic vein, and associated proptosis (Fig. 12.9). Ultrasound doppler may show arterialized low resistance retrograde flow in the superior ophthalmic vein, within the cavernous plexus, and even the middle cerebral vein. Symptoms vary since they depend on the flow pattern and venous drainage, but usually include proptosis, chemosis, orbital bruits, headache, red eye, chemosis, orbital pain, and even CN VI ophthalmoplegia [50].

Temporal Bone Fractures

Temporal bone fractures in the pediatric population pose a serious risk due the proximity of these fractures to the delicate ear structures, cranial nerves, and dural venous sinus. Temporal bone fractures can result in facial nerve injury, cerebrospinal fluid leak, conductive or sensorineural hearing loss, perilymphatic fistulas, hemotympanum, tympanic membrane perforation, ossicular chain dissociation, labyrinthine concussion, and even brainstem injury [51]. Traumatic perilymphatic fistulas are abnormal middle and inner ear connections that can cause vestibular or cochlear symptoms. High-resolution CT (HRCT) can show pneumolabyrinth in the vestibules and semicircular canals (Fig. 12.10). HRCT is important since these tiny structures may be missed with a normal 5 mm slice thickness [52]. Examples of ossicular chain dislocations include incudostapedial, incudomalleolar, and stapediovestibular subluxations.

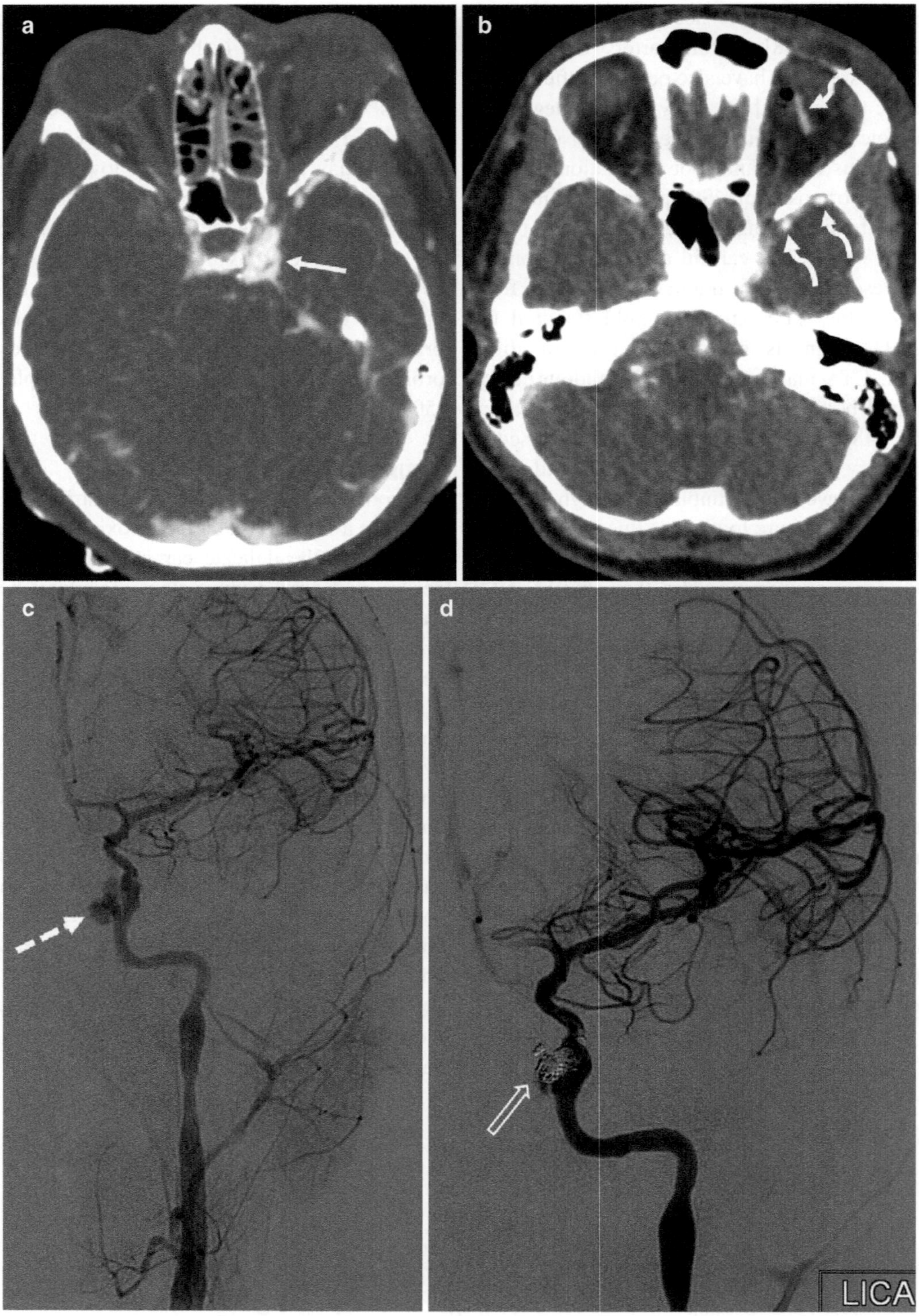

Fig. 12.9 CT angiogram (**a**, **b**), Digital subtraction angiogram (**c**, **d**): 13-year-old girl with traumatic brain injury due to gunshot wound: Abnormal appearance of the left cavernous carotid artery with large area of surrounding high attenuation consistent with arterial injury and active hemorrhage (arrow). In addition, there is increased enhancement of left superior ophthalmic and left middle cranial fossa cortical veins (curved arrows) supporting carotid cavernous fistula. DSA demonstrates left carotid cavernous fistula (dashed arrow). Successful treatment of the fistula using balloon-assisted coiling (open arrow)

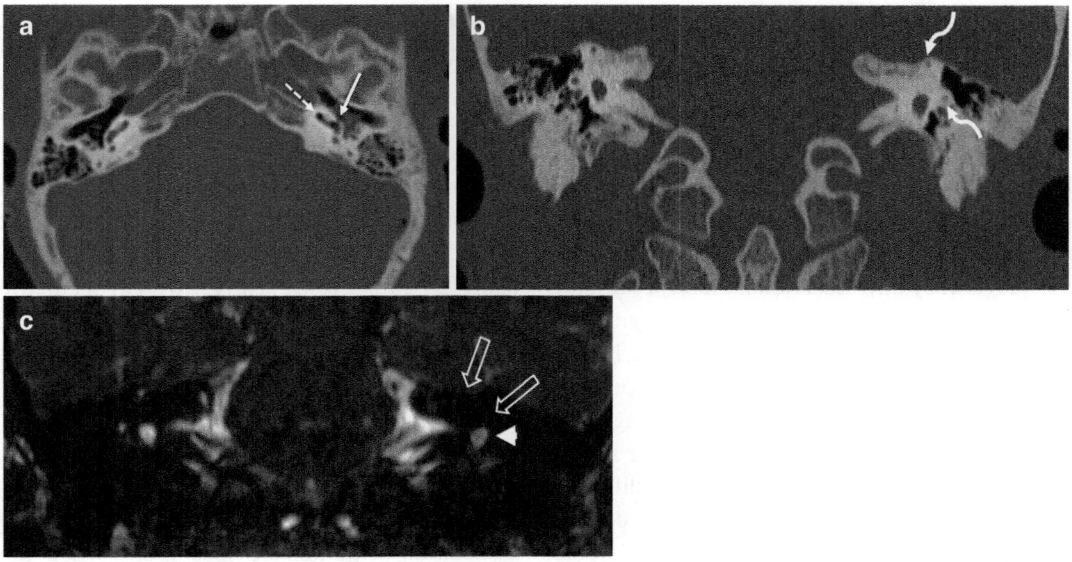

Fig. 12.10 Initial axial CT (**a**), 4-month follow-up coronal CT (**b**) and coronal FIESTA (**c**): 12-year-old female with left-sided sensorineural hearing loss following left temporal bone fracture. There is subtle osseous lucency with associated hematoma along the basal turn of the cochlea, just anterior to the round window (arrow). In addition, foci of air are seen within the left basal turn of cochlea and vestibule [pneumolabyrinth] (dashed arrow). Subtle mineralization of left lateral and superior semicircular canals (curved arrows) compared to the right. Asymmetrical loss of normal T2 hyperintense signal of the left lateral, and superior semicircular canals (open arrows). The left vestibule appears asymmetrically slightly less hyperintense on heavily T2 weighted imaging (arrowhead). The findings represent posttraumatic labyrinthitis ossificans

Pediatric Chest and Abdominal Trauma

Blunt injuries account for nearly 85% of traumatic injuries in children. Only 15% of injuries are penetrating injuries, most often from stab wounds or gunshot wounds [53]. Children are more susceptible to intrabdominal injury from blunt trauma than adults. Children have a smaller torso and larger organ size creating a larger surface area for potential solid organ impact and multi-organ injury. Additionally, there is less intra-abdominal or extra-abdominal fat to protect the solid organs. The clinical decision to obtain CT in a pediatric trauma patient is based on physical examination and laboratory findings and may include abdominal wall tenderness, seatbelt sign, hematuria, elevated transaminases, drop in hemoglobin or positive FAST scan [6, 53, 54]. The "seatbelt sign" is an important sign for potential intrabdominal injury after a motor vehicle crash. In children, the lap belt often sits too high over the abdomen rather than over the pelvic bones, transmitting the blunt force impact to the abdominal organs rather than the pelvis [53]. Intravenous contrast-enhanced CT remains the gold standard for diagnosing solid organ injuries, though should be used judiciously in children. The AAST grading for solid organ injuries is the same for both pediatric and adult patients.

Spleen and Liver Injuries

The spleen and liver are the most commonly injured organs in blunt abdominal trauma[54]. The elasticity of the rib cage in children transmits more force to the intrabdominal organs including the liver and spleen [55]. Grading of liver and spleen injuries follows the AAST grading scale. Fortunately, regardless of the AAST grading, a vast majority of liver and spleen injuries can be managed non-operatively.

Splenic injuries include lacerations, hematomas, or a fracture, which is defined as a laceration extending through two surfaces of the spleen. If the splenic capsule remains intact, hematoma will be confined to the parenchyma or contained beneath the capsule. Hemoperitoneum only occurs once there is a capsular tear and usually extends along the left paracolic gutter and into the pelvis [55, 56]. Lacerations have a variable appearance from linear to branching regions of low attenuation in the spleen (Fig. 12.11). A potential pitfall that may lead to false positive identification of a splenic laceration is imaging in arterial phase, where the spleen may have a marbled or striated appearance owing to the different enhancement pattern of the white and red pulp. Splenic clefts may also mimic laceration but are smoothly marginated whereas lacerations should be more irregular [54]. A contrast blush is indicative of contrast extravasation and indicates active bleeding. However, children have enhanced vasoconstriction response and a thicker splenic capsule, so bleeding is more likely to spontaneously stop than in adults. Contrast extravasation has traditionally been an indication for embolization and is more common in adults, but children can often be managed non-operatively using hemodynamic stability as the primary determinant [54–58]. Now, nearly 90% of pediatric splenic injuries are managed non-operatively.

Liver injuries include lacerations, hematomas, and vascular injuries. The posterior right hepatic lobe is most frequently injured, owing to its greater ligamentous fixation than the remaining portions of the liver, resulting in localized shearing injuries [54]. Hemoperitoneum occurs in association with hepatic lacerations when the laceration reaches the margin of the liver and disrupts the capsule. The largest pocket of hemoperitoneum is often away from the liver in the

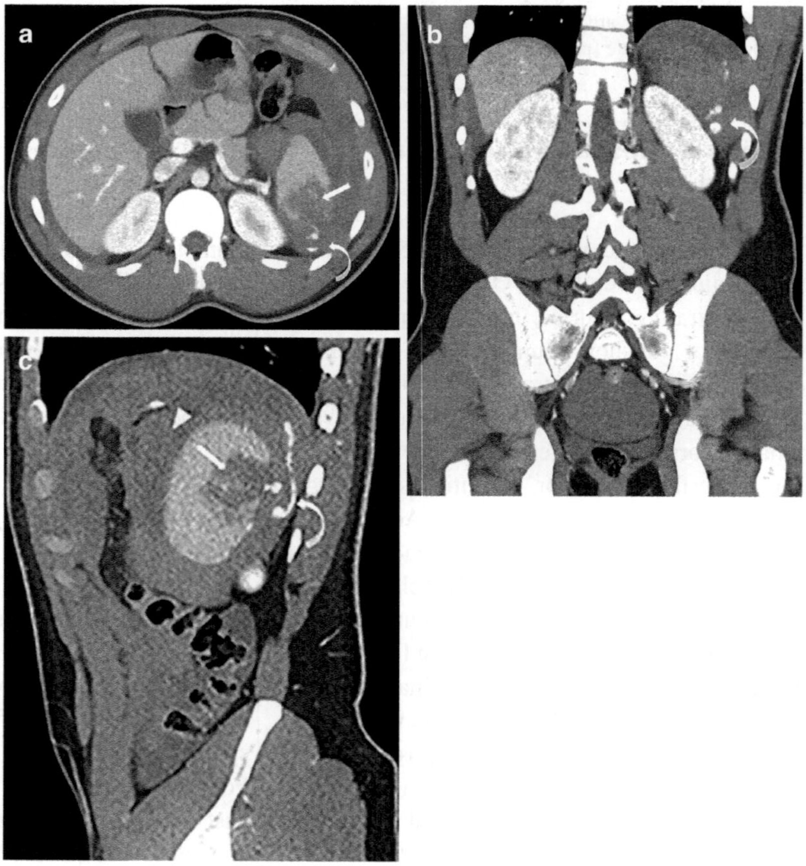

Fig. 12.11 Axial (**a**), Coronal (**b**), and Sagittal (**c**) contrast-enhanced CT abdomen and pelvis in a child injured in a sledding accident shows a high-grade splenic injury. There is a large parenchymal laceration >3 cm in depth in the inferior aspect of the spleen (arrow). Extravasated contrast is pooling dependently, indicating vascular injury (curved arrow). There is a subcapsular hematoma with hemoperitoneum, indicating splenic capsular disruption (arrowhead)

pelvis [54]. In contrast, retroperitoneal hematomas can occur when the injury affects the bare area of the liver [54, 59]. Periportal low attenuation zones have been reported in both traumatic and non-traumatic conditions. Studies have found that they are nonspecific and most likely represent fluid losses and distension of periportal lymphatics after aggressive fluid resuscitation and are not clinically significant as an isolated finding [60, 61].

Pancreatic Injuries

Pancreatic injuries are rare, representing only 0.3% of pediatric traumas. A vast majority of pancreatic injuries occur in conjunction with other organ injuries, most commonly liver and lung [62]. Despite the rarity of these injuries, these injuries can carry a 5% mortality rate and nearly 25% complication rate [63]. Complications include pancreatitis, pseudocyst formation, abscess, duct injuries, fistulas, or pancreatic insufficiency [62].

Pancreatic injuries are more commonly associated with high impact blunt injuries, including handlebar injuries and non-accidental trauma [64–66]. Because the pancreas is retroperitoneal and is better protected than other abdominal organs by retroperitoneal fat, it is less commonly injured with minor trauma. However, children are overall more susceptible than adults because of their thinner body habitus. The body of the pancreas is the most common site of injury, owing to compression of the pancreas against the vertebral column during blunt impact (Figs. 12.12 and 12.13). Detection of pancreatic duct injuries is an important determinant of injury severity and management. The presence of pancreatic duct injury indicates a high-grade injury of at least grade III and is an important determinant in the management [64, 67]. However, visualization of duct injuries, especially by CT, can be challenging. Multiple studies have found that MRI/MRCP is superior to CT in visualization of the pancreatic duct and detection of duct injuries, though ERCP remains the gold standard [62, 67]. Indirect signs of duct disruption on CT include a laceration of greater than 50% in short axis, free intraperitoneal fluid, or loculated peripancreatic fluid [64, 67].

Urinary Tract Injuries

The kidney is the most common urinary system injury in children and occurs in 10–20% of children with blunt abdominal trauma [68]. Like

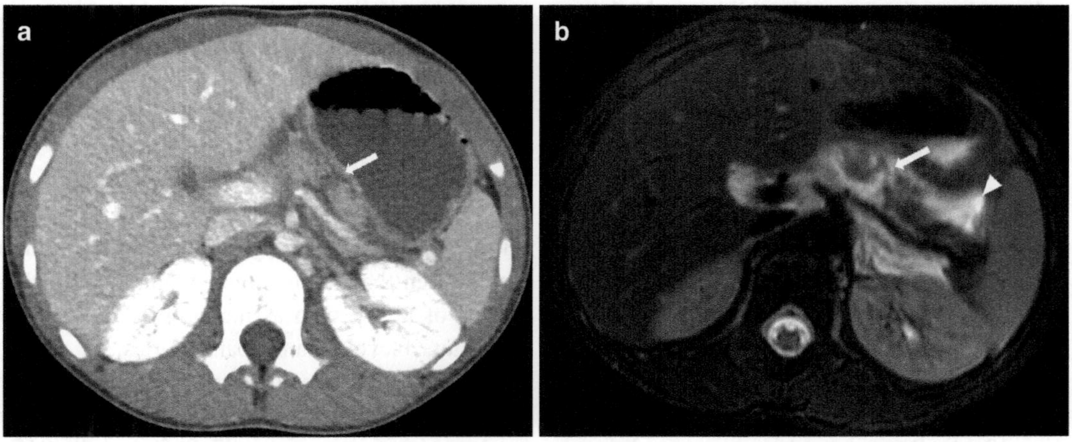

Fig. 12.12 Axial contrast enhanced CT images (**a**) and axial T2 fat saturated MRI images (**b**) of a child who fell from a bicycle and sustained a handlebar injury, with elevated lipase. There is a complete transection of the body of the pancreas (arrows). The is edema in the injured portion of the pancreas with peripancreatic fluid (arrowheads). The pancreatic duct was not seen

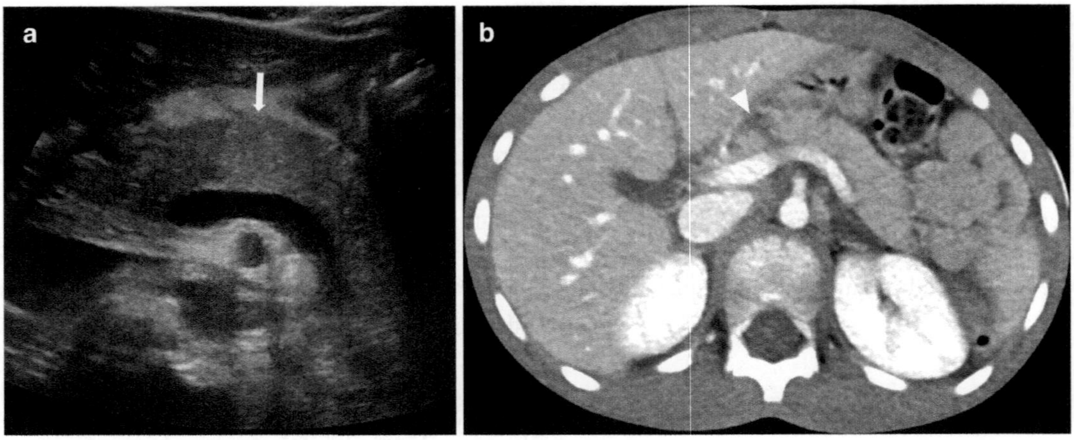

Fig. 12.13 Transverse ultrasound image (**a**) and axial contrast-enhanced CT (**b**) of the abdomen in a child who fell from a bicycle and sustained a handlebar injury shows focal edema in the body of the pancreas (arrow), corresponding to a complete transection of the pancreas (arrowhead). The patient was treated with distal pancreatectomy

other solid organs, children are at increased risk for renal injuries than adults due to less retroperitoneal fat, incompletely ossified ribs, weaker abdominal wall musculature, lower position and proportionally larger size of the kidneys [68, 69]. Contrast-enhanced CT with delayed urographic phase is the gold standard for diagnosing and grading renal injuries with a negative predictive value of over 99% [68]. However, contrast-enhanced ultrasound has emerged as an alternative imaging modality in children and can be used in hemodynamically stable children with low to moderate blunt trauma to diagnose renal injuries, avoiding ionizing radiation [69].

Renal contusions are most common and represent focal areas of hemorrhage and edema, manifesting as areas of delayed enhancement [54]. Lacerations appear as linear hypo-enhancing areas in the kidney and can be large with branching patterns. Large lacerations may involve the renal collecting system, resulting in urine leakage and extravasation of intravenous contrast. Delayed urographic phase imaging is critical for diagnosing these types of injuries [54, 59] (Fig. 12.14). Parenchymal injuries may be associated with perirenal hematomas, which can be subcapsular or perinephric. Subcapsular hematomas are confined by the renal capsule and therefore exert greater mass effect on the adjacent kidney (Fig. 12.15) [54].

Bladder injuries are the second most commonly affected of the urinary tract [68]. Most bladder injuries are extraperitoneal, occurring in relation to pelvic fractures. Intraperitoneal bladder injuries usually result from shearing injury of the distended bladder from a lap belt [54]. CT cystography is the gold standard for diagnosing bladder rupture and the location of extravasated contrast can help differentiate extraperitoneal and intraperitoneal ruptures, which has important implications for management [54, 59].

Bowel and Mesentery Injuries

Bowel and mesentery injuries are more common in children than adults, owing to unique mechanisms of injury such as inappropriate passenger restraint, bicycle handlebar injuries, or abuse. Bowel and mesentery injuries often occur together but can be difficult to detect by CT. Specificity and sensitivity vary from 87–95% and 48–84%, respectively [70]. Diagnosis must be based on clinical findings in conjunction with imaging findings. The small intestine is most injured, most

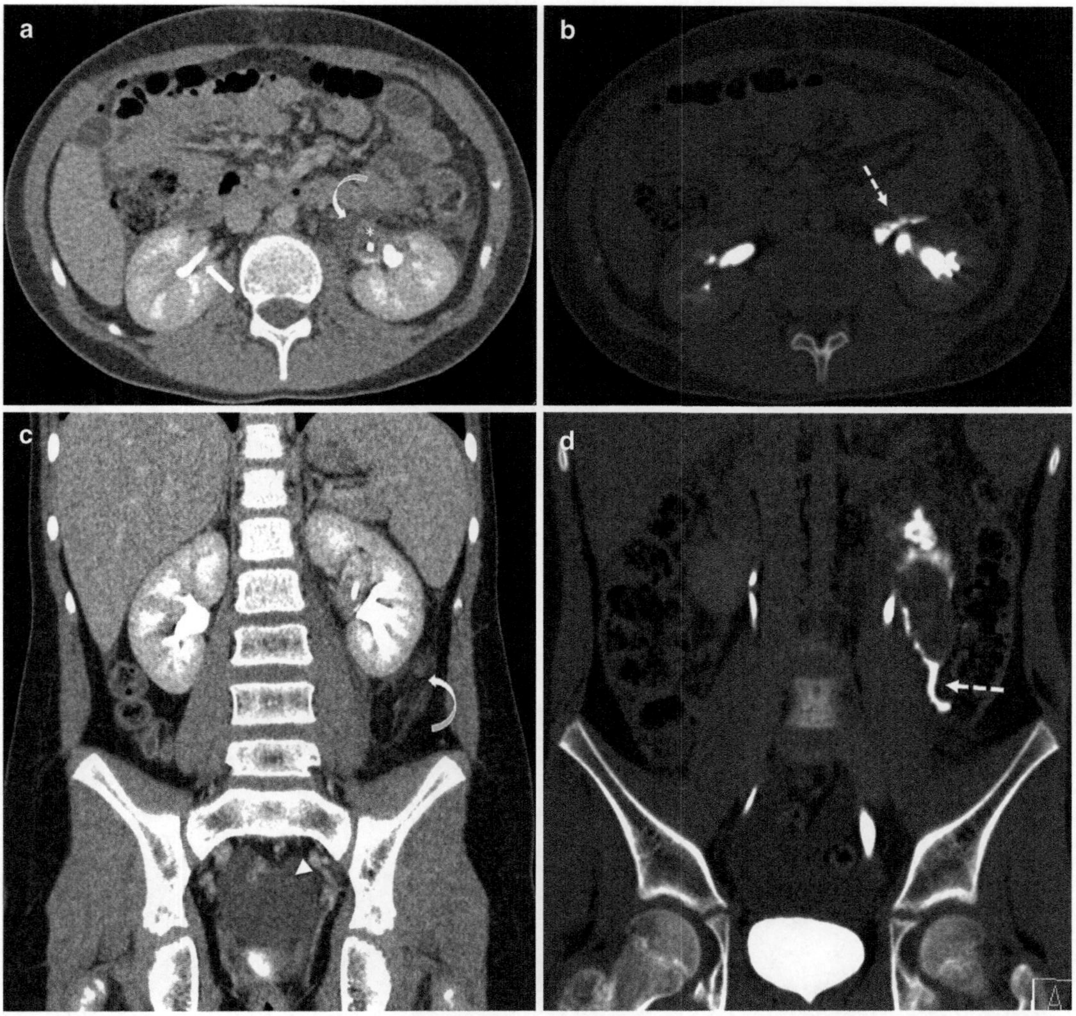

Fig. 12.14 Axial and coronal split bolus contrast-enhanced CT in early excretory (**a**, **c**) and late excretory (**b**, **d**) phases of a child who sustained an iatrogenic renal injury after nephroureteral stent placement for renal stones. Initial split bolus CT with early excretory phase shows contrast starting to fill the collecting system (arrow). The nephroureteral stent is seen in the proximal ureter (asterisk). There is perinephric edema but no early contrast extravasation (curved arrow). Contrast extravasation confirming a ureteral injury is only seen on delayed excretory phase (dashed arrow). Urinoma is seen in the pelvis (arrowhead)

frequently the proximal jejunum or distal ileum. CT findings suggestive of bowel injury include bowel wall thickening, free fluid, abnormal bowel wall enhancement (either increased or decreased enhancement). The presence of interloop fluid or free air in association with bowel wall thickening is more sensitive for bowel injury [71]. Diffuse bowel wall hyperenhancement may be due to hypoperfusion complex rather than focal bowel wall injury. Bowel wall discontinuity, extraluminal contrast, or free intraperitoneal air are specific signs [70, 71]. Mesenteric findings include stranding, hematoma, pseudoaneurysm, contrast extravasation, or vascular disruption [70] (Figs. 12.16 and 12.17). Isolated free intraperitoneal fluid seen on CT performed for trauma is commonly encountered and can present a diagnostic challenge. The presence of free fluid should raise suspicion for a bowel or mesentery injury, though rarely occurs in isolation; other associated imag-

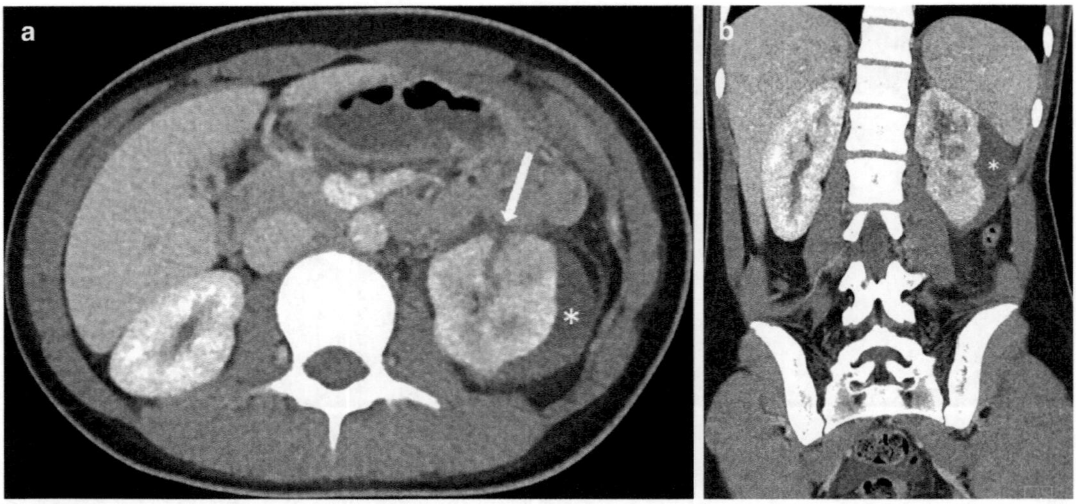

Fig. 12.15 Axial (**a**) and coronal (**b**) contrast-enhanced CT images of the abdomen in a child who fell from a skateboard shows a linear laceration in the inferior pole of the kidney (arrow), extending to the surface of the kidney with subcapsular hematoma (asterisk), consistent with a grade III injury. There was no associated injury to the main renal vasculature or the collecting system

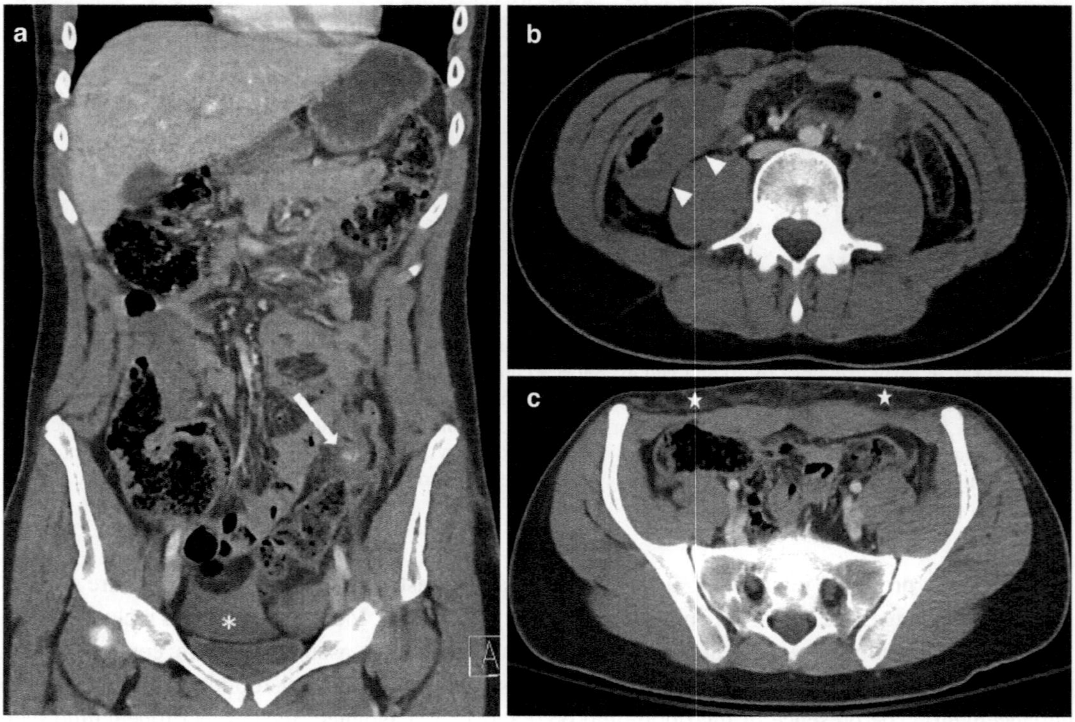

Fig. 12.16 Coronal (**a**) and axial (**b**, **c**) contrast-enhanced CT of the abdomen and pelvis in a child with abdominal pain after motor vehicle crash. There is a focal injury of the descending colon with wall thickening and small mural hematoma with active contrast extravasation (arrow). Additional larger mural hematoma is seen along the descending colon (arrowheads). There is a small amount of free intraperitoneal fluid (asterisk). Linear subcutaneous edema in the lower abdominal wall is seen along the lap belt injury (star)

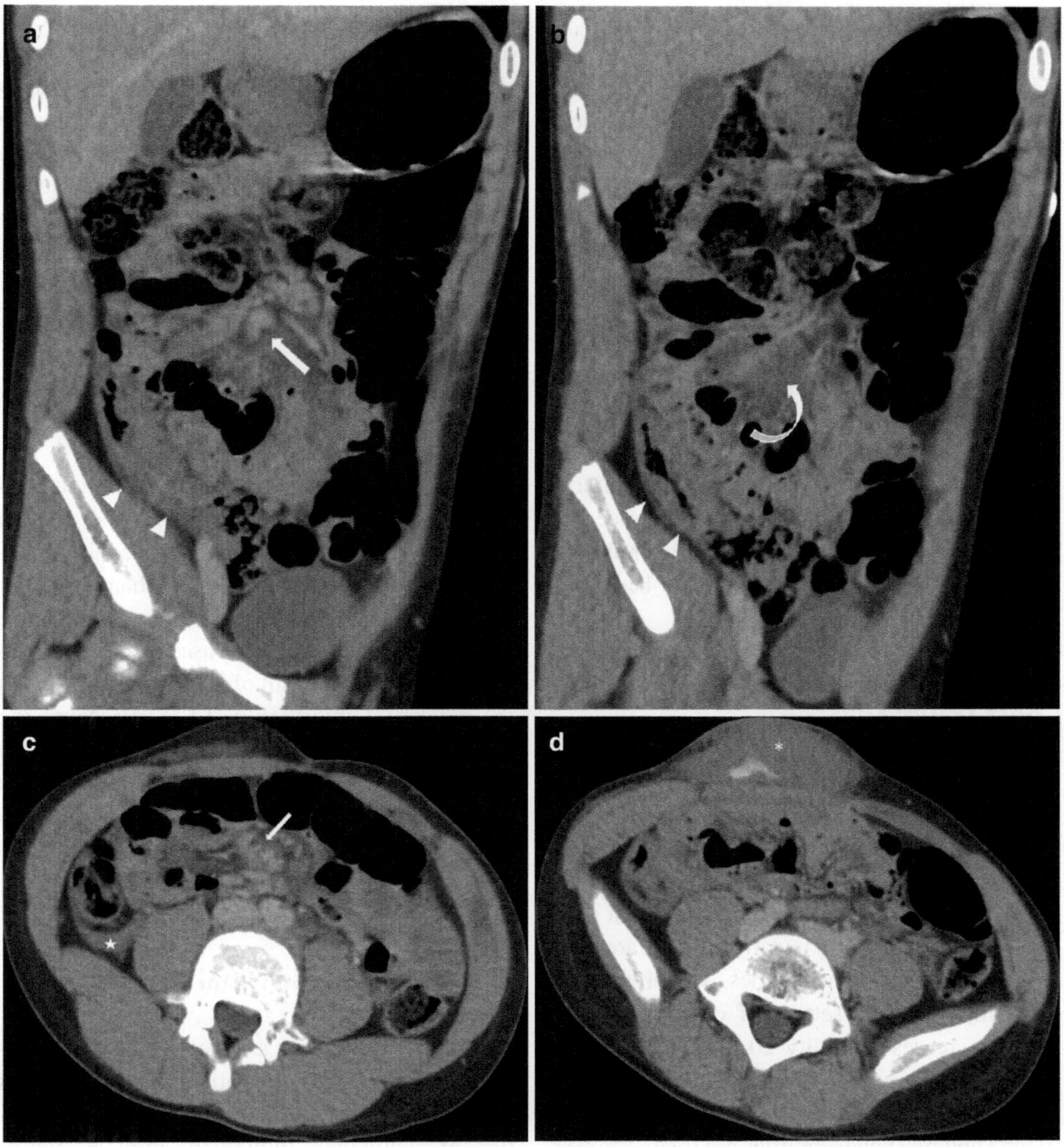

Fig. 12.17 Coronal (**a**, **b**) and axial (**c**, **d**) contrast-enhanced CT images in a child presenting with abdominal pain after motor vehicle crash with lap belt injury. There is localized infiltration of the mesentery (curved arrow) with focal mesenteric hematoma (arrow). There is a short segment circumferential wall thickening of the ascending colon indicating a bowel injury (arrowhead). A large abdominal wall hematoma with active contrast extravasation is present at the site of the lap belt (asterisk). Small amount of free intraperitoneal fluid layers along the right paracolic gutter (star)

ing findings are often present. Multiple recent studies have shown that isolated free intraperitoneal fluid in hemodynamically stable female or male pediatric patients has not been shown to associated with significant intrabdominal injury [59, 72–74]. Lack of free fluid has a high negative predictive value in excluding bowel/mesentery injuries [71].

Handlebar Injuries

Handlebar injuries are a unique mechanism of injury in children. There are two main categories of bicycle injuries. First, the child may fall or be thrown from the bike, most often resulting in head injuries, facial trauma, or extremity fractures. Second, the child may the strike the bicycle handlebar and fall over the bicycle, most often resulting in blunt abdominal or chest trauma, or abdominal wall injuries [67, 75]. Handlebar injuries are difficult to diagnose. There may be minimal outward signs of trauma such as bruising, and complaints are often vague, leading to delayed diagnosis. The most common injuries include parenchymal injuries to liver, spleen, or pancreas, bowel or mesentery injuries, or abdominal wall injuries including traumatic hernias or hematomas [67, 76].

Chest Trauma

Like abdominal trauma, a vast majority of chest trauma results from blunt force injuries. The most common injury mechanisms include motor vehicle crashes, abuse, falls, auto versus pedestrian accidents, or bicycle accidents. Most chest injuries do not occur in isolation, rather are associated with other organ injuries. The presence of chest injury in the setting of other multiorgan injury increases mortality 20-fold, owing to the severity of the overall trauma [77, 78]. However, most mortality is not a direct result of the chest trauma and most chest injuries are treated conservatively [78]. Chest injury patterns differ in children than adults. In children, there is greater flexibility of the rib cage resulting in fewer rib fractures, but more pulmonary contusions. The mediastinum is also more mobile with greater potential for a large pneumothorax or hemothorax causing cardiac or respiratory failure [77]. Aortic injuries occur less frequently due to greater elasticity of arterial structures in children [77, 78]. The most encountered chest injuries are pulmonary contusions, pneumothorax, hemothorax, and rib fractures [78].

Chest CT should be used cautiously in children. Several studies have found that actionable chest findings are usually detected on radiographs alone or included in the lower chest on abdomen and pelvic CT [79–81]. Chest CT in the presence of a normal chest radiograph does not usually change clinical management [82]. Others have suggested limiting CT to trauma patients with abnormal mediastinal silhouette to evaluate for vascular injury [83].

Pleural and Rib Injuries

Rib fractures, while still frequent, occur less commonly in children than adults and tend to occur in the posterior ribs, as opposed to the lateral ribs in adults. In children less than 3 years of age, the presence of rib fractures should raise strong suspicion for child abuse, especially when the reported mechanism of injury does not match the pattern of injury (Fig. 12.18). Because the mediastinum in children is more mobile, children are more prone to cardiovascular compromise from a large hemothorax or pneumothorax [77, 78]. Tension pneumothorax occurs three times more frequently in children than adults [78].

Pulmonary Parenchymal Injuries

Pulmonary contusions are most common, occurring in about half of all patients [77, 84]. CT is more sensitive than radiographs for identification of contusions, though the clinical significance of these radiographically occult contusions is questionable. Contusions classically appear as peripheral opacities, most commonly at the posterior lung bases, with characteristic subpleural sparing [77, 78, 84]. The presence of subpleural sparing helps differentiate contusions form other parenchymal abnormalities, including atelectasis or pneumonia. Contusions typically have a ground glass appearance representing edema, hemorrhage and consolidation [78]. Adjacent rib fractures may or may not be present. Pneumatoceles are

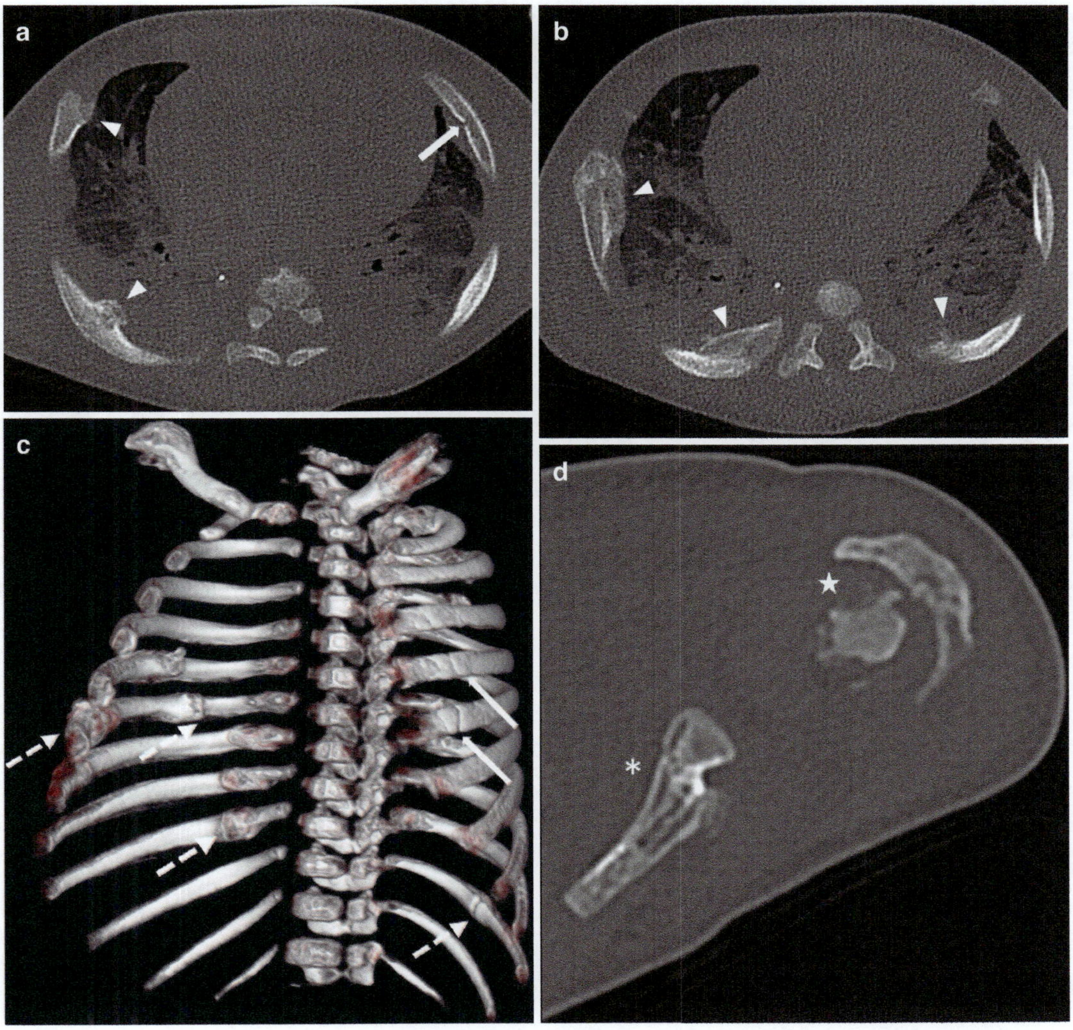

Fig. 12.18 Post-mortem CT in an infant found unresponsive. Axial CT images of the chest (**a**, **b**) show multiple bilateral rib fractures in various stages of healing. Both healing rib fractures (arrowheads) and acute rib fractures (arrow) are present. (**c**) 3D Volume rendered images of the ribcage depicts the multiple rib fractures in various stages of healing (some depicted with dashed arrows and arrows) and healing clavicle fractures. Axial images through the left shoulder (**d**) show additional healing fractures of the scapula (asterisk) and proximal humerus (star). The pattern of fractures is consistent with non-accidental trauma

collections of air within the lung that result from rupture of the distal airways often surrounded by pulmonary contusion [84].

Mediastinal and Vascular Injuries

Pneumomediastinum occurs in up to 10% of children with blunt thoracic trauma; the mechanism being large airway injury, esophageal rupture, alveolar rupture with air dissecting along the interstitium to the mediastinum, or subdiaphragmatic air dissecting to the mediastinum [78, 84]. In young children, one unique sign of pneumomediastinum is the spinnaker sail sign, where air uplifts the thymic lobes [84]. Aortic injuries are less common in children due to increased elasticity of the arterial structures [77]. These injuries most commonly occur at the ligamentum arteriosum just distal to the left subcla-

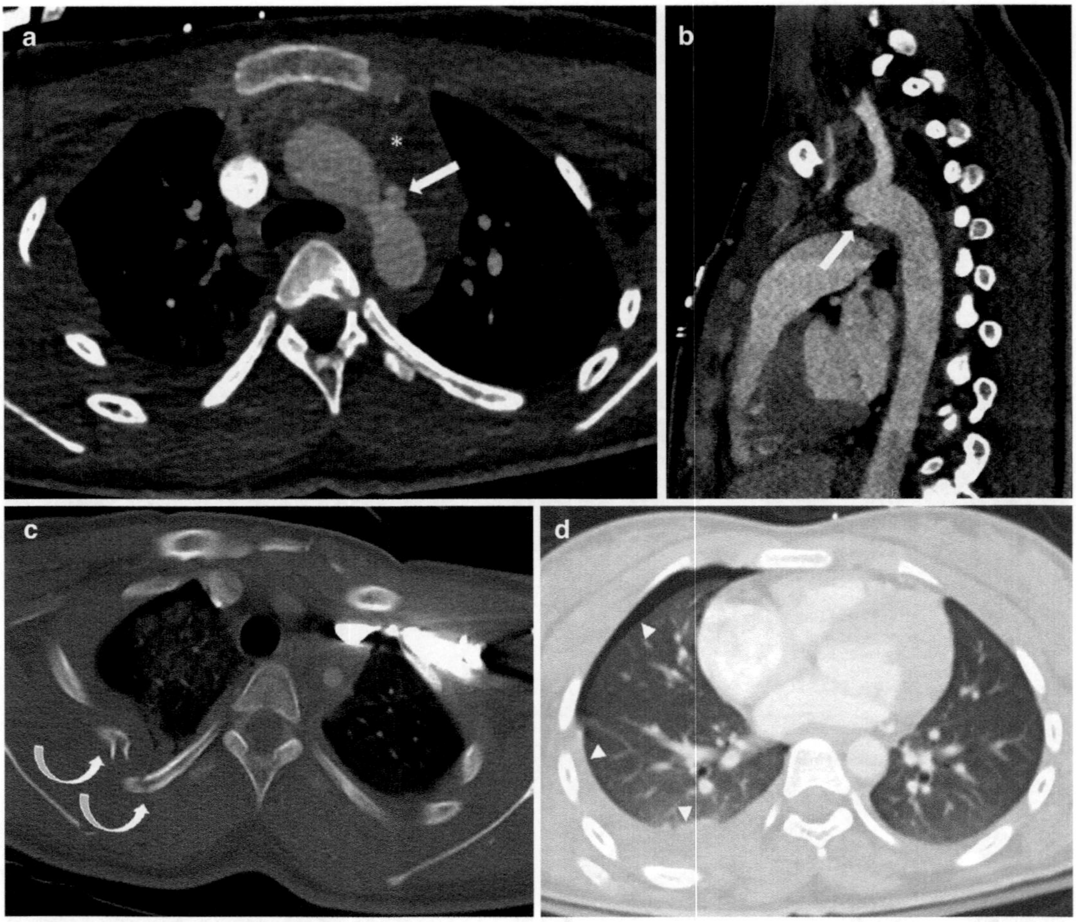

Fig. 12.19 Axial (**a**) and coronal (**b**) CT angiogram of the chest in a teenager after motor vehicle accident shows a pseudoaneurysm of the thoracic aorta in the typical location at the aortic isthmus (arrows) with adjacent mediastinal hematoma (asterisk). Bone (**c**) window reformats show multiple right upper rib fractures (curved arrows) with adjacent pulmonary contusion. The lung window of the same CT (**d**) shows a small right pneumothorax and hemothorax (arrowheads)

vian artery where the relatively mobile aortic arch becomes fixed at the descending thoracic aorta [78, 84] (Fig. 12.19).

Musculoskeletal Trauma

Pediatric musculoskeletal injuries often differ from adults owing to differences in the growing skeleton that creates unique strengths and vulnerabilities. The primary physis is where long bone growth occurs from cartilaginous precursors and is the weakest portion of the growing long bones. As a result, many pediatric fractures involve the growth plate and are classified according to the Salter Harris classification. Fractures involving the physes can result in premature physeal fusion, resulting in growth disturbances. The apophyses are secondary ossification centers and are attachment sites for tendons. The adjacent physis that attaches the apophyses to the parent bone is the weakest point, resulting in avulsion of the apophysis with acute or chronic myotendinous injuries. The bony cortex in children is more pliable and can buckle and bend before fracturing creating bowing, incomplete, or torus type fractures [85,

86]. The periosteum plays an important role in the enhanced fracture healing potential in children. Undifferentiated cells in the periosteum can differentiate and produce periosteal new bone. The periosteum is also thicker, tightly adhered, and more vascular in children and so is less often disrupted [86]. A vast majority of fractures are result of sports injuries or falls. Radiographs are the mainstay of imaging for diagnosis and follow-up. However, CT plays an important role in the classification of some fractures, pre-surgical planning for complex fractures, and for assessment of complications. 3D volume rendered reconstructions can be especially helpful in visualizing complex fracture patterns for surgical planning.

Salter Harris Fractures

Long bone growth occurs at the physis, where cartilaginous precusors contribute to endochondral ossification and growth. The cartilaginous physis is weaker than the surrounding bone, and most susceptible to fracture. Physeal involvement is seen in 15–18% of all pediatric fractures [87]. The distal radius and ulna are the most common site of fracture. Injuries to the physis can result in later growth disturbances, including angular deformities or limb length discrepancies [86]. Most Salter Harris fractures are not routinely assessed by CT.

Ankle fractures are one of the most common types of pediatric fractures (Fig. 12.20). Transitional fractures occur during physeal closure and result in characteristic fracture patterns. Triplane fractures are Salter Harris type IV fractures with a sagittal fracture through the epiphysis, axial fracture through the physis and coronal fracture through the posterior metaphysis. Tillaux fractures are a Salter Harris type III type fracture that characteristically involves the anterolateral tibial physis, which is the last portion of the physis to fuse. Owing to the growth potential of the tibia and intra-articular fracture components, these fractures must be carefully managed and monitored to minimize risk of growth disturbance or arthritis. Operative treatment of these fractures may be needed depending on degree of displacement. One study found poor reliability in determining degree of displacement and classification of Triplane fractures based on radiographs. With the addition of CT, there was significant change in the description of the fracture pattern, classification, and management. The treatment plan changed from non-operative to operative in 27% of cases [88]. This study highlights the importance of routine CT in the management of ankle fractures. CT may also be used after attempted reduction and casting of Salter Harris fractures to confirm adequate reduction and identify barriers to reduction and healing, such as periosteal entrapment [89].

Premature physeal fusion is most often post-traumatic related to fractures. The physes of the distal femur, proximal tibia, and distal tibia contribute the greatest growth potential and are most prone to growth disturbances. The clinical implications of growth arrest depend on the age of the patient, remaining growth potential, bone affected, and portion of bone affected [86]. CT or MRI can be used to assess for the presence, location, and extent of physeal bars (Fig. 12.21). Central physeal bars restrict longitudinal growth, resulting in limb length discrepancies. Peripheral bars result in angular deformities [86, 87].

Pelvic Fractures

CT plays an important role in diagnosis of pelvic fractures in adults and has been shown to be more sensitive in detecting posterior ring fractures involving the sacrum and sacroiliac joints than radiographs. However, these types of posterior pelvic fractures are reported less commonly in children. Furthermore, most children with pelvic fractures can be treated non-operatively. Several studies have concluded that radiographs can be used to classify and manage most pediatric pelvic fractures and that the addition of CT for pelvic fractures does not significantly change management [90, 91]. CT should be reserved for complex fractures, operative planning, or when adequate radiographs cannot be obtained [90].

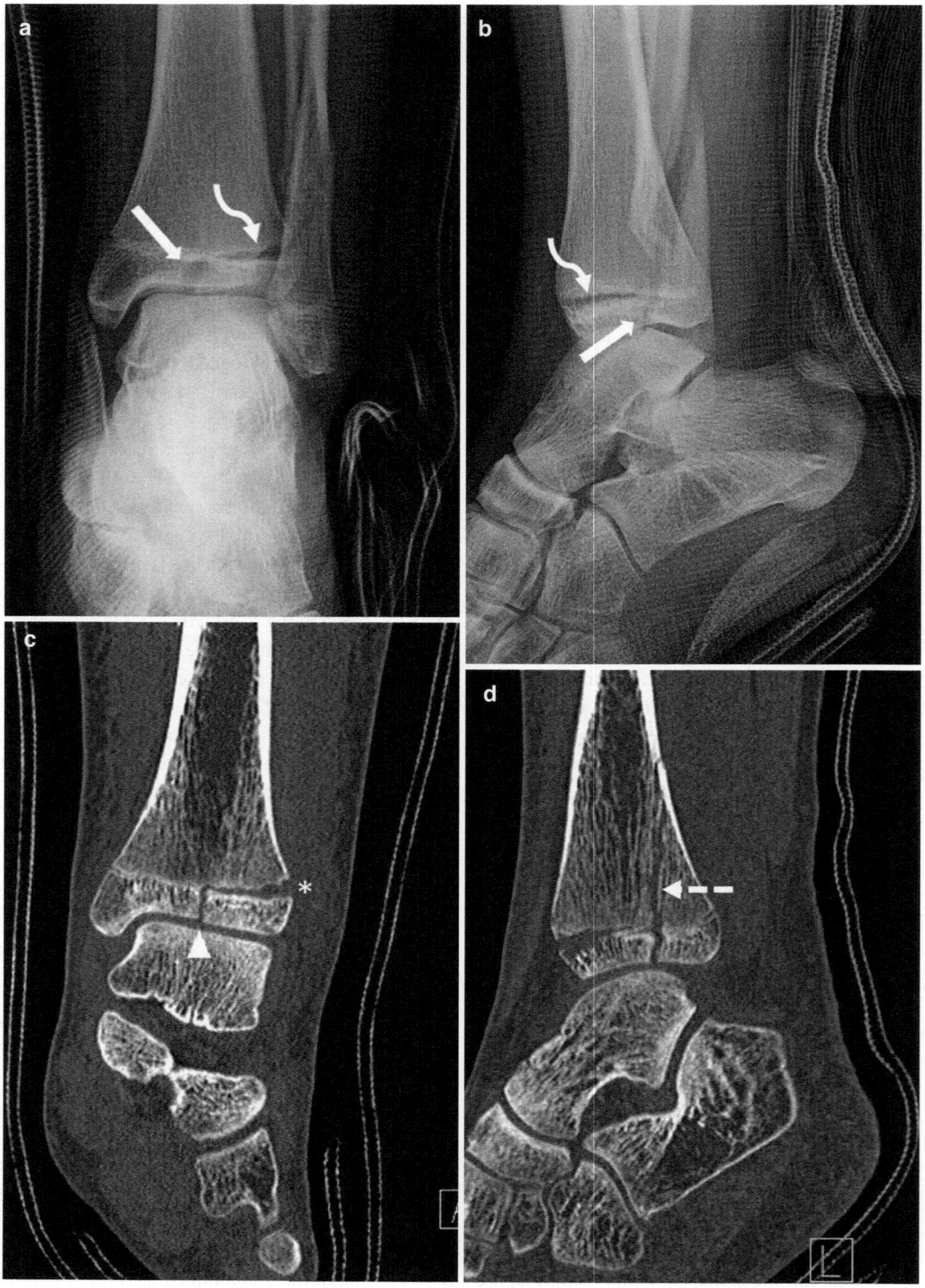

Fig. 12.20 AP (**a**) and sagittal (**b**) radiographs of the ankle show fractures of both distal tibia and fibula. On AP view, the fracture extending through the distal tibial epiphysis (arrows) and physis is well seen (curved arrows), however the posterior metaphyseal component is harder to visualize. Coronal (**c**) and sagittal (**d**) non-contrast CT of the ankle better shows the characteristic triplane fracture pattern with a sagittal fracture through the epiphysis (arrowhead), axial fracture through the lateral tibial physis (asterisk), and coronal fracture through the posterior metaphysis (dashed arrow)

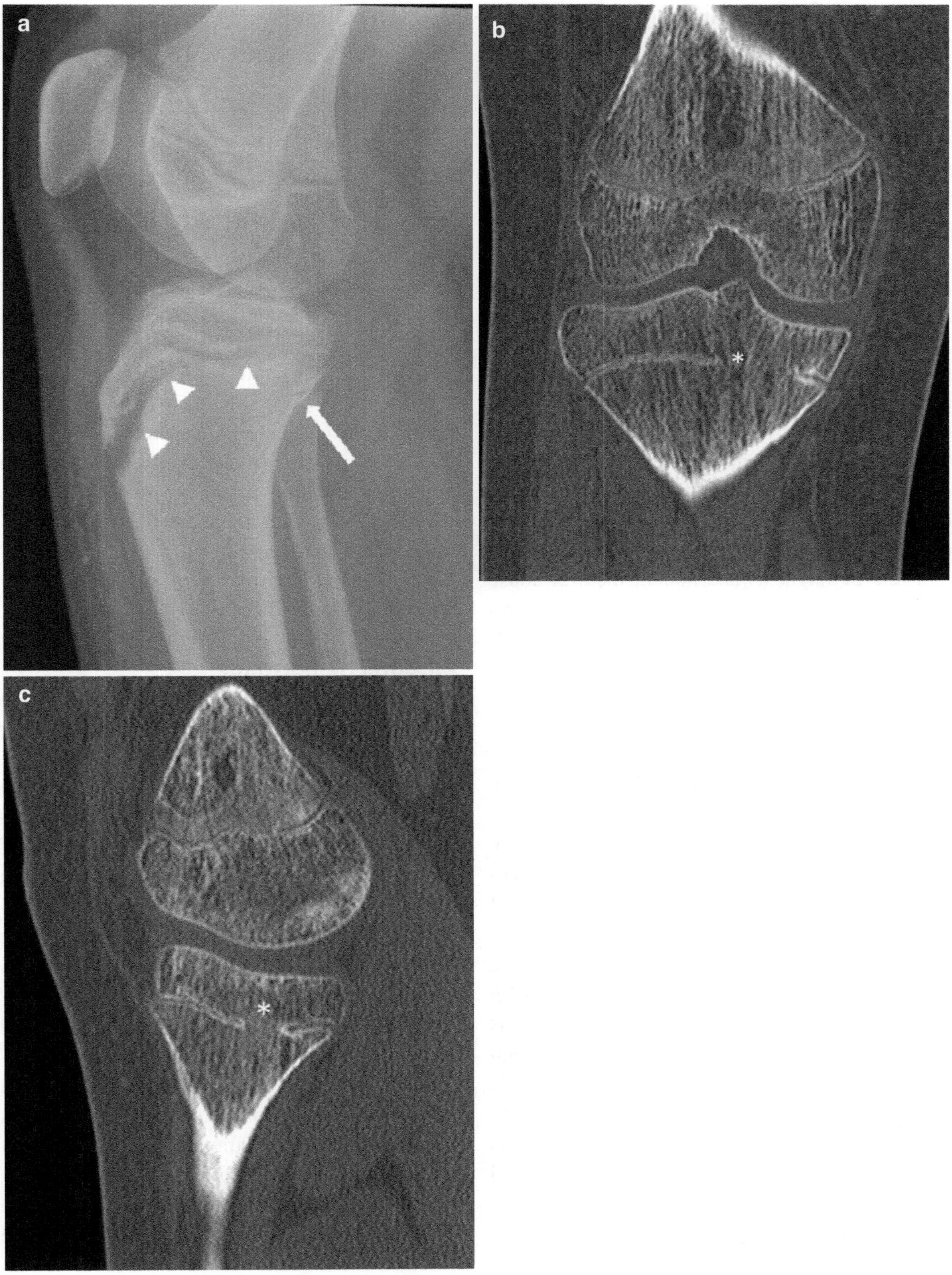

Fig. 12.21 (**a**) Initial sagittal radiograph of the knee shows an acute Salter-Harris Type II fracture of the proximal tibial physis (arrowhead) extending through the posterior tibial metaphysis (arrow). Coronal (**b**) and sagittal (**c**) CT of the same knee 1 year later shows the development of a physeal bar across the posteromedial aspect of the proximal tibial physis (asterisk)

Non-accidental Trauma

Introduction

Non-accidental trauma represents a significant cause of morbidity and mortality in pediatric population. According to the latest edition of the annual child maltreatment report "*Child Maltreatment 2021*" [92], approximately 3.01 million children received a child protective services investigation response or alternative response, with the national estimate of victims who succumbed to abuse and neglect being 1820 and a child fatality rate of 2.46 per 100,000 children. In addition, the survivors of abusive head trauma show severe disability (e.g., tetraplegia, epilepsy or blindness) in 34%, and moderate disability (e.g., hemiplegia, memory and attention deficits) in 25% of the cases. Imaging plays a pivotal role in diagnosis and management of abuse as the physical signs of abuse are not always identifiable or may nonspecific such as irritability, lethargy, altered mental status, seizures, respiratory compromise, or apnea.

Imaging Appropriateness Criteria

The American College of Radiology Appropriateness Criteria rates imaging procedures for specific clinical situations on a scale of 1–9, with 1 being not at all appropriate and 9 being highly appropriate. These criteria can be used to guide imaging decisions. In a child with suspected physical abuse but no apparent signs of neurological or visceral injuries, a skeletal survey (or focused X-ray in an older child) is highly appropriate (9), while NECT and non-contrast brain MRI *may* be appropriate. NECT is highly appropriate in the setting of neurological signs/symptoms, apnea, complex skull fracture, other fractures, or highly suspicious injuries. Non-contrast MRI of the brain and spine is also highly appropriate for these patients, in the non-emergent setting. In a child with suspected thoracic or abdominopelvic injuries based on bruising, tenderness, or lab abnormalities, a skeletal survey with contrast-enhanced abdomen and pelvis CT are highly appropriate. CT chest with IV contrast and NECT *may* be appropriate in these patients [93].

Abusive Head Trauma

Abusive head trauma (AHT) is a leading cause of fatal head injuries in children younger than 2 years of age and is responsible for 53% of the serious or fatal traumatic brain injuries [94]. Fatal AHT has a peak incidence at 1–2 months of age [94]. Multitude of injury mechanisms underlie AHT including shaking (change in momentum of the force by acceleration or deceleration), blunt impact, whiplash-shaking injury, strangulation injury, and stabbing. Common imaging findings in abusive head trauma include subdural hemorrhage, parenchymal brain injuries, retinal hemorrhages, spine injury, and spinal subdural hemorrhage detailed below.

Subdural Hemorrhage

Subdural hemorrhage/hematoma (SDH) is the most common intracranial abnormality in young infants with AHT, seen in up to 90% of cases. Most commonly parafalcine in location, SDH is a result of shearing forces on the convexity bridging veins leading to the tears at the junction of bridging veins and superior sagittal sinus. In addition, shearing forces may also result in rupture of the arachnoid membrane, e.g., in the vicinity of strained blood vessels or at Pacchionian granulations, resulting in inter-mixing of cerebrospinal fluid with subdural blood and mixed attenuation subdural hematomas (hematohygroma) (Fig. 12.22). Such mixed-attenuation subdural hematomas are found with greater prevalence in abusive head trauma than in accidental head trauma [95]. Bradford et al., in a cohort of 115 children with abusive head trauma reported a 92% incidence of SDH on initial CT scans. The collections were homogeneously hyperdense in 27.8%, mixed density in 57.7% and were homogeneously hypodense in 14.4% of cases [96]. Precise dating of subdural collections based on neuroimaging alone is unrealistic. Not infrequently, the differentiation of subdural hygroma

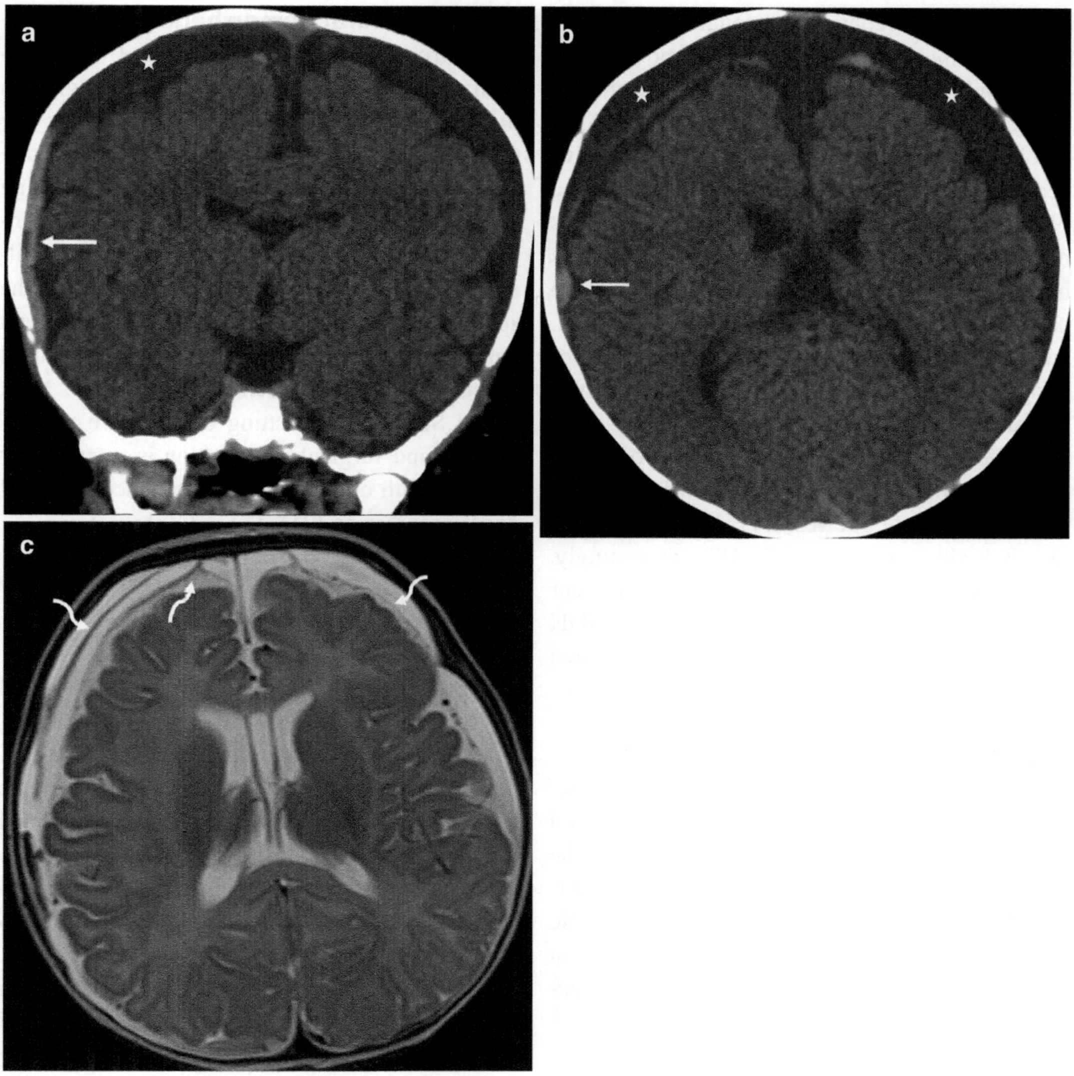

Fig. 12.22 Coronal (**a**) and axial (**b**) CT scan, axial T2 (**c**) MRI: 4-month-old boy with altered mental status and clinical suspicion for abusive head trauma: there is a small right sided subdural hemorrhage adjacent to the temporal bone (arrow). In addition, there are bilateral hematohygromas slightly hyperdense compared to the CSF (star). Multiple neomembranes are seen in the frontal convexities (curved arrows) favoring chronic subdural hemorrhages

from chronic subdural hemorrhage poses a diagnostic challenge due to quite similar attenuation, while the former is compatible with both a rapid and a delayed process, the latter suggests a traumatic event that occurred a few weeks ago. The most important criterion aiding in differentiation is the presence of subdural neomembranes, septa, or chamber like formations characteristic of chronic SDH, typically described after 2–4 weeks. Their radiologic detection is challenging and often warrants contrast enhanced MRI [97].

Parenchymal Injuries

Parenchymal brain injury represents the most significant cause of morbidity and mortality in AHT and includes a spectrum of abnormalities as a result of direct (contusion, axonal injury, parenchymal hematoma) and indirect (hypoxic ischemic) injury mechanisms. Hypoxic ischemic injury is seen in about 1/3rd of patients with AHT and is up to four times more common in abusive head trauma (37%) than in accidental trauma (9%) [98]. The cause is multifactorial, and is most likely a combination of apnea, secondary hypotension, reactive vasospasm adjacent to hemorrhage, respiratory distress, strangulation, and oxidative stress. The common pattern of hypoxic ischemic injury in AHT are diffuse supratentorial and supratentorial parasagittal watershed territory distribution. Diffuse or multifocal ischemia not in an arterial distribution, and in the absence of large vessel occlusion or dissection is highly suggestive of AHT. Interestingly, unilateral hypoxic ischemic injuries often occur ipsilateral to an asymmetric or unilateral SDH and have a strong association with confirmed abuse (Fig. 12.23).

Ocular Hemorrhage

One systematic review showed that intraocular hemorrhage (IOH) had a sensitivity of 75% and specificity of 94% for abusive head trauma. The most common finding was intraretinal hemorrhages at the posterior pole (Fig. 12.24). Optic nerve sheath hemorrhages can also be seen in AHT but have a much lower sensitivity and specificity [99].

Spinal Injuries

Radiographs and CT often underestimate spinal injuries in AHT because ligamentous injuries are much more common than osseous injuries. Injuries commonly involve posterior occipital-atlanto-axial, nuchal and interspinous ligaments and are best evaluated on spinal MRI (Fig. 12.25). 78% of the AHT patients and 46% of the accidental trauma patients had cervical spine ligamentous injuries in a retrospective study [100]. There is a strong correlation between ligamentous injury of occipitocervical region and hypoxic ischemic brain injury. Not commonly, vertebral compression fractures can also be seen in NAT (Fig. 12.26).

Spinal Subdural Hemorrhage

One retrospective study found that 60% of children who underwent thoracolumbar imaging in the setting of AHT had spinal SDH [21]. The mechanism is unclear and is likely not the same as intracranial SDH due to the lack of bridging vessels. The association of spinal subdural hemorrhage and intracranial SDH raises the possibility of tracking of intracranial hemorrhage into the spinal canal by gravity. Although CT can detect hemorrhage as a hyperdensity in the subdural space, MR SWI is much more sensitive. Most spinal SDHs in the setting of AHT are asymptomatic and surgical intervention is reserved for patients with clinical or MRI evidence of spinal cord compression [21] (Fig. 12.27).

Mimics of Abusive Head Trauma

The pattern of brain injury, clinical history, and physical examination are all important when considering abusive head trauma. Erroneously diagnosing abusive head trauma can have grave consequences for the child and family, and legal repercussions for both the family and clinicians. Imaging plays a vital role in the workup of abusive head trauma as clinical information regarding mechanism or timing of injury is often vague. While SDH is one of the hallmark intracranial findings of AHT and is present in nearly 90% of cases of AHT, there is significant overlap in the presence of SDH with accidental head trauma. Therefore, it is imperative to consider other clinical and imaging findings including the pattern of SDH. Interhemispheric, convexity, and posterior fossa SDHs are significantly associated with AHT especially in the setting of brain parenchymal injuries and retinal hemorrhages [23]. An isolated finding of subarachnoid hemorrhage is non-discriminatory in differentiating accidental from abusive head trauma [23, 101]. An epidural hemorrhage with a skull fracture and scalp swelling is associated with accidental head trauma [23, 102]. Birth related hemorrhage, discussed earlier in the chapter is an important mimic to consider in neonates. It is important to note that a majority

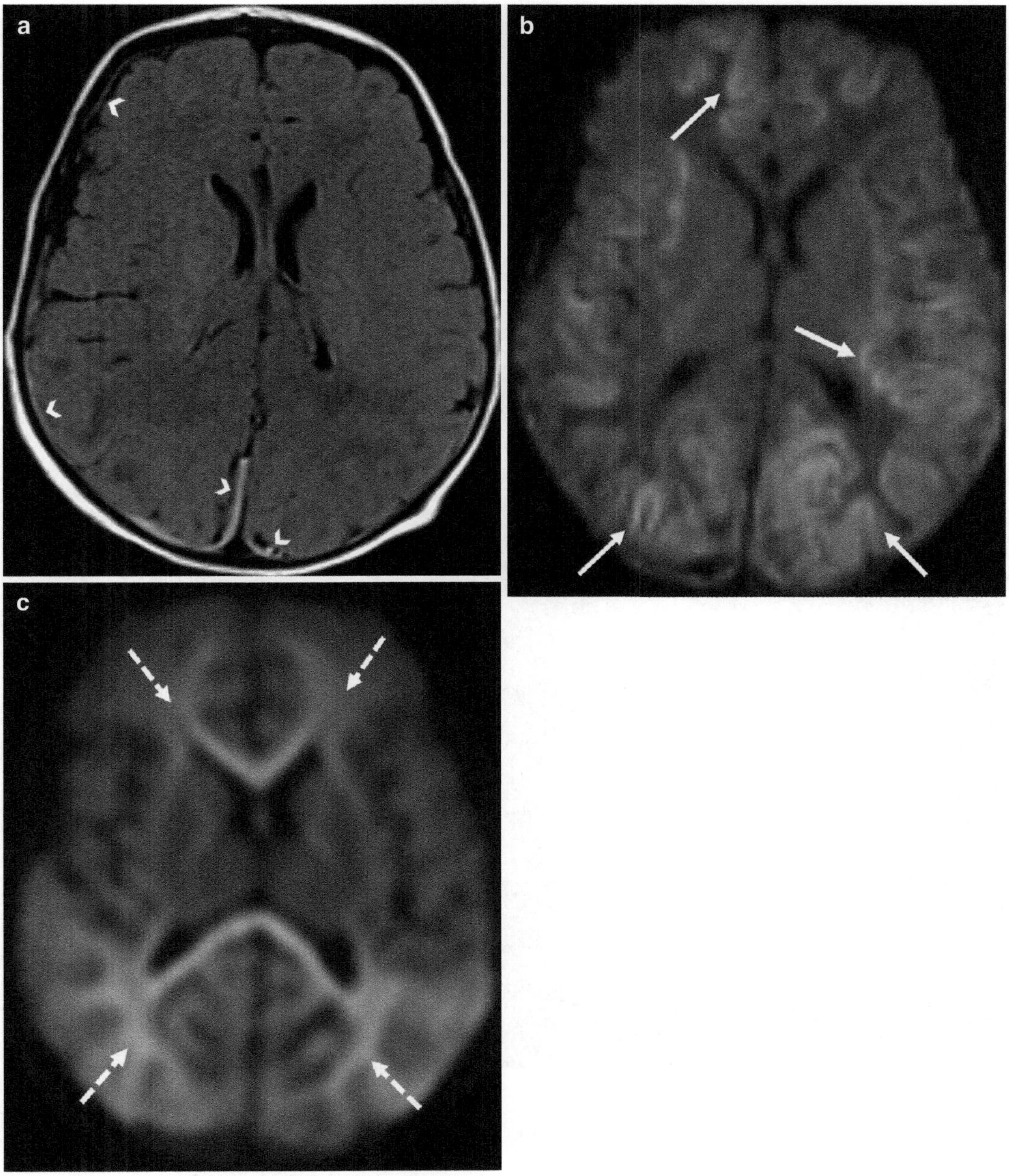

Fig. 12.23 Axial FLAIR (**a**), axial DWI (**b**), follow-up DWI 5 days later (**c**): 7-week-old boy with suspicion for non-accidental trauma: Bilateral supratentorial subdural hemorrhages are seen, right greater than left (chevron arrows). Extensive hypoxic ischemic injury of the supratentorial cortex is demonstrated including the frontal, parietal, and occipital lobes (arrows) with relative sparing of the temporal lobes. Follow-up DWI shows delayed white matter injury (postanoxic leukoencephalopathy) (dashed arrows)

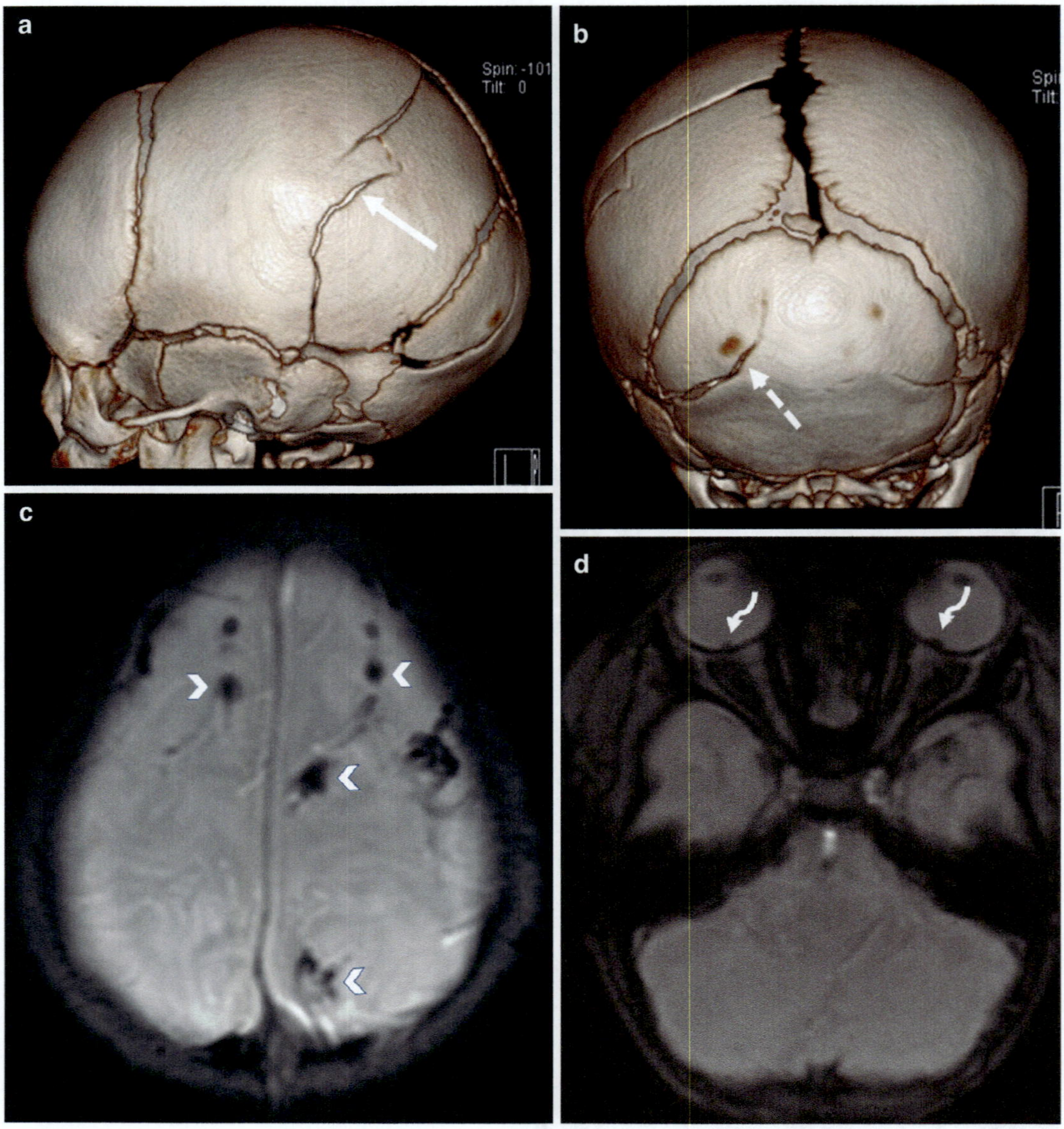

Fig. 12.24 3D reconstruction of calvarium (**a**, **b**), axial gradient (**c**, **d**) images: 5-month-old female with concern for nonaccidental trauma: There is a complex nondepressed fracture of the right parietal bone (arrow) and right occipital bone (dashed arrow). Multiple areas of curvilinear susceptibility are seen particularly at the vertex, representing thrombosed bridging veins "lollipop sign" (chevron arrows) along with bilateral subdural hemorrhages (not shown). Additionally, bilateral retinal hemorrhages are identified (curved arrows)

of birth related hemorrhage should resolve by 4 weeks [23].

Infection may also mimic AHT. Intracranial infection may present with encephalopathy with cerebral edema and SDH, mimicking AHT. Although uncommon, herpes simplex virus associated with encephalitis in infants can show intraparenchymal hemorrhage [23]. Vitamin K deficiency can also present with intraparenchymal bleeding, fractures and skin bruising either spontaneously or with minor trauma mimicking child abuse [103].

Knowledge of normal cranial bone formation is crucial to make the correct diagnosis of a skull fracture. Accessory sutures are common anatomic variants that occur due to anomalous

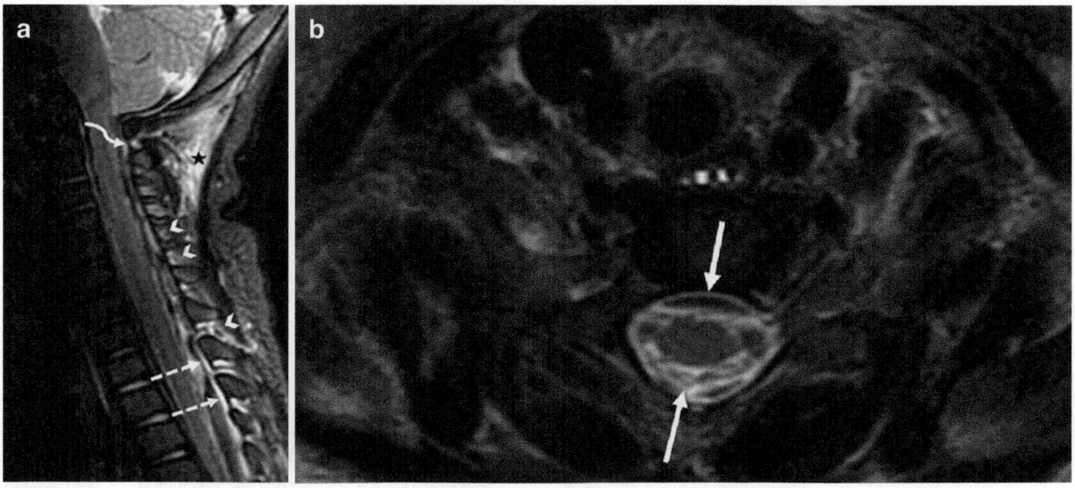

Fig. 12.25 Sagittal STIR (**a**) and axial T2 (**b**): 10-month-old with suspected non accidental trauma and intracranial injury: There is edema in the posterior paraspinal soft tissues (star). The interspinous ligaments are increased in signal suggestive of injury (chevron arrows). Edema is identified along the ligamentum flava at the cervicothoracic junction (dashed arrow) consistent with partial tears. In addition, the posterior atlantoaxial ligament is bright in signal concerning for injury (curved arrow). The anterior and posterior longitudinal ligaments are intact. Trace epidural hemorrhage is noted anteriorly and posteriorly within the epidural space (arrows)

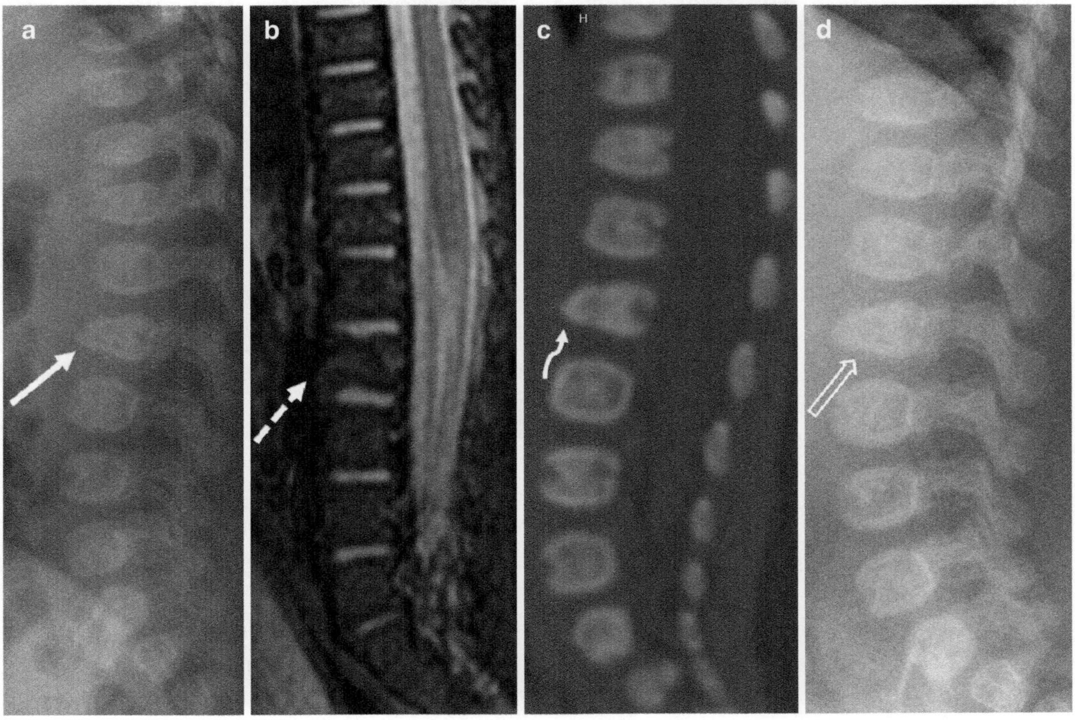

Fig. 12.26 Lateral X-ray lumbar spine (**a**), sagittal STIR MRI (**b**), sagittal CT (**c**), Latera X-ray 3-week follow-up (**d**): 3-month-old bcy with suspected NAT: abnormal L3 vertebral body morphology suspicious for compression deformity (arrow). Correspondingly there is loss of height of L3 vertebral body with minimal marrow edema (dashed arrow), which may represent a healing fracture. No additional information on CT scan suggesting healing fracture (curved arrow). Follow up X-ray shows increased sclerosis (open arrow)

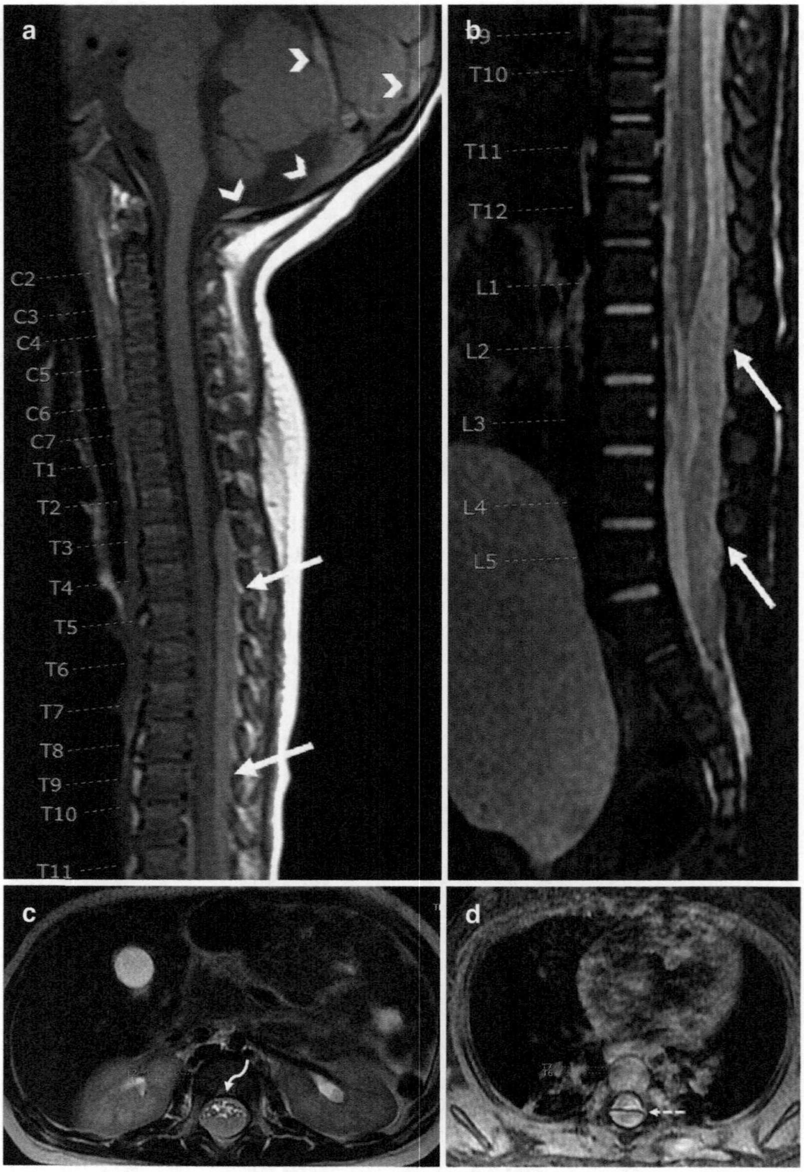

Fig. 12.27 Sagittal T1 (**a**), sagittal T2 (**b**), axial T2 (**c**), and axial gradient (**d**): 5-month-old female with suspected child abuse: large amount of posterior dependent subdural hemorrhage (arrows) is seen extending from T3 to the end of thecal sac tracking from the cerebral extra-axial hemorrhage (chevron arrows) along the tentorium and posterior fossa. This is causing mild anterior displacement of the cord and cauda equina nerve fibers (curved arrow). Axial gradient demonstrates fluid level in the thoracic spine (dashed arrow)

fusion and separation of ossification centers, within the calvarium and skull base, which can be a diagnostic challenge. In general, sutures usually have sclerotic borders with interdigitating, zig-zagging margins and do not extend across another suture, whereas fractures tend to have sharp margins and non-sclerotic edges and cross sutures [23, 104]. Surface-rendered 3D CT reconstructions are extremely helpful in differentiating between fractures, accessory sutures, and wormian bones.

Incidental findings on imaging in infants can also mimic child abuse. One such finding is benign enlargement of subarachnoid space in infancy (BESS) [105]. Small incidental SDHs, either spontaneously or due to minor trauma may be seen in the setting of BESS. It is thought that the bridging veins are more susceptible to tearing due to the longer distance traversed through the enlarged subarachnoid space. SDH in infants with BESS are not pathognomonic for AHT, but should be carefully scrutinized [106].

Abusive Body and Musculoskeletal Injuries

Abusive intra-abdominal injuries are less common than abusive head injuries or fractures and are found in only 2–3% of children being evaluated for abuse. No single abdominal injury is indicative of abuse. Abdominal injuries must be assessed in the context of other injuries, bruising, and the plausibility of reported mechanism of injury. Falls from a low height is the most common reported mechanism of injury in children being evaluated for blunt abdominal trauma that ultimately are found to have abusive trauma [66]. Studies have shown that hollow viscus injuries including duodenal injuries, and pancreatic injuries are more commonly seen in abuse than accidental trauma (Fig. 12.28) [66, 107]. Moreover, children with abusive abdominal injuries are likely to be younger, have more severe injuries, multiple injuries, or delayed presentation for care [23, 65]. CT abdomen and pelvis with IV contrast has a rating of 9 (highly appropriate) in the ACR Appropriateness Criteria in children with suspected thoracic or abdominopelvic injuries in the setting of abuse, and may combined with chest CT when there is concern for chest trauma [93].

Fractures occur in over half of abused children [108]. Skeletal survey radiographs remain a cornerstone in the workup and follow-up for fractures non-accidental trauma, have a rating of 9 (highly appropriate) on the ACR Appropriateness Criteria [93]. Rib fractures are one of the most common and specific injuries for non-accidental trauma. They may be the only fractures present and unfortunately may be difficult to visualize by radiographs due to lack of displacement or callous formation. One study showed a 17% miss rate of rib fractures on skeletal surveys when compared to CT, most often acute rib fractures [108]. These misses can have important safety and legal implications. Low dose CT has recently been advocated for better detection of rib fractures with studies showing significant increased detection of acute or healing rib fractures by low dose CT as compared to skeletal survey [108, 109] (Fig. 12.18). Furthermore, 3D print models can be made as a visual aid for physicians or legal experts [110]. Despite the lower ACR Appropriateness Criteria rating, low dose CT chest can be considered for better detection of rib fractures when clinically warranted.

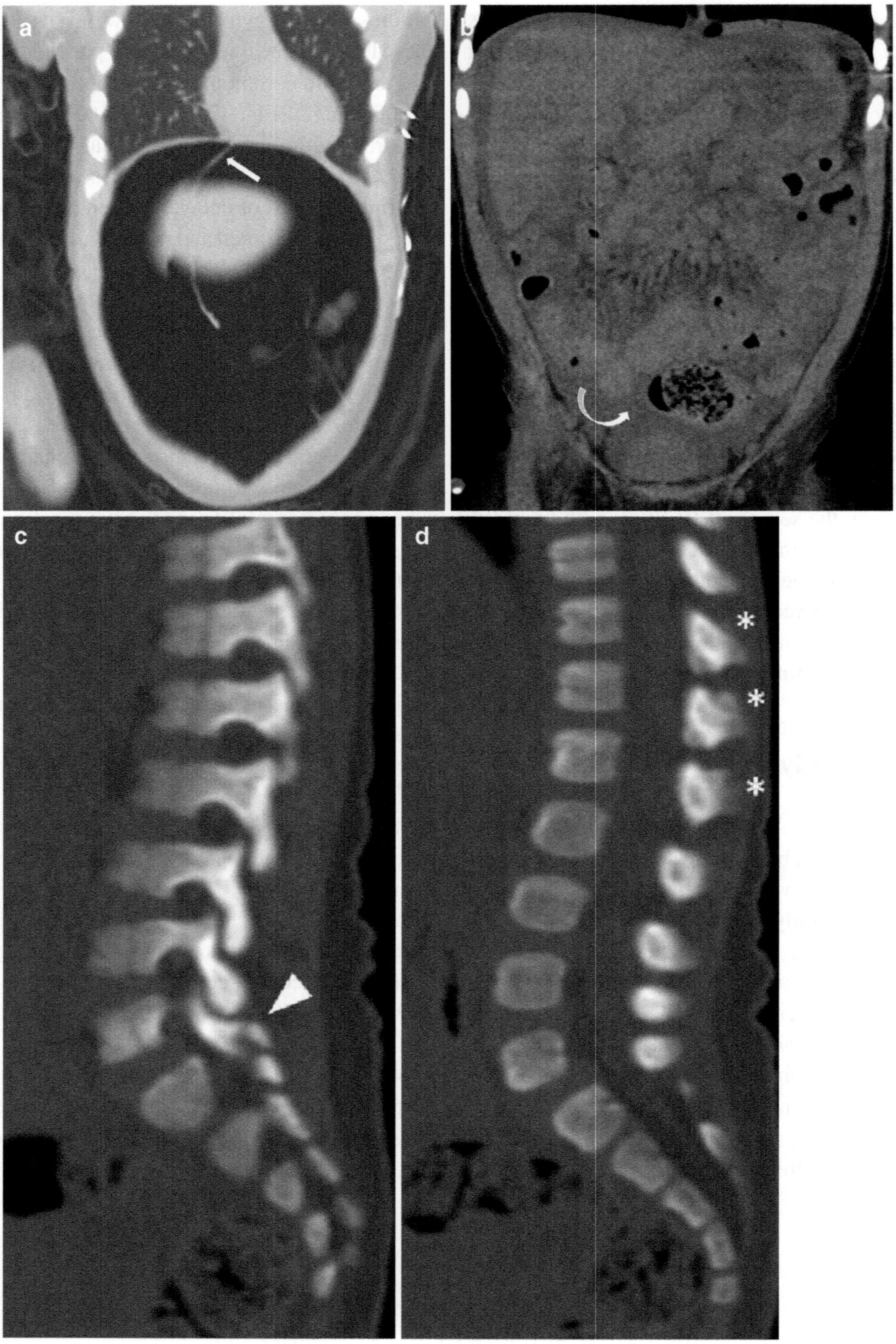

Fig. 12.28 Coronal (**a**, **b**) and sagittal (**c**, **d**) non-contrast CT performed at an outside hospital in a toddler with altered mental status shows large volume pneumoperitoneum outlining the falciform ligament (arrow) with free intraperitoneal fluid (curved arrow). There are healing spinous process fractures in the lower thoracic and lumbar spine (asterisks) and more recent fractures of the L5 pars interarticularis with spondylolisthesis (arrowhead). Constellation of findings including perforated hollow viscus, spinous process fractures, and fractures of various stages of healing is highly suspicious for non-accidental trauma. Gastric perforation was found intra-operatively

References

1. Centers for Disease Control and Prevention, National Center for Health Statistics. National vital statistics system, mortality 2018-2021 on CDC WONDER online database, released in 2021. Accessed at http://wonder.cdc.gov/ucd-icd10-expanded.html.
2. Goodman TR, Mustafa A, Rowe E. Pediatric CT radiation exposure: where we were, and where we are now. Pediatr Radiol. 2019;49(4):469–78.
3. Goske MJ, Applegate KE, Boylan J, Butler PF, Callahan MJ, Coley BD, Farley S, Frush DP, Hernanz-Schulman M, Jaramillo D, Johnson ND, Kaste SC, Morrison G, Strauss KJ, Tuggle N. The image gently campaign: working together to change practice. AJR Am J Roentgenol. 2008;190(2):273–4.
4. Pediatric Radiology & Imaging. Radiation safety – image gently. www.imagegently.org.
5. Ohana O, Soffer S, Zimlichman E, Klang E. Overuse of CT and MRI in paediatric emergency departments. Br J Radiol. 2018;91(1085):20170434.
6. Gaffley M, Neff LP, Sieren LM, Zeller KA, Pranikoff T, Rush T, Petty JK. Evaluation of an evidence-based guideline to reduce CT use in the assessment of blunt pediatric abdominal trauma. J Pediatr Surg. 2021;56(2):297–301.
7. Arbra CA, Vogel AM, Plumblee L, Zhang J, Mauldin PD, Dassinger MS, Russell RT, Blakely ML, Streck CJ. External validation of a five-variable clinical prediction rule for identifying children at very low risk for intra-abdominal injury after blunt abdominal trauma. J Trauma Acute Care Surg. 2018;85(1):71–7.
8. Streck CJ, Vogel AM, Zhang J, Huang EY, Santore MT, Tsao K, Falcone RA, Dassinger MS, Russell RT, Blakely ML, Pediatric Surgery Research Collaborative. Identifying children at very low risk for blunt intra-abdominal injury in whom CT of the abdomen can be avoided safely. J Am Coll Surg. 2017;224(4):449–58.
9. Sathya C, Alali AS, Wales PW, Langer JC, Kenney BD, Burd RS, Nance ML, Nathens AB. Computed tomography rates and estimated radiation-associated cancer risk among injured children treated at different trauma center types. Injury. 2019;50(1):142–8.
10. Kim YH, Kim MJ, Shin HJ, Yoon H, Lee MJ. Simplified split-bolus intravenous contrast injection technique for pediatric abdominal CT. Clin Imaging. 2017;46:28–32.
11. Thomas KE, Mann EH, Padfield N, et al. Dual bolus intravenous contrast injection technique for multiregion paediatric body CT. Eur Radiol. 2015;25:1014–22.
12. Siegel MJ, Ramirez-Giraldo JC. Dual-energy CT in children: imaging algorithms and clinical applications. Radiology. 2019;291(2):286–97. https://doi.org/10.1148/radiol.2019182289.
13. Vogl TJ, Schulz B, Bauer RW, Stöver T, Sader R, Tawfik AM. Dual-energy CT applications in head and neck imaging. AJR Am J Roentgenol. 2012;199(5):34–9. https://doi.org/10.2214/AJR.12.9113.
14. Naruto N, Tannai H, Nishikawa K, et al. Dual-energy bone removal computed tomography (BRCT): preliminary report of efficacy of acute intracranial hemorrhage detection. Emerg Radiol. 2018;25(1):29–33. https://doi.org/10.1007/s10140-017-1558-7.
15. Katsura M, Sato J, Akahane M, Kunimatsu A, Abe O. Current and novel techniques for metal artifact reduction at CT: practical guide for radiologists. Radiographics. 2018;38(2):450–61. https://doi.org/10.1148/rg.2018170102.
16. Ryan ME, Pruthi S, et al. ACR appropriateness criteria® head trauma-child. J Am Coll Radiol. 2020;17(5S):S125–37. https://doi.org/10.1016/j.jacr.2020.01.026.
17. Kuppermann N, Holmes JF, Dayan PS, et al. Identification of children at very low risk of clinically-important brain injuries after head trauma: a prospective cohort study. Lancet. 2009;374(9696):1160–70. https://doi.org/10.1016/S0140-6736(09)61558-0.
18. Hodges H, Epstein KN, Retrouvey M, et al. Pitfalls in the interpretation of pediatric head CTs: what the emergency radiologist needs to know. Emerg Radiol. 2022;29(4):729–42. https://doi.org/10.1007/s10140-022-02042-4.
19. Looney CB, Smith JK, Merck LH, et al. Intracranial hemorrhage in asymptomatic neonates: prevalence on MR images and relationship to obstetric and neonatal risk factors. Radiology. 2007;242(2):535–41. https://doi.org/10.1148/radiol.2422060133.
20. Nikam RM, Kandula VV, Yue X, et al. Birth-related subdural hemorrhage: prevalence and imaging morphology. Pediatr Radiol. 2021;51(6):939–46. https://doi.org/10.1007/s00247-021-05060-5.
21. Choudhary AK, Bradford RK, Dias MS, Moore GJ, Boal DKB. Spinal subdural hemorrhage in abusive head trauma: a retrospective study. Radiology. 2012;262(1):216–23. https://doi.org/10.1148/radiol.11102390.
22. Squier W. The "Shaken Baby" syndrome: pathology and mechanisms. Acta Neuropathol. 2011;122(5):519–42. https://doi.org/10.1007/s00401-011-0875-2.
23. Mankad K, Chhabda S, Lim W, et al. The neuroimaging mimics of abusive head trauma. Eur J Paediatr Neurol. 2019;23(1):19–30. https://doi.org/10.1016/j.ejpn.2018.11.006.
24. Chaturvedi A, Chaturvedi A, Stanescu AL, Blickman JG, Meyers SP. Mechanical birth-related trauma to the neonate: an imaging perspective. Insights Imaging. 2018;9(1):103–18. https://doi.org/10.1007/s13244-017-0586-x.
25. Acuña J, Adhikari S. Point-of-care ultrasound to distinguish subgaleal and cephalohematoma: case report. Clin Pract Cases Emerg Med. 2021;5(2):198–201.
26. Schweitzer AD, Niogi SN, Whitlow CT, Tsiouris AJ. Traumatic brain injury: imaging patterns and

complications. Radiographics. 2019;39(6):1571–95. https://doi.org/10.1148/rg.2019190076.
27. Janas AM, Qin F, Hamilton S, et al. Diffuse axonal injury grade on early MRI is associated with worse outcome in children with moderate-severe traumatic brain injury. Neurocrit Care. 2022;36(2):492–503. https://doi.org/10.1007/s12028-021-01336-8.
28. Dreizin D, Kim W, Kim JS, Boscak AR, Bodanapally UK, Munera F, Stein DM. Will the real SCIWORA please stand up? Exploring clinicoradiologic mismatch in closed spinal cord injuries. AJR Am J Roentgenol. 2015;205(4):853–60.
29. McAllister AS, Nagaraj U, Radhakrishnan R. Emergent imaging of pediatric cervical spine trauma. Radiographics. 2019;39(4):1126–42. https://doi.org/10.1148/rg.2019180100.
30. Copley PC, Tilliridou V, Kirby A, Jones J, Kandasamy J. Management of cervical spine trauma in children. Eur J Trauma Emerg Surg. 2019;45(5):777–89. https://doi.org/10.1007/s00068-018-0992-x. Epub 2018 Aug 24.
31. Pang D, Nemzek WR, Zovickian J. Atlanto-occipital dislocation–part 2: The clinical use of (occipital) condyle-C1 interval, comparison with other diagnostic methods, and the manifestation, management, and outcome of atlanto-occipital dislocation in children. Neurosurgery. 2007;61(5):995–1015; discussion 1015. https://doi.org/10.1227/01.neu.0000303196.87672.78.
32. Pang D. Spinal cord injury without radiographic abnormality in children, 2 decades later. Neurosurgery. 2004;55(6):1325–42; discussion 1342. https://doi.org/10.1227/01.neu.0000143030.85589.e6.
33. Smith P, Linscott LL, Vadivelu S, Zhang B, Leach JL. Normal development and measurements of the occipital condyle-C1 interval in children and young adults. AJNR Am J Neuroradiol. 2016;37(5):952–7. https://doi.org/10.3174/ajnr.A4543.
34. Konovalov N, Peev N, Zileli M, Sharif S, Kaprovoy S, Timonin S. Pediatric cervical spine injuries and SCIWORA: WFNS spine committee recommendations. Neurospine. 2020;17(4):797–808. https://doi.org/10.14245/ns.2040404.202.
35. Rao RD, Tang S, Lim C, Yoganandan N. Developmental morphology and ossification patterns of the C1 vertebra. J Bone Joint Surg Am. 2013;95(17):e1241–7. https://doi.org/10.2106/JBJS.L.01035.
36. Kobets AJ, Nakhla J, Biswas A, Kinon MD, Yassari R, Abbott IR. Isolated synchondrosis fracture of the atlas presenting as rotatory fixation of the neck: case report and review of literature. Surg Neurol Int. 2016;7(Suppl 42):S1092–5. https://doi.org/10.4103/2152-7806.196768.
37. Alvarez Caro F, Pumarada Prieto M, Alvarez BF. Congenital defect of the atlas and axis. A cause of misdiagnose when evaluating an acute neck trauma. Am J Emerg Med. 2008;26(7):840. https://doi.org/10.1016/j.ajem.2008.01.038.
38. Sharifi G, Lotfinia M, Rahmanzade R, et al. Congenital absence of the posterior element of C1, C2, and C3 along with bilateral absence of C4 pedicles: case report and review of the literature. World Neurosurg. 2018;111:395–401. https://doi.org/10.1016/j.wneu.2017.12.070.
39. Karwacki GM, Schneider JF. Normal ossification patterns of atlas and axis: a CT study. AJNR Am J Neuroradiol. 2012;33(10):1882–7. https://doi.org/10.3174/ajnr.A3105.
40. Mistry D, Munjal H, Ellika S, Chaturvedi A. Pediatric spine trauma: a comprehensive review. Clin Imaging. 2022;87:61–76. https://doi.org/10.1016/j.clinimag.2022.04.012.
41. Rusin JA, Ruess L, Daulton RS. New C2 synchondrosal fracture classification system. Pediatr Radiol. 2015;45(6):872–81. https://doi.org/10.1007/s00247-014-3224-5.
42. Hedequist DJ, Mo AZ. Os odontoideum in children. J Am Acad Orthop Surg. 2020;28(3):e100–7. https://doi.org/10.5435/JAAOS-D-18-00637.
43. Singhal A, Mitra A, Cochrane D, Steinbok P. Ring apophysis fracture in pediatric lumbar disc herniation: a common entity. Pediatr Neurosurg. 2013;49(1):16–20. https://doi.org/10.1159/000355127.
44. Le TV, Baaj AA, Deukmedjian A, Uribe JS, Vale FL. Chance fractures in the pediatric population. J Neurosurg Pediatr. 2011;8(2):189–97. https://doi.org/10.3171/2011.5.PEDS10538.
45. Hazen BJ, Keane OA, Vandewalle RJ, et al. Difference in presentation and concomitant intra-abdominal injury with chance fracture in pediatric and adult populations. Am Surg. 2022;2022:31348221102607. https://doi.org/10.1177/00031348221102607.
46. Durel R, Rudman E, Milburn J. Clinical images - a quarterly column: chance fracture of the lumbar spine. Ochsner J. 2014;14(1):9–11.
47. Nash M, Rafay MF. Craniocervical arterial dissection in children: pathophysiology and management. Pediatr Neurol. 2019;95:9–18.
48. Bent C, Shen P, Dahlin B, Coulter K. Blunt intraoral trauma resulting in internal carotid artery dissection and infarction in a child. Pediatr Emerg Care. 2016;32(8):534–5. https://doi.org/10.1097/PEC.0000000000000321.
49. Al Ali A, Ganesan R, Nouri M, Shayna Z, Ranger A, Tay K. 736: chiropractic treatments and stroke with arterial dissection in an infant. Crit Care Med. 2021;49(1):364. https://doi.org/10.1097/01.ccm.0000728832.27003.18.
50. Yang Y, Kapasi M, Abdeen N, Dos Santos MP, O'Connor MD. Traumatic carotid cavernous fistula in a pediatric patient. Can J Ophthalmol. 2015;50(4):318–21. https://doi.org/10.1016/j.jcjo.2015.05.014.
51. Dunklebarger J, Branstetter B, Lincoln A, et al. Pediatric temporal bone fractures: current trends and comparison of classification schemes. Laryngoscope. 2014;124(3):781–4. https://doi.org/10.1002/lary.21891.

52. Prisman E, Ramsden JD, Blaser S, Papsin B. Traumatic perilymphatic fistula with pneumolabyrinth: diagnosis and management. Laryngoscope. 2011;121(4):856–9. https://doi.org/10.1002/lary.21439.
53. Drexel S, Azarow K, Jafri MA. Abdominal trauma evaluation for the pediatric surgeon. Surg Clin North Am. 2017;97(1):59–74.
54. Sivit CJ. Imaging children with abdominal trauma. AJR Am J Roentgenol. 2009;192(5):1179–89.
55. Coccolini F, Montori G, Catena F, et al. Splenic trauma: WSES classification and guidelines for adult and pediatric patients. World J Emerg Surg. 2017;12:40.
56. Lynn KN, Werder GM, Callaghan RM, Sullivan AN, Jafri ZH, Bloom DA. Pediatric blunt splenic trauma: a comprehensive review. Pediatr Radiol. 2009;39(9):904–16; quiz 1029–30. https://doi.org/10.1007/s00247-009-1336-0.
57. Bansal S, Karrer FM, Hansen K, Partrick DA. Contrast blush in pediatric blunt splenic trauma does not warrant the routine use of angiography and embolization. Am J Surg. 2015;210(2):345–50.
58. Davies DA, Ein SH, Pearl R, Langer JC, Traubici J, Mikrogianakis A, Wales PW. What is the significance of contrast "blush" in pediatric blunt splenic trauma? J Pediatr Surg. 2010;45(5):916–20.
59. Soto JA, Anderson SW. Multidetector CT of blunt abdominal trauma. Radiology. 2012;265(3):678–93.
60. Patrick LE, Ball TI, Atkinson GO, Winn KJ. Pediatric blunt abdominal trauma: periportal tracking at CT. Radiology. 1992;183(3):689–91.
61. Sivit CJ, Taylor GA, Eichelberger MR, Bulas DI, Gotschall CS, Kushner DC. Significance of periportal low-attenuation zones following blunt trauma in children. Pediatr Radiol. 1993;23(5):388–90.
62. Ibrahim A, Wales PW, Aquino MR, Chavhan GB. CT and MRI findings in pancreatic trauma in children and correlation with outcome. Pediatr Radiol. 2020;50(7):943–52. https://doi.org/10.1007/s00247-020-04642-z. Epub 2020 Mar 14. PMID: 32172401.
63. Englum BR, Gulack BC, Rice HE, Scarborough JE, Adibe OO. Management of blunt pancreatic trauma in children: review of the National Trauma Data Bank. J Pediatr Surg. 2016;51(9):1526–31.
64. Biyyam DR, Hwang S, Patel MC, Bardo DME, Bailey SS, Youssfi M. CT findings of pediatric handlebar injuries. Radiographics. 2020;40(3):815–26.
65. Wood J, Rubin DM, Nance ML, Christian CW. Distinguishing inflicted versus accidental abdominal injuries in young children. J Trauma. 2005;59(5):1203–8.
66. Carter KW, Moulton SL. Pediatric abdominal injury patterns caused by "falls": a comparison between nonaccidental and accidental trauma. J Pediatr Surg. 2016;51(2):326–8.
67. Rosenfeld EH, Vogel A, Russell RT, Maizlin I, Klinkner DB, Polites S, Gaines B, Leeper C, Anthony S, Waddell M, St Peter S, Juang D, Thakkar R, Drews J, Behrens B, Jafri M, Burd RS, Beaudin M, Carmant L, Falcone RA Jr, Moody S, Naik-Mathuria BJ. Comparison of diagnostic imaging modalities for the evaluation of pancreatic duct injury in children: a multi-institutional analysis from the Pancreatic Trauma Study Group. Pediatr Surg Int. 2018;34(9):961–6.
68. Singer G, Arneitz C, Tschauner S, Castellani C, Till H. Trauma in pediatric urology. Semin Pediatr Surg. 2021;30(4):151085.
69. Paltiel HJ, Barth RA, Bruno C, et al. Contrast-enhanced ultrasound of blunt abdominal trauma in children. Pediatr Radiol. 2021;51:2253–69.
70. Chatoorgoon K, Brown RL, Garcia VF, Falcone RA Jr. Role of computed tomography and clinical findings in pediatric blunt intestinal injury: a multicenter study. Pediatr Emerg Care. 2012;28(12):1338–42.
71. Khasawneh R, Ramakrishnaiah RH, Singh S, Hegde SV. CT findings in pediatric blunt intestinal injury. Emerg Radiol. 2013;20(6):545–52.
72. Perea LL, San Roman J, Gaughan JP, Gefen R, Hazelton JP. Low-density isolated intraperitoneal free fluid in pediatric blunt trauma is not associated with abdominal injury. Pediatr Emerg Care. 2022;38(1):e143–6.
73. Berona K, Kang T, Rose E. Pelvic free fluid in asymptomatic pediatric blunt abdominal trauma patients: a case series and review of the literature. J Emerg Med. 2016;50(5):753–8. https://doi.org/10.1016/j.jemermed.2016.01.003. Epub 2016 Feb 13. PMID: 26884127.
74. Yu J, Fulcher AS, Wang DB, Turner MA, Ha JD, McCulloch M, Kennedy RM, Malhotra AK, Halvorsen RA. Frequency and importance of small amount of isolated pelvic free fluid detected with multidetector CT in male patients with blunt trauma. Radiology. 2010;256(3):799–805.
75. Vandewalle RJ, Barker SJ, Raymond JL, Brown BP, Rouse TM. Pediatric handlebar injuries: more than meets the abdomen. Pediatr Emerg Care. 2021;37(9):e517–23.
76. Klimek PM, Lutz T, Stranzinger E, Zachariou Z, Kessler U, Berger S. Handlebar injuries in children. Pediatr Surg Int. 2013;29(3):269–73.
77. Donnelly LF. Imaging issues in CT of blunt trauma to the chest and abdomen. Pediatr Radiol. 2009;39(3):406–13.
78. Moore MA, Wallace EC, Westra SJ. The imaging of paediatric thoracic trauma. Pediatr Radiol. 2009;39(5):485–96.
79. Stephens CQ, Boulos MC, Connelly CR, Gee A, Jafri M, Krishnaswami S. Limiting thoracic CT: a rule for use during initial pediatric trauma evaluation. J Pediatr Surg. 2017;52(12):2031–7.
80. Holl EM, Marek AP, Nygaard RM, Richardson CJ, Hess DJ. Use of chest computed tomography for blunt pediatric chest trauma: does it change clinical course? Pediatr Emerg Care. 2020;36(2):81–6.
81. Patel RP, Hernanz-Schulman M, Hilmes MA, Yu C, Ray J, Kan JH. Pediatric chest CT after trauma:

impact on surgical and clinical management. Pediatr Radiol. 2010;40(7):1246–53.
82. Azari S, Hoover T, Dunstan M, Harrison TJ, Browne M. Review, monitor, educate: a quality improvement initiative for sustained chest radiation reduction in pediatric trauma patients. Am J Surg. 2020;220(5):1327–32.
83. Golden J, Isani M, Bowling J, et al. Limiting chest computed tomography in the evaluation of pediatric thoracic trauma. J Trauma Acute Care Surg. 2016;81(2):271–7.
84. Hammer MR, Dillman JR, Chong ST, Strouse PJ. Imaging of pediatric thoracic trauma. Semin Roentgenol. 2012;47(2):135–46.
85. Samet JD. Pediatric sports injuries. Clin Sports Med. 2021;40(4):781–99.
86. Ho-Fung VM, Zapala MA, Lee EY. Musculoskeletal traumatic injuries in children. Radiol Clin N Am. 2017;55(4):785–802.
87. Brian JM, Choi DH, Moore MM. The primary physis. Semin Musculoskelet Radiol. 2018;22(1):095–103.
88. Eismann EA, Stephan ZA, Mehlman CT, Denning J, Mehlman T, Parikh SN, Tamai J, Zbojniewicz A. Pediatric triplane ankle fractures: impact of radiographs and computed tomography on fracture classification and treatment planning. J Bone Joint Surg Am. 2015;97(12):995–1002.
89. Olgun ZD, Maestre S. Management of pediatric ankle fractures. Curr Rev Musculoskelet Med. 2018;11(3):475–84.
90. Silber JS, Flynn JM, Katz MA, Ganley TJ, Koffler KM, Drummond DS. Role of computed tomography in the classification and management of pediatric pelvic fractures. J Pediatr Orthop. 2001;21(2):148–51.
91. Bent MA, Hennrikus WL, Latorre JE, Armstrong DG, Shaw B, Jones KC, Segal LS. Role of computed tomography in the classification of pediatric pelvic fractures-revisited. J Orthop Trauma. 2017;31(7):e200–4.
92. https://www.acf.hhs.gov/cb/report/child-maltreatment-2021.
93. Wootton-Gorges SL, Soares BP, Alazraki AL, Anupindi SA, Blount JP, Booth TN, Dempsey ME, Falcone RA Jr, Hayes LL, Kulkarni AV, Partap S, Rigsby CK, Ryan ME, Safdar NM, Trout AT, Widmann RF, Karmazyn BK, Palasis S, Expert Panel on Pediatric Imaging. ACR appropriateness Criteria® suspected physical abuse-child. J Am Coll Radiol. 2017;14(5S):S338–49.
94. Choudhary AK, Servaes S, Slovis TL, Palusci VJ, Hedlund GL, Narang SK, Moreno JA, Dias MS, Christian CW, Nelson MD Jr, Silvera VM, Palasis S, Raissaki M, Rossi A, Offiah AC. Consensus statement on abusive head trauma in infants and young children. Pediatr Radiol. 2018;48(8):1048–65. https://doi.org/10.1007/s00247-018-4149-1.
95. Hedlund G. Abusive head trauma: extra-axial hemorrhage and nonhemic collections. In: Kleinman P, editor. Diagnostic imaging of child abuse. Cambridge: Cambridge University Press; 2015. p. 394–452.
96. Bradford R, Choudhary AK, Dias MS. Serial neuroimaging in infants with abusive head trauma: timing abusive injuries. J Neurosurg Pediatr. 2013;12(2):110–9. https://doi.org/10.3171/2013.4.PEDS12596.
97. Wittschieber D, Karger B, Pfeiffer H, Hahnemann ML. Understanding subdural collections in pediatric abusive head trauma. AJNR Am J Neuroradiol. 2019;40(3):388–95. https://doi.org/10.3174/ajnr.A5855. Epub 2018 Dec 6. PMID: 30523144; PMCID: PMC7028666.
98. Ichord RN, Naim M, Pollock AN, Nance ML, Margulies SS, Christian CW. Hypoxic-ischemic injury complicates inflicted and accidental traumatic brain injury in young children: the role of diffusion-weighted imaging. J Neurotrauma. 2007;24(1):106–18. https://doi.org/10.1089/neu.2006.0087.
99. Bhardwaj G, Chowdhury V, Jacobs MB, Moran KT, Martin FJ, Coroneo MT. A systematic review of the diagnostic accuracy of ocular signs in pediatric abusive head trauma. Ophthalmology. 2010;117(5):983–992.e17. https://doi.org/10.1016/j.ophtha.2009.09.040.
100. Choudhary AK, Ishak R, Zacharia TT, Dias MS. Imaging of spinal injury in abusive head trauma: a retrospective study. Pediatr Radiol. 2014;44(9):1130–40. https://doi.org/10.1007/s00247-014-2959-3.
101. Piteau SJ, Ward MGK, Barrowman NJ, Plint AC. Clinical and radiographic characteristics associated with abusive and nonabusive head trauma: a systematic review. Pediatrics. 2012;130(2):315–23. https://doi.org/10.1542/peds.2011-1545.
102. Kemp AM, Jaspan T, Griffiths J, et al. Neuroimaging: what neuroradiological features distinguish abusive from non-abusive head trauma? A systematic review. Arch Dis Child. 2011;96(12):1103–12. https://doi.org/10.1136/archdischild-2011-300630.
103. Brousseau TJ, Kissoon N, McIntosh B. Vitamin K deficiency mimicking child abuse. J Emerg Med. 2005;29(3):283–8. https://doi.org/10.1016/j.jemermed.2005.02.009.
104. Idriz S, Patel JH, Ameli Renani S, Allan R, Vlahos I. CT of normal developmental and variant anatomy of the pediatric skull: distinguishing trauma from normality. Radiographics. 2015;35(5):1585–601. https://doi.org/10.1148/rg.2015140177.
105. Khosroshahi N, Nikkhah A. Benign enlargement of subarachnoid space in infancy: "a review with emphasis on diagnostic work-up". Iran J Child Neurol. 2018;12(4):7–15.
106. McNeely PD, Atkinson JD, Saigal G, O'Gorman AM, Farmer JP. Subdural hematomas in infants with benign enlargement of the subarachnoid spaces are not pathognomonic for child abuse. AJNR Am J Neuroradiol. 2006;27(8):1725–8.
107. Henry MK, Bennett CE, Wood JN, Servaes S. Evaluation of the abdomen in the setting of suspected child abuse. Pediatr Radiol. 2021;51(6):1044–50.

108. Pomeranz CB, Barrera CA, Servaes SE. Value of chest CT over skeletal surveys in detection of rib fractures in pediatric patients. Clin Imaging. 2022;82:103–9.
109. Sanchez TR, Lee JS, Coulter KP, Seibert JA, Stein-Wexler R. CT of the chest in suspected child abuse using submillisievert radiation dose. Pediatr Radiol. 2015;45(7):1072–6.
110. Barrera CA, Silvestro E, Calle-Toro JS, Scribano PV, Wood JN, Henry MK, Andronikou S. Three-dimensional printed models of the rib cage in children with non-accidental injury as an effective visual-aid tool. Pediatr Radiol. 2019;49(7):965–70.

Contrast-Associated Acute Kidney Injury in Trauma

13

Michael R. Rudnick and Ryan Spiardi

Abbreviations

AKI	Acute kidney injury
CA-AKI	Contrast-associated acute kidney injury
CECT	Contrast-enhanced computed tomography
CI-AKI	Contrast-induced acute kidney injury
CIN	Contrast-induced nephropathy
CKD	Chronic kidney disease
CT	Computed tomography
DM	Diabetes mellitus
eGFR	Estimated glomerular filtration rate
KDIGO	Kidney disease improving global outcomes
NaCl	Sodium chloride
SCr	Serum creatinine

M. R. Rudnick (✉) · R. Spiardi
Renal-Electrolyte and Hypertension Division, Perelman School of Medicine, University of Pennsylvania, Philadelphia, PA, USA
e-mail: michael.rudnick@pennmedicine.upenn.edu; ryan.spiardi@pennmedicine.upenn.edu

Introduction

Acute kidney injury (AKI) is a heterogenous entity defined by an acute increase in serum creatinine (SCr) or reduction in urine output, and is associated with progression to chronic kidney disease (CKD), end-stage kidney disease, and increased mortality [1]. AKI is common in trauma patients, afflicting up to 24% of patients admitted to the intensive care unit for trauma or traumatic brain injuries, and associated with an over three-fold increase in mortality compared to trauma patients who do not suffer AKI [2]. Various pathophysiologic mechanisms may underlie the development of trauma-associated AKI, which often are not related to direct renal trauma. These include abrupt changes in volume status and circulation, crush injury leading to directly nephrotoxic myoglobin release, use of vasopressors, exposure to iodinated contrast or other potentially nephrotoxic medications, and production of reactive oxygen species after perfusion is restored. Additionally, polytrauma may lead to damage-associated molecular patterns, facilitating a downstream activation of the coagulation cascade and complement systems, as well as production of inflammatory markers, all of which may promote renal injury [3]. AKI may be more common in trauma patients, particularly those who are older, or have a history of diabetes or hypertension. Other presentation-specific risk factors associated with AKI in trauma admissions

F. Knollmann (ed.), *Trauma Computed Tomography*, https://doi.org/10.1007/978-3-031-45746-3_13

include those with shock, higher injury severity scores, abdominal injuries, or sepsis [2].

Contrast-associated acute kidney injury (CA-AKI) was previously defined as an increase in SCr of 25% of baseline, or 0.5 mg/dL, 48 h or more after a contrast-enhanced study [4]. This definition of AKI has now been replaced by a holistic, consensus definition developed by the Kidney Disease Improving Global Outcomes (KDIGO) AKI Workgroup: an increase in SCr by ≥0.3 mg/dL or ≥1.5 times baseline SCr within 48 h, or urine volume <0.5 mL/kg/h for 6 h [5].

Terminology of contrast nephrotoxicity has also evolved. Initially the term *contrast-induced nephropathy* (CIN) was used to define AKI caused by contrast media. However, multiple studies have demonstrated that AKI following contrast exposure should not be assumed to be caused by contrast media [6, 7]. As such, the American College of Radiology has proposed new terminology. The term *contrast-associated acute kidney injury* (CA-AKI) should be used for AKI following contrast exposure in which the etiology of AKI is unclear, as the clinical events surrounding contrast exposure often creates a favorable milieu for other causes of kidney injury. The term *contrast-induced acute kidney injury* (CI-AKI) is reserved for cases in which a careful review of clinical information demonstrates that the AKI is likely due to contrast media per se [8]. Since most publications involve observational data in which it is uncertain if contrast media was the primary cause of the AKI, we will use the term CA-AKI for this chapter. CA-AKI typically is characterized by a non-oliguric rise in SCr 24–72 h post-contrast exposure with a variable, but often low (< 1%), fractional excretion of sodium [9]. The pathophysiology of CA-AKI is due to both direct renal nephrotoxicity and hypoxic injury to the kidney, particularly in the low oxygen environment of the outer medulla [9–11].

There are multiple patient-centered, independent risk factors for CA-AKI that have been previously established in the literature. The primary risk factor for CA-AKI is chronic kidney disease. The degree of risk is directly proportional to the severity of the CKD, which is usually defined by the estimated glomerular filtration rate (eGFR). CA-AKI rarely occurs in patients with normal renal function (eGFR ≥60 mL/min/1.73 m^2) or mild CKD (eGFR 45–59 mL/min/1.73 m^2). Diabetes mellitus (DM) by itself is not a risk factor but becomes a risk factor when coupled with CKD. Thus, a patient with CKD and DM is more at risk for CA-AKI than patient with the same degree of CKD without DM. Other risk factors such as hypotension, congestive heart failure, elderly age, and anemia have been reported but it is likely these risk factors are epiphenomena for a reduced eGFR [12–14]. There are currently risk score models, used primarily in cardiac angiography, which can be used to predict the risk of CA-AKI [15].

CA-AKI: What Is the Risk?

It is clinically important to determine the *true risk* of CA-AKI for each patient. If the risk is overestimated, the patient may not be offered contrast-enhanced computed tomography (CECT) resulting in a failure to identify critical diagnostic information, which in turn increases the clinical risk to the patient. On the other hand, if the risk of CA-AKI is underestimated, patients may needlessly be exposed to contrast media and the risks of AKI. For example, in a study of patients undergoing coronary angiography after myocardial infarction, the use of angiography was 50% less in patients with abnormal renal function compared to patients with normal renal function, despite similar indications for angiography in both groups. In turn, this reduced exposure to contrast media was associated with a higher mortality in the patients with abnormal renal function [16]. The term "renalism" has been used to describe this change in standard practice due to fear of CI-AKI.

Due to inconsistencies in reporting and methodological flaws of early reports evaluating contrast and AKI, which included absence of a control group or selection bias despite a control group present, the true risk of CA-AKI was previously overstated. In an early prospective non-randomized study, the incidence of CA-AKI was determined in patients undergoing CECT compared to patients (controls) undergoing unenhanced CT or ultrasound [14]. In diabetic patients without CKD the incidence of CA-AKI was 2.4% in contrast exposed and 3.4% in control patients. In nondiabetic patients with CKD, the incidence of CA-AKI was 12.9% in contrast exposed and 7.6% in the controls. Finally, in patients with diabetes and CKD, the incidence of CA-AKI was 8.8% in contrast exposed and 1.6% in controls. This study demonstrated that diabetes by itself without CKD did not increase the risk of CA-AKI, but that CKD increased the risk of CA-AKI. This study again demonstrated that CKD is a powerful risk factor for CA-AKI, and more importantly suggested not all AKI in patients following a contrast-enhanced radiologic study can be attributed to contrast exposure [14].

The long-held notion that AKI following contrast exposure was due to contrast nephrotoxicity has been questioned by more recent studies. In 2008, Newhouse et al. performed a retrospective analysis of approximately 32,000 hospitalized patients who had serial SCr values on 5 consecutive days and had no contrast media exposure [6]. During the 5-day period, a significant portion of these patients developed AKI, leading the authors to conclude AKI following contrast exposure is a *post hoc, ergo propter hoc* (after this, therefore because of this) logical fallacy. In 2009, Bruce et al. performed a retrospective study in >11,000 patients comparing the AKI incidence in patients who underwent either CECT or unenhanced CT and demonstrated that AKI occurred in 4% of CECT and 5.9% of unenhanced CT, again suggesting that AKI following contrast exposure cannot automatically be assumed due to contrast media nephrotoxicity [7].

Numerous other studies comparing AKI incidences between patients undergoing CECT to patients undergoing unenhanced CT demonstrate similar results—equivalent rates of AKI between contrast exposed and unexposed groups. A meta-analysis of 28 controlled studies, examining only intravenous contrast patients compared to non-contrast controls, found similar rates of AKI between the two groups [17]. However, all of these controlled studies have major limitations, including a higher prevalence of CKD in the control groups indicating *selection bias*, lack of adjustment between the two groups for confounding factors, and limited numbers of patients at high-risk for CA-AKI [18].

Given these limitations of controlled studies, the ideal way to determine the true risk of CA-AKI would be to perform a prospective randomized trial between contrast exposed and unexposed patients. However, ethical and logistical considerations make the performance of such a trial not possible. Recognizing this, researchers examined the question of true CA-AKI incidence following intravenous contrast using propensity score matching methodology. Propensity scoring is an advanced statistical method used to control confounding in observational research based on known confounders. This method takes into account, and adjusts for, a subject's likelihood (or propensity) of receiving one treatment compared to another. Davenport et al. examined over 20,000 patients exposed to low osmolar contrast media. Patients were matched 1:1 on propensity scores. Overall, there was no association between contrast media exposure and AKI. However, at all baseline serum creatinine levels ≥1.6 mg/dL, there was a statistically significant association between the exposure and outcome by a variety of CA-AKI definitions [19]. A propensity-matched analysis, published by the same group and including 17,652 patients stratified by eGFR, showed a similar association between contrast exposure and CA-AKI in those with eGFR <30 mL/min/1.73 m^2 [20].

The finding of increased risk of AKI following contrast exposure compared to controls in patients with eGFR <30 mL/min/1.73 m^2, however, was not confirmed in several studies published by McDonald and colleagues [21–24]. A recent meta-analysis of propensity score studies examining CA-AKI in CECT compared to nonenhanced CT supports the findings of the initial propensity score studies [25]. This analysis demonstrated an increased risk of CA-AKI in contrast exposed patients with eGFR ≤30 mL/min/1.73 m^2 (odds ratio 1.68, 95% confidence interval 1.29–2.19, $p = 0.0001$).

These findings led to the American College of Radiology and others to conclude that true contrast-induced acute kidney injury is a "real, albeit rare, entity" [8, 26]. However, these conclusions of a low or non-existent risk of CA-AKI based on the propensity score studies may be premature. The propensity score studies of CA-AKI have multiple limitations. Most importantly, these studies are not equivalent to prospective randomized controlled trials, and as such cannot completely eliminate the potential for selection bias or residual confounding. In propensity score studies, there remains a risk of unmeasured confounders which are unadjusted for and the continued presence of selection bias despite propensity matching. In the CA-AKI propensity score matched studies, presence of prior AKI at time of contrast exposure and use or non-use of prophylactic strategies such as volume expansion with intravenous fluids, were not adjusted for. In one study, the incidence of AKI was higher in patients not exposed to contrast media, while in another there was an increased odds for emergent dialysis in the contrast exposed patients; both observations could suggest residual selection bias [27, 28]. In addition, despite very robust numbers of patients evaluated in these propensity score studies, only a small number of these patients were truly at risk for CA-AKI [18]. Finally, patients with eGFRs between 30 to 44 mL/min/1.73 m^2 were, for the most part, not studied as a separate risk group when stratifying the severity of CKD.

In summary, based on the controlled and propensity-matched trials examining CA-AKI, it is fair to state that the incidences of CA-AKI previously reported, especially in uncontrolled studies, have been overstated. Recent studies confirm the long-held observation that CA-AKI rarely occurs in patients with normal renal function (eGFR $\geq$60 mL/min/1.73 m^2), or in patients with mild impairment of renal function (eGFR 45–59 mL/min/1.73 m^2). There is also consensus that patients with severe renal impairment (eGFR <30 mL/min/1.73 m^2) have an increased risk of CA-AKI. For patients with moderate renal impairment (eGFR 30–44 mL/min/1.73 m^2) it currently remains unclear whether this group has an increased risk of CA-AKI. Until this group is evaluated in more detail in future studies, we recommend treating this group as having an increased risk of CA-AKI, especially if diabetes mellitus is concomitantly present.

CA-AKI: Prevention and Therapeutic Options

Multiple preventive strategies have been suggested to prevent CA-AKI. One of the initial prevention strategies was the use of non-ionic, or low osmolar, contrast media, which was demonstrated to possess a significantly lower risk of CA-AKI compared to high osmolar contrast media in patients at higher risk for CA-AKI [13]. The use of non-ionic contrast media is now standard of care due to lower adverse reactions overall [29]. There have also been multiple pharmacologic preventive strategies which have been proposed, but for the most part have not been either consistently effective or targeted to patients at highest risk of CA-AKI. Another accepted strategy for reducing CA-AKI risk is reducing the dose of contrast given at a time [30]. However, significant contrast dose reduction is more applicable in coronary angiography than CECT.

Administration of intravenous isotonic fluids has been the primary preventive strategy for CA-AKI for the past 40 years [31]. The justification for intravenous fluids as a prophylactic strategy is multifaceted. Benefits include a decrease in tubuloglomerular feedback and reduction in vasoactive hormones such as angiotensin and endothelin. Intravenous fluids might prevent both obstruction and direct toxicity to tubules by contrast media, and provide protection from reactive oxygen species.

Despite the widespread use of intravenous fluids, prospective randomized studies comparing intravenous fluids to no fluids to prevent CA-AKI are limited. A commonly cited study, the AMACING trial, was an open-label noninferiority trial comparing intravenous isotonic fluid using 0.9% sodium chloride (NaCl) and no fluids. Approximately 50% of patients in this study underwent CECT. The results of the trial demonstrated that no fluid administration was non-inferior to intravenous fluid administration. However, there were several limitations of this trial. Notably, this study did not include patients with eGFR <30 mL/min/1.73 m^2, and only about 1/3 of patients overall had a baseline eGFR between 30–45 mL/min/1.73 m^2 [32]. Additionally, some patients had serum creatinine measurement up to 6 days post-procedure, raising concerns that earlier transient increases in serum creatinine may have been undetected. In summary, the results of the AMACING trial cannot be generalized to patients at highest risk for CA-AKI. In contrast, a meta-analysis of three randomized, controlled trials comparing intravenous fluids to no fluids in patients undergoing coronary angiography demonstrated a 34% reduction in CA-AKI risk in patients receiving volume expansion with intravenous fluids [33]. In a more recent meta-analysis of studies comparing intravenous fluids to no fluids or only oral fluids, there was a 38% risk reduction for CA-AKI in the intravenous fluid patients [34].

Several studies have evaluated the use of different solutions on CA-AKI. Initial regimens previously consisted of 0.45% NaCl. However, a randomized, open-label trial in 2002 showed that 0.9% NaCl was superior to 0.45% NaCl in prevention of CA-AKI [35]. PRESERVE, a 2018 randomized trial evaluating 0.9% NaCl solution compared with 1.26% sodium bicarbonate, included many patients at higher risk of CA-AKI. There was no difference in the primary endpoint of death, dialysis, or >50% increase in SCr at 90 days from intervention. Additionally, there was no difference in risk of CA-AKI between the two solutions [36]. Studies comparing long to short periods of intravenous fluid administration are limited. Long periods of intravenous fluid volume expansion are usually 0.9% NaCl at 1 mL/kg/h for 8–12 h both pre- and post-contrast administration. Short periods of intravenous fluid volume expansion are 0.9% NaCl given at 3 mL/kg for the hour preceding contrast and then 1 mL/kg/h for the 6-h period post-contrast. As a result of practical considerations, short volume expansion periods are generally used even though there are no definitive studies demonstrating short expansion periods to be more or equally efficacious as long expansion periods. Pragmatically, short periods of volume expansion are most likely to be utilized in the setting of trauma.

Oral hydration has gained popularity due to the current practice of performing intravascular contrast studies in the outpatient setting for patients who are medically stable. In general, studies evaluating oral hydration show equivalent rates of CA-AKI compared to patients who receive intravenous fluids [31]. However, any conclusions about equal effectiveness between oral hydration and intravenous fluids must be tempered by limitation of the trials comparing these two preventive strategies—small number of patients studied, inclusion primarily of patients at low risk for CA-AKI, and in several trials, confounding by inclusion of patients who got some intravenous fluids or oral sodium in the oral fluid group. In general, due to these study limitations, we recommend intravenous fluids over oral hydration in patients at the highest risk for CA-AKI (eGFR ≤30 mL/min/1.73 m^2).

Conclusion

In summary, the development of CA-AKI following intravenous contrast remains a concern in patients who present with lower eGFR (≤30 mL/min/1.73 m^2), or patients who have eGFR between 30–45 mL/min/1.73 m^2 and have other established risk factors, such as diabetes mellitus. The risk for CA-AKI in patients with eGFR >45 mL/min/1.73 m^2 is minimal and should not prompt variation in medically necessary CT scanning contrast protocols. As previously discussed, patients presenting with trauma may have active bleeding, hemodynamic instability, crush injuries, developing sepsis, or inflammatory mediators that may potentiate the risk for AKI in general, and CA-AKI in particular. Because of this, it is encouraged to attempt to estimate baseline eGFR in patients who are in need of CECT. However, it should be acknowledged that occasionally these decisions must be made on a solitary SCr, which may not reflect the current severity of renal injury due to the development of AKI prior to or at time of presentation.

In patients at the highest risk for CA-AKI (eGFR ≤30 ml/min/1.73 m^2), the first approach is to evaluate if the diagnostic information from a CECT can be accomplished with an alternative imaging procedure that does not involve iodinated contrast. If so, we recommend that imaging studies without contrast are preferable. However, we recognize that imaging studies in trauma patients often necessitate intravenous contrast to provide the most precise and useful clinical information. In these cases, a fear of CA-AKI *should not negate* administration of intravenous contrast media since the adverse clinical consequences of inadequate imaging outweigh the risk and clinical consequences of CA-AKI. When CECT is required in patients at high-risk of CA-AKI, intravenous fluid administration with 0.9% NaCl should be administered both pre- and post-contrast administration. When clinically feasible, we recommend longer over shorter periods of intravenous fluid administration.

References

1. Coca SG, Singanamala S, Parikh CR. Chronic kidney disease after acute kidney injury: a systematic review and meta-analysis. Kidney Int. 2012;81(5):442–8.
2. Søvik S, Isachsen MS, Nordhuus KM, Tveiten CK, Eken T, Sunde K, et al. Acute kidney injury in trauma patients admitted to the ICU: a systematic review and meta-analysis. Intensive Care Med. 2019;45(4):407–19.
3. Messerer DAC, Halbgebauer R, Nilsson B, Pavenstädt H, Radermacher P, Huber-Lang M. Immunopathophysiology of trauma-related acute kidney injury. Nat Rev Nephrol. 2021;17(2):91–111.
4. Kellum JA, Lameire N, Aspelin P, Barsoum RS, Burdmann EA, Goldstein SL, et al. Kidney disease: improving global outcomes (KDIGO) acute kidney injury work group. KDIGO clinical practice guideline for acute kidney injury. Kidney Int Suppl. 2012;2(1):1–138.
5. Lameire N, Kellum JA. Contrast-induced acute kidney injury and renal support for acute kidney injury: a KDIGO summary (part 2). Crit Care. 2013;17(1):205.
6. Newhouse JH, Kho D, Rao QA, Starren J. Frequency of serum creatinine changes in the absence of iodinated contrast material: implications for studies of contrast nephrotoxicity. AJR Am J Roentgenol. 2008;191(2):376–82.
7. Bruce RJ, Djamali A, Shinki K, Michel SJ, Fine JP, Pozniak MA. Background fluctuation of kidney function versus contrast-induced nephrotoxicity. AJR Am J Roentgenol. 2009;192(3):711–8.
8. ACR Committee on Drugs and Contrast Media. ACR manual on contrast media. Reston: American College of Radiology; 2022.
9. Yu AS, Chertow GM, Luyckx VA, Marsden PA, Skorecki K, Taal MW, editors. Brenner & Rector's the kidney. 11th ed. Philadelphia: Saunders; 2011.
10. Mehran R, Dangas GD, Weisbord SD. Contrast-associated acute kidney injury. N Engl J Med. 2019;380(22):2146–55.
11. Persson PB, Tepel M. Contrast medium-induced nephropathy: the pathophysiology. Kidney Int. 2006;69:S8–S10.
12. Tsai TT, Patel UD, Chang TI, Kennedy KF, Masoudi FA, Matheny ME, et al. Contemporary incidence, predictors, and outcomes of acute kidney injury in patients undergoing percutaneous coronary interventions: insights from the NCDR Cath-PCI registry. JACC Cardiovasc Interv. 2014;7(1):1–9.
13. Rudnick MR, Goldfarb S, Wexler L, Ludbrook PA, Murphy MJ, Halpern EF, et al. Nephrotoxicity of ionic and nonionic contrast media in 1196 patients: a randomized trial. The Iohexol Cooperative Study. Kidney Int. 1995;47(1):254–61.
14. Parfrey PS, Griffiths SM, Barrett BJ, Paul MD, Genge M, Withers J, et al. Contrast material-induced renal failure in patients with diabetes mellitus, renal insufficiency, or both. N Engl J Med. 1989;320(3):143–9.
15. Mehran R, Aymong ED, Nikolsky E, Lasic Z, Iakovou I, Fahy M, et al. A simple risk score for prediction of contrast-induced nephropathy after percutaneous coronary intervention: development and initial validation. J Am Coll Cardiol. 2004;44(7):1393–9.
16. Chertow GM, Normand SL, McNeil BJ. "Renalism": inappropriately low rates of coronary angiography in elderly individuals with renal insufficiency. J Am Soc Nephrol. 2004;15(9):2462–8.
17. Aycock RD, Westafer LM, Boxen JL, Majlesi N, Schoenfeld EM, Bannuru RR. Acute kidney injury after computed tomography: a meta-analysis. Ann Emerg Med. 2018;71(1):44–53.e4.
18. Rudnick MR, Leonberg-Yoo AK, Litt HI, Cohen RM, Hilton S, Reese PP. The controversy of contrast-induced nephropathy with intravenous contrast: what is the risk? Am J Kidney Dis. 2020;75(1):105–13.
19. Davenport MS, Khalatbari S, Dillman JR, Cohan RH, Caoili EM, Ellis JH. Contrast material-induced nephrotoxicity and intravenous low-osmolality iodinated contrast material. Radiology. 2013;267(1):94–105.
20. Davenport MS, Khalatbari S, Cohan RH, Dillman JR, Myles JD, Ellis JH. Contrast material-induced nephrotoxicity and intravenous low-osmolality iodinated contrast material: risk stratification by using

estimated glomerular filtration rate. Radiology. 2013;268(3):719–28.
21. McDonald RJ, McDonald JS, Bida JP, Carter RE, Fleming CJ, Misra S, et al. Intravenous contrast material-induced nephropathy: causal or coincident phenomenon? Radiology. 2013;267(1):106–18.
22. McDonald JS, McDonald RJ, Carter RE, Katzberg RW, Kallmes DF, Williamson EE. Risk of intravenous contrast material-mediated acute kidney injury: a propensity score-matched study stratified by baseline-estimated glomerular filtration rate. Radiology. 2014;271(1):65–73.
23. McDonald JS, McDonald RJ, Lieske JC, Carter RE, Katzberg RW, Williamson EE, et al. Risk of acute kidney injury, dialysis, and mortality in patients with chronic kidney disease after intravenous contrast material exposure. Mayo Clin Proc. 2015;90(8):1046–53.
24. McDonald JS, McDonald RJ, Williamson EE, Kallmes DF. Is intravenous administration of iodixanol associated with increased risk of acute kidney injury, dialysis, or mortality? A propensity score-adjusted study. Radiology. 2017;285(2):414–24.
25. Obed M, Gabriel MM, Dumann E, Vollmer Barbosa C, Weißenborn K, Schmidt BMW. Risk of acute kidney injury after contrast-enhanced computerized tomography: a systematic review and meta-analysis of 21 propensity score-matched cohort studies. Eur Radiol. 2022;32(12):8432–42.
26. Davenport MS, Perazella MA, Yee J, Dillman JR, Fine D, McDonald RJ, et al. Use of intravenous iodinated contrast media in patients with kidney disease: consensus statements from the American College of Radiology and the National Kidney Foundation. Radiology. 2020;294(3):660–8.
27. McDonald JS, McDonald RJ, Williamson EE, Kallmes DF, Kashani K. Post-contrast acute kidney injury in intensive care unit patients: a propensity score-adjusted study. Intensive Care Med. 2017;43(6):774–84.
28. Wilhelm-Leen E, Montez-Rath ME, Chertow G. Estimating the risk of radiocontrast-associated nephropathy. J Am Soc Nephrol. 2017;28(2):653–9.
29. Baerlocher MO, Asch M, Myers A. The use of contrast media. CMAJ. 2010;182(7):697.
30. Brown JR, Robb JF, Block CA, Schoolwerth AC, Kaplan AV, O'Connor GT, et al. Does safe dosing of iodinated contrast prevent contrast-induced acute kidney injury? Circ Cardiovasc Interv. 2010;3(4):346–50.
31. Rudnick MR, Fay K, Wahba IM. Fluid administration strategies for the prevention of contrast-associated acute kidney injury. Curr Opin Nephrol Hypertens. 2022;31(5):414–24.
32. Nijssen EC, Rennenberg RJ, Nelemans PJ, Essers BA, Janssen MM, Vermeeren MA, et al. Prophylactic hydration to protect renal function from intravascular iodinated contrast material in patients at high risk of contrast-induced nephropathy (AMACING): a prospective, randomised, phase 3, controlled, open-label, non-inferiority trial. Lancet. 2017;389(10076):1312–22.
33. Wang Z, Song Y, Geru A, Li Y. Role of hydration in contrast-induced nephropathy in patients who underwent primary percutaneous coronary intervention. Int Heart J. 2019;60(5):1077–82.
34. Michel P, Amione-Guerra J, Sheikh O, Jameson LC, Bansal S, Prasad A. Meta-analysis of intravascular volume expansion strategies to prevent contrast-associated acute kidney injury following invasive angiography. Catheter Cardiovasc Interv. 2021;98(6):1120–32.
35. Mueller C, Buerkle G, Buettner HJ, Petersen J, Perruchoud AP, Eriksson U, et al. Prevention of contrast media-associated nephropathy: randomized comparison of 2 hydration regimens in 1620 patients undergoing coronary angioplasty. Arch Intern Med. 2002;162(3):329–36.
36. Weisbord SD, Gallagher M, Jneid H, Garcia S, Cass A, Thwin SS, et al. Outcomes after angiography with sodium bicarbonate and acetylcysteine. N Engl J Med. 2018;378(7):603–14.

Artificial Intelligence in Trauma Imaging

14

Mohamed Elbanan and Hersh Sagreiya

Medical imaging, and in particular computed tomography (CT), plays a crucial role in routine trauma care. As discussed in other chapters throughout this book, CT aids in the early detection of traumatic injuries in various body parts, leading to early diagnosis and improved patient survival. In this chapter, we will discuss the role of the new emerging technology of artificial intelligence in trauma imaging. We will start with a gentle introduction to artificial intelligence followed by a detailed discussion of artificial intelligence applications in trauma imaging. Finally, we touch on some future directions and additional resources.

Artificial Intelligence

Artificial intelligence (AI) or machine learning (ML) is a branch of computer science that aims at creating computer algorithms that simulate human intelligence and can solve problems efficiently without being explicitly programmed [1]. Current applications of artificial intelligence are narrow in scope, i.e., focusing on solving a specific problem, rather than general AI, which deals with general non-specific day-to-day problems in a human-like manner, drawing upon multiple sources of knowledge and experience in an integrative fashion (Fig. 14.1).

Depending on the nature of the problem and the available data and resources, machine learning can be divided into:

1. Supervised learning
2. Unsupervised learning
3. Reinforcement learning

Most medical imaging applications fall into the category of supervised ML. In supervised ML, the algorithm learns from labeled data or medical images [2]. Examples of applications of supervised ML include

Medical Imaging

1. *Image classification:* Classification of an image into a certain set of pre-defined classes or labels, e.g., determining if a chest radiograph contains pneumothorax or not (Fig. 14.2).
2. *Object detection:* Focuses on the identification of the exact location of the object of interest within a given image, e.g., providing a bounding box locating pneumothorax in a chest radiograph (Fig. 14.3).

M. Elbanan
Division of Abdominal Imaging, Department of Radiology, Hospital of the University of Pennsylvania, Philadelphia, PA, USA

Division of Abdominal Imaging, Department of Radiology, University of Missouri, Columbia, MO, USA
e-mail: mohamed.elbanan@health.missouri.edu

H. Sagreiya (✉)
Division of Abdominal Imaging, Department of Radiology, Hospital of the University of Pennsylvania, Philadelphia, PA, USA
e-mail: hersh.sagreiya@pennmedicine.upenn.edu

F. Knollmann (ed.), *Trauma Computed Tomography*, https://doi.org/10.1007/978-3-031-45746-3_14

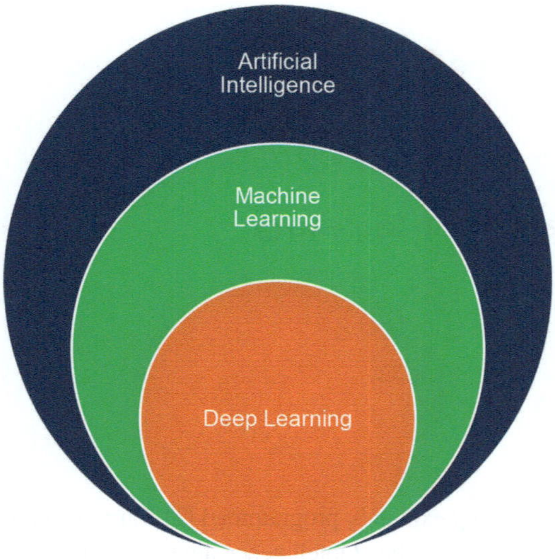

Fig. 14.1 Machine learning. Machine learning (ML) is a subset of the general concept of artificial intelligence that aims at creating computer algorithms that simulate human intelligence and can solve problems efficiently by learning patterns in the data without explicit pre-programmed instructions. Deep learning, a subset of machine learning, relies on artificial neural networks that perform both image feature extraction and classification automatically

3. *Object segmentation:* Outlining the exact boundaries of the object of interest within the given image, e.g., providing the boundaries around the area of pneumothorax within a chest radiograph. In this type of problem, all instances of the object of interest are treated as one label/object (Fig. 14.4).
4. *Semantic segmentation:* Outlining each instance of the object of interest within an image, e.g., outlining each site of pneumothorax within the chest radiograph as a separate object.

Natural Language Processing

1. *Named entity recognition:* extraction and identification of key information (entities) within unstructured text, e.g., identification of incidental findings in radiology reports for follow-up.
2. *Sentiment Analysis:* classification of the emotion or direction of a text, e.g., classifying a

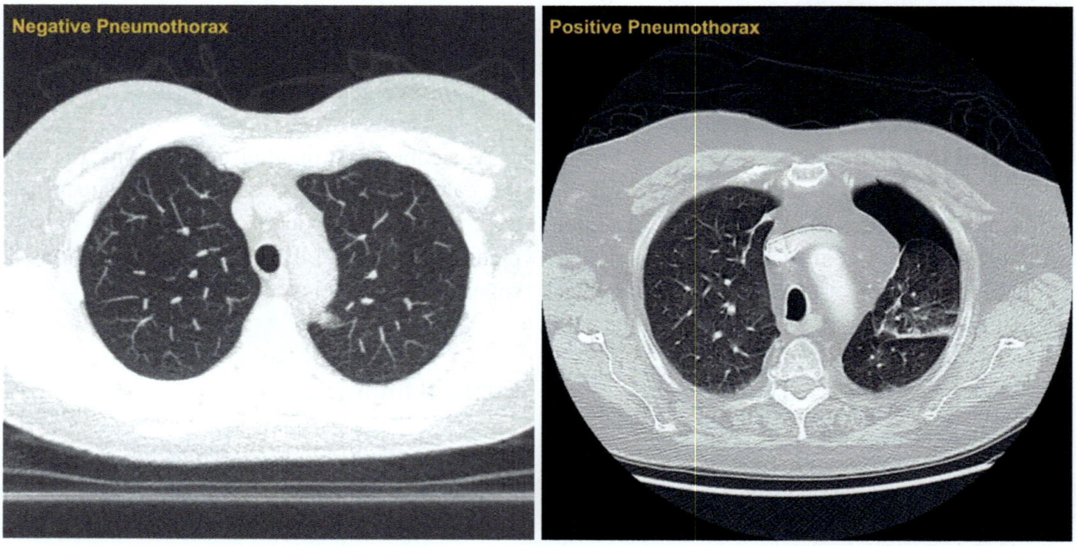

Fig. 14.2 Binary classification of pneumothorax. Two axial chest CT images, left: negative for pneumothorax and right: positive for pneumothorax. The binary classification algorithm would classify each of the images as 1 or 0 for the presence of pneumothorax with 1 meaning positive and 0 meaning negative

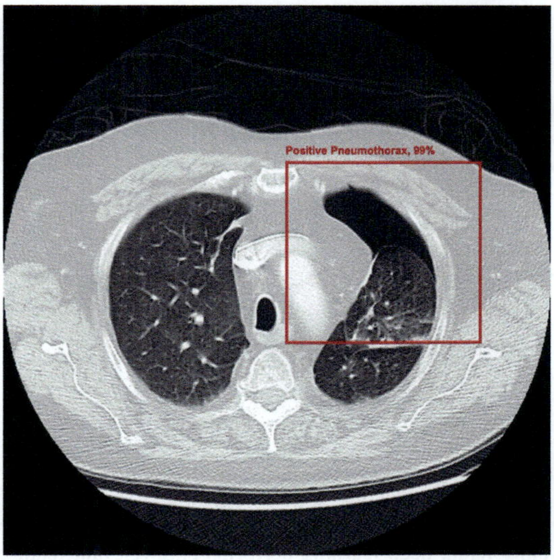

Fig. 14.3 Object detection. Axial chest CT image demonstrating a bounding box surrounding the region of the image that the machine learning or deep learning algorithm selects with the highest probability of having the object of interest, pneumothorax in this example. This example shows a probability of 99% in that region

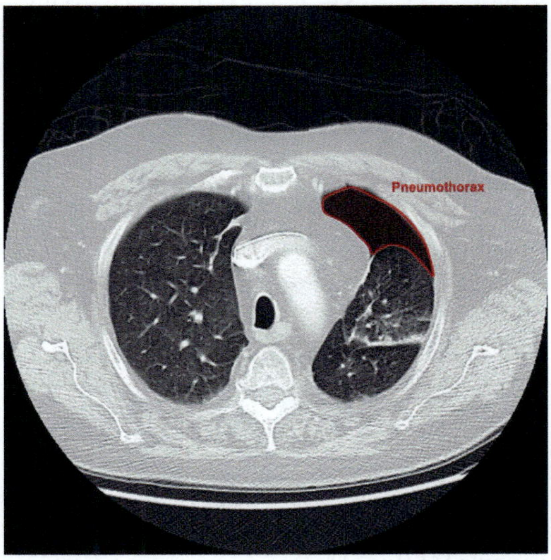

Fig. 14.4 Object segmentation. Axial chest CT image demonstrating the region of the image that the machine learning or deep learning algorithm selects with the highest probability of having the object of interest, pneumothorax in this example, outlined in red

medical imaging report as positive or negative.

3. *Text Summarization:* extraction of meaningful information from a block of text and returning a summary of this information, e.g., summarizing relevant clinical notes from the electronic medical record.

Depending on the available data and the nature of the problem, supervised machine learning can be further subclassified into traditional machine learning and deep learning (DL).

In traditional machine learning, relevant or meaningful features are pre-determined by individuals with domain expertise, e.g., radiologists. These features are then extracted from medical imaging and fed into a machine-learning statistical model that performs the classification task. One example is classifying adrenal masses on CT based on attenuation values and size into benign versus malignant. In this scenario, attenuation values and size represent the relevant pre-determined features which will then be fed into a machine learning algorithm, e.g., support vector machines (SVM) or K-nearest neighbors (KNN), to learn and perform the classification task (Fig. 14.5).

On the other hand, in many of the more complex problems, no reliable domain expert features can be pre-defined. Even when this has previously been attempted, as in CAD for mammography, it is difficult to pre-program all the forms in which pathology can present itself, especially with scanner, protocol, and patient heterogeneity. In these cases, deep learning comes into action. In deep learning, the ML algorithms perform relevant feature extraction and training at the same time [1, 3]. This is performed through a series of stacked layers (thus the name deep) within artificial neural networks, which take inspiration from the natural neural networks found in human brains. The most widely used network architecture in imaging tasks is the convolutional neural network (CNN), e.g., ResNet152, InceptionV3, and DenseNet121 (Fig. 14.6).

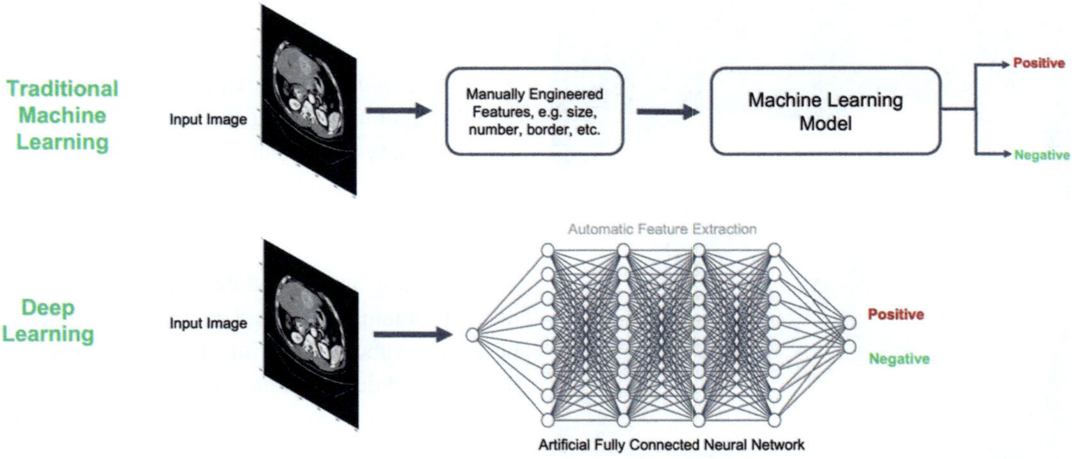

Fig. 14.5 Machine learning and deep learning. In traditional machine learning, a statical model performs the classification/regression task utilizing a set of features that are pre-defined in advance by domain experts. On the other hand, deep learning performs both relevant feature extraction and classification/regression automatically

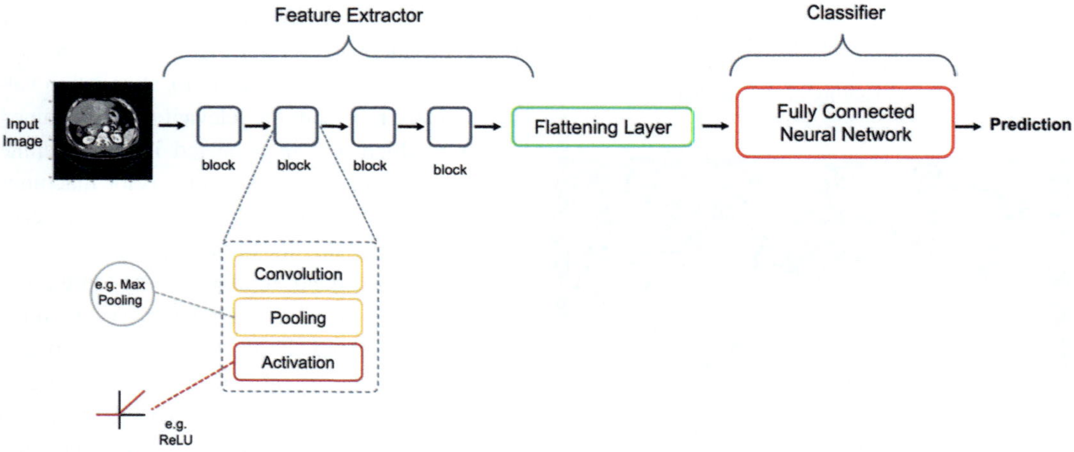

Fig. 14.6 Convolutional neural network (CNN). A CNN consists of two parts: a feature extractor and a classifier. The feature extractor consists of building blocks made of a convolutional layer, a pooling layer, and an activation function. A flattening layer is needed between the two parts of the network. The classifier is a typical fully connected neural network

Due to recent computational advances, the availability of training resources, and the large amounts of labeled data, deep learning has achieved a super-human level in several imaging classification and object detection tasks. This has enabled deep learning to currently become the most used ML technique in medical imaging and other image-related tasks. In particular, a popular deep neural network architecture for segmenting medical images is the U-Net and its different variants [4] (Fig. 14.7).

However, training a deep learning algorithm typically requires vast amounts of labeled data/images, which are not easy to obtain in healthcare applications due to privacy and legal regulations, or in some instances the scarcity of imaging for rare diseases. In these scenarios, a common technique known as "Transfer

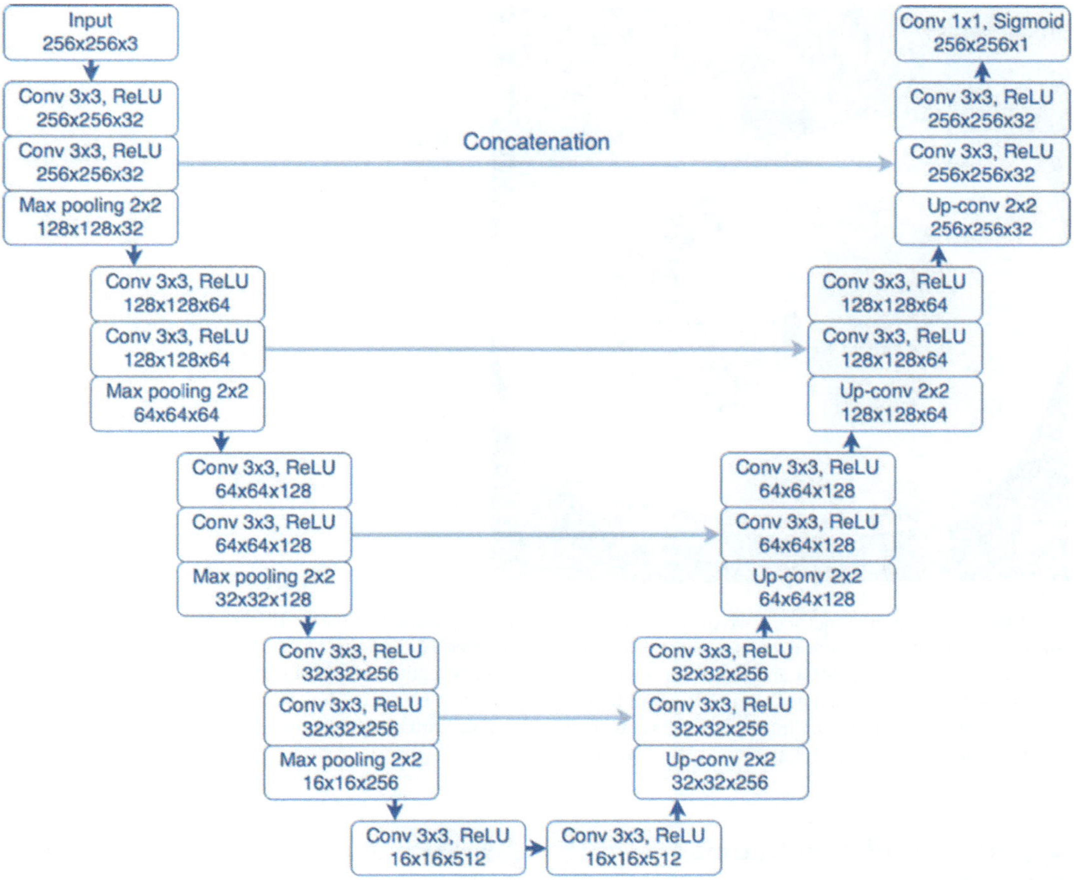

Fig. 14.7 U-Net. An illustration showing the architecture of the U-Net neural network. The network contains two segments composed of a convolution encoder (left side) and a deconvolution decoder (right side). These segments are connected through skip connections to maintain spatial information

Learning" is used [5–7]. Transfer Learning involves using algorithms that have typically been trained on non-medical images and have demonstrated a high level of accuracy to perform the medical imaging tasks described earlier. Transfer learning is based on the notion that basic low-level features, such as edges, shapes, corners, and intensity, can be shared across different domains, and thus knowledge transfer among tasks is possible [5].

Training a DL or ML algorithm is followed by the critical step of examining the performance of the trained algorithm on new unseen instances of data or images that the algorithm has not been introduced to during the training step. This process is known as "Validation" and some authors also refer to it as "Testing." "External Validation" refers to testing the trained algorithm on new data from a different institution to avoid inherent bias in the original training dataset that the algorithm was trained on. The performance metric used to evaluate the trained model depends on the nature of the problem or the task itself. For image classification tasks, sensitivity, specificity, and positive and negative predictive value are commonly used metrics. For object detection and segmentation tasks, commonly used metrics include Intersection-over-Union (IoU or Jaccard Index) and DICE coefficient (Fig. 14.8).

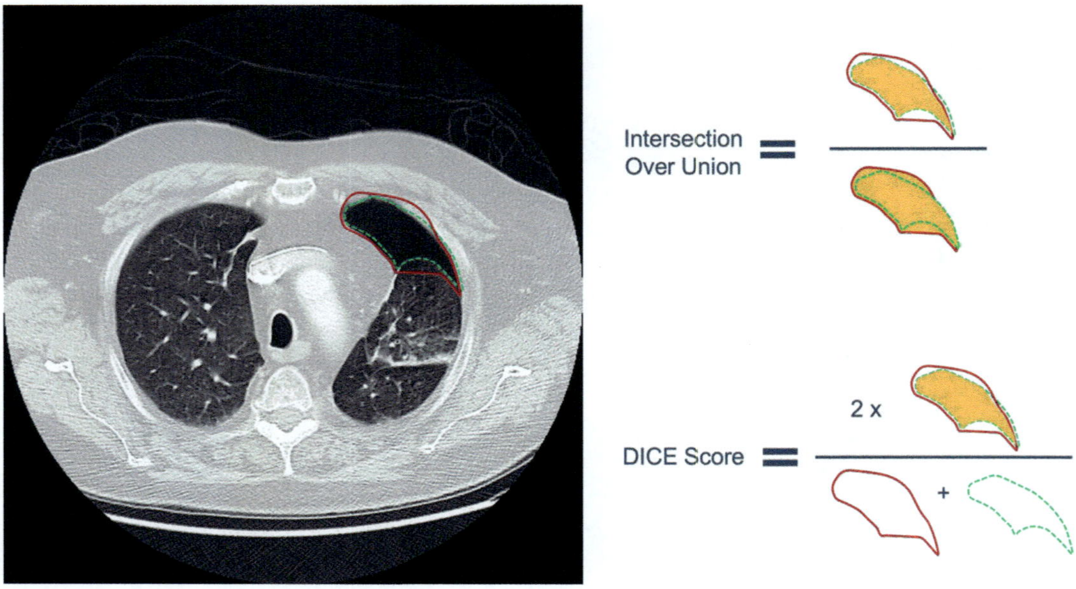

Fig. 14.8 Segmentation metrics. Two of the most important metrics in object detection and segmentation include Intersection over Union (IoU) and DICE score. The IoU (also known as the Jaccard index) is a measure of how the predicted segmentation/bounding box overlaps with the ground truth region. It is calculated by dividing the area of the intersection of the prediction and the ground truth by the area of the union of both areas. The DICE score is another method of measuring segmentation accuracy and is calculated by dividing twice the intersection area by the sum of ground truth and predicted areas

Applications of AI in Trauma Imaging

In the following sections of this chapter, we will explore examples of the different applications of AI in trauma imaging. These include, for example, the detection of pneumothorax, pneumoperitoneum, liver and splenic lacerations, intracranial hemorrhage, and skeletal fractures.

Abdominal Imaging

Hemoperitoneum/Intra-abdominal Free Fluid

The presence of intra-abdominal free fluid, including hemoperitoneum, in the setting of either blunt or penetrating trauma is an indicator of occult solid organ laceration, bowel injury, or active bleeding, which are often difficult to detect through physical examination. The amount of free fluid has been established as an independent factor in determining therapeutic approaches, including watchful waiting for small-volume fluid versus surgical hemostasis or angioembolization for large-volume fluid. Focused assessment with sonography for trauma (FAST) is a non-invasive and fast imaging technique for detecting intra-abdominal free fluid. Studies have shown that early detection of fluid using FAST has a significant role in decreasing the time to surgical intervention and improving patient outcomes. Thus, FAST has been used as part of the standard of care for trauma patients [8].

However, as with all ultrasound examinations, results are largely dependent on the experience of the performing sonographer. Artificial intelligence algorithms have demonstrated a promising role in the automatic identification of intra-abdominal free fluid on FAST examinations, thus reducing inter-observer variability [9–12]. For example, utilizing transfer learning, the classification of FAST images as positive or negative for intra-abdominal free fluid reached an accuracy of 97.8% for FAST video clips and 93.4% for still frames [10].

On the other hand, segmenting areas of free fluid within FAST images has been investigated using the U-Net neural network architecture, which achieved an area under the ROC curve (ROC-AUC) of 0.91, as well as a high sensitivity and specificity of 97.1% and 86.3%, respectively [11].

Compared to ultrasound, computed tomography provides higher sensitivity and specificity, not only for detecting the amount and type of intra-abdominal free fluid but also for detecting associated injuries and sources of bleeding. As mentioned earlier, the amount of free fluid is an independent factor in determining the swift need for surgical intervention and patient outcomes. However, manual segmentation of intra-abdominal fluid is both labor-intensive and time-consuming and thus is not cost-effective in the trauma setting. U-Net neural networks and multiscale attentional networks (MSAN) can accurately and promptly estimate free fluid volume [13]. Compared to a mean manual segmentation time ranging from 3 to 49 min (mean 21 min), these algorithms provided an inference time of 2.5 min, thus allowing rapid estimation of the free fluid volume.

Pneumoperitoneum

In the absence of recent surgical history, the presence of pneumoperitoneum in the setting of nonpenetrating trauma is a strong indication of underlying bowel perforation [14]. Recently, several commercially available solutions have been introduced, aiming at the automatic detection of pneumoperitoneum, that have been externally validated at different institutions [15–17].

In a single institution external validation of a commercial algorithm for the detection of acute abdominal findings using 188 cases, the algorithm achieved a 93% sensitivity and 97% specificity for the detection of acute abdominal findings on CT images and 92% sensitivity and 93% specificity in the detection of intra-abdominal free air [16]. Besides computed tomography, automatic detection of intra-abdominal free air on abdominal and chest radiographs has been explored [18–20]. For example, utilizing a dataset of 1287 chest radiographs, Goyal et al. explored the sensitivity and specificity of different deep neural network architectures that were previously trained on ImageNet and finetuned for detecting pneumoperitoneum through transfer learning [20]. Their work demonstrated the superior performance of DenseNet161 compared to InceptionV3, ResNet101, and ResNeXt101 with accuracy, sensitivity, specificity and AUC of 0.908, 0.916, 0.899, and 0.957, respectively. These results were comparable to those achieved by Su et al. whose results also proved the superior performance of DenseNet121 compared to InceptionV4 and Inception ResNet V2 [18].

Liver Injuries

Due to its relatively large size, anterior location, and unique parenchyma, the liver is one of the most commonly injured abdominal organs in blunt abdominal trauma. In severe blunt trauma patients who undergo CT evaluation, blunt hepatic injuries are identified in up to 25%. Thus, early detection and management are crucial to patient survival and improved outcomes.

Computed tomography is the current gold standard for the identification and classification of traumatic hepatic injuries with the CT-based American Association for the Surgery of Trauma (AAST) liver injury scale being the main tool to assess the extent of liver trauma and guide subsequent management [21]. Therefore, prompt identification, quantification, and reporting of hepatic injuries or lacerations on computed tomography are crucial for improving patient survival and guiding management.

However, manual grading of hepatic injuries suffers from inter- and intra-observer variability even with experienced readers. Moreover, swift real-time reporting of CT exams is not always feasible, particularly in areas with limited 24-h radiologist coverage. In these situations, automatic detection and quantification of traumatic injuries has the potential to provide prompt results to help guide patient management in a timely manner.

A proposed approach by Farzaneh et al. included utilizing U-Net deep neural networks to provide automatic segmentation of the whole

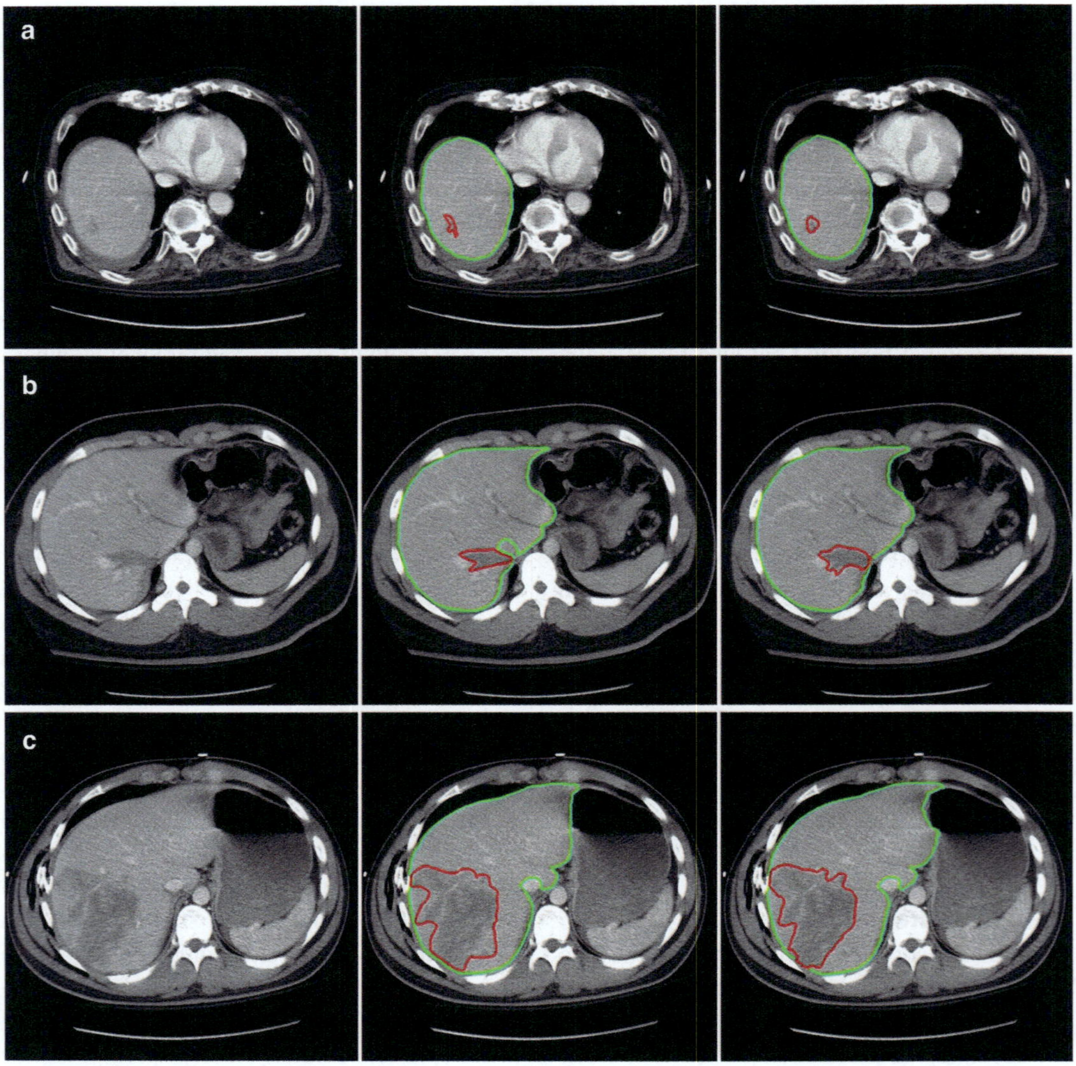

Fig. 14.9 Liver laceration detection with AI. Examples of liver trauma and organ segmentation results, along with ground truth annotations in three separate patients, labeled with **a**, **b**, and **c**, with progressively increasing levels of liver injury. The first column corresponds to the original CT image; the second column corresponds to the ground truth annotations; and the third column corresponds to the automated segmentation results. In both the ground truth annotations and the segmentation results, the green line shows the liver contour while the red line marks the contour of trauma regions. Figure reused under the Creative Commons License from reference [22]

liver and areas of parenchymal injury on single-phase computed tomography exams to provide automated reporting of the volume of parenchymal injury [22]. The proposed pipeline was able to segment the liver and parenchymal injuries with DICE coefficient, recall, and precision of 96.1%, 96.0%, and 96.4% for the liver, and 51.2%, 53.2%, and 56.8% for parenchymal injury. Interestingly, a combination of traditional machine learning models and deep learning algorithms demonstrated high accuracy in detecting hepatic artery injuries associated with trauma (e.g., pseudoaneurysm, AVF, or predicted active contrast extravasation on digital subtraction angiography) on pre-angiography CT imaging and thus can help in triaging patients who would benefit from angiography and intervention [23] (Fig. 14.9).

Splenic Injuries

Splenic injuries are yet another common type of injury frequently encountered in blunt trauma, particularly those associated with rib fractures. Like hepatic injuries, the CT-based AAST grading system for traumatic splenic injuries has established a critical role in the quantification of splenic injuries and guiding further management [21]. However, this grading system also suffers from inter-reader variability and lack of widespread adoption by radiologists owing to different factors, including required fast turn-around-time in the traumatic setting. Thus, the need for automated identification and AAST grading of traumatic splenic injuries holds the potential for improving patient outcomes and helping reduce radiologists' time pressures.

Deep learning algorithms exhibited favorable results for automatically grading splenic injuries, including a combination of a 3D U-Net deep neural network for splenic segmentation, an nnU-Net ensemble (2D U-Net, low-resolution 3D U-Net, high-resolution 3D U-Net, and a low- and high-resolution cascaded 3D U-Net) for identifying splenic parenchymal disruption, and a Faster-Recurrent neural network (F-RCNN) for detecting pseudoaneurysm and active bleeding [24]. This proposed pipeline achieved an AUC, accuracy, sensitivity, and specificity of 0.84, 88%, 82%, and 91% for active bleeding detection and 0.79, 83%, 91%, and 78% for pseudoaneurysm detection. Overall, this pipeline achieved an accuracy, sensitivity, and specificity of 92%, 93%, and 92% in diagnosing high-grade (IV and V) splenic injuries, which require immediate intervention for bleeding control.

Thoracic Imaging

Pneumothorax

Pneumothorax, particularly in the traumatic setting, is a life-threatening condition that can interfere with normal hemodynamic functions, requiring immediate identification and intervention. As mentioned earlier in the book, computed tomography is the current cornerstone in thoracic trauma imaging. Computed tomography demonstrates high sensitivity and specificity for detecting even trace-volume pneumothorax. However, in routine daily practice, since studies might not be read in real-time, the need for an automated system to identify urgent critical findings, like pneumothorax, for priority interpretation has emerged.

Utilizing an eight-layer convolutional neural network that previously exhibited high performance for classifying interstitial lung disease, Li et al. investigated using such a deep neural network for identifying pneumothorax on chest CT [25]. With a rapid processing and detection time of less than 151 s per study, their proposed algorithm achieved a sensitivity and specificity of 100% and 82.5%, respectively, on a testing dataset of 200 CT exams. False positive classifications in that study were reportedly related to emphysema and/or artifacts in the test images. More recently, a deep residual U-Net neural network architecture was proposed for automated detection, volume-level grading, and pixel-level classification of pneumothorax. This methodology achieved an ROC-AUC of 0.98 and a DICE similarity coefficient of 0.94, which was comparable to the inter-rater segmentation accuracy of two radiologists, who achieved a DICE score of 0.92 [26] (Fig. 14.4).

Beyond computed tomography, the detection of pneumothorax on chest radiographs, and even ultrasound, has been the focus of numerous investigators over the past few years [27–31]. These exams are less expensive than CT and are useful for serial monitoring. One of the most notable initiatives is the pneumothorax detection challenge organized by the Society for Imaging Informatics in Medicine (SIIM) in 2019 on Kaggle. Several innovative approaches to enable rapid and automated deep learning identification of pneumothorax were demonstrated over the period of the challenge. Details of this large dataset and the methodologies proposed by the different participants have been discussed by Tolkachev et al. [32].

Hemothorax

Hemothorax, especially the rapid accumulation of blood in the pleural space in a traumatic setting, can be fatal. Accordingly, immediate identification and management is essential and plays a significant role in patient outcome. Recently, a pipeline that utilized an ensemble U-net neural network architecture achieved a mean DICE score of 0.75 and a mean volume similarity of 0.91 in the detection and quantification of hemothorax volume on computed tomography images [33]. Interestingly, not only was the pipeline able to detect and quantify hemothorax, but automated volume cut-offs of 77 mL and 334 mL predicted outcomes, such as the need for massive transfusion, with 93% sensitivity and 90% specificity. It is worth mentioning that automatic detection and quantification was achieved in less than 2 minutes per exam, as compared to a 25–30 min routine turn-around time.

Rib Fractures

Rib fractures are one of the most encountered injuries in trauma settings either blunt or penetrating. The number, nature, and severity of rib fractures, particularly displaced ones, are strongly associated with patient outcomes and the development of possible complications including pneumothorax and atelectasis. Thus, accurate identification of rib fractures is of utmost importance. CT imaging is considered the gold standard for the detection of rib fractures due to its superior specificity and sensitivity over chest radiographs. CT imaging also allows the discovery of other thoracic injuries, as well as rib fracture-associated complications. However, identifying rib fractures on CT remains challenging due to the large number of images that need to be reviewed in a timely manner, the complex shape of the ribs, and the subtle nature of some rib fractures. The exceptional performance of novel artificial intelligence algorithms in image classification and object detection has paved the path for these algorithms to hold a promising role in swift rib fracture detection [34–41] (Fig. 14.10).

RB-Net is a customized 3D U-Net deep neural network trained on a dataset of 8289 patients with a total of 39,659 fractures in 31,461 ribs [34]. This algorithm demonstrated superior overall sensitivity in detecting per-patient level rib fractures (93.1%) compared to experienced radiologists (75.2%) upon external validation. Particularly, the algorithm showed higher sensitivity in detecting non-displaced and old fractures compared to experienced radiologists with a sensitivity of 85.3% and 92%, respectively, for the algorithm, compared to 67.3% and 71%, respectively, for the radiologists. However, the algorithm showed a lower specificity compared to the experienced radiologists (85.9% vs. 93.7%). Consequently, RB-Net could serve as a fast triaging or additional screening tool for radiologists to improve turn-around time in time-sensitive trauma cases.

A more complex pipeline for rib fracture detection and segmentation was proposed utilizing a combination of 3D U-Net and Faster-RNN with a ResNet50 backbone trained on the ImageNet dataset [39]. The proposed pipeline achieved a detection performance (precision, 82.2%; sensitivity, 84.9%) comparable to three experienced radiologists (mean precision, 90.6%; mean sensitivity, 79.7%). Interestingly, when the radiologists used the algorithm, the mean sensitivity demonstrated an improvement (from 79.7% to 89.2%), with a comparable precision (from 90.6% to 88.4%). This highlights the robust potential synergistic role of deep learning algorithms as digital assistants to radiologists, resulting in enhanced performance and timeliness.

Pulmonary Contusions

Pulmonary contusions commonly occur in approximately 75% of blunt chest trauma cases and are mostly associated with rib fractures [42]. Computed tomography plays a cornerstone role in the early identification of pulmonary contusion in the first few hours following trauma when pulmonary contusions might not be visible on chest radiographs [42]. Pulmonary contusions remain a predictor of ARDS and have a high mortality rate in post-traumatic patients. Therefore, timely identification and management are vital to patient outcomes in the trauma setting. Deep learning has been investigated for the detection and quantification of traumatic pulmonary contusions. A multi-model pipeline, composed of a previously trained U-net architecture to segment lung

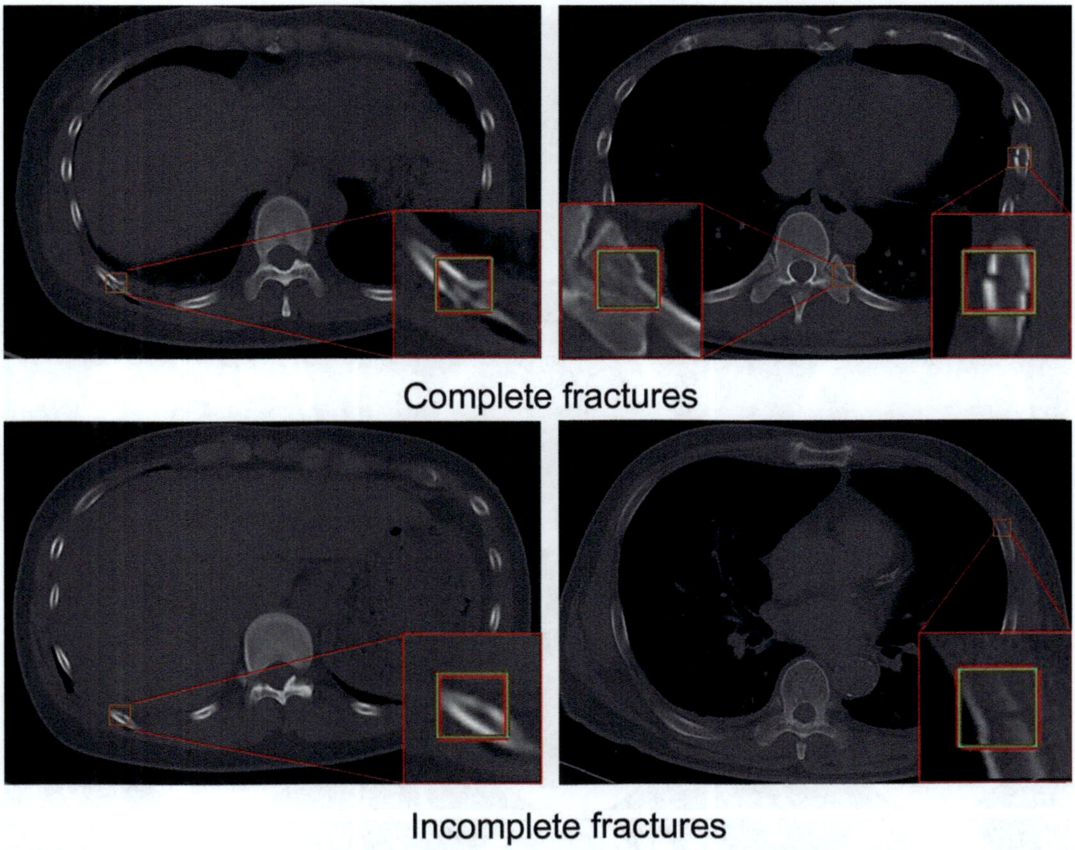

Fig. 14.10 Rib fracture detection with AI. Examples of complete and incomplete rib fractures identified on CT images using deep learning. Figure reused under the Creative Commons License from [35]

volumes, Hessian matrix to subtract blood vessels, and binary thresholding to segment lung contusion, was able to accurately identify lung parenchymal contusions, including blood vessels, within 1% of the manually labeled contusions [43].

Neuroimaging

Intracranial Hemorrhage

Intracranial hemorrhage (ICH) is one of the most critical and dreadful injuries in both traumatic and non-traumatic settings. Due to associated high mortality and functional impairment, urgent identification and intervention within the first few hours of onset are imperative for patient survival and outcomes. Non-contrast CT (NCCT) imaging of the head is regarded as the gold standard for the detection of ICH. As discussed in other chapters of this book, not only does CT imaging detect ICH accurately, but it also helps to identify associated traumatic injuries including skull fractures and foreign bodies. After initial detection, additional CT examinations provide an accurate means of both qualitative and quantitative follow-up of ICH to alert for critical life-threatening changes, including expanding hematomas and brain herniation. Accordingly, a rapid automated tool for fast detection and quantification of ICH has become the focus of multiple scholars, institutions, and research teams [44, 45] (Fig. 14.11).

Dimension reduction U-Net (DR-UNet) is a novel deep learning algorithm for ICH detection, segmentation, and volume measurements [46]. This algorithm achieved performance similar to that of experts in internal testing (DICE score of 0.861) and external testing (DICE score of 0.874)

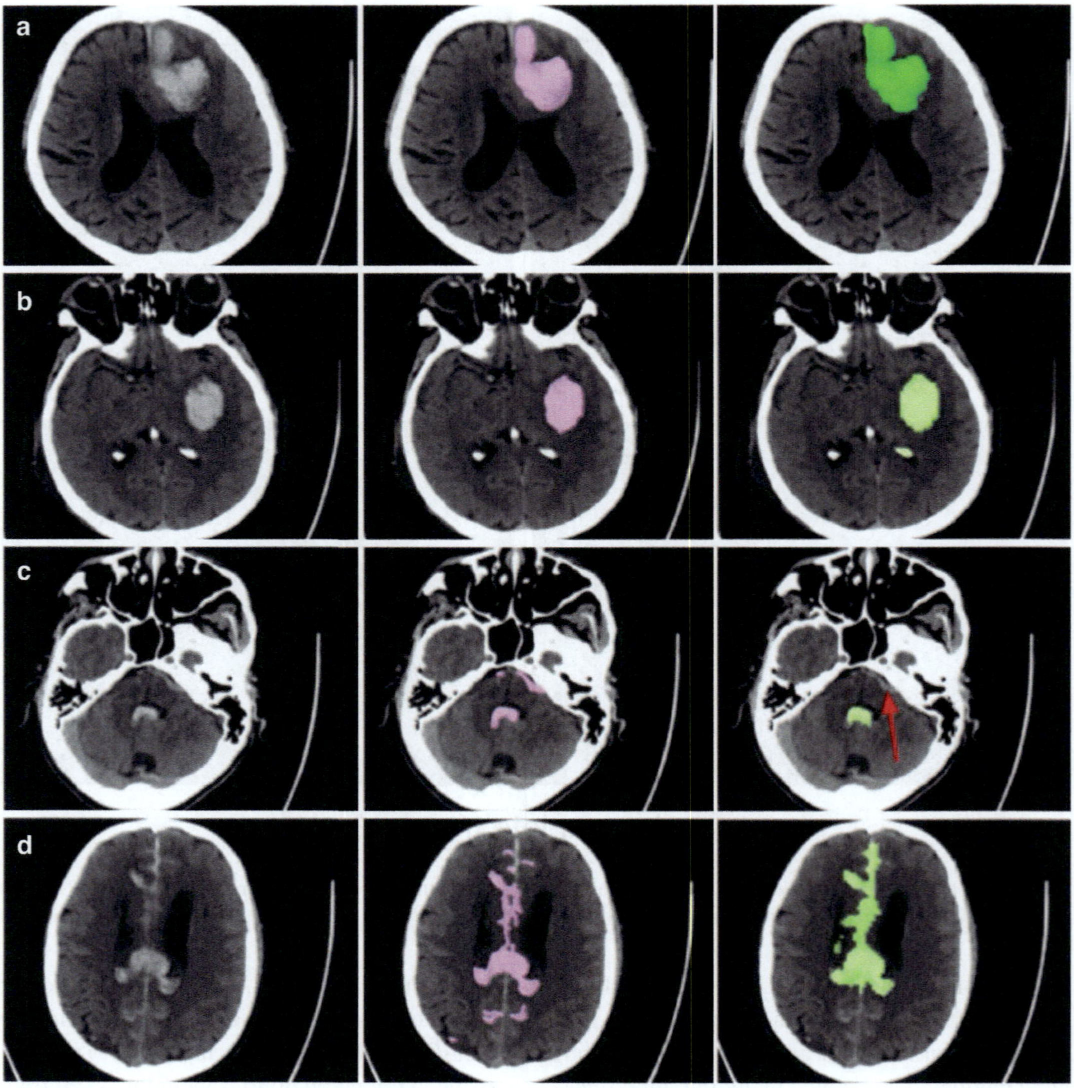

Fig. 14.11 ICH Segmentation with Deep Learning. In each panel, the left, middle, and right images are the original CT slice, the "ground truth" label, and the CNN-predicted segmentation, respectively. The pointing arrow indicates the error. (**a**) CNN method demonstrates an expert-level performance. (**b**) A false positive instance where a calcified structure is labeled as a hemorrhagic area. (**c**) A false negative example in which the CNN method identified part of the hemorrhage but missed some blood close to the bone. (**d**) A complex hemorrhage where the discrepancies between the "ground truth" and the predicted segmentation cannot necessarily be attributed to erroneous prediction. Figure reused under Creative Commons License from [45]

datasets. Moreover, the volume measurements derived from DR-UNet strongly correlated with manual segmentation (R^2 = 0.9979). A more complex pipeline consisting of an EfficientNet neural network and a custom convolutional neural network architecture known as "DeepMedic" achieved an overall accuracy of 96.2% in the detection of ICH [47, 48].

Several commercially available solutions are currently available for automated ICH detection and worklist prioritization. A number of these solutions have been externally validated to establish their accuracy and potential benefit. One commercially available solution was examined at a single institution for 2 months during which the software flagged 373 NCCT for possible ICH out of the 2011 scans surveyed [49]. Among these, 144 CT examinations were flagged for new ICH, including 66 positive cases (44.4%), of which 39 (58.2%) were trauma/emergency cases. The sensitivity, specificity, positive predictive value, negative predictive value, and accuracy of the software were 88.7%, 94.2%, 73.7%, 97.7%, and 93.4%, respectively. Moreover, the accuracy of ICH detection was significantly higher for emergency cases than for inpatient cases (96.5% versus 89.4%).

In another study, commercially available software reported the presence of ICH in 28 NCCT head examinations that were previously reported by radiologists as negative for ICH [50]. 16 out of these 28 examinations were confirmed through neuroradiologists' consensus. Thus, FDA-approved deep learning solutions have the potential to help radiologists diagnose ICH and decrease the error rate [50].

However, these available solutions do not come without several limitations. For example, non-hemorrhagic entities were falsely identified as ICH including calcifications, postoperative and postischemic defects, tumors, thrombosis, and artifacts [49]. On the other hand, false negative or missed ICH included subacute subdural hematomas, small subdural and epidural hematomas (2–3 mm), as well as small intraparenchymal hematomas (3–5 mm) [49, 51]. This highlights the need for radiologists and AI algorithms to work in tandem, leveraging each other's strengths.

An exciting application of deep learning algorithms is the enhancement of CT image quality. Trauma head NCCT images reconstructed utilizing deep learning algorithms have demonstrated lower noise and superior signal-to-noise ratio compared to those produced through the adaptive iterative reconstruction technique [52]. Moreover, deep learning image reconstruction can contribute to a reduction in the radiation dose associated with CT exams [53, 54]. This is particularly useful in the pediatric population where exposure to radiation that accompanies CT examinations poses a significant challenge.

Spine Fractures and Cord Injuries

Spinal fractures and spinal cord injuries are severely devastating injuries associated with both blunt and penetrating trauma, and they can result in major consequences ranging from severe neurological dysfunction, lifelong disability, or even mortality. Medical imaging, including CT and MRI, play an imperative role in the identification of spinal fractures and cord injuries and help guide management and improve patient outcomes. Details of different types of fractures and injuries are discussed in other chapters of this book. In this section, we explore the different applications of artificial intelligence in the identification of spinal fractures and cord injuries.

Vertebral morphology and posterior ligamentous complex (PLC) integrity are two critical predictors of outcomes and the need for surgical intervention in thoracolumbar traumatic injuries. A state-of-the-art faster R-CNN trained on CT images of 111 patients, including a total of 129 injuries, achieved outstanding performance in vertebral localization and PLC integrity classification with DICE scores of 0.92 and 0.88, respectively [55]. The algorithm performed remarkably in binary classification between non-injured and injured vertebral morphological scores (including compression fracture, burst fracture, translational/rotational injury, or distraction injury) with an accuracy of 95.1%. This showed that artificial intelligence tools can help streamline the management of patients with traumatic spinal fractures and identify those in need of urgent surgical intervention. An additional critical component in vertebral fracture management is differentiating benign causes of vertebral fractures from malignant etiologies. A pre-trained ResNet-50 neural network demonstrated promising results in classifying vertebral fractures into benign versus malignant by utilizing coronal reformatted CT images [56]. The model's per-slice sensitivity, specificity, and accuracy in differentiating benign vs. malignant vertebral fractures were 0.90, 0.79, and 85%, respectively, while its per-patient performance demonstrated sensitivity, specificity, and accuracy of 0.95, 0.80, and 88%.

It is worth mentioning that several studies have investigated the use of artificial intelligence algorithms for the detection of spinal fractures from radiographs [57–61]. For example, Chen et al. proposed an ensemble model based on a ResNet-50 backbone to differentiate between old and fresh lumbar vertebral compression fractures on radiographs [60]. The proposed pipeline achieved a sensitivity, specificity, and accuracy of 80%, 68%, and 74%, respectively.

On the other hand, early automated detection of traumatic cord injuries is an ongoing challenge. Literature on cord injury identification using CT imaging is scarce. Thus, we will touch on the most recent advances in traumatic spinal cord injury detection using MR imaging. For example, a traditional ML algorithm (KNN and SVM) that utilized fractional anisotropy obtained from axial diffusion tensor imaging (DTI) MR images of the spine was able to predict whether the spinal cord in a particular image slice was injured or normal with specificity and sensitivity of 0.952 and 0.912, respectively [62]. Similarly, U-Net-based models for segmenting regions of traumatic spinal cord injuries on MR images achieved a DICE score of up to 0.93, indicating outstanding potential [63].

Skeletal Fractures

Skeletal fractures are by far the most common traumatic injuries with an estimated volume of 9.4 million cases per year in the United States [64]. Medical imaging, including radiography, CT, and MRI, is the cornerstone of identifying fractures and triaging those who need immediate surgical intervention. However, a substantial number of these fractures are missed, in part due to the large volume of studies and radiologists' workload. Artificial intelligence algorithms have promising potential for automated fracture detection and worklist prioritization, potentially reducing radiologists' workload and fatigue.

Most of the published literature on AI musculoskeletal trauma imaging focused on radiographs with only a few looking into CT and MRI. In this section, we will explore the most recent advances in automated fracture detection predominantly on CT imaging.

Whole body CT, including of the chest, abdomen, and pelvis, is commonly acquired in the trauma setting. Deep learning algorithms can rapidly detect fractures on these exams and alert radiologists and clinicians to the need for urgent patient care. For example, a Faster-RCNN-Inception-V2 deep neural network that was trained on CT examinations from 189 patients achieved a mean sensitivity and precision of 0.786 and 0.648, respectively, for automatic localization and classification of fractures [65]. The highest sensitivity was for detecting pelvis fractures (0.839) while the lowest was for detecting rib fractures (0.713) (Fig. 14.12).

Pelvic fractures are potentially life-threatening due to the associated risk of vascular injury and large-volume bleeding. It is estimated that in patients with unstable pelvic fractures, hemodynamic instability can lead to up to 20–50% mortality [66]. The Orthopedic Trauma Association (OTA) and AO Foundation imaging-based Tile classification system is the most widely-adopted system for pelvic instability grading. A novel approach utilizing the ResNeXt-50 neural network architecture to identify and grade pelvic fractures on full-thickness multiplanar reconstructions from whole body CT images has been proposed by Dreizin et al. [67]. The proposed algorithm achieved an accuracy of 74% in identifying rotationally unstable fractures and 85% in identifying translationally unstable fractures. Comparatively, radiologists achieved an accuracy of 76% and 75%, respectively. On the other hand, a pipeline using a 3-D CNN based on the YOLOv3 architecture was able to achieve an ROC-AUC of 0.824 and IoU of 10% for detecting and segmenting pelvic fractures on CT [68].

Intertrochanteric femoral fractures are common, particularly in elderly patients where they carry a significant risk of immobility, disability, and complication-associated mortality. CT imaging is crucial for the identification and surgical planning of IT fractures. An automated multiclass faster R-CNN algorithm for intertrochanteric fracture identification and grading from CT imaging was proposed by Yoon et al. [69]. The algorithm achieved outstanding results with an average accuracy of 0.97 and an intersection over

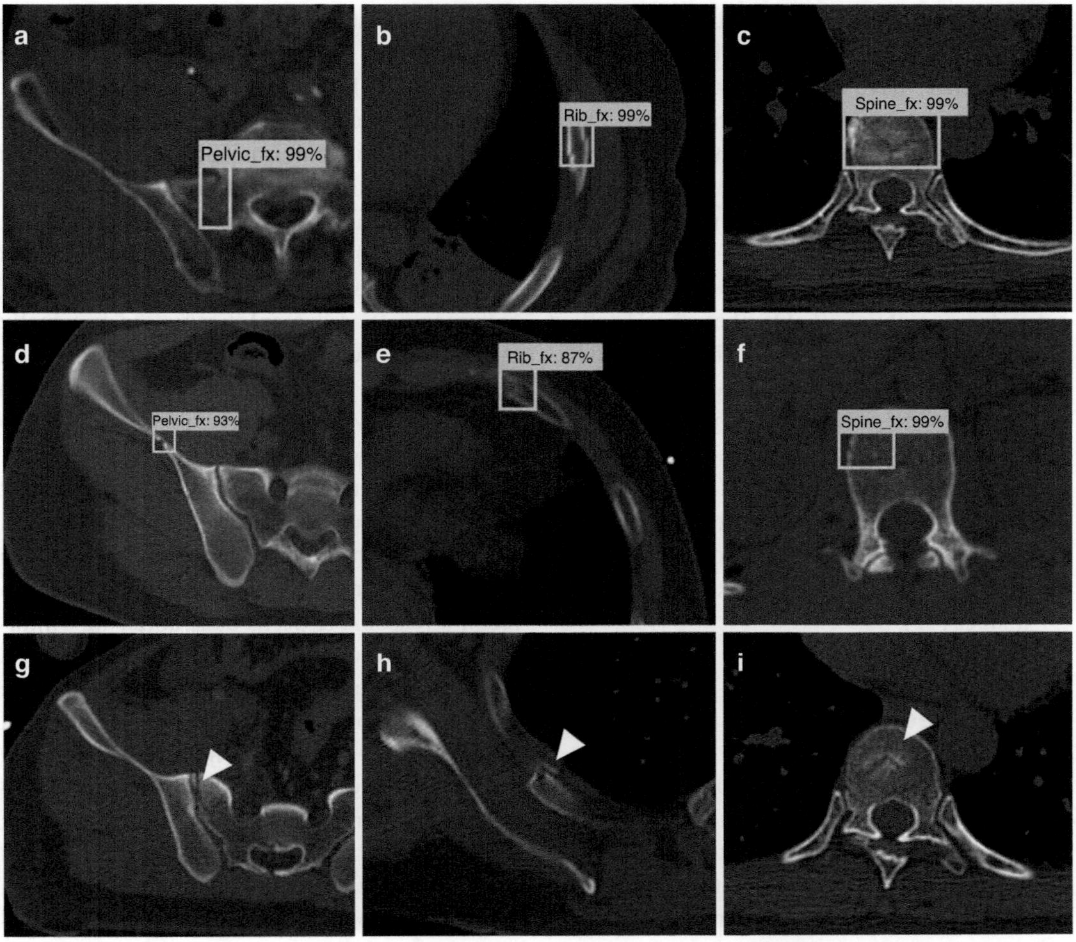

Fig. 14.12 Fracture detection on whole body CT. Representative images of true positive, false positive, and false negative examples. (**a–c**) CT axial slices detected and diagnosed correctly by the CNN model as representing three fractures (true positives). (**d–f**) CT axial slices of a misdiagnosed fracture (false positives). The vascular groove was mistaken for a pelvic fracture (**d**); the boundary between the costal cartilage and rib was mistaken for a rib fracture (**e**); the vascular groove was mistaken for a spine fracture (**f**). (**g–i**) CT axial slices of a missed fracture (false negatives are indicated by arrowheads). Figure reused under the Creative Commons License from reference [65]

union value of 0.87. Deep learning algorithms have also shown promising potential in automated 3D CT segmentation of intertrochanteric fractures which is essential for presurgical planning [70].

Literature on artificial intelligence applications for upper extremity fracture identification on CT imaging is insufficient. Most of the published literature focuses mainly on radiograph-based automatic detection, including proximal humeral, radial, wrist, and hand fractures [71–75]. CT imaging in extremity fractures is mostly used in regions of complex anatomy where plain radiographs are not sufficient to exclude subtle fractures. An example of these are foot fractures, particularly calcaneal fractures. In a study by Pranata et al. a combination pipeline of a CNN (ResNet-152) to classify CT images into "fracture" or "no fracture" was followed by a speeded-up robust features (SURF) algorithm, Canny edge detection, and contour tracing for fracture localization [76]. ResNet-152 demonstrated an accuracy of 98% in the automated classification of calcaneal fractures on CT images.

Within a similar realm, facial and skull fractures are frequently encountered in trauma settings and may have a significant role in patient outcome and survival. Deep learning algorithms have been investigated for the automated, robust, and timely identification of different facial fractures. For example, U-Net based neural networks were able to achieve a DICE score of 0.943 in identifying mandibular fractures on spiral computed tomography [77]. On the other hand, a 3D-ResNet34 neural network achieved an ROC-AUC, sensitivity, and specificity of 0.94, 0.87, and 0.87, respectively, in classifying nasal fractures on CT images [78]. In another study, Fracture R-CNN, an anchor-efficient anti-interference deep learning framework, demonstrated superior performance to Faster R-CNN algorithms in the detection of skull fractures on CT images [79].

Future Directions

Throughout this chapter, we explored various applications of artificial intelligence in trauma imaging, particularly computed tomography. We demonstrated how the incorporation of artificial intelligence solutions in trauma imaging can help to streamline the workflow by providing robust and fast preliminary results that can improve patient outcomes and reduce radiologist workload and burnout.

Owing to this significant and promising role of artificial intelligence, multiple initiatives have been proposed by major radiological and imaging societies to promote research and external validation of available solutions. Examples of these include the RSNA intracranial hemorrhage detection challenge, the RSNA cervical spine fracture AI Challenge, the SIIM-ACR pneumothorax segmentation challenge, as well as multiple Grand-Challenge competitions [80–82]. Front-runners in these challenges were required to share their proposed algorithms and solutions to ensure fairness and encourage future research. Additionally, multiple open-source datasets are available to promote further research and external validation. Examples include FracNet, an open-source dataset of CT images for rib fracture detection, and the NIH Chest X-ray Dataset, a dataset of 112,120 chest radiographs of different pathologies including pneumothorax.

It is worth mentioning that there are multiple challenges that hinder the routine application of artificial learning algorithms in medical imaging and patient care. First, the nature of medical images itself is different from other non-medical images. For example, radiologists usually evaluate different MRI sequences or CT series to characterize a lesion of interest. Thus, building a model would require taking all of these sequences and phases into consideration. Additionally, most lesions are not simply 2-D structures, but 3-D volumetric objects. Accordingly, the models need to incorporate the information form multiple contiguous images to reach a reasonable performance. Second, training these artificial intelligence algorithms typically requires large amounts of images and data, on the order of thousands or even millions of images. In the medical domain, this is highly challenging due to institutional polices and regulations preventing data sharing. This is even more challenging particularly in instances when the disease of interest is rare. To overcome that, there are on-going efforts to create shared multi-institutional datasets like those mentioned earlier. In addition, techniques such as transfer learning can mitigate this issue, taking advantage of knowledge from one dataset and transferring it to another one. Additional challenges include selecting the gold standard against which the performance of the algorithm will be compared to, necessary for supervised learning algorithms, as well as creating curated datasets that reflect the disease prevalence in the general population.

Several additional important applications of artificial intelligence in the trauma setting were not discussed in this chapter, although the reader is encouraged to explore them. These include worklist prioritization, prediction of trauma volume for resource optimization, outcome prediction, as well as identification of incidental findings on trauma imaging reports for appropriate follow-up [83–86].

References

1. Erickson BJ, et al. Machine learning for medical imaging. RadioGraphics. 2017;37(2):505–15.
2. Cheng PM, et al. Deep learning: an update for radiologists. Radiographics. 2021;41(5):1427–45.
3. Chartrand G, et al. Deep learning: a primer for radiologists. Radiographics. 2017;37(7):2113–31.
4. Ronneberger O, Fischer P, Brox T. U-net: convolutional networks for biomedical image segmentation. In: International conference on medical image computing and computer-assisted intervention. Cham: Springer; 2015.
5. Raghu M, et al. Transfusion: understanding transfer learning for medical imaging. Adv Neural Inf Proces Syst. 2019;32:3347–57.
6. Kim HE, et al. Transfer learning for medical image classification: a literature review. BMC Med Imaging. 2022;22(1):69.
7. Sellergren AB, et al. Simplified transfer learning for chest radiography models using less data. Radiology. 2022;305(2):454–65.
8. Savatmongkorngul S, Wongwaisayawan S, Kaewlai R. Focused assessment with sonography for trauma: current perspectives. Open Access Emerg Med. 2017;9:57–62.
9. Cheng CY, et al. Deep learning assisted detection of abdominal free fluid in Morison's pouch during focused assessment with sonography in trauma. Front Med. 2021;8:707437.
10. Kornblith AE, et al. Development and validation of a deep learning strategy for automated view classification of pediatric focused assessment with sonography for trauma. J Ultrasound Med. 2022;41(8):1915–24.
11. Lin Z, et al. Deep learning for emergency ascites diagnosis using ultrasonography images. J Appl Clin Med Phys. 2022;23(7):e13695.
12. Sjogren AR, et al. Image segmentation and machine learning for detection of abdominal free fluid in focused assessment with sonography for trauma examinations: a pilot study. J Ultrasound Med. 2016;35(11):2501–9.
13. Dreizin D, et al. Performance of a deep learning algorithm for automated segmentation and quantification of traumatic pelvic hematomas on CT. J Digit Imaging. 2020;33(1):243–51.
14. Kane NM, et al. Traumatic pneumoperitoneum. Implications of computed tomography diagnosis. Investig Radiol. 1991;26(6):574–8.
15. Brejnebøl MW, et al. Artificial Intelligence based detection of pneumoperitoneum on CT scans in patients presenting with acute abdominal pain: a clinical diagnostic test accuracy study. Eur J Radiol. 2022;150:110216.
16. Winkel DJ, et al. Evaluation of an AI-based detection software for acute findings in abdominal computed tomography scans: toward an automated work list prioritization of routine CT examinations. Investig Radiol. 2019;54(1):55–9.
17. Taubmann O, et al. Automatic detection of free intra-abdominal air in computed tomography. In: Medical image computing and computer assisted intervention – MICCAI 2020. Cham: Springer; 2020.
18. Su C-Y, et al. A deep learning method for alerting emergency physicians about the presence of subphrenic free air on chest radiographs. J Clin Med. 2021;10(2):254.
19. Kim M, et al. Detection of pneumoperitoneum in the abdominal radiograph images using artificial neural networks. Eur J Radiol Open. 2021;8:100316.
20. Goyal M, et al. Sensitivity and specificity evaluation of deep learning models for detection of pneumoperitoneum on chest radiographs. 2020.
21. Kozar RA, et al. Organ injury scaling 2018 update: spleen, liver, and kidney. J Trauma Acute Care Surg. 2018;85(6):1119–22.
22. Farzaneh N, et al. A deep learning framework for automated detection and quantitative assessment of liver trauma. BMC Med Imaging. 2022;22(1):39.
23. Dreizin D, et al. Added value of deep learning-based liver parenchymal CT volumetry for predicting major arterial injury after blunt hepatic trauma: a decision tree analysis. Abdom Radiol. 2021;46(6):2556–66.
24. Chen H, Unberath M, Dreizin D. Toward automated interpretable AAST grading for blunt splenic injury. Emerg Radiol. 2022;30(1):41–50.
25. Li X, et al. Deep learning-enabled system for rapid pneumothorax screening on chest CT. Eur J Radiol. 2019;120:108692.
26. Röhrich S, et al. Deep learning detection and quantification of pneumothorax in heterogeneous routine chest computed tomography. Eur Radiol Exp. 2020;4(1):26.
27. Malhotra P, et al. Deep learning-based computer-aided pneumothorax detection using chest X-ray images. Sensors. 2022;22(6):2278.
28. Hillis JM, et al. Evaluation of an artificial intelligence model for detection of pneumothorax and tension pneumothorax in chest radiographs. JAMA Netw Open. 2022;5(12):e2247172.
29. Boice EN, et al. Training ultrasound image classification deep-learning algorithms for pneumothorax detection using a synthetic tissue phantom apparatus. J Imaging. 2022;8(9):249.
30. Thian YL, et al. Deep learning systems for pneumothorax detection on chest radiographs: a multicenter external validation study. Radiol Artif Intell. 2021;3(4):e200190.
31. Kitamura G, Deible C. Retraining an open-source pneumothorax detecting machine learning algorithm for improved performance to medical images. Clin Imaging. 2020;61:15–9.
32. Tolkachev A, et al. Deep learning for diagnosis and segmentation of pneumothorax: the results on the kaggle competition and validation against radiologists. IEEE J Biomed Health Inform. 2021;25(5):1660–72.
33. Dreizin D, et al. A pilot study of deep learning-based CT volumetry for traumatic hemothorax. Emerg Radiol. 2022;29(6):995–1002.

34. Wang S, et al. Assessment of automatic rib fracture detection on chest CT using a deep learning algorithm. Eur Radiol. 2022;33(3):1824–34.
35. Niiya A, et al. Development of an artificial intelligence-assisted computed tomography diagnosis technology for rib fracture and evaluation of its clinical usefulness. Sci Rep. 2022;12(1):8363.
36. Gao Y, et al. Deep learning-based framework for segmentation of multiclass rib fractures in CT utilizing a multi-angle projection network. Int J Comput Assist Radiol Surg. 2022;17(6):1115–24.
37. Zhang B, et al. Improving rib fracture detection accuracy and reading efficiency with deep learning-based detection software: a clinical evaluation. Br J Radiol. 2021;94(1118):20200870.
38. Yao L, et al. Rib fracture detection system based on deep learning. Sci Rep. 2021;11(1):23513.
39. Wu M, et al. Development and evaluation of a deep learning algorithm for rib segmentation and fracture detection from multicenter chest CT images. Radiol Artif Intell. 2021;3(5):e200248.
40. Meng XH, et al. A fully automated rib fracture detection system on chest CT images and its impact on radiologist performance. Skelet Radiol. 2021;50(9):1821–8.
41. Kaiume M, et al. Rib fracture detection in computed tomography images using deep convolutional neural networks. Medicine. 2021;100(20):e26024.
42. Lewis BT, et al. Imaging manifestations of chest trauma. Radiographics. 2021;41(5):1321–34.
43. Choi J, et al. Scalable deep learning algorithm to compute percent pulmonary contusion among patients with rib fractures. J Trauma Acute Care Surg. 2022;93(4):461–6.
44. Tanioka S, et al. Machine learning prediction of hematoma expansion in acute intracerebral hemorrhage. Sci Rep. 2022;12(1):12452.
45. Arab A, et al. A fast and fully-automated deep-learning approach for accurate hemorrhage segmentation and volume quantification in non-contrast whole-head CT. Sci Rep. 2020;10(1):19389.
46. Yu N, et al. A robust deep learning segmentation method for hematoma volumetric detection in intracerebral hemorrhage. Stroke. 2022;53(1):167–76.
47. Phaphuangwittayakul A, et al. An optimal deep learning framework for multi-type hemorrhagic lesions detection and quantification in head CT images for traumatic brain injury. Appl Intell. 2022;52(7):7320–38.
48. Kamnitsas K, et al. Efficient multi-scale 3D CNN with fully connected CRF for accurate brain lesion segmentation. Med Image Anal. 2017;36:61–78.
49. Ginat DT. Analysis of head CT scans flagged by deep learning software for acute intracranial hemorrhage. Neuroradiology. 2020;62(3):335–40.
50. Rao B, et al. Utility of artificial intelligence tool as a prospective radiology peer reviewer - detection of unreported intracranial hemorrhage. Acad Radiol. 2021;28(1):85–93.
51. Seyam M, et al. Utilization of artificial intelligence-based intracranial hemorrhage detection on emergent noncontrast CT images in clinical workflow. Radiol Artif Intell. 2022;4(2):e210168.
52. Alagic Z, et al. Deep learning versus iterative image reconstruction algorithm for head CT in trauma. Emerg Radiol. 2022;29(2):339–52.
53. Nagayama Y, et al. Deep learning-based reconstruction for lower-dose pediatric CT: technical principles, image characteristics, and clinical implementations. Radiographics. 2021;41(7):1936–53.
54. Immonen E, et al. The use of deep learning towards dose optimization in low-dose computed tomography: a scoping review. Radiography. 2022;28(1):208–14.
55. Doerr SA, et al. Automated prediction of the thoracolumbar injury classification and severity score from CT using a novel deep learning algorithm. Neurosurg Focus. 2022;52(4):E5.
56. Li Y, et al. Differential diagnosis of benign and malignant vertebral fracture on CT using deep learning. Eur Radiol. 2021;31(12):9612–9.
57. Rosenberg GS, et al. Artificial intelligence accurately detects traumatic thoracolumbar fractures on sagittal radiographs. Medicina. 2022;58(8):998.
58. Kong SH, et al. Development of a spine X-ray-based fracture prediction model using a deep learning algorithm. Endocrinol Metab. 2022;37(4):674–83.
59. Chen X, Liu Y. A classification method for thoracolumbar vertebral fractures due to basketball sports injury based on deep learning. Comput Math Methods Med. 2022;2022:8747487.
60. Chen W, et al. A deep-learning model for identifying fresh vertebral compression fractures on digital radiography. Eur Radiol. 2022;32(3):1496–505.
61. Boonrod A, et al. Diagnostic accuracy of deep learning for evaluation of C-spine injury from lateral neck radiographs. Heliyon. 2022;8(8):e10372.
62. Tay B, Hyun JK, Oh S. A machine learning approach for specification of spinal cord injuries using fractional anisotropy values obtained from diffusion tensor images. Comput Math Methods Med. 2014;2014:276589.
63. McCoy DB, et al. Convolutional neural network-based automated segmentation of the spinal cord and contusion injury: deep learning biomarker correlates of motor impairment in acute spinal cord injury. AJNR Am J Neuroradiol. 2019;40(4):737–44.
64. Collaborators GBDF. Global, regional, and national burden of bone fractures in 204 countries and territories, 1990-2019: a systematic analysis from the Global Burden of Disease Study 2019. Lancet Healthy Longev. 2021;2(9):e580–92.
65. Inoue T, et al. Automated fracture screening using an object detection algorithm on whole-body trauma computed tomography. Sci Rep. 2022;12(1):16549.
66. Costantini TW, et al. Current management of hemorrhage from severe pelvic fractures: Results of an American Association for the Surgery of Trauma multi-institutional trial. J Trauma Acute Care Surg. 2016;80(5):717–23; discussion 723-5.

67. Dreizin D, et al. An automated deep learning method for Tile AO/OTA pelvic fracture severity grading from trauma whole-body CT. J Digit Imaging. 2021;34(1):53–65.
68. Ukai K, et al. Detecting pelvic fracture on 3D-CT using deep convolutional neural networks with multi-orientated slab images. Sci Rep. 2021;11(1): 11716.
69. Yoon SJ, et al. Automatic multi-class intertrochanteric femur fracture detection from CT images based on AO/OTA classification using faster R-CNN-BO method. J Appl Biomed. 2020;18(4):97–105.
70. Wang D, et al. Accuracy and reliability analysis of a machine learning based segmentation tool for intertrochanteric femoral fracture CT. Front Surg. 2022;9:913385.
71. Ozkaya E, et al. Evaluation of an artificial intelligence system for diagnosing scaphoid fracture on direct radiography. Eur J Trauma Emerg Surg. 2022;48(1):585–92.
72. Cohen M, et al. Artificial intelligence vs. radiologist: accuracy of wrist fracture detection on radiographs. Eur Radiol. 2022;33(6):3974–83.
73. Raisuddin AM, et al. Critical evaluation of deep neural networks for wrist fracture detection. Sci Rep. 2021;11(1):6006.
74. Oka K, et al. Artificial intelligence to diagnosis distal radius fracture using biplane plain X-rays. J Orthop Surg Res. 2021;16(1):694.
75. Chung SW, et al. Automated detection and classification of the proximal humerus fracture by using deep learning algorithm. Acta Orthop. 2018;89(4): 468–73.
76. Pranata YD, et al. Deep learning and SURF for automated classification and detection of calcaneus fractures in CT images. Comput Methods Prog Biomed. 2019;171:27–37.
77. Wang X, et al. Detection and classification of mandibular fracture on CT scan using deep convolutional neural network. Clin Oral Investig. 2022;26(6):4593–601.
78. Seol YJ, et al. A study on 3D deep learning-based automatic diagnosis of nasal fractures. Sensors. 2022;22(2):506.
79. Lin X, et al. Fracture R-CNN: an anchor-efficient anti-interference framework for skull fracture detection in CT images. Med Phys. 2022;49(11):7179–92.
80. SIIM. The pneumothorax challenge - society for imaging informatics in medicine. 2023. Available at https://siim.org/page/pneumothorax_challenge.
81. RSNA. RSNA cervical spine fracture AI challenge. 2022. Available at https://www.rsna.org/education/ai-resources-and-training/ai-image-challenge/cervical-spine-fractures-ai-detection-challenge-2022.
82. RSNA. RSNA intracranial hemorrhage detection challenge. 2019. Available at https://www.rsna.org/education/ai-resources-and-training/ai-image-challenge/RSNA-Intracranial-Hemorrhage-Detection-Challenge-2019.
83. Pease M, et al. Outcome prediction in patients with severe traumatic brain injury using deep learning from head CT scans. Radiology. 2022;304(2):385–94.
84. Evans CS, et al. A natural language processing and machine learning approach to identification of incidental radiology findings in trauma patients discharged from the emergency department. Ann Emerg Med. 2022;81(3):262–9.
85. O'Neill TJ, et al. Active reprioritization of the reading worklist using artificial intelligence has a beneficial effect on the turnaround time for interpretation of head CT with intracranial hemorrhage. Radiol Artif Intell. 2021;3(2):e200024.
86. Stonko DP, et al. Artificial intelligence can predict daily trauma volume and average acuity. J Trauma Acute Care Surg. 2018;85(2):393–7.

Index

F. Knollmann (ed.), *Trauma Computed Tomography*, https://doi.org/10.1007/978-3-031-45746-3

C

D

E

F

GPSR Compliance

The European Union's (EU) General Product Safety Regulation (GPSR) is a set of rules that requires consumer products to be safe and our obligations to ensure this.

If you have any concerns about our products, you can contact us on ProductSafety@springernature.com

In case Publisher is established outside the EU, the EU authorized representative is:

Springer Nature Customer Service Center GmbH
Europaplatz 3
69115 Heidelberg, Germany

Batch number: 10732809

Printed by Printforce, the Netherlands